坎贝尔骨科手术学
足踝外科

Campbell's Operative Orthopaedics

第 14 版
（影印版）

Frederick M. Azar, MD

James H. Beaty, MD

人民卫生出版社
·北 京·

图书在版编目（CIP）数据

坎贝尔骨科手术学 . 足踝外科：英文 /（美）弗雷德里克·M. 阿扎尔（Frederick M. Azar),（美）詹姆斯·H. 比蒂（James H. Beaty）主编 . —影印本 . —北京：人民卫生出版社，2021.12

ISBN 978-7-117-32517-2

Ⅰ. ①坎…　Ⅱ. ①弗…　②詹…　Ⅲ. ①骨科学 – 外科手术 – 英文②足 – 外科手术 – 英文③踝关节 – 外科手术 – 英文　Ⅳ. ①R68②R658.3

中国版本图书馆 CIP 数据核字（2021）第 241416 号

| 人卫智网 | www.ipmph.com | 医学教育、学术、考试、健康，购书智慧智能综合服务平台 |
| 人卫官网 | www.pmph.com | 人卫官方资讯发布平台 |

图字：01–2021–6747 号

坎贝尔骨科手术学

足踝外科

Kanbeier Guke Shoushuxue

Zuhuai Waike

主　　编：Frederick M. Azar　James H. Beaty

出版发行：人民卫生出版社（中继线 010-59780011）

地　　址：北京市朝阳区潘家园南里 19 号

邮　　编：100021

E - mail：pmph @ pmph.com

购书热线：010-59787592　010-59787584　010-65264830

印　　刷：三河市宏达印刷有限公司（胜利）

经　　销：新华书店

开　　本：889×1194　1/16　印张：32.5

字　　数：1548 千字

版　　次：2021 年 12 月第 1 版

印　　次：2022 年 1 月第 1 次印刷

标准书号：ISBN 978-7-117-32517-2

定　　价：429.00 元

打击盗版举报电话：010-59787491　E-mail：WQ @ pmph.com

质量问题联系电话：010-59787234　E-mail：zhiliang @ pmph.com

坎贝尔骨科手术学
足踝外科

Campbell's Operative Orthopaedics

第 14 版
（影印版）

Frederick M. Azar, MD

Professor

Department of Orthopaedic Surgery and Biomedical Engineering University of Tennessee–Campbell Clinic

Chief of Staff, Campbell Clinic

Memphis, Tennessee

James H. Beaty, MD

Harold B. Boyd Professor and Chair

Department of Orthopaedic Surgery and Biomedical Engineering University of Tennessee–Campbell Clinic

Memphis, Tennessee

Editorial Assistance

Kay Daugherty *and* **Linda Jones**

人民卫生出版社
·北 京·

Elsevier (Singapore) Pte Ltd.
3 Killiney Road,
#08–01 Winsland House I,
Singapore 239519
Tel: (65) 6349–0200; Fax:(65) 6733–1817

Campbell's Operative Orthopaedics, 14E

Copyright © 2021 by Elsevier Inc. All rights reserved.

Previous editions copyrighted © 2017, 2013, 2008, 2003, 1998, 1992, 1987, 1980, 1971, 1963, 1956, 1949, 1939.

ISBN: 978–0–323–67217–7

This English Reprint of Part XIX from Campbell's Operative Orthopaedics, 14E by Frederick M. Azar and James H. Beaty was undertaken by People's Medical Publishing House and is published by arrangement with Elsevier (Singapore) Pte Ltd.

Part XIX from Campbell's Operative Orthopaedics, 14E by Frederick M. Azar and James H. Beaty由人民卫生出版社进行影印，并根据人民卫生出版社与爱思唯尔（新加坡）私人有限公司的协议约定出版。

ISBN: 978–7–117–32517–2

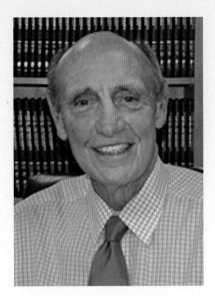

S. Terry Canale, MD

It is with humble appreciation and admiration that we dedicate this edition of *Campbell's Operative Orthopaedics* to Dr. S. Terry Canale, who served as editor or co-editor of five editions. He took great pride in this position and worked tirelessly to continue to improve "The Book." As noted by one of his co-editors, "Terry is probably the only person in the world who has read every word of multiple editions of *Campbell's Operative Orthopaedics*." He considered *Campbell's Operative Orthopaedics* an opportunity for worldwide orthopaedic education and made it a priority to ensure that each edition provided valuable and up-to-date information. His commitment to and enthusiasm for this work will continue to influence and inspire every future edition.

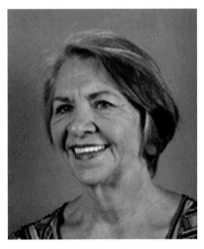

Kay C. Daugherty

It is with equal appreciation and regard that we dedicate this edition to Kay C. Daugherty, the managing editor of the last nine editions *Campbell's Operative Orthopaedics*. Over the last 40 years, she has faithfully and tirelessly edited, reshaped, and overseen all aspects of publication from manuscript preparation to proofing. She has a profound talent to put ideas and disjointed words into comprehensible text, ensuring that each revision maintains the gold standard in readability. Each edition is a testament to her dedication to excellence in writing and education. A favorite quote of Mrs. Daugherty to one of our late authors was, "I'll make a deal. I won't operate if you won't punctuate." We are grateful for her many years of continual service to the Campbell Foundation and for the publications yet to come.

CONTRIBUTORS

FREDERICK M. AZAR, MD
Professor
Director, Sports Medicine Fellowship
University of Tennessee–Campbell Clinic
Department of Orthopaedic Surgery and
    Biomedical Engineering
Chief-of-Staff, Campbell Clinic
Memphis, Tennessee

JAMES H. BEATY, MD
Harold B. Boyd Professor and Chair
University of Tennessee–Campbell Clinic
Department of Orthopaedic Surgery and
    Biomedical Engineering
Memphis, Tennessee

MICHAEL J. BEEBE, MD
Instructor
University of Tennessee–Campbell Clinic
Department of Orthopaedic Surgery and
    Biomedical Engineering
Memphis, Tennessee

CLAYTON C. BETTIN, MD
Assistant Professor
Director, Foot and Ankle Fellowship
Associate Residency Program Director
University of Tennessee–Campbell Clinic
Department of Orthopaedic Surgery and
    Biomedical Engineering
Memphis, Tennessee

TYLER J. BROLIN, MD
Assistant Professor
University of Tennessee–Campbell Clinic
Department of Orthopaedic Surgery and
    Biomedical Engineering
Memphis, Tennessee

JAMES H. CALANDRUCCIO, MD
Associate Professor
Director, Hand Fellowship
University of Tennessee–Campbell Clinic
Department of Orthopaedic Surgery and
    Biomedical Engineering
Memphis, Tennessee

DAVID L. CANNON, MD
Associate Professor
University of Tennessee–Campbell Clinic
Department of Orthopaedic Surgery and
    Biomedical Engineering
Memphis, Tennessee

KEVIN B. CLEVELAND, MD
Instructor
University of Tennessee–Campbell Clinic
Department of Orthopaedic Surgery and
    Biomedical Engineering
Memphis, Tennessee

ANDREW H. CRENSHAW JR., MD
Professor Emeritus
University of Tennessee–Campbell Clinic
Department of Orthopaedic Surgery and
    Biomedical Engineering
Memphis, Tennessee

JOHN R. CROCKARELL, MD
Professor
University of Tennessee–Campbell Clinic
Department of Orthopaedic Surgery and
    Biomedical Engineering
Memphis, Tennessee

GREGORY D. DABOV, MD
Assistant Professor
University of Tennessee–Campbell Clinic
Department of Orthopaedic Surgery and
    Biomedical Engineering
Memphis, Tennessee

MARCUS C. FORD, MD
Instructor
University of Tennessee–Campbell Clinic
Department of Orthopaedic Surgery and
    Biomedical Engineering
Memphis, Tennessee

RAYMOND J. GARDOCKI, MD
Assistant Professor
University of Tennessee–Campbell Clinic
Department of Orthopaedic Surgery and
    Biomedical Engineering
Memphis, Tennessee

BENJAMIN J. GREAR, MD
Instructor
University of Tennessee–Campbell Clinic
Department of Orthopaedic Surgery and
    Biomedical Engineering
Memphis, Tennessee

JAMES L. GUYTON, MD
Associate Professor
University of Tennessee–Campbell Clinic
Department of Orthopaedic Surgery and
    Biomedical Engineering
Memphis, Tennessee

JAMES W. HARKESS, MD
Associate Professor
University of Tennessee–Campbell Clinic
Department of Orthopaedic Surgery and
    Biomedical Engineering
Memphis, Tennessee

ROBERT K. HECK JR., MD
Associate Professor
University of Tennessee–Campbell Clinic
Department of Orthopaedic Surgery and
    Biomedical Engineering
Memphis, Tennessee

MARK T. JOBE, MD
Associate Professor
University of Tennessee–Campbell Clinic
Department of Orthopaedic Surgery and
    Biomedical Engineering
Memphis, Tennessee

DEREK M. KELLY, MD
Professor
Director, Pediatric Orthopaedic Fellowship
Director, Resident Education
University of Tennessee–Campbell Clinic
Department of Orthopaedic Surgery and
    Biomedical Engineering
Memphis, Tennessee

SANTOS F. MARTINEZ, MD
Assistant Professor
University of Tennessee–Campbell Clinic
Department of Orthopaedic Surgery and
    Biomedical Engineering
Memphis, Tennessee

ANTHONY A. MASCIOLI, MD
Assistant Professor
University of Tennessee–Campbell Clinic
Department of Orthopaedic Surgery and
    Biomedical Engineering
Memphis, Tennessee

BENJAMIN M. MAUCK, MD
Assistant Professor
Director, Hand Fellowship
University of Tennessee–Campbell Clinic
Department of Orthopaedic Surgery and
    Biomedical Engineering
Memphis, Tennessee

MARC J. MIHALKO, MD
Assistant Professor
University of Tennessee–Campbell Clinic
Department of Orthopaedic Surgery and
    Biomedical Engineering
Memphis, Tennessee

WILLIAM M. MIHALKO, MD PhD
Professor, H.R. Hyde Chair of Excellence in
    Rehabilitation Engineering
Director, Biomedical Engineering
University of Tennessee–Campbell Clinic
Department of Orthopaedic Surgery and
    Biomedical Engineering
Memphis, Tennessee

ROBERT H. MILLER III, MD
Associate Professor
University of Tennessee–Campbell Clinic
Department of Orthopaedic Surgery and
   Biomedical Engineering
Memphis, Tennessee

G. ANDREW MURPHY, MD
Associate Professor
University of Tennessee–Campbell Clinic
Department of Orthopaedic Surgery and
   Biomedical Engineering
Memphis, Tennessee

ASHLEY L. PARK, MD
Clinical Assistant Professor
University of Tennessee–Campbell Clinic
Department of Orthopaedic Surgery and
   Biomedical Engineering
Memphis, Tennessee

EDWARD A. PEREZ, MD
Associate Professor
University of Tennessee–Campbell Clinic
Department of Orthopaedic Surgery and
   Biomedical Engineering
Memphis, Tennessee

BARRY B. PHILLIPS, MD
Professor
University of Tennessee–Campbell Clinic
Department of Orthopaedic Surgery and
   Biomedical Engineering
Memphis, Tennessee

DAVID R. RICHARDSON, MD
Associate Professor
University of Tennessee–Campbell Clinic
Department of Orthopaedic Surgery and
   Biomedical Engineering
Memphis, Tennessee

MATTHEW I. RUDLOFF, MD
Assistant Professor
Co-Director, Trauma Fellowship
University of Tennessee–Campbell Clinic
Department of Orthopaedic Surgery and
   Biomedical Engineering
Memphis, Tennessee

JEFFREY R. SAWYER, MD
Professor
Co-Director, Pediatric Orthopaedic
   Fellowship
University of Tennessee–Campbell Clinic
Department of Orthopaedic Surgery and
   Biomedical Engineering
Memphis, Tennessee

BENJAMIN W. SHEFFER, MD
Assistant Professor
University of Tennessee–Campbell Clinic
Department of Orthopaedic Surgery and
   Biomedical Engineering
Memphis, Tennessee

DAVID D. SPENCE, MD
Assistant Professor
University of Tennessee–Campbell Clinic
Department of Orthopaedic Surgery and
   Biomedical Engineering
Memphis, Tennessee

NORFLEET B. THOMPSON, MD
Instructor
University of Tennessee–Campbell Clinic
Department of Orthopaedic Surgery and
   Biomedical Engineering
Memphis, Tennessee

THOMAS W. THROCKMORTON, MD
Professor
Co-Director, Sports Medicine Fellowship
University of Tennessee–Campbell Clinic
Department of Orthopaedic Surgery and
   Biomedical Engineering
Memphis, Tennessee

PATRICK C. TOY, MD
Associate Professor
University of Tennessee–Campbell Clinic
Department of Orthopaedic Surgery and
   Biomedical Engineering
Memphis, Tennessee

WILLIAM C. WARNER JR., MD
Professor
University of Tennessee–Campbell Clinic
Department of Orthopaedic Surgery and
   Biomedical Engineering
Memphis, Tennessee

JOHN C. WEINLEIN, MD
Assistant Professor
Director, Trauma Fellowship
University of Tennessee–Campbell Clinic
Department of Orthopaedic Surgery and
   Biomedical Engineering
Memphis, Tennessee

WILLIAM J. WELLER, MD
Instructor
University of Tennessee–Campbell Clinic
Department of Orthopaedic Surgery and
   Biomedical Engineering
Memphis, Tennessee

A. PAIGE WHITTLE, MD
Associate Professor
University of Tennessee–Campbell Clinic
Department of Orthopaedic Surgery and
   Biomedical Engineering
Memphis, Tennessee

KEITH D. WILLIAMS, MD
Associate Professor
University of Tennessee–Campbell Clinic
Department of Orthopaedic Surgery and
   Biomedical Engineering
Memphis, Tennessee

DEXTER H. WITTE III, MD
Clinical Assistant Professor in
   Radiology
University of Tennessee–Campbell Clinic
Department of Orthopaedic Surgery and
   Biomedical Engineering
Memphis, Tennessee

PREFACE

When Dr. Willis Campbell published the first edition of *Campbell's Operative Orthopaedics* in 1939, he could not have envisioned that over 80 years later it would have evolved into a four-volume text and earned the accolade of the "bible of orthopaedics" as a mainstay in orthopaedic practices and educational institutions all over the world. This expansion from some 400 pages in the first edition to over 4,500 pages in this 14th edition has not changed Dr. Campbell's original intent: "to present to the student, the general practitioner, and the surgeon the subject of orthopaedic surgery in a simple and comprehensive manner." In each edition since the first, authors and editors have worked diligently to fulfill these objectives. This would have not been possible without the hard work of our contributors who always strive to present the most up-to-date information while retaining "tried and true" techniques and tips. The scope of this text continues to expand in the hope that the information will be relevant to physicians no matter their location or resources.

As always, this edition also is the result of the collaboration of a group of "behind the scenes" individuals who are involved in the actual production process. The Campbell Foundation staff—Kay Daugherty, Linda Jones, and Tonya Priggel—contributed their considerable talents to editing often confusing and complex author contributions, searching the literature for obscure references, and, in general, "herding the cats." Special thanks to Kay and Linda who have worked on multiple editions of *Campbell's Operative Orthopaedics* (nine editions for Kay and six for Linda). They probably know more about orthopaedics than most of us, and they certainly know how to make it more understandable. Thanks, too, to the Elsevier personnel who provided guidance and assistance throughout the publication process: John Casey, Senior Project Manager; Jennifer Ehlers, Senior Content Development Specialist; and Belinda Kuhn, Senior Content Strategist.

We are especially appreciative of our spouses, Julie Azar and Terry Beaty, and our families for their patience and support as we worked through this project.

The preparation and publication of this 14th edition was fraught with difficulties because of the worldwide pandemic and social unrest, but our contributors and other personnel worked tirelessly, often in creative and innovative ways, to bring it to fruition. It is our hope that these efforts have provided a text that is informative and valuable to all orthopaedists as they continue to refine and improve methods that will ensure the best outcomes for their patients.

Frederick M. Azar, MD
James H. Beaty, MD

CONTENTS

CHAPTER 1

SURGICAL TECHNIQUES

Benjamin J. Grear

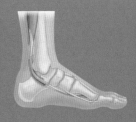

PREOPERATIVE PREPARATION

Careful preoperative planning, a thorough knowledge of the pertinent anatomy, good surgical exposure, skill in the use of equipment, and elimination of distraction reduce the likelihood of an undesirable outcome after foot surgery. Careful preoperative planning requires knowledge of the indications and operative techniques, but it also consists of instrument selection, patient positioning, antiseptic preparation, prophylactic antibiotics, tourniquet use, anesthesia, risk factor optimization, and postoperative anticoagulation.

INSTRUMENTS

Two trays of instruments, designated as "foot tray—soft tissue" and "foot tray—bone," are helpful. The instruments in the soft-tissue foot tray should include delicate forceps with and without teeth for soft-tissue handling (i.e., Adson and Brown-Adson forceps). Fine, two-tooth skin hooks, narrow and wide-neck mini-Hohmann retractors, and small double-ended, right-angle retractors (i.e., Ragnell and Senn retractors) allow the assistant's hand to be positioned outside the field of dissection, and yet afford excellent exposure. A No. 15 Bard-Parker blade attached to a multisided handle facilitates quick changes during dissection. Sharp dissection is indicated whenever practical to prevent tearing of the tissue and the edematous reaction that follows indelicate dissection. When blunt dissection is required, small scissors (i.e., Metzenbaum scissors) with gently curved and slightly blunted tips are helpful. Mosquito hemostats for small vessel occlusion, Webster needle holders with smooth jaws for grasping fine suture, and a freer elevator complete the foot tray for use in soft tissues.

The foot tray for bony procedures has many of the same instruments but on a larger scale. Heavier blades, forceps, dissecting scissors, retractors, and needle holders may be required for procedures that include bone and large tendon surgery. Thin osteotomes, a small mallet, small curettes, heavy-duty two-tooth retractors, a wide dissecting probe, and an Inge retractor, with arms that have been thinned and teeth that have been narrowed, all facilitate bony procedures.

Two power instruments are helpful in surgery of the foot. A power drill with varying chucks (wire driver, AO chuck, and key chuck) allows versatility for bone drilling, screw advancement, and efficient Kirschner wire placement. A power oscillating saw with thin, narrow blades is also helpful for osteotomies and other bony procedures.

Lighting that reduces shadows and focuses sharply on the foot is necessary. A high-intensity headlight is useful, especially during deep plantar dissections. Magnification with loupes may also improve visualization. Last, a camera that is simple and easy to use by the operating room personnel is recommended for recording key findings before, during, and after surgery.

PATIENT POSITIONING

The level of exposure required will generally guide patient positioning, but positioning should always maintain patient safety and comfort. Usually, patients are secured in a lateral decubitus position, either supine or prone. All bony prominences should be well padded, and the patient and his extremities should be secured to the operative table. Superficial nerves, such as the ulnar nerve or superficial peroneal nerve, should be well padded or floated. Chest rolls should be used when the patient is prone to allow adequate chest wall expansion. Other less common positions may include "sloppy lateral," which allows medial and posterolateral hindfoot access through hip rotation. Soft bumps under the ipsilateral or contralateral hip assist with fine-tuning the rotation of the leg. Elevating the operative leg on a stack of linen or "bone foam" facilitates keeping the contralateral limb out of the way, which improves access to the operative field and aids with imaging.

TOURNIQUET

The use of a tourniquet allows dissection in a bloodless field, thereby improving visualization and efficiency while decreasing the likelihood of injury to nerves, vessels, and tendons. However, adequate surgery of the foot can be performed without a tourniquet and, in selected patients, a tourniquet might be contraindicated. When the blood supply to the foot is questionable, a tourniquet is not recommended. Deleterious effects of prolonged tourniquet time have been well documented. To prevent chemical burns, care must be taken to avoid accumulation of skin preparation under the tourniquet. Patients undergoing open reduction and internal fixation of an ankle fracture with a tourniquet demonstrated greater pain and swelling up to 6 weeks postoperatively, but no differences in length of hospital stay or complication rates were reported with the use of a tourniquet. Other authors have noted that tourniquet use over 90 minutes is a risk factor for wound healing complications in elective foot and ankle surgery. In a systematic review analyzing the available clinical and basic science data, Fitzgibbons et al. reported that typical tourniquet usage in orthopaedic surgery is safe without significant risk of complications but noted that each case must be analyzed individually. Optimal tourniquet pressures and durations remain unknown. Most surgeons consider blood pressure, limb size, or both in determining the amount of cuff pressure to apply. For calf and ankle cuffs, the pressures most commonly used by surgeons in a survey of members of the American Orthopaedic Foot and Ankle Society (AOFAS) ranged from 201 to 250 mm Hg, and thigh cuff pressures most commonly used ranged from 251 to 351 mm Hg. Fitzgibbons et al. recommended that tourniquet duration be assessed at 2 hours. If a tourniquet time of more than 2.5 hours is anticipated, then a 10-minute deflation interval should be employed every hour. If the tourniquet time is anticipated to be less than 2.5 hours, the pressure should remain lower than 300 mm Hg, and if over 2.5 hours, then 50 to 75 mm Hg above the limb occlusion pressure should be considered.

Rather than using a pneumatic thigh cuff, an ankle cuff or elastic wrap around the ankle permits most forefoot and midfoot procedures to be performed in a bloodless field. The patient experiences little tourniquet discomfort provided the tourniquet does not reach the musculotendinous junction at the middle third of the leg, allowing for the use of regional anesthesia instead of general anesthesia. However, the surgeon must be aware that an ankle tourniquet will affect the passive soft-tissue balance of the forefoot. Just as the position of the ankle (neutral, plantarflexion, or dorsiflexion) affects the forefoot, tourniquet compression essentially shortens the long flexor and extensor tendons around the ankle, causing increased toe clawing. Hence, releasing an ankle tourniquet or using a thigh tourniquet may be necessary for soft-tissue balancing procedures. Rudkin et al. audited 1000 patients who had undergone foot and ankle surgery with ankle block anesthesia and an ankle cuff tourniquet. Only eight of the 1000 patients had significant tourniquet pain that interrupted surgery without any significant complications. The safety and efficacy of elastic wrap ankle tourniquets was evaluated by Grebing and Coughlin. They evaluated pressures beneath 4- and 6-inch elastic rubber bandages (Esmarch), applied using three and four tensioned wraps around the ankle, followed by tucking the remainder of the bandage beneath the proximal end of the wrap. Three wraps with a tuck produced an average pressure of 222 mm Hg (range, 146 to 319 mm Hg), and four wraps around the ankle with a tuck generated an average pressure of 288 mm Hg (range, 202 to 405 mm Hg). The investigators concluded that the clinical experience has shown this technique of exsanguination to be safe and effective. A survey of 140 members of the AOFAS showed that 20% of surgeons use an elastic wrap for ankle tourniquets. Ankle tourniquets, whether pneumatic cuffs or elastic wraps, are safe and convenient for procedures on the foot.

APPLICATION OF A TOURNIQUET

TECHNIQUE 1.1

- Instruct an assistant to hold the end of the wrap at a 45-degree angle to the foot and to place tension on the free end while the surgeon's thumb holds the wrap firmly against the skin.
- Do not overlap each turn more than half the width of the tourniquet. Wrap the tourniquet above the ankle, taking care not to leave any skin uncovered and not to allow the edges to roll back on themselves.
- When above the ankle, proceed proximally, no more than 8 to 10 cm proximal to the malleoli, staying distal to the muscle mass. Do not continue proximally because this will increase the discomfort caused by the tourniquet.
- Complete the exsanguination with no more than three or four "cinches" around the ankle, followed by a tuck.

SURGICAL ANTISEPTIC

Due to the normally high bacterial flora residing on the foot, particularly in the web spaces, the extremity to be operated on is scrubbed for 8 to 10 minutes from toes to knee with an antibacterial soap of the surgeon's choice that the patient's skin can tolerate, followed by application of an antiseptic solution. Particular attention is directed to the web spaces. Quantitative analysis of positive cultures has shown significant reductions in heavy bacterial growth when bristled brushes or toe cleft scrubbing are employed with an antiseptic before surgery.

Presently, no consensus has been reached regarding the best skin preparation in foot and ankle surgery, although several studies have compared different types of solutions and preparation methods (Table 1.1). In Yammine and Harvey's meta-analysis of randomized and quasi-randomized controlled trials, using a modified version of the Cochrane Collaboration's tool, 716 feet evaluated across eight trials met the study criteria. Analysis of the postpreparation culture data revealed that alcohol-based chlorhexidine had better efficacy than alcoholic povidone-iodine at the hallux nail fold. Furthermore, povidone-iodine followed by an alcohol application or chlorhexidine scrub followed by an alcohol application was better than povidone-iodine (scrub and paint) alone. More recently, Shadid et al. and Hunter et al. demonstrated similar conclusions that both chlorhexidine/alcohol and iodine/alcohol solutions provide similar reduction in bacterial cultures. In hindfoot procedures, Goucher and Coughlin found no benefit in covering the toes after the forefoot had been prepped with chlorhexidine gluconate and isopropyl alcohol. Only 2 of 40 patients had positive cultures after surgery, and neither patient developed an infection. Hence, foot and ankle surgical preparation should include toe cleft scrubbing using isopropyl alcohol with either chlorhexidine gluconate or povidone-iodine solutions.

PERIOPERATIVE MEDICAL MANAGEMENT

Appreciating and optimizing patient risk factors are critical for improving surgical outcomes. Complicated and poorly controlled diabetes worsens surgical outcomes. Increased hemoglobin A1c (>7.5 mg/dL) and peripheral neuropathy (diabetic or nondiabetic neuropathy) increase the risk for surgical site infections after foot and ankle surgery. In patients with rheumatic diseases, disease-modifying antirheumatic drugs (DMARDs) and chronic corticosteroids must be

TABLE 1.1

Studies of Different Skin Preparation Methods

CHARACTERISTICS	CHENG ET AL.	KEBLISH ET AL.	BIBBO ET AL.	OSTRANDER ET AL.
No. of subjects	50	50	127	125
Age (years), mean ± SD	51.1 ± 17.4	—	46 (16-85)	48 (19-78)
Healthy volunteers or patients	Patients	Healthy volunteers*	Patients	Patients
Solutions used 1	Povidone-iodine (1%) with isopropyl alcohol (23%)	Povidone-iodine	Povidone-iodine (7.5%-10%)	Povidone-iodine (0.7%) with isopropyl alcohol (74%)
Solutions used 2	Chlorhexidine gluconate (0.5%) with isopropyl alcohol (70%)	Alcohol prewash then povidone-iodine	Chlorhexidine gluconate (4%) with isopropyl alcohol (70%)	Chlorhexidine gluconate (2%) with isopropyl alcohol (70%)
Solutions used 3	—	Alcohol only	—	Chloroxylenol (3%)
Preparation methods	Comparison of scrubbing and painting with painting only	Comparison of scrubbing and painting with painting only	Scrubbing only	Painting only
Duration of scrub (min)	3	5	7	—
Type of analysis	Quantitative and qualitative	Quantitative and qualitative	Qualitative	Qualitative
Postoperative infection rate (%)	0	—	0	7.5

*Swabbed after skin preparation to determine rates of positive cultures at various sites in the foot and ankle.

Modified from Cheng K, Robertson H, St. Mart JP, et al: Quantitative analysis of bacteria in forefoot surgery: a comparison of skin preparation techniques, *Foot Ankle Int* 30:992–997, 2009.

managed prudently. These medications impair wound healing and increase infection risks. The American College of Rheumatology (ACR) and American Association of Hip and Knee Surgeons (AAHKS) published guidelines recommending DMARDs be halted prior to an elective total joint arthroplasty, based on their half-life, and resumed after complete wound healing. These same guidelines should be applied to elective foot and ankle surgery.

Similarly, tobacco use has been associated with worse surgical outcomes. Smoking cigarettes increases the risks for wound complications, bony nonunions, persistent narcotic use, and pain. The harmful effects of smoking tobacco should be included in patient counseling and surgical decision-making. Finally, the increased frequency of vitamin D deficiency and its negative effect on bone healing should prompt surgeons to consider prescribing vitamin D supplementation after procedures that require bony union.

PROPHYLACTIC ANTIBIOTICS

Prophylactic antibiotics are used routinely in foot and ankle procedures, but few studies have examined the effect of antibiotics on surgical site infection rates exclusively in the foot and ankle. Currently, we follow the American Academy of Orthopaedic Surgeons (AAOS), American Society of Health-System Pharmacists (ASHP), and Surgical Care Improvement Project (SCIP) guidelines, which recommend administration of cefazolin or cefuroxime within 1 hour of incision, with no postoperative prophylaxis. If the patient is allergic to penicillin or cephalosporin, then clindamycin is the recommended antibiotic. Lachman et al. retrospectively compared patients receiving 24 hours of intravenous antibiotics after surgery with patients receiving 24 hours of oral antibiotics after surgery and with those receiving no antibiotics after ankle fracture surgery. No differences in the frequency of cellulitis or return to the operating room for infection were found between the groups. When surveying members of AOFAS, 75% of respondents reported the use of postoperative prophylactic antibiotics. Of these, only 16% routinely prescribed postoperative antibiotics. The data are insufficient to support or refute the use of postoperative antibiotics. Although not routinely prescribed, postoperative prophylactic antibiotics are administered in special circumstances.

PROPHYLACTIC ANTICOAGULATION

Although routine prophylactic postoperative anticoagulation is often recommended after hip or knee surgery, especially after joint replacement surgery, its use after foot and ankle surgery is not as widespread. In large populations undergoing elective or nonelective foot and ankle surgery, rates of deep venous thrombosis (DVT) have been reported to range from 0.6% to 34%, but the rates of symptomatic DVT and pulmonary embolism are low (<1%). Patients with increased risk factors should receive prophylaxis, but significant risk factors have varied within the literature. Obesity, current history of smoking, history of a thromboembolic event, neoplasia, hormone use, immobilization, and age have been suggested to increase the risk of thromboembolic events. With simple toe exercises or full weight bearing, popliteal vein flow is maintained despite immobilization in below-knee casts. For patients without risk factors, we do not routinely use prophylactic anticoagulation after foot and ankle surgery at our institution, but the use of prophylaxis should be determined on an individual basis.

PERIOPERATIVE PAIN MANAGEMENT

Pain control plays an important role in patient satisfaction and outcomes. In the past 2 decades, pain control relied heavily on the use of narcotic pain medications; however, more recently, the recognition of the ever-increasing opioid dependence and opioid-related deaths has forced physicians and law makers to reevaluate the use of narcotics. From 1999 to 2017, nearly 400,000 opioid-related deaths occurred in the United States. Opioids still play an important role in acute, postsurgical pain management, but the adjunct of other modalities is important to minimize the use of opioids.

In patients with ankle and hindfoot fusion the use of multimodal pain protocols has decreased the lengths of hospital stay and narcotic consumption. These protocols typically consist of nonsteroidal antiinflammatory drugs (NSAIDs) such as celecoxib, pregabalin, acetaminophen, and prednisone with adjustments as needed for sensitivities and allergies. Selective COX-2 inhibitors do not significantly affect platelet function and do not increase the risk of intraoperative or postoperative bleeding, making them appropriate for perioperative pain management. On the other hand, the frequent and persistent use of NSAIDs remains controversial for bone healing. Animal studies have demonstrated increased rates of nonunions and weaker unions, but Giannoudis et al. suggested that NSAIDs can be considered safe when primary healing is anticipated and/or during the first week of secondary bone healing. Perioperative ketorolac has not had an effect on bone healing in operatively treated ankle fractures.

Unintentional overprescribing of narcotics has contributed to the opioid epidemic. Each patient must be evaluated individually, but several authors suggest 20 to 30 opioid pills should be a sufficient quantity after outpatient foot and ankle surgery. Identifying preoperative risk factors for increased pain can help improve patients' expectations and improve pain management strategies. The use of narcotics preoperatively, chronic pain, mood disorders, and use of tobacco products significantly increase the risk of postoperative pain after ankle and hindfoot reconstruction. A comprehensive approach to pain relief after surgery should include optimizing psychologic disorders, coping strategies, and multimodal therapy in addition to more traditional treatments (opioids, ice, elevation, and compression).

REGIONAL ANESTHESIA

Regional anesthesia has many advantages and is gaining interest and use by surgeons. It decreases length of hospital stay without increasing complication rates. Furthermore, it improves patient pain control, improves patient satisfaction and recovery times, reduces postoperative narcotic use, and reduces the need for general anesthesia.

Depending on the location and involvement of the procedure, varying types of regional anesthesia are used, such as forefoot blocks, ankle blocks, or more proximal popliteal and saphenous blocks. Details on differing techniques for regional anesthesia within the literature are beyond the scope of this

chapter. However, we include some techniques commonly used by foot and ankle surgeons.

The patient should always be counseled regarding the use of general anesthesia if the block fails. Anesthesia personnel should be present in the operating room to sedate and monitor the patient during procedures completed under local or regional anesthesia. The same precautions are used in foot surgery performed with local anesthesia as with general anesthesia; appropriate laboratory data, history, and physical examination are all documented, and the patient is required to abstain from food or drink at least 8 hours before surgery.

◼ FOREFOOT BLOCK AND ANKLE BLOCK

The forefoot block is safe and effective for distal forefoot procedures, including first metatarsal osteotomies, arthrodeses, and lesser toe procedures. Ptaszek et al. prospectively reported 50 patients undergoing elective forefoot surgery. The forefoot block was successful in 92% of the patients, and no complications related to the block were reported.

Likewise, numerous hindfoot procedures can be performed with ankle block anesthesia. Rudkin et al. reported a 95% success rate in a prospective analysis of 1000 patients who had undergone foot or ankle surgery with ankle block anesthesia. White et al. compared intraarticular block with conscious sedation and found that the intraarticular block provided sufficient analgesia for closed reduction of ankle fracture-dislocations. The average time for reduction and splinting was 63.8 minutes for the block group and 81.5 minutes for the sedation group.

A mixture of short- and long-acting anesthetic agents given in a recommended volume provides adequate anesthesia for most forefoot and hindfoot surgeries. The dose for each patient must be calculated and must remain less than the maximum recommended dosage, but in most adults, 30 mL of 1% lidocaine with 0.25% bupivacaine is usually a safe and effective volume (Ptaszek et al.). Once the block has been administered, the time it takes to prepare and drape the patient is usually long enough to allow the block to take effect.

◼ POPLITEAL SCIATIC NERVE BLOCK (PRONE)

For procedures above the hindfoot, a popliteal sciatic nerve block has been reported to be safe and effective. Provenzano et al. reported no neurapraxia or other complications with the use of popliteal fossa nerve blocks in 439 patients. Others have reported rare complications with peripheral blocks, including infection, nerve injury, and systemic toxicity. Nerve injury is the most commonly reported complication, with rates ranging from 0% to 24%, and smokers may have an increased risk for neuropathy symptoms. The use of a nerve stimulator or ultrasound to guide the injection improves block success. Evidence suggests that ultrasound decreases the procedure time and procedure-related pain when compared with nerve stimulation techniques for popliteal blocks, but both techniques offer effective analgesia. The use of continuous catheters increases the longevity of the popliteal block, but visual analog pain scores do not significantly differ until the third postoperative day when compared with single bolus blocks. Furthermore, catheters are associated with minor complications, including leakage, bubble blockage, and inadvertent removal. Thus the small improvement in pain scores may not justify the cost and complications associated with catheters. Multiple factors affect block longevity, but single bolus popliteal blocks last approximately 18 hours.

■ LATERAL POPLITEAL NERVE BLOCK

Grosser et al. recommended a preoperative lateral popliteal nerve block in sedated patients in the operating room for postoperative pain control. Patients reported no pain immediately postoperatively. The average time the block lasted was 14 hours. They reported no complications following use of this technique.

FOREFOOT BLOCK

TECHNIQUE 1.2

- Palpate the dorsalis pedis artery as it reaches the first intermetatarsal space (Fig. 1.1A). The deep peroneal nerve to the first web space accompanies this artery.
- Using a 25-gauge needle and avoiding the artery, inject 2 to 3 mL of a mixture of short- and long-acting local anesthetic agents subcutaneously.
- If a second or third hammer toe procedure is planned, direct the needle laterally just beneath the dorsal veins from the same entrance point and block the common digital branches of the superficial peroneal nerve to the second (and, if required, the third) intermetatarsal space (Fig. 1.1B). Injection of another 2 to 3 mL should be adequate.
- Return to the same entrance point, but direct the needle medially. Stay immediately beneath the dorsal veins and superficial to the extensor hallucis longus tendon to block the medial hallucal branch of the dorsomedial superficial peroneal nerve. This is the nerve commonly encountered dorsal and medial to the "bunion" during surgery for hallux valgus.
- Conclude the dorsal sensory block at the dorsomedial aspect of the forefoot approximately 1 cm distal to the first metatarsomedial cuneiform articulation. By this time, 6 to 8 mL of anesthetic agents have been administered (Fig. 1.1C).
- Entering the anesthetized area on the dorsomedial aspect of the forefoot, proceed plantarward in the subcutaneous space superficial to the abductor hallucis muscle until the plantar surface of the medial side of the foot is reached (Fig. 1.1D). Inserting a small amount of anesthetic agent as the needle progresses plantarward lessens the discomfort.
- The proper plantar branch to the medial side of the hallux is superficial at that level, having penetrated the deep fascia over the abductor hallucis and flexor hallucis brevis at about the level of the first metatarsomedial cuneiform articulation.
- Palpate the tip of the needle subcutaneously and withdraw it 2 to 3 mm. Instill 2 to 3 mL of anesthetic agent.
- Complete the block by anesthetizing the common digital branch of the medial plantar nerve to the first web space as follows (Fig. 1.1E and F):
  - Return to the dorsal surface of the base of the first intermetatarsal space.
  - The dorsalis pedis artery bifurcates at this point into the first dorsal intermetatarsal artery and the plantar penetrating branch, which turns immediately plantarward,

almost at a right angle to its origin, to communicate with the deep plantar arch (Fig. 1.1G). This is similar to the dorsal branch of the radial artery in the hand. To avoid this arterial bifurcation, move the entrance point distally 1 to 1.5 cm, and, angling obliquely 10 to 20 degrees to the skin, pass the 1.5-inch, 25-gauge needle plantarward between the first and second metatarsals until its tip can be felt subcutaneously on the plantar surface of the foot. Instilling a small amount of the anesthetic agent as the needle passes plantarward and moving slowly lessens the discomfort. Withdraw the needle tip 2 to 3 mm, and instill 4 to 5 mL of solution.
  - If a hammer toe procedure is planned, repeat the same technique between the second and third metatarsals. This should provide adequate anesthesia for the third toe, if required. Supplementing the block with 1 mL of anesthetic agent at the base of the third toe near the web space may be necessary.
- The recommended total maximal dose of anesthetic agents should be calculated for each patient. The patient should have no history of allergy to a local anesthetic agent.

ANKLE BLOCK

TECHNIQUE 1.3

SUPERFICIAL PERONEAL NERVE
- Palpate the tip of the lateral malleolus, and proceed proximally 8 to 10 cm anterior to the subcutaneous border of the shaft of the fibula (Fig. 1.2A).
- Instill 5 to 7 mL of local anesthetic agent subcutaneously. The superficial peroneal nerve will have penetrated the deep fascia and lies subcutaneously at this level in most patients. It may have divided into medial and lateral branches, but their proximity to one another ensures that both will be reached with this volume of agent.

DEEP PERONEAL NERVE
- The anterior tibial artery can usually be palpated beneath the superior extensor retinaculum 4 to 5 cm proximal to the distal articular surface of the tibia. This artery and the deep peroneal nerve that accompanies it lie between the tendons of the anterior tibial and the extensor digitorum longus, and just lateral to the extensor hallucis longus, which is more deeply situated. The nerve usually lies just lateral to the artery.
- If the artery is not palpable, the tendon of the anterior tibia, which is large and lies adjacent to the subcutaneous border of the tibia, can serve as a landmark. Enter the skin just lateral to this tendon; the nerve is located at a depth of 1 to 1.5 cm into the skin (Fig. 1.2B and C).
- The anesthetic agent should flow freely. If not, reposition the needle slightly and insert 3 to 5 mL of the agent, being careful to aspirate before the injection.

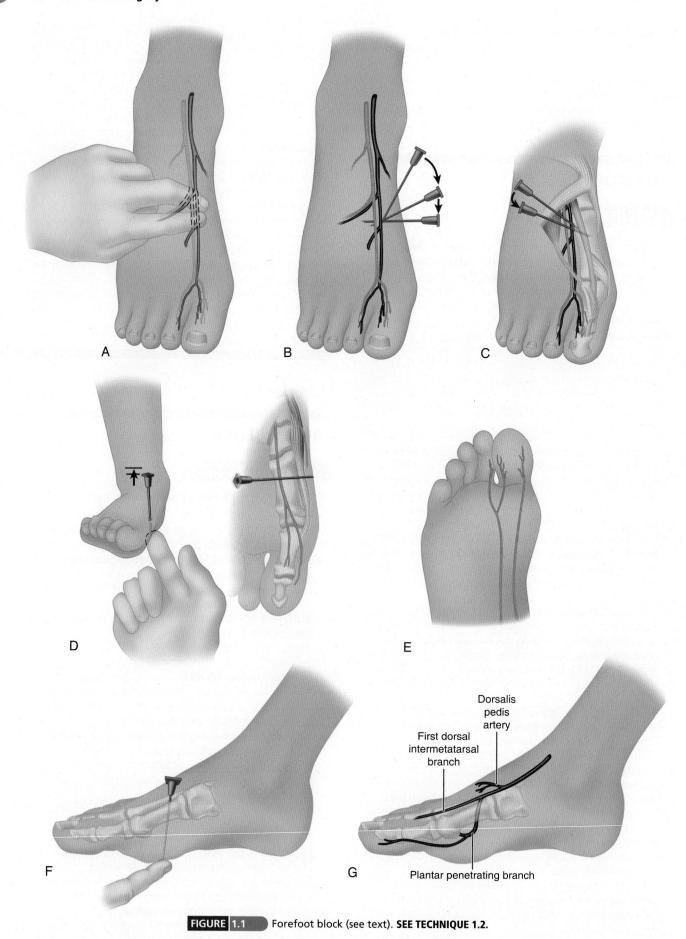

Dorsalis
pedis
artery

First dorsal
intermetatarsal
branch

Plantar penetrating branch

FIGURE 1.1   Forefoot block (see text). **SEE TECHNIQUE 1.2.**

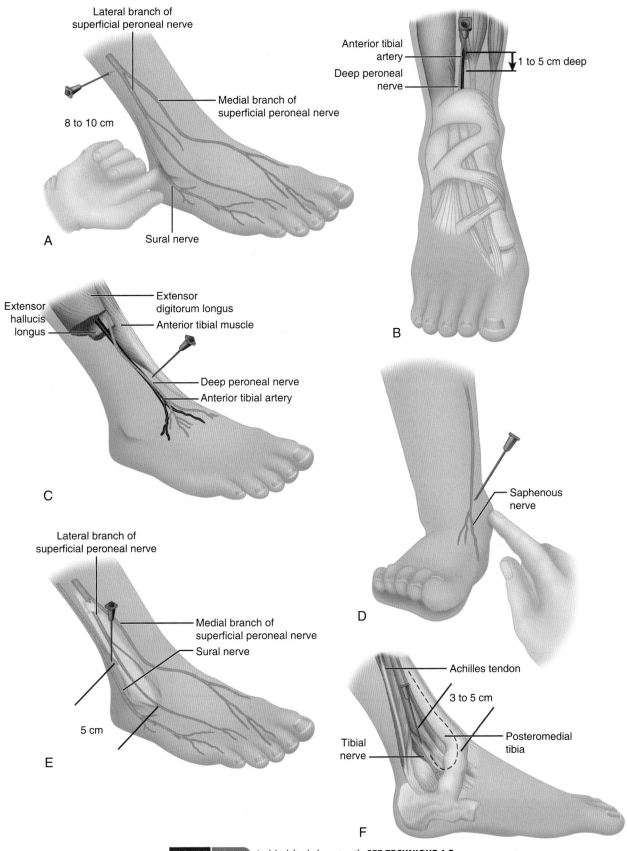

FIGURE 1.2 Ankle block (see text). **SEE TECHNIQUE 1.3.**

SAPHENOUS NERVE

- Palpate the tip of the medial malleolus and 3 to 5 cm proximal to this landmark, and enter the subcutaneous space, directing the needle anteriorly (Fig. 1.2D). The saphenous nerve is located just medial or posterior to the saphenous vein and in a slightly deeper plane.
- Aspirate and inject 2 mL of the anesthetic agent.

SURAL NERVE

- Palpate the tip of the lateral malleolus, and at 5 cm proximal to this point, palpate the peroneus longus tendon along the posterior subcutaneous border of the fibula (Fig. 1.2E). Approximately half way between this tendon and the lateral border of the Achilles tendon, the sural nerve passes just anterolateral to the small saphenous vein. These two structures usually cross one another behind the lateral malleolus such that the nerve lies posterior to the vein.
- Inject 2 to 3 mL of solution subcutaneously at this point.

TIBIAL NERVE

- The tibial nerve is the most difficult but most important nerve to block to ensure adequate surgical anesthesia.
- Palpate the posteromedial border of the tibia approximately 5 cm proximal to the tip of the medial malleolus. Allow the index and middle fingers to slide over the flexor digitorum longus and (deeper) posterior tibial tendons. At the posterior border of these tendons, mark a point of reference with a pen.
- Palpate the medial border of the Achilles tendon. Half way between these two points lies the tibial artery, which is palpable at this level and serves as a helpful landmark.
- Point the needle inferiorly at about 60 degrees to the skin, penetrating 1 to 1.5 cm (Fig. 1.2F).
- Aspirate to ensure that the posterior tibial artery or veins have not been entered, and then instill 8 to 10 mL of the anesthetic agent.

POPLITEAL SCIATIC NERVE BLOCK (PRONE)

TECHNIQUE 1.4

- With the patient prone, draw a line across the popliteal crease, extending between the tendons of the biceps femoris and the semitendinosus muscles, and identify the midline of the crease. The popliteal fossa triangle is bordered by the semitendinosus-semimembranosus, the biceps femoris, and the popliteal crease.
- Measure exactly 7 cm cephalad along a midline axis and 1 cm lateral to the axis (Fig. 1.3A).
- After sterile preparation, raise a skin wheal with 1% plain lidocaine.
- Attach a nerve simulator in accordance with the manufacturer's instructions, placing the negative lead on the involved leg and the positive lead on the ipsilateral leg. Direct the needle cephalad and parallel to the femur, at a 45-degree angle to the skin, and advance it slowly with continuous aspiration (Fig. 1.3B).
- Apply an electrical current of 1 mA at 1 Hz until a brisk contraction of the gastrocnemius is observed, and then decrease the current to 0.3 mA.
- Slowly advance the needle until a brisk muscle twitch is visible, and inject a test dose of 1 mL of local anesthetic.
- Following cessation of the twitch and confirmation that the patient did not experience any pain with the injection, administer 35 mL of local anesthetic in 5-mL increments.
- With the patient supine, use an additional 5 mL of anesthetic to block the saphenous nerve and its infrapatellar branches at the level of the tibial tuberosity.
- Postoperatively, patients should not be allowed to bear weight on the operated limb for 12 to 18 hours to allow return of neurologic function in the foot and ankle.

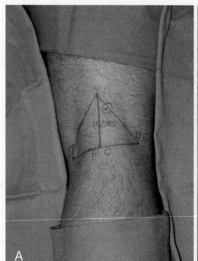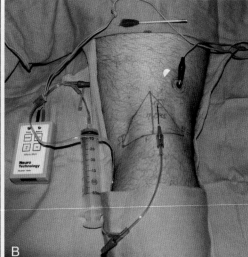

FIGURE 1.3   **A,** Posterior view of popliteal fossa of right knee, with popliteal triangle outlined; *circle* indicates injection site for sciatic nerve block. **B,** Nerve stimulator used to aid in locating sciatic nerve before injection. **SEE TECHNIQUE 1.4.**

LATERAL POPLITEAL NERVE BLOCK

TECHNIQUE 1.5

(GROSSER)

- Place the patient supine, with a 10-lb sandbag placed under the proximal calf as a fulcrum to increase tension on the biceps femoris.
- Instruct an assistant to stabilize the ankle and keep the patella in a neutral position to about 10 degrees of internal rotation.
- Use 30 mL of 0.5% bupivacaine with epinephrine: 20 mL for the peroneal and tibial injection sites and 10 mL for the saphenous nerve site.
- Identify the proximal pole of the patella and the fibular head.
- Draw an axial line from the proximal pole of the patella posteriorly to bisect another line drawn horizontally from the fibular head proximally. The intersection of these two lines is the point of initial needle insertion to anesthetize the peroneal and tibial divisions of the sciatic nerve.

- Direct the needle 30 degrees proximally. Set a nerve stimulator at 5 mA, and advance the needle slowly until the biceps twitch is encountered, and insert further until the peroneal division is localized in eversion and dorsiflexion, and then until the tibial division is in inversion and plantarflexion of the foot (Fig. 1.4).
- When both nerve branch contractions are demonstrated, decrease the nerve stimulator level until the toes are no longer in plantarflexion. A level of more than 1.0 mA is optimal for twitch absence. In a sedated patient who cannot provide feedback, it is concerning if the amplitude drops below 1 mA.
- To localize the nerves, withdraw the needle from the skin to redirect the needle in an anteroposterior plane. In a larger leg, judging the depth of the needle may be difficult, but the tibial division typically is 0.5 to 1 cm lateral to the midline and 1.5 to 2 cm posterior to the femur.
- When the needle is in the proper location, turn the stimulator back up to 3 to 4 mA to elicit twitches and, after negative aspiration for blood, inject 20 mL of anesthetic. Anesthesia is adequate when the contractions cease.
- Disconnect the stimulator and remove the needle.

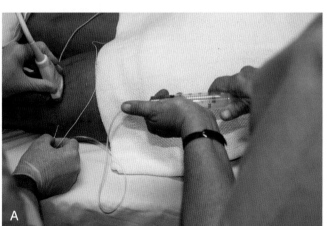

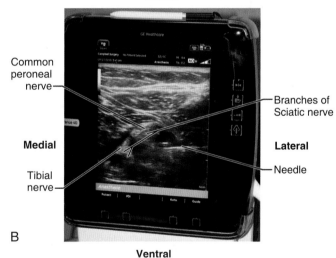

Dorsal

Common peroneal nerve

Branches of Sciatic nerve

Medial **Lateral**

Needle

Tibial nerve

Ventral

A

B

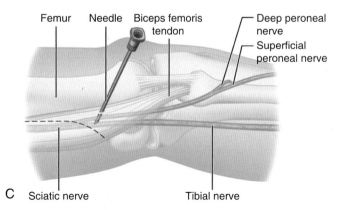

Femur   Needle   Biceps femoris tendon

Deep peroneal nerve

Superficial peroneal nerve

C   Sciatic nerve   Tibial nerve

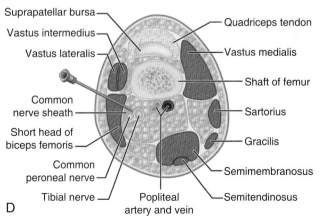

Suprapatellar bursa

Quadriceps tendon

Vastus intermedius

Vastus lateralis

Vastus medialis

Shaft of femur

Common nerve sheath

Sartorius

Short head of biceps femoris

Gracilis

Common peroneal nerve

Semimembranosus

Tibial nerve   Popliteal artery and vein

Semitendinosus

D

FIGURE 1.4   Lateral popliteal nerve block. **SEE TECHNIQUE 1.5.**

- If saphenous nerve anesthesia is required, identify the tibial tubercle and sterilize the medial aspect of the knee with povidone-iodine.
- Insert the needle subdermally, and inject the remaining 10 mL while advancing the needle medially, creating a wheal around the saphenous nerve course.
- Remove the needle and rub the wheal to disperse the anesthetic (McLeod maneuver).

REFERENCES

Bendtsen TF, Nielsen TD, Rohde CV, et al.: Ultrasound guidance improves a continuous popliteal sciatic nerve block when compared with nerve stimulation, *Reg Anesth Pain Med* 36:181, 2011.

Cancienne JM, Cooper MT, Laroche KA, et al.: Hemoglobin A1c as a predictor of postoperative infection following elective forefoot surgery, *Foot Ankle Int* 38:832, 2017.

Chin KJ, Wong NW, Macfarlane AJ, Chan VW: Ultrasound-guided versus anatomic landmark-guided ankle blocks: a 6-year retrospective review, *Reg Anesth Pain Med* 36:611, 2011.

Craik JD, clark A, Hendry J, Hamilton PD: The effect of ankle joint immobilization on lower limb venous flow, *Foot Ankle Int* 36:18, 2015.

Cunningham DJ, DeOrio JK, Nunley JA, et al.: The effect of patient characterisitics on 1 to 2 year and minimum 5-year outcomes after total ankle arthroplasty, *J Bone Joint Surg Am* 101:199, 2019.

Elliot R, Pearce CJ, Seifert C, Calder JD: Continuous infusion versus single bolus popliteal block following major ankle and hindfoot surgery: a prospective, randomized trial, *Foot Ankle Int* 12:1043, 2010.

Finger A, Teunis T, Hageman MG, et al.: Association between opioid intake and disability after surgical management of ankle fractures, *J Am Acad Orthop Surg* 25:519, 2017.

Fitzgibbons PG, Digiovanni C, Hares S, Akelman E: Safe tourniquet use: review of the evidence, *J Am Acad Orthop Surg* 20:310, 2012.

Gartke K, Portner O, Taljaard M: Neuropathic symptoms following continuous popliteal block after foot and ankle surgery, *Foot Ankle Int* 33:267, 2012.

Giannoudis PV, Hak D, Sanders D, et al.: Inflammation, bone healing, and anti-inflammatory drugs: an update, *J Orthop Trauma* 29:S6, 2015.

Goodman SM, Springer B, Guyatt G, et al.: 2017 American College of Rheuamatology/American Association of Hip and Knee Surgeons guideline for the perioperative management of antirheumatic medication in patients with rheumatic diseases undergoing elective total hip or total knee arthroplasty, *J Arthroplasty* 32:2628, 2017.

Griffiths JT, Matthews L, Pearce CJ, Calder JD: Incidence of venous thromboembolism in elective foot and ankle surgery with and without aspirin prophylaxis, *J Bone Joint Surg Br* 94B:210, 2012.

Guichard L, Vanhaesebrouck A, Fletcher D, et al.: Pain trajectory after ankle surgeries for osteoarthritis, *Foot Ankle Int* 40:367, 2019.

Gupta A, Kumar K, Roberts MM, et al.: Pain management after outpatient foot and ankle surgery, *Foot Ankle Int* 39:149, 2018.

Hickey BA, Morgan A, Pugh N, Perera A: The effect of lower limb cast immobilization on calf muscle pump fuction: a simple strategy of exercises can maintain flow, *Foot Ankle Int* 35:429, 2014.

Horne PH, Jennings JM, DeOrio JK, et al.: Low incidence of symptomatic thromboembolic events after total ankle arthroplasty without routine use of chemoprophylaxis, *Foot Ankle Int* 36:611, 2015.

Hunter JG, Dawson LK, Soin SP, Baumhauer JF: Randomized, prospective study of the order of preoperative preparation solutions for patietns undergoing foot and ankle orthopedic surgery, *Foot Ankle Int* 37:478, 2016.

Jameson SS, Augustine A, James P, et al.: Venous thromboembolic events following foot and ankle surgery in the English National Health Service, *J Bone Joint Surg Br* 93B:490, 2011.

Konrad G, Markmiller M, Lenich A, et al.: Tourniquets may increase postoperative swelling and pain after internal fixation of ankle fractures, *Clin Orthop Related Res* 433:189, 2005.

Lachman RJ, Elkrief JI, Pipitone PS, Haydel CL: Comparison of surgical site infections in ankle fracture surgery with or without the use of postoperative antibiotics, *Foot Ankle Int* 39:1278, 2018.

Lam NC, Petersen TR, Gerstein NS, et al.: A randomized clinical trial comparing the effectiveness of ultrasound guidance versus nerve stimulation for lateral popliteal-sciatic nerve blocks in obese patients, *J Ultrasound Med* 33:1057, 2014.

Luiten WE, Schepers T, Luitse JS, et al.: Comparison of continuous nerve block versus patient-controlled analgesis for postoperative pain and outcome afte talar and calcaneal fractures, *Foot Ankle Int* 35:1116, 2014.

Maalouf D, Liu SS, Movahedi R, et al.: Nerve stimulator versus ultrasound guidance for placement of popliteal catheters for foot and ankle surgery, *J Clin Anesth* 24:44, 2012.

McDonald E, Winters B, Nicholson K, et al.: Effect of postoperative ketorolac administration on bone healing in ankle fracture surgery, *Foot Ankle Int* 39:1135, 2018.

Merrill HM, Dean DM, Mottla JL, et al.: Opiod consumption following foot and ankle surgery, *Foot Ankle Int* 39:649, 2018.

Mulligan RP, McCarthy KJ, Grear BJ, et al.: Psychosocial risk factors for postoperative pain in ankle and hindfoot reconstruction, *Foot Ankle Int* 37:1065, 2016.

Mulligan RP, McCarthy KJ, Grear BJ, et al.: Preoperative risk factors for complications in elective ankle and hindfoot reconstruction, *Foot Ankle Spec* 11:54, 2018.

Nasell H, Ottosson C, Tornqvist H, et al.: The impact of smoking on complications after operatively treated ankle fractures—a follow-up study of 906 patients, *J Orthop Trauma* 25:748, 2011.

Patel A, Ogawa B, Charlton T, Thordarson D: Incidence of deep vein thrombosis and pulmonary embolism after Achilles tendon rupture, *Clin Orthop Relat Res* 470:270, 2012.

Pelet S, Roger ME, Belzile EL, Bouchard M: The incidence of thromboembolic events in surgically treated ankle fracture, *J Bone Joint Surg Am* 94:502, 2012.

Richey JM, Weintraub MLR, Schuberth JM: Incidence and risk factors of symptomatic venous thromboembolism following foot and ankle surgery, *Foot Ankle Int* 40:98, 2019.

Robbins J, Green CL, Parekh SG: Liposomal bupivacaine in forefoot surgery, *Foot Ankle Int* 36:503, 2015.

Ruta DJ, Kadakia AR, Irwin TA: What are the patterns of prophylactic postoperative oral antibiotic use after foot and ankle surgery? *Clin Orthop Relat Res* 472:3204, 2014.

Saini S, McDonald EL, Shakked R, et al.: Prospective evaluation of utilization patterns and prescribing guidelines of opioid consumption following orthopedic foot and ankle surgery, *Foot Ankle Int* 39:1257, 2018.

Sanders A, Gupta A, Jones M, et al.: Pain management after outpatient foot and ankle surgery, *Foot Ankle Orthopaedics* 2, 2017.

Saporito A, Sturini E, Borgeat A, Aguirre J: The effect of continuous popliteal sciatic nerve block on unplanned postoperative visits and readmissions after foot surgery – a randomized, controlled study comparing day-care and inpatient management, *Anaesthesia* 69:1197, 2014.

Selby R, Geerts WH, Kreder HJ, et al.: Symptomatic venous thromboembolism uncommon without thromboprophylaxis after isolated lower-limb fracture, *J Bone Joint Surg Am* 96:83, 2014.

Shadid MB, Speth MJGM, Voorn GP, Wolterbeek N: Chlorhexidine 0.5%/70% Alcohol and Iodine 1%/70% alcohol both reduce bacterial load in clean foot surgery: a randomized, controlled trial, *J Foot Ankle Surg* 58:278, 2019.

Shah A, Huntley S, Harshadkumar P, et al.: Incidence of venous thromboembolism in orthopaedic foot and ankle surgeries, *Foot Ankle Orthopeadics* 2018.

Sim J, Grocott N, Majeed H, McClelland D: Effect of hospital length of stay on tourniquet use during internal fixation of ankle fractures: randomized control trial, *J Foot and Ankle Surg* 58:114, 2019.

Sindhu K, Cohen B, Gil J: Perioperative management of rheumatoid medications in orthopedic surgery, *Orthopedics* 40:282, 2017.

Smith JT, Halim K, Palms DA, et al.: Prevalence of Vitamin D deficiency in patients with foot and ankle injuries, *Foot Ankle Int* 35:8, 2014.

Smith TO, Hing CB: The efficacy of the tourniquet in foot and ankle surgery? A systematic review and meta-analysis, *Foot Ankle Surg* 16:3, 2010.

White BJ, Walsh M, Egol KA, Tejwani NC: Intra-articular block compared with conscious sedation for closed reduction of ankle fracture-dislocations, *J Bone Joint Surg* 90(A):731, 2008.

Wiewiorski M, Barg A, Hoerterer H, et al.: Risk factors for wound complications in patients after elective orthopedic foot and ankle surgery, *Foot Ankle Int* 36:479, 2015.

Wukich DK, Crim BE, Frykberg RG, Rosario BL: Neuropathy and poorly controlled diabetes increase the rate of surgical site infection after foot and ankle surgery, *J Bone Joint Surg Am* 96:832, 2014.

Yammine K, Harvey A: Efficacy of preparation solutions and cleansing techniques on contamination of the skin in foot and ankle surgery, *J Bone Joint Br* 95B:498, 2013.

Yeganeh MH, Kheir MM, Shahi A, Parvizi J: Rheumatoid arthritis, disease modifying agents, and periprosthetic joint infection: what does a joint surgeon need to know? *J Arthroplasty* 33:1258, 2018.

The complete list of references is available online at ExpertConsult.com.

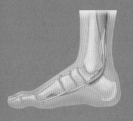

HALLUX VALGUS (BUNION)

Hallux valgus (lateral deviation of the great toe) is not a single disorder, as the name implies, but a complex deformity of the first ray that frequently is accompanied by deformity and symptoms in the lesser toes. Often the angle between the first and second metatarsals is more than the 8 to 9 degrees usually considered to be the upper limits of normal. The valgus angle of the first metatarsophalangeal joint also is more than the 15 to 20 degrees considered to be the upper limits of normal (Fig. 2.1). If the valgus angle of the first metatarsophalangeal joint exceeds 30 to 35 degrees, pronation of the great toe usually results. With this abnormal rotation, the abductor hallucis, which is normally plantar to the flexion-extension axis of the first metatarsophalangeal joint, moves farther plantarward (Fig. 2.2). In this case, the only restraining medial structure is the medial capsular ligament with its capsulosesamoid portion (inserting into the base of the proximal phalanx) and capsulophalangeal portion (inserting into the plantar plate). The adductor hallucis, which is unopposed by the abductor hallucis, pulls the great toe farther into valgus, stretching the medial capsular ligament (particularly the capsulosesamoid), attenuating this structure, and allowing the metatarsal head to drift medially from the sesamoids. In addition, the flexor hallucis brevis, flexor hallucis longus, adductor hallucis, and extensor hallucis longus increase the valgus moment at the metatarsophalangeal joint, further deforming the first ray. The deep transverse intermetatarsal ligament runs between the plantar plates at the metatarsophalangeal joints and does not insert into bone on the adjacent sides of the metatarsal heads. Finally, the sesamoid ridge on the plantar surface of the first metatarsal head (the crista) flattens because of

pressure (abutment) from the tibial sesamoid (Fig. 2.3). With this restraint lost, the fibular sesamoid displaces partially or completely into the first intermetatarsal space (see Fig. 2.1). In this situation, the patient is bearing less weight on the first ray and more on the lesser metatarsal heads, increasing the likelihood of transfer metatarsalgia, callosities, and stress fracture of a lesser metatarsal.

Two other anatomic variants involving the articular surface of the first metatarsophalangeal joint can lead to hallux valgus. In the first variant, the articular surface of the metatarsal head is offset, resembling a scoop of ice cream sitting at an angle on a cone (Fig. 2.4). This has been described as the distal metatarsal articular angle (Fig. 2.5). In the second, the articular angle of the base of the proximal phalanx in relation to its longitudinal axis is offset. This has been described as the phalangeal articular angle (Fig. 2.6). Although the normal range of these angles is generally considered to be 7 to 10 degrees for the phalangeal articular angle and 10 to 15 degrees for the distal metatarsal articular angle, exact measurements are difficult to reproduce because of the variability of radiographic and measurement techniques (see Fig. 2.6). Increasing evidence indicates, however, that the failure to correct these two deformities, especially the distal metatarsal articular angle, can cause unsatisfactory results after surgery in some patients. Forceful straightening of the hallux should be avoided if it sacrifices a congruent metatarsophalangeal articulation; phalangeal osteotomy or distal metatarsal osteotomy, rather than tightening of the medial capsular repair, should be used for further correction.

The valgus posture of the great toe frequently causes a hammer toe–like deformity of the second toe (Fig. 2.7).

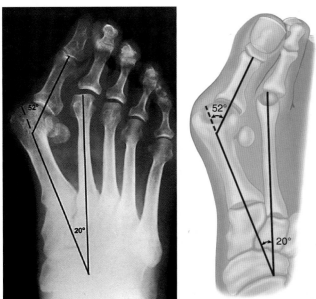

FIGURE 2.1 Hallux valgus complex. Note increase in inter-metatarsal angle, lateral dislocation of sesamoids, subluxation of first metatarsophalangeal joint (leaving metatarsal head uncovered), and pronation of great toe associated with marked hallux valgus.

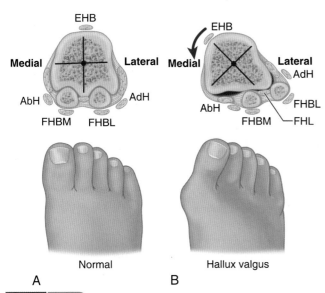

FIGURE 2.2 Pronation of hallux. **A,** Normal. **B,** Note plantar shift of abductor hallucis and lateral shift of sesamoids with associated intrinsic muscles of hallux. *AbH,* Abductor hallucis; *AdH,* adductor hallucis; *EHB,* extensor hallucis brevis; *FHBL,* flexor hallucis brevis lateral; *FHBM,* flexor hallucis brevis medial. (Redrawn from Miller J: Acquired hallux varus a preventable and correctable disorder, *J Bone Joint Surg* 57A:183, 1975.)

In addition, the splaying of the forefoot makes the wearing of shoes more difficult; with shoes that have a narrow toe box, corns often develop, as does bursal hypertrophy over the medial eminence of the first metatarsal head (bunion). With valgus subluxation of the first metatarsophalangeal joint, osteoarthritis frequently develops. In this case, the entire spectrum of hallux valgus is present: varus deformity of the first metatarsal, valgus of the great toe, bunion formation, arthritis of the first metatarsophalangeal joint, hammer toe of one or more toes, corns, calluses, and metatarsalgia. The entire forefoot must be evaluated for these multiple components of hallux valgus before surgical planning is complete and recommendations can be made to the patient.

The controversy continues over which deformity is the essential lesion in hallux valgus: metatarsus primus varus or lateral deviation of the great toe. Each is incriminated as the cause of the other. The strongest data probably support lateral deviation of the great toe as the primary deformity in most patients, followed by medial angulation of the first metatarsal, but metatarsus primus varus may be the principal cause in adolescents. Further controversy surrounds the role of footwear as the prime offender in the development of hallux valgus. Most orthopaedic surgeons have seen unilateral hallux valgus when both feet are clinically and radiographically the same structurally except that one foot has a bunion deformity and the other foot is normal. Evidence supports that hallux valgus may be familial, especially when it occurs in adolescents. Although no study of shod and unshod societies has implicated inappropriate footwear as the sole cause of hallux valgus, after genetic factors and binding, unphysiologically designed footwear probably is the major cause in modern societies.

Hypermobility of the first ray also has been suggested as a causative factor in the development of hallux valgus and first metatarsal varus, but this is controversial. Dietz et al. reviewed pedobarographic studies, clinical examinations, and standard weight-bearing radiographs in patients with hallux valgus, correlating the findings with radiokinematic first ray instability in the sagittal plane. Their analysis showed an association between a wide intermetatarsal angle and increased maximal dorsiflexion of the first ray during walking. They noted that first tarsometatarsal joint instability increased the maximum transfer of force to the central forefoot, which increases the risk of metatarsalgia.

Finally, anatomic and structural abnormalities almost certainly play a causative role in hallux valgus. Pronated flatfeet, abnormal insertion of the posterior tibial tendon, increased obliquity of the first metatarsomedial-cuneiform joint, an abnormally long first ray, incongruous articular surfaces of the first metatarsophalangeal joint, and excessive valgus tilt of the articular surface of the first metatarsal head and proximal phalangeal articular surface may contribute alone or in combination to the deformity and influence the recommended treatment. Hypertrophy of the medial eminence has been described as a component of hallux valgus deformity since the earliest reports; however, more recent investigations have found that bony proliferation is not a component of the pathoanatomy of hallux valgus and that the prominence of the medial eminence results from the combination of metatarsus primus varus and medial deviation that uncovers the articular surface.

With more than 130 operations recommended for the treatment of hallux valgus, it is practical to describe only a few. Although Spiers made the following observation in 1920, most procedures to correct hallux valgus still use one or more of the components he described:

An operative attempt to relieve the pain and disability accompanying hallux valgus is far from a new procedure.

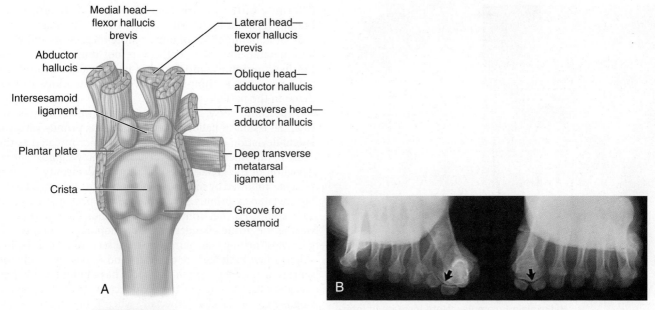

FIGURE 2.3   **A,** Plantar surface of first metatarsal head. Entire sesamoid sling with attached intrinsic musculature has been rotated distally off metatarsal head to present schematically relationships of muscle, tendon, capsule, ligaments, and articular configuration of first metatarsophalangeal joint. **B,** As metatarsal head moves medially, sesamoid sling apparatus becomes valgus deforming force, and metatarsal rotates (pronates) on its longitudinal axis. Intrinsic and extrinsic muscle balance is lost, and deformity increases. (**A** after Beverly Kessler; courtesy LTI Medica and The Upjohn Company.)

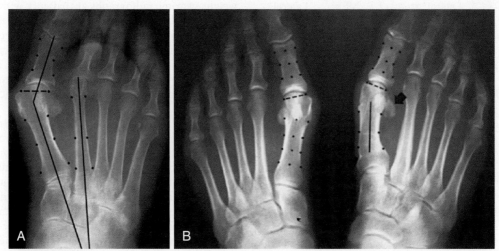

FIGURE 2.4   **A,** Note valgus orientation of articular surface of first metatarsal head. **B,** After proximal metatarsal osteotomy on right foot. Sesamoid sling remains dislocated, articular surface of metatarsal head maintains valgus posture, and joint is congruous in valgus. Double osteotomy of first metatarsal (proximally for varus correction and distally for valgus correction of articular surface) and soft-tissue realignment are necessary. Alternatively, arthrodesis of first metatarsophalangeal joint or distal metatarsal osteotomy (chevron) can be performed. Without anatomic reduction of sesamoid sling apparatus, distal metatarsal osteotomy would fail.

Removal of the exostosis, dissection of the bursa, tenotomy and transplantation of the tendons, removal of the sesamoids, partial and complete removal of the head of the first metatarsal, and removal of the proximal end of the proximal phalanx, together with numerous combinations of the foregoing, have all been advocated and practiced.

This chapter presents in detail the soft-tissue procedures, bony procedures, and procedures combining soft-tissue and bony correction that have endured the clinical test of adequate numbers of patients, lengthy and detailed review, and reports by multiple observers using essentially the same techniques. Different groups of procedures are successful

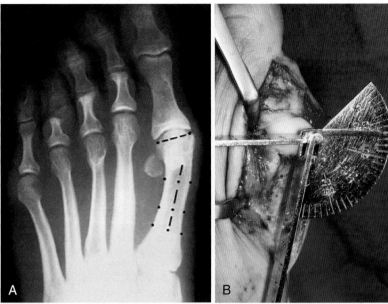

FIGURE 2.5   **A,** Determination of position of articular surface of metatarsal head in relation to longitudinal axis of first metatarsal. **B,** Measurement of distal metatarsal articular angle at time of surgery. Markings are at medial and lateral margins of articular surface of first metatarsal head and longitudinal axis of first metatarsal shaft.

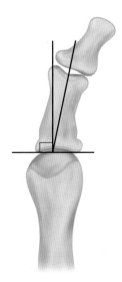

FIGURE 2.6   Proximal phalangeal articular angle.

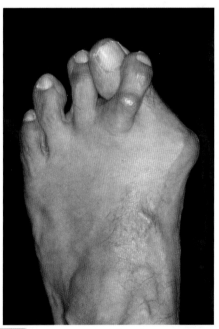

FIGURE 2.7   Hammer toe deformity. Note severe crossover-toe deformity of second toe associated with severe hallux valgus. Primary complaint frequently is not severe hallux valgus deformity but pain beneath second metatarsal head.

for different surgeons, and none of the following treatment recommendations is meant to be the conclusive opinion on "bunion surgery." Surgeons should be technically comfortable with several different procedures for the correction of hallux valgus, including one or more bony, soft-tissue, or combined procedures. Several authors have described algorithms for selecting the appropriate operative procedure in the treatment of hallux valgus and hallux rigidus (Fig. 2.8). Regardless, without surgery the quality of life in patients with symptomatic hallux valgus is lower than in the general population. The decision on whether to proceed with correction, as well as the type of surgery to perform, should be based not only on the severity of the deformity but also on the patient's symptoms.

PREOPERATIVE ASSESSMENT AND MANAGEMENT

No procedure should be recommended until the entire foot, not just the first ray, is thoroughly examined clinically while the patient is standing, sitting, and lying supine and prone (if practical). Particular attention should be given to the remainder of the forefoot, and corns, calluses, warts, interdigital neuromas, bunionettes, hammer toes, and claw toes should

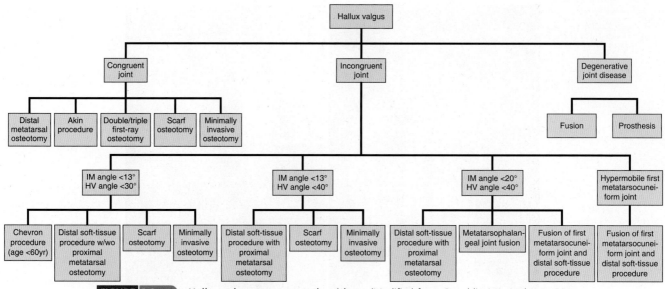

FIGURE 2.8 **Hallux valgus treatment algorithm.** (Modified from Coughlin MJ, Anderson RB: Hallux valgus. In Coughlin MJ, Saltzman CL, Anderson RB, editors: *Mann's Surgery of the Foot and Ankle*, Philadelphia, Elsevier, 2014, pp 202–204.)

be identified. Although pain and deformity may be relieved after correction of the hallux valgus, the result can be marred if symptoms in the lesser toes or the metatarsals remain. This should be explained carefully to the patient before surgery to avoid false expectations and disappointment. Finally, the midfoot and hindfoot must be examined carefully before making treatment recommendations for forefoot surgery.

Initially, most patients can be treated nonoperatively with appropriate shoe modifications, exercises, and activity adjustments. Operative treatment of hallux valgus for cosmetic reasons alone is seldom indicated except in an adolescent with a significant progressive deformity. Even the mildest symptoms in an adolescent often worsen, especially when there is a family history of hallux valgus. Correction of hallux valgus in adolescents can be difficult and often disappointing.

Any procedure chosen must take into account the following physical examination components:

1. Patient desires for activity and shoe requirements
2. Morphology of the toe (i.e., a short, wide toe as opposed to a long, thin toe)
3. Lesser toe deformities, especially varus or valgus of the second toe (quality-of-life measures are significantly worse with lesser toe deformity or metatarsalgia than with hallux valgus alone)
4. Plantar callosities of the forefoot or tenderness under the lesser metatarsal heads
5. Arch height
6. Clinical pronation of the great toe
7. Range of motion of the toe (the toe pronates as it is extended, an indication of intrinsic malalignment)
8. Sensation about the toe, especially the dorsal medial hallucal nerve (terminal branch of the dorsal medial cutaneous nerve)
9. Contracture of the gastrocsoleus complex
10. Smoking status
11. Patient weight
12. Patient age and sex (men and adolescents commonly have congruent joints)

13. Generalized hypermobility (Fig. 2.9)

The following radiographic parameters should be taken into account:

1. Valgus deviation of the great toe (hallux valgus)
2. Varus deviation of the first metatarsal
3. Pronation of the hallux or first metatarsal, or both
4. Hallux valgus interphalangeus
5. Arthritis and limitation of motion of the first metatarsophalangeal joint
6. Length of the first metatarsal relative to lesser metatarsals
7. Excessive mobility or obliquity of the first metatarsomedial cuneiform joint
8. The medial eminence (bunion)
9. The location of the sesamoid apparatus
10. Intrinsic and extrinsic muscle-tendon balance and synchrony
11. Presence of metatarsus adductus
12. Width of the first metatarsal (wider metatarsal in the presence of the same intermetatarsal angle will allow greater lateral translation of a distal osteotomy)
13. Deformity of the lesser toes

Inadequate vascularity or sensibility should be investigated thoroughly before bunion surgery is considered. In addition, the position of the articular surface of the metatarsal head in relation to the longitudinal axis of the first metatarsal should be determined (see Fig. 2.5).

Standard preoperative radiographs should include standing dorsoplantar and lateral views, a nonstanding lateral oblique view, and axial sesamoid views. Some authors have found a discrepancy between anteroposterior and axial views in determining the tibial sesamoid position, especially in sesamoid positions 4 and 5 of the Hardy and Clapham scale. We believe that an axial sesamoid view helps to determine the extent of intrinsic malalignment, especially if the tibial sesamoid is in position 4 or 5 on an anteroposterior view. The hallux valgus angle and the first-second intermetatarsal angle should first be drawn on the standing dorsoplantar view by

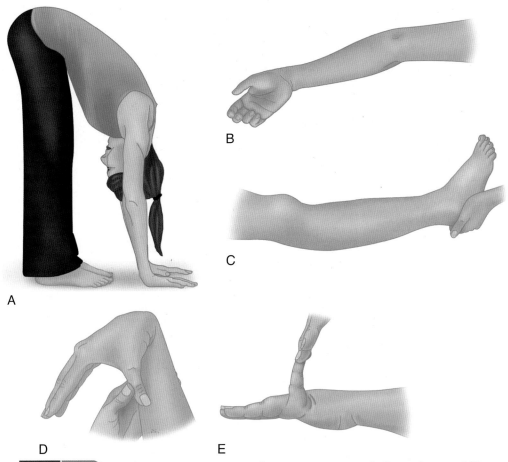

FIGURE 2.9 Beighton score. An answer of yes to two or more indicates hypermobility. **A,** 1 point if while forward bending and legs straight palms can be placed on ground. **B,** 1 point for each elbow that can bend backward. **C,** 1 point for each knee that can bend backward. **D,** 1 point for each thumb that can touch the forearm when forward bending. **E,** 1 point for each finger that can bend more than 90 degrees backward.

bisecting the shafts of the bones (Fig. 2.10), with an awareness of the normal ranges. These angles are most frequently cited as guidelines for treatment decisions, but Donnelly et al. reported that interobserver measurements of the hallux valgus angle varied by approximately 6 degrees and those of the intermetatarsal angle by 4 degrees. They cautioned that potential errors in measurement should be considered when these parameters are used to make treatment decisions. Ortiz et al. defined a new angular measurement that they termed "angle to be corrected (ATC)" in which a line is drawn from the first metatarsal head center to the center of the first metatarsal base and a second line from the metatarsal base through the sesamoid complex midpoint (Fig. 2.11). They found this measurement angle to be as reliable as the intermetatarsal angle.

The hallux valgus interphalangeus angle and any evidence of degenerative arthritic changes at the first metatarsophalangeal or metatarsocuneiform joints should be documented. Oddities may be present and, if overlooked, may compromise a technically well-done procedure. The presence of an os intermetatarseum between the bases of the first and second metatarsals might preclude the effectiveness of a soft-tissue procedure alone to provide sufficient correction of the increased intermetatarsal angle. Likewise, accessory

sesamoids and prominent ungual tuberosities at the interphalangeal joint contribute to a painful callus at the tibial side of this joint. An os tibiale externum frequently is associated with excessive hallux valgus interphalangeus. Varus of the first metatarsal might be a significant part of the overall deformity of the foot even with an intermetatarsal angle of less than 10 degrees. Metatarsus varus with a relatively small hallux valgus angle (15 to 20 degrees) may produce significant deformity even though the angles are not excessive.

The usefulness of computer-assisted compared with manual measurement of the intermetatarsal angle, hallux valgus angle, and distal metatarsal articular angle is still uncertain. Both methods have closer interobserver and intraobserver correlation in measurement of the intermetatarsal angle and hallux valgus angle than in measurement of the distal metatarsal articular angle. The reliability of either method has such a wide range (5 degrees). Measurements of these angles, although useful as a guide, do not provide a completely reliable indication of the magnitude of deformity. Schneider et al. reported two methods of determining angular measurements based on distinctly different reference points: (1) a longitudinal axis of the first metatarsal using middiaphyseal reference points and (2) a center-head technique using a center head (center of the articular surface) and center base (center

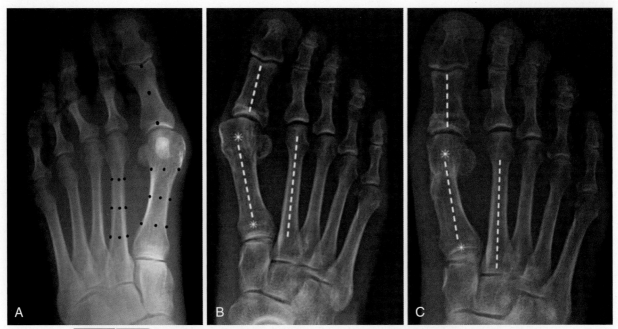

FIGURE 2.10   Method of measuring hallux valgus angle and intermetatarsal angle. **A,** Center points are connected; if lines are extended, angles are defined. Most current Picture Archiving and Communication Systems (PACS) have functions that determine angles. **B** and **C,** Center-head technique of intermetatarsal angle measurement versus preoperative shaft measurement technique.

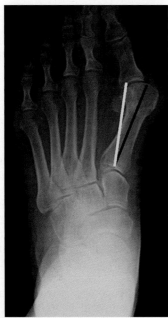

FIGURE 2.11   Angle to be corrected (ATC). Black line (metatarsal bone axis) passes through midline of base of metatarsal head. Yellow line begins at same point as metatarsal bone axis but ends at midpoint of sesamoid complex, mid-distance between medial and lateral sesamoid. (From Ortiz et al: "Angle to be corrected" in preoperative evaluation for hallux valgus surgery: analysis of a new angular measurement, *Foot Ankle Int* 37:172, 2016.)

of the proximal diaphysis) as reference points. They found that measured correction of the hallux valgus and intermetatarsal angles varied by approximately 9 degrees depending on which reference points were used. Recommendations of

Coughlin, Saltzman, and Nunley (American Orthopaedic Foot and Ankle Society Ad Hoc Committee on Angular Measurements) included standardized radiographic technique, specific placement of reference points, use of a protractor rather than a goniometer for measurements, and, after distal osteotomies, dual measurements using a center-head technique and a Mose sphere. Farber et al. determined that the use of a computer-assisted angle measurement on digital radiographs provided more reliable results than use of a goniometer and plain films: interobserver and intraobserver agreement improved from 66% to 80% (Box 2.1).

Kimura et al. recommended evaluating the hallux valgus deformity using a weight-bearing CT image because it can provide detail in three dimensions. They created a loading device that can be used in conventional scanners to simulate a weight-bearing state. Standing radiographic measurements of the hallux valgus angle, the first–second intermetatarsal angle, the lateral talo–first metatarsal angle, and the calcaneal angle correlated well with those measured using their device, indicating that this may be a suitable substitute for standing radiographs when measuring three-dimensional joint angles.

First ray pronation may have a role in the development and progression of hallux valgus as well as treatment. Although pronation of the first ray is frequently present, especially in patients with severe deformities, it remains technically difficult to measure. Eustace et al. described a method of detecting pronation in a cadaver model and found significant correlations between pronation of the proximal phalanx and the intermetatarsal angle, as well as between pronation of the first metatarsal and pronation of the proximal phalanx. As the intermetatarsal angle increased so did first metatarsal pronation. They concluded that pronation and varus deviation of the first metatarsal are linked. Saltzman et al. also found a weak relationship between first metatarsal pronation and the

Observations on Weight-Bearing Anteroposterior Views

Varus of first metatarsal (normal intermetatarsal angle is ≤9 degrees)

Severity of valgus of hallux (normal hallux valgus angle is ≤15 degrees)

Congruity or incongruity of first metatarsophalangeal joint (hallux valgus deformity can exist even in a congruous joint)

Length of first metatarsal relative to second (is second metatarsal >6-7 mm longer than first?)

Subluxation of sesamoid bones (if present, to what extent?)

Well-developed facet between first and second metatarsals, suggesting difficulty displacing first metatarsal laterally at first metatarsocuneiform joint

Sloping of first metatarsocuneiform articulation laterally to medially at a severe angle

Degenerative arthritic changes at interphalangeal, metatarsophalangeal, or metatarsocuneiform articulations

Hallux valgus interphalangeus of ≤10 degrees in neutral flexion and extension of interphalangeal joint

Excessive distal metatarsal articular angle (normal distal metatarsal angle is ≤15 degrees)

Convex medial bowing of proximal phalanx

hallux valgus angle, and Gómez Galván et al. noted a relation between hallux valgus severity and pronation of the proximal phalanx. A study by Campbell et al. using CT and a three-dimensional computer-aided design geometric method did not find a significant correlation between the intermetatarsal angle or hallux valgus angle and the severity of pronation of the first metatarsal; however, pronation of the first metatarsal relative to the second metatarsal was significantly larger in patients with hallux valgus. They noted, however, that this lack of correlation could have been the result of differences in bunions, as they did not classify patients by the type of bunion. Nevertheless, they concluded that surgical correction must take into account the triplanar deformity involved in hallux valgus, including pronation of the great toe and pronation of the first metatarsal. They advised caution using any clinical or radiographic measures until these have been more clearly defined.

Although the use of radiographic angles is important when deciding treatment for patients with hallux valgus, Matthews et al. found that the angles do not correlate well with patient-reported outcomes and suggested that too much emphasis is being placed on these preoperative and postoperative values. Using weight-bearing radiographs and correct foot positioning are necessary to obtain correct angle measurements. According to Kuyucu et al., the hallux valgus angle was more susceptible to false weight-bearing radiographs obtained in different positions than the intermetatarsal angle.

POSTOPERATIVE CONSIDERATIONS

Hallux valgus correction is one of the most frequently performed surgeries in the United States. Most patients benefit in terms of pain and function after surgery; however, as many as a third of patients continue to have some degree of pain

for 6 to 18 months postoperatively, with most being pain free by 2 years. Postoperative pain management can be challenging, especially as it pertains to opioid prescriptions. With the opioid epidemic, it is necessary to individualize prescriptions for pain by patient and type of procedure. Finney et al., in a review of 36,562 patients who underwent correction for hallux valgus, found that persistent opioid use affected a large number of patients (6.2%). Patients who had first metatarsal–cuneiform arthrodesis were more likely to persistently use opioids compared with patients who had a distal metatarsal osteotomy. Other associated factors included surgeon prescribing patterns and coexisting mental health and pain disorders in patients. Rogero et al. compared four different procedures and found no significant differences between prolonged opioid use and surgery, although they did find significant associations between prolonged opioid consumption and preoperative visual analog pain scores and younger patient age.

Shakked et al. studied the relationship between depression and outcomes after hallux valgus surgery in 239 patients. Although patients with depressive symptoms had more pain at baseline and less pain after surgery than patients without depression, their satisfaction scores and functional outcomes were lower. The reasons for this were unclear but should be considered when counseling patients regarding outcomes. Lai et al. evaluated the role that mental health status has on postoperative outcomes after the scarf osteotomy. They found that patients with preoperative mental component scores (MCS) of more than 50 had significantly higher postoperative functional scores than patients with preoperative MCS of less than 50.

Return to driving after hallux valgus surgery is a frequent question posed by patients, especially when the surgery involves the right lower extremity. Studies on lower extremity fractures have cited 6 weeks after initial weight bearing for safe return to driving. McDonald et al. conducted a study in 60 patients after first metatarsal osteotomy for hallux valgus correction, assessing their driving readiness by visual analog scale survey and testing of reaction times. They determined that some patients can return as early as 6 weeks, depending on their readiness survey, and most were able to return to driving at 8 weeks postoperatively.

SOFT-TISSUE PROCEDURES

The usual candidate for soft-tissue correction of the hallux valgus complex is a 30- to 50-year-old woman with clinical symptoms and a valgus angle at the metatarsophalangeal joint of 15 to 25 degrees, an intermetatarsal angle of less than 13 degrees, valgus of the interphalangeal joint of less than 15 degrees, no degenerative changes at the metatarsophalangeal joint, and a history of conservative management failure. The modified McBride procedure is basically a combination of the procedures described by Silver in 1923 and McBride in 1928 and later modified by DuVries and popularized by Mann. The results of this procedure are successful in properly selected patients (Fig. 2.12). Stress view radiographs can help determine which patients can be treated with a modified McBride procedure. "Booking open" of the medial side of the metatarsocuneiform joint on stress views may indicate incongruous motion, lateral impingement, and loss of bony support and the medial capsule acting as a spring on stretch. Osteotomy usually is indicated in patients with this medial

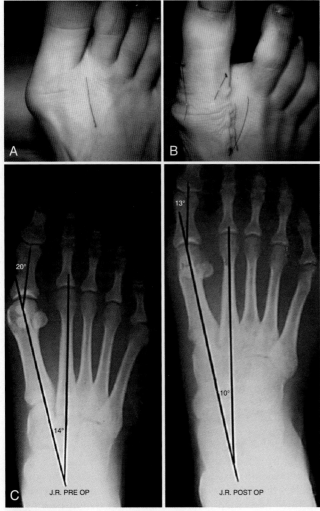

A

B

13°

20°

10°

14°

C   J.R. PRE OP   J.R. POST OP

FIGURE **2.12**   Hallux valgus treated by modified McBride procedure. **A,** Preoperative deformity in 30-year-old patient. **B,** Correction obtained at surgery. **C,** Preoperative and postoperative radiographs (note fibular sesamoid was not removed). More deformity can be corrected by fibular sesamoidectomy, but overcorrection (hallux varus) is a risk. If fibular sesamoid is excised, medial capsule should be closed while holding hallux in 5 to 10 degrees valgus and kept in that position until capsular healing.

wedged opening of the joint. If a firm forefoot wrap reduces the intermetatarsal angle to a normal value and decreases the hallux valgus angle, however, while congruously rotating the base of the first metatarsal on the medial cuneiform without levering the joint open medially, the McBride procedure can correct the deformity. Correction is improved by excision of the fibular (lateral) sesamoid because the adductor hallucis and lateral head of the flexor hallucis brevis are released, markedly reducing the valgus moment at the first metatarsophalangeal joint. In addition, the pull of the fibular sesamoid on the flexor hallucis longus through its tendon sheath and pulley system is prevented, reducing another important valgus-producing force on the hallux at the metatarsophalangeal joint. If the fibular sesamoid is excised, the medial capsule should be repaired with the hallux held in 10 to 15 degrees of valgus. This position must be maintained by a postoperative dressing for 3 or 4 weeks. It seems convincing that correction of the sesamoid position in hallux valgus surgery occurs by

placing the metatarsal head over the sesamoid rather than by reducing the sesamoids by pulling them under the metatarsal head. A study by Huang et al. of 165 patients with hallux valgus treated with reconstruction found that sesamoid correction correlated with first to second intermetatarsal correction. Their results did not support the concept that medial plication pulls the sesamoids under the first metatarsal.

MODIFIED MCBRIDE BUNIONECTOMY

TECHNIQUE 2.1

ANESTHESIA
- For a mild or moderate deformity, a regional anesthetic can be used. For severe deformity, the patient should be placed under general anesthesia with a supplemental block given.

TOURNIQUET
- For a mild or moderate deformity, an ankle tourniquet can be used; however, it should be released before final closure of the capsule because the tension on the long flexor and extensor to the toe limit the assessment of the final position of the toe. For severe deformity, we advise using a thigh tourniquet so that intraoperative decision making and technique are not influenced by the ankle tourniquet producing contracture of the flexor hallucis longus or extensor hallucis longus.

SKIN AND CAPSULAR INCISION
- With the patient supine and a tourniquet on the limb, extend a midline, straight, medial incision from the middle of the proximal phalanx to 2 cm proximal to the junction of the medial eminence with the metatarsal shaft (Fig. 2.13). This incision usually is in an internervous plane between the most medial branches of the superficial peroneal nerve dorsally and the medial proper digital branch of the medial plantar nerve plantarward. (McBride recommended a single incision beginning at the first web space and extending proximally and medially across the metatarsal, ending on the medial side of the first metatarsal proximal to the exostosis.)
- Mobilize the skin 2 to 3 mm dorsally and plantarward to ensure that no sensory nerve would be injured by the capsular incision.
- Coagulate the superficial veins as encountered to minimize postoperative bleeding.
- Use delicate, two-tooth retractors and 1.5-mm forceps in this initial dissection to avoid unnecessary skin trauma.
- Make a longitudinal capsular incision (the original McBride capsular incision was transverse) 3 to 4 mm plantar to the line of the skin incision (Fig. 2.14).
- By sharp dissection, raise the periosteum and the capsule dorsally and plantarward from the base of the proximal phalanx to the proximal edge of the medial eminence (Fig. 2.15). At the proximal end of the medial eminence, avoid releasing the proximal bony attachments of the medial capsule on the metatarsal neck (especially in the dorsal direction) in an attempt to expose the medial eminence.

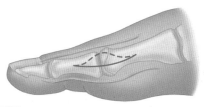

FIGURE 2.13 Modified McBride procedure: first incision. *Dashed line* denotes dorsally curved incision; *solid line* indicates preferred incision (internervous plane). **SEE TECHNIQUE 2.1.**

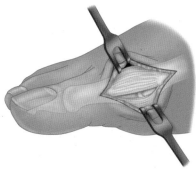

FIGURE 2.14 Modified McBride procedure. Longitudinal capsular incision is 3 to 4 mm plantar to skin incision. **SEE TECHNIQUE 2.1.**

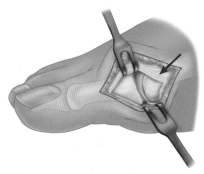

FIGURE 2.15 Modified McBride procedure. Capsule is opened, and attachment of capsule on metatarsal neck *(arrow)* is carefully preserved. **SEE TECHNIQUE 2.1.**

To ensure adequate exposure without disruption of this proximal attachment, a longitudinal capsular incision is suggested.
- Elevate the capsule by sharp dissection dorsalward and plantarward to expose the dorsal aspect of the metatarsal head, the entire medial eminence, and the plantar plate. A periosteal elevator is not recommended because of the possibility that the proximal attachments of the capsule may be released.

L-SHAPED CAPSULAR INCISION
- Alternatively, a capsular incision in an inverted-L shape can be made (Fig. 2.16A).
- Make an incision (Fig. 2.16A) and raise the dorsal flap deep to the nerve and veins until the accessory slip of the extensor hallucis longus tendon is seen in the proximal portion of the incision where it is easier to identify

(Fig. 2.16B). The tendon almost always can be located with careful searching. If it is not seen at the dorsomedial aspect of the first metatarsal, however, begin the longitudinal limb of the incision at this slope of the metatarsal from dorsal to medial.
- Begin the incision proximally on the dorsomedial side of the first metatarsal shaft and 2 to 3 mm medial to the accessory slip of the extensor hallucis longus tendon. Carry the incision to the bone at the level of the first metatarsal joint, extending proximally 4 to 6 cm (Fig. 2.16C).
- Make the transverse limb of the capsular incision at the level of the joint, stopping 2 to 3 mm from the tibial sesamoid bone; this limb transects the capsular insertion of the abductor hallucis muscle (see Fig. 2.16C).
- Beginning on the plantar aspect of the incision, remove the capsule from the medial eminence from the inside out. Avoid buttonholing the capsule at the junction of the medial eminence and the metatarsal by directing the small-bladed knife down the slope of the eminence.
- Free the capsule subperiosteally on its dorsomedial surface and retract it proximally and plantarward (Fig. 2.16D).
- Insert one small Hohmann retractor over the dorsolateral surface of the metatarsal head and another beneath the head at the head and neck junction, while distracting and plantarflexing the hallux to expose the articular surface of the metatarsal head for evaluation of its condition and orientation. Reduce the hallux congruently on the metatarsal head.
- If the hallux is in more than 15 degrees of valgus after reduction, a distal metatarsal osteotomy is needed.

MEDIAL EMINENCE REMOVAL
- After inspecting the metatarsophalangeal joint for degenerative changes, loose bodies, or synovial abnormalities, remove the medial eminence by first scoring with an osteotome its proximal edge where the eminence meets the shaft. Always consult the preoperative radiographs to determine how much of the medial eminence should be removed.
- Using the same osteotome or a power saw, begin the exostectomy distally at the parasagittal groove and direct it medially toward the scored area on the metatarsal shaft (Fig. 2.17). If a power saw is used, a 9-mm blade, rather than a 4- to 5-mm blade, is preferred. The medial direction of the osteotomy prevents splitting of the metatarsal shaft, especially if the proximal edge of the osteotomy has been scored as recommended.
- After the medial eminence has been removed, use a small rongeur to round off the dorsal and plantar edges of the medial aspect of the metatarsal head. Rasping the raw bone concludes the initial stage of the procedure. Use bone wax on the raw surfaces of bone of the metatarsal head.

ADDUCTOR TENDON AND LATERAL CAPSULAR RELEASE
- Begin the second stage with a dorsal longitudinal incision beginning 2 to 3 mm proximal to the dorsal aspect of the first web space to avoid web contracture postoperatively; extend it proximally between the first and second metatarsal heads for 3 to 4 cm (Fig. 2.18). This allows adequate exposure of the adductor insertion into the base of the

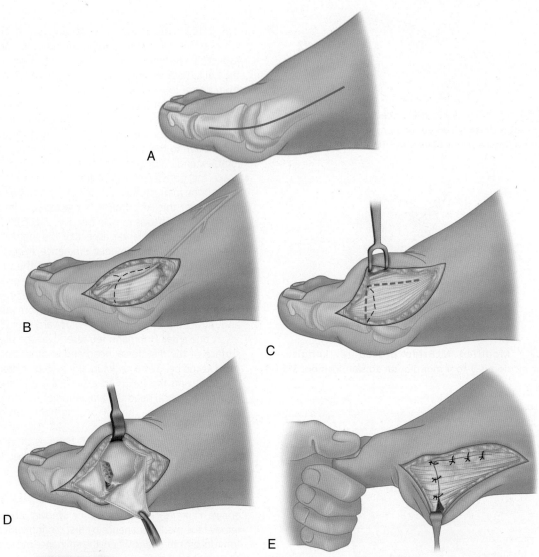

FIGURE 2.16   Inverted-L capsulotomy. **A,** Skin incision. **B,** Most medial branch of superficial peroneal nerve. **C,** Limits of capsulotomy with medial-based wedge. **D,** Capsule raised to expose articular surface of metatarsal head for assessment of orientation on metatarsal head. **E,** Closure of L-shaped capsulotomy holding first metatarsophalangeal joint reduced. **SEE TECHNIQUE 2.1.**

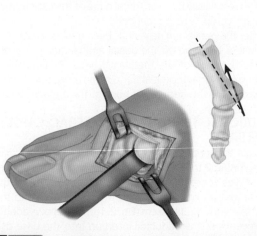

FIGURE 2.17   Modified McBride procedure. Medial eminence is removed. **SEE TECHNIQUE 2.1.**

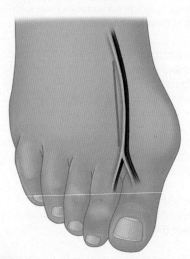

FIGURE 2.18   Modified McBride procedure: second incision. Deep peroneal nerve branch to first web space is avoided, and terminal portion of first dorsal intermetatarsal artery is exposed. **SEE TECHNIQUE 2.1.**

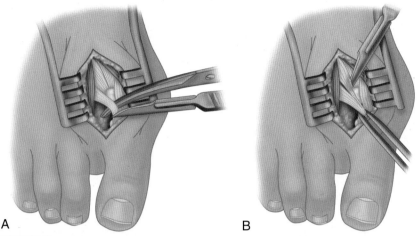

FIGURE 2.19 Modified McBride procedure. **A** and **B,** Adductor hallucis is exposed and released (see text). **SEE TECHNIQUE 2.1.**

proximal phalanx, the lateral head of the flexor hallucis brevis muscle converging on the fibular sesamoid, and the entire lateral capsule from the extensor hallucis longus muscle to the plantar plate.

- Delicate retraction of the skin exposes the dorsal digital branches of the veins, which should be cauterized if they obscure the deeper dissection. The terminal branches of the first dorsal intermetatarsal artery may be encountered at a location adjacent to the proper digital branches of the deep peroneal nerve to the first web space.

- The main portion of the adductor tendon inserts into the base of the proximal phalanx just plantar to the longitudinal axis of the phalanx. It also has a smaller insertion, along with the lateral head of the flexor hallucis brevis muscle, into the fibular sesamoid. The simplest technique to identify the insertion of the adductor hallucis tendon is to place a small, pointed, curved hemostat on the dorsolateral base of the proximal phalanx, slide it firmly plantarward, and lift the hemostat dorsally and laterally; the tip of the instrument usually rests in the axilla of the insertion of the adductor tendon (Fig. 2.19A). This is comparable to securing the iliopsoas tendon for tenotomy at the lesser trochanter.

- When the primary insertion is released, grasp the tendon with forceps or a hemostat and, with traction, displace it dorsally and laterally toward the second metatarsal so that further dissection is on the medial side of the adductor, or push the sesamoid sling laterally through the previously placed medial incision to aid exposure.

- While spreading the first and second metatarsal heads with a small Inge retractor, heavy-duty two-tooth retractors, or a Weitlaner retractor, hold the adductor tendon under tension, which facilitates exposure. The lateral head of the flexor hallucis brevis muscle, the lateral border of the fibular sesamoid, and the slip of the adductor tendon (confluent with the lateral head of the flexor hallucis brevis muscle) come into view in the depths of the wound.

- All attachments of the adductor into its conjoined insertion with the lateral head of the flexor hallucis brevis muscle into the fibular sesamoid must be severed; with trac-

tion on the adductor, it freely and independently moves without tethering the fibular sesamoid (Fig. 2.19B).

- This deep transverse intermetatarsal ligament, which lies just plantar to the adductor, may be released by the incision along the lateral border of the sesamoid. If not, release this ligament, carefully preserving the neurovascular bundle immediately beneath it and incise the lateral capsule. Mann emphasized that release of the deep transverse metatarsal ligament endangers the neurovascular bundle to the first web space, which lies immediately beneath this ligament. Sliding a small Freer elevator between this ligament and the neurovascular bundle would protect the latter structures.

FIBULAR (LATERAL) SESAMOIDECTOMY: DORSAL APPROACH

- If after complete adductor hallucis release, and preferably after a lateral capsular release, a fibular sesamoidectomy is needed to correct the valgus deformity of the great toe fully, it should be done at this time.

- Adequately separate the first and second metatarsal heads for exposure.

- Plantarflex the metatarsophalangeal joint 10 to 20 degrees, which reduces tension on the sesamoids.

- Grasp the fibular sesamoid with a small Kocher clamp or sturdy tissue forceps and pull it laterally into the intermetatarsal space (Fig. 2.20).

- Release the intersesamoid ligament. When this ligament has been incised, bring the fibular sesamoid into the intermetatarsal space, where its removal is straightforward. Care must be taken when incising the intersesamoid ligament to avoid severing the flexor hallucis longus tendon immediately plantar to it. If the tendon is severed, it probably should not be repaired at this level; loss of the tendon causes little if any functional impairment, and repair may result in a fixed flexion contracture of the interphalangeal joint.

- An alternative to fibular sesamoidectomy was recommended by Mauldin, Sanders, and Whitmer, who released part or all of the flexor hallucis brevis lateral head at its insertion into the fibular sesamoid. This release of the

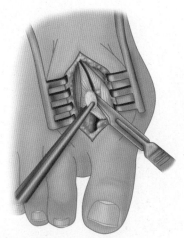

FIGURE 2.20 Modified McBride procedure. Fibular sesamoid is removed. **SEE TECHNIQUE 2.1.**

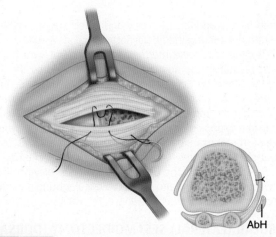

FIGURE 2.21 Modified McBride procedure. Medial capsule is imbricated, with plantar flap over dorsal flap. *Inset,* Cross section through metatarsal head. AbH, abductor hallucis. **SEE TECHNIQUE 2.1.**

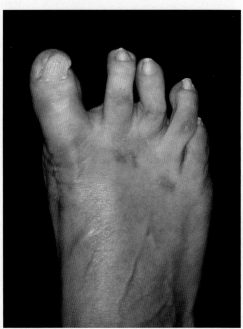

FIGURE 2.22 Hallux varus deformity after McBride bunionectomy and fibular sesamoidectomy through plantar incision. **SEE TECHNIQUE 2.1.**

sesamoid is needed only if fixed valgus remains after the adductor hallucis has been released, a lateral capsulotomy has been performed, and the fibular sesamoid has been mobilized. Also, in this situation, a metatarsal osteotomy may be needed, rather than a fibular sesamoidectomy. Performing both may cause hallux varus.

MEDIAL CAPSULAR IMBRICATION AND WOUND CLOSURE

- With an assistant holding the metatarsophalangeal joint in a congruously reduced position in the varus-valgus and flexion-extension planes, imbricate the medial capsule in the following manner (Fig. 2.21).
- Using absorbable 3-0 or interrupted sutures, place the initial suture through the plantar flap of the capsule at a point 4 to 5 mm medial to the proximal medial border of the medial (tibial) sesamoid and in an outside-to-inside direction.
- Turn the needle on itself and pass it through the dorsal flap at the same level in an outside-to-inside direction. Immediately pass the suture back through the dorsal flap

from inside out and finally through the plantar flap from inside out (a swedged-on needle would suffice, but a small cutting needle is recommended).

- With the hallux held in the desired position, tie this suture, bringing the plantar flap over the dorsal flap and pulling the plantar-displaced abductor hallucis toward the midline of the longitudinal axis of the proximal phalanx and first metatarsal.
- Allow the toe to rest unassisted to judge its resting posture and the tension on the capsular repair.
- If the fibular sesamoid has been removed, do not imbricate the medial capsule to avoid pulling the tibial sesamoid medial to the metatarsal head (Fig. 2.22). If a large medial eminence has persisted for many years with increased capsular reaction and redundancy, a portion of the dorsal flap may need to be excised before closure.
- It is imperative to avoid pulling the medial side of the tibial sesamoid medial to the articular surface of the first metatarsal head; do not uncover the tibial sesamoid (Fig. 2.23).
- If the resting posture of the hallux is acceptable, close the remaining portion of the capsule with interrupted 2-0 or 3-0 absorbable sutures.

CLOSURE OF THE INVERTED-L CAPSULOTOMY

- Begin the closure proximally using 3-0 sutures on a small swedged-on needle; bending the needle to increase the curve makes passage easier in a small wound (see Fig. 2.16E).
- While an assistant applies tension distally on the free corner of the capsule, place the most proximal suture in the longitudinal limb of the capsular incision; place two or three sutures at 5-mm intervals. Do *not* place the corner suture.

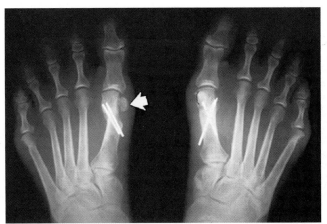

FIGURE 2.23 Dislocation of tibial sesamoid caused by over-tightening of medial capsule and too much lateral shift of capital fragment *(left)*. Right foot has correct sesamoid position. **SEE TECHNIQUE 2.1.**

- Begin to close the transverse limb of the incision at the medial plantar corner.
- Hold the hallux reduced on the metatarsal head while tying all sutures.
- Unless the capsule is redundant, do not imbricate the medial capsule over the area of eminence removal. Close this portion of the transverse limb with side-to-side sutures and place the imbricating suture in the dorsomedial corner of the capsulotomy.
- Begin this final suture distally on the transverse limb of the inverted L, passing the needle from the outside in.
- Reverse the needle and enter the capsular flap from the outside in on the transverse limb.
- Reverse the needle and reenter the capsular flap from the inside out on the longitudinal limb of the flap.
- Make the final pass of the needle from the inside out on the dorsal side of the longitudinal limb of the incision. Holding the joint in its reduced position, tie the suture.
- If the joint reduction is congruent but the hallux is still in an unacceptable valgus position, metatarsal osteotomy should be considered.
- If the transverse limb of the capsular repair is too loose, allowing the hallux to slide into valgus, remove the midline medial suture in the transverse limb. While holding the hallux in the proper position, place the suture 2 to 3 mm farther away from the incision or excise more capsule from the proximal portion. Take care in removing any extra capsule because removal of even a small portion results in a significant correction of capsular laxity and may cause varus of the hallux.
- At the conclusion of the procedure, the hallux should rest on the metatarsal head in about 5 degrees of valgus and 10 degrees of extension.
- If an elastic wrap has been used as a tourniquet, remove it and have the patient flex and extend the toe (if a local anesthetic has been used) to assess function and congruence of the repositioned hallux.
- Lavage the wound, secure hemostasis, and close the skin with interrupted or simple mattress sutures. If simple sutures are used, ensure that the skin edges are not inverted or overlapped. If everted mattress sutures are used, do not evert the edges so much that they do not approximate evenly.

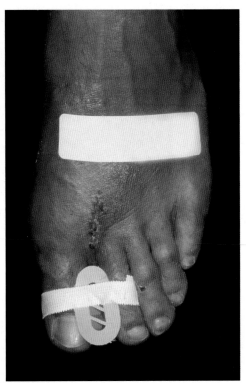

FIGURE 2.24 Toe spacer is worn for 6 weeks after surgery to maintain medial capsular stabilization.

POSTOPERATIVE CARE A bulky compression dressing is applied to the forefoot, and the foot is placed in a position of maximal elevation for 48 to 72 hours. Bathroom privileges only are allowed, and the patient must wear a wooden-soled shoe. Increased ambulation after 72 hours is allowed as tolerated by the patient. The need for crutches or a walker varies, but assisted ambulation is not encouraged unless the patient is unsteady. At 3 weeks, if the wounds are healed, the sutures are removed and adhesive strips are applied if needed; leaving the sutures in longer has no untoward effect. Some type of immobilizer or toe spacer to hold the toe in proper alignment is used (Fig. 2.24). The wooden-soled shoe is used for 3 to 4 weeks, at which time a deep shoe with a wide toe box is recommended; a jogging shoe is sufficient; an extra-depth orthopaedic shoe with a soft toe box also is permissible. The toe spacer is worn for 6 weeks. At 12 to 14 weeks, a reasonably attractive shoe usually can be worn. The period of postoperative edema varies, however, and it may take 4 to 6 months before this type of shoe is tolerated. This is explained to the patient before surgery.

DuVries and Mann made major modifications in the McBride bunionectomy, including the following:
1. Reattach the adductor hallucis muscle to the periosteal cuff on the lateral aspect of the first metatarsal head.
2. Suture the medial capsule of the second metatarsal head to the lateral capsule of the first metatarsal, with interposition of the released adductor hallucis tendon.
3. Perform a coronal or vertical medial capsulotomy beginning 2 to 3 mm proximal to the base of the proximal phalanx. This initial capsular incision is the most distal limb of a partial capsulectomy. The proximal incision is

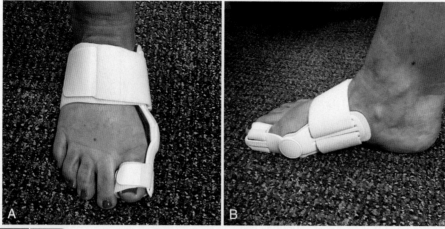

FIGURE 2.25   **A** and **B,** Hallux valgus night splint to be worn for 6 to 8 weeks after dressing changes are completed.

parallel to the first and 5 to 8 mm proximal to it. The two parallel incisions are joined by an inverted-V incision made dorsally with its apex ending 5 mm medial to the extensor hallucis longus tendon. The plantar V incision, joining the plantar ends of the parallel incisions, ends at the medial margin of the tibial sesamoid. The intervening capsule is removed and rarely exceeds 8 mm in width.

4. Close the capsule while the hallux is held in a varus angle of 5 degrees.
5. Weekly postoperative dressing changes for 6 to 8 weeks are emphasized, followed by use of a night splint that holds the hallux in position until the end of the third month (Fig. 2.25).

The McBride procedure rarely is used alone (10% to 15% of patients) for hallux valgus correction. The decision is made intraoperatively by checking reduction of the intermetatarsal angle with manual lateral displacement of the first metatarsal. If the reduction is secure, no proximal metatarsal osteotomy is necessary; if it is not secure, proximal crescentic first metatarsal osteotomy is done in addition to the distal soft-tissue realignment.

COMBINED SOFT-TISSUE AND BONY PROCEDURES

KELLER RESECTION ARTHROPLASTY

The Keller procedure combines resection hemiarthroplasty of the first metatarsophalangeal joint with removal of the medial eminence of the first metatarsal (Fig. 2.26). Although removing the base of the proximal phalanx decompresses the joint and mobilizes the hallux, allowing marked correction of valgus, the varus of the first metatarsal is not corrected and therefore maintaining correction of the valgus of the hallux is difficult. Other complications of the Keller procedure have been emphasized in the literature to such an extent (with neither the incidence nor the severity of such complications clearly documented) that the indications for this procedure have been limited severely. In our experience, however, complications are uncommon if patients are selected carefully. Modifications in the original

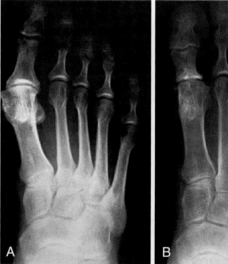
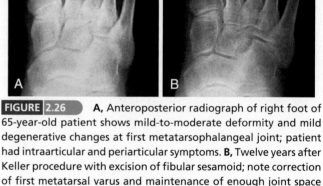

FIGURE 2.26   **A,** Anteroposterior radiograph of right foot of 65-year-old patient shows mild-to-moderate deformity and mild degenerative changes at first metatarsophalangeal joint; patient had intraarticular and periarticular symptoms. **B,** Twelve years after Keller procedure with excision of fibular sesamoid; note correction of first metatarsal varus and maintenance of enough joint space to allow functional range of motion.

technique also have allowed expansion of the indications for the Keller bunionectomy.

Candidates for the Keller procedure are generally over the physiologic age of 70 years, have a more sedentary lifestyle, have a hallux valgus angle of over 30 degrees, have a moderate intermetatarsal angle (13 to 16 degrees), and often have mild to moderate arthritis of the first metatarsophalangeal joint. An incongruous first metatarsophalangeal joint caused by lateral subluxation of the phalanx on the metatarsal head, severe lateral displacement of the sesamoids, and any evidence of degenerative cartilage changes in the joint all are radiographic indications for the Keller procedure.

Two modifications in technique can expand these indications, however, to include patients with more severe deformities (Fig. 2.27) (but not to include younger patients):

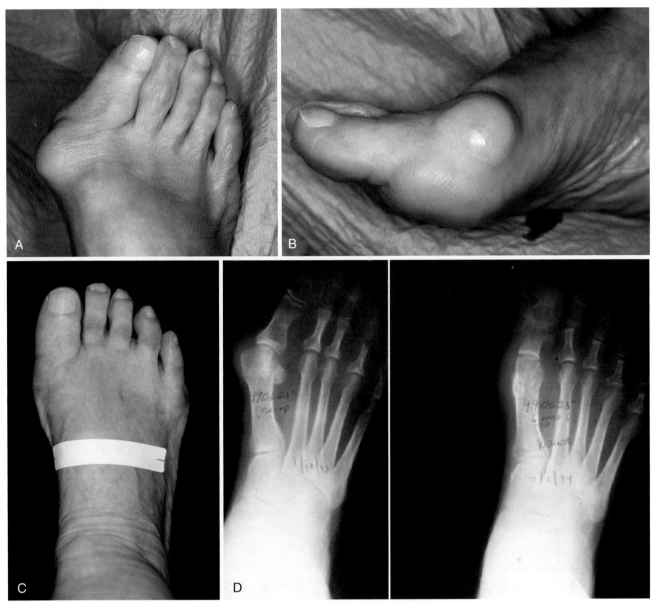

FIGURE 2.27   Severe hallux valgus with bursa formation in 70-year-old woman. **A** and **B,** Anteroposterior and lateral clinical photographs of patient's right foot. **C,** Correction of deformity by modified Keller procedure. **D,** Preoperative and postoperative weight-bearing radiographs of same patient.

fibular sesamoidectomy and lateral displacement of the first metatarsal. Patients with 50 degrees or more of valgus of the hallux (18 to 20 degrees of varus of the first metatarsal), complete lateral dislocation of the sesamoids, marked degenerative changes, and severe pronation of the hallux may benefit functionally and cosmetically from alterations of the standard technique.

Whether the Keller resection arthroplasty is useful in patients with hallux valgus and hallux rigidus is still undetermined. Putti et al., in a retrospective review of 32 patients, reported excellent and good subjective results in 39% and 37% of patients, respectively. They did have a significant number of complications; however, these did not affect the final result. Their study suggests a role for Keller arthroplasty in patients with hallux valgus and hallux rigidus.

TECHNIQUE 2.2

- If pedal pulses are good, use an Esmarch wrap tourniquet (see Technique 2.1 for tourniquet use and anesthetic).
- Use 1% lidocaine (Xylocaine) and 0.5% bupivacaine (Marcaine) in equal portions within standard dose limits for the forefoot block.
- Make a straight midline medial incision 1 cm proximal to the interphalangeal joint of the hallux and extend it proximally to the junction of the distal and middle thirds of the first metatarsal. This lengthy incision is made to avoid excessive traction tension on the skin.
- By blunt dissection, locate the most medial branch of the superficial peroneal nerve at the proximal-dorsal edge of the medial eminence and retract it for protection.

- Carry the dissection to the first metatarsal in the midline medially, beginning in the proximal limit of the wound and extending distally across the midline of the medial eminence and along the proximal phalanx to the distal extent of the wound.
- Raise the deep flap of tissue by sharp dissection dorsally, beginning at the junction of the medial eminence and shaft of the first metatarsal.
- Raise the periosteum and capsule dorsally up to one third to one half the width of the metatarsal.
- At the joint, continue the capsular elevation along the extensor hallucis brevis insertion until the proximal third of the proximal phalanx is exposed as far laterally as possible under direct vision. To make exposure easier, have an assistant pronate the hallux as the dissection proceeds laterally. Subperiosteal dissection should expose only the portion of the proximal phalanx that is to be removed.
- Plantarly dissect just enough to expose the plantar aspect of the medial eminence proximally, the tibial sesamoid in the center of the wound, and the plantar-medial corner of the proximal phalanx.
- Supinate the proximal phalanx to expose the plantar corner and proximal third of the shaft for the sharp dissection. The proximal phalanx is round on three sides, but its plantar surface is flat and even concave in the midline where the flexor hallucis longus tendon passes. This change in contour must be taken into account when dissecting to avoid injury of the flexor hallucis longus tendon.
- By blunt dissection, identify the flexor hallucis longus tendon and retract it plantarward with a small right-angle retractor to protect it throughout the dissection of the proximal phalanx.
- Resect the medial eminence at the sagittal groove, beginning dorsally at its distal edge and directing a 9-mm oscillating blade (or osteotome) plantarward and slightly medially (5 to 10 degrees).
- Remove the base of the proximal phalanx at the metaphyseal-diaphyseal junction, which usually constitutes the proximal third of the phalanx (Fig. 2.28A,B). To prevent damage to the flexor hallucis longus and the neurovascular bundles, place a retractor over the bone dorsally and plantarward and rotate the phalanx into view. Also, do not allow the saw blade to exit bone more than 1 to 2 mm.
- When the osteotomy has been completed, grasp the basilar fragment with a small Kocher clamp or towel clip and rotate the fragment while applying medial pull to excise it. Lift it away from its lateral attachments, which are primarily the lateral collateral ligaments and the adductor muscle tendinous insertion (Fig. 2.28C).
- With the ankle at 90 degrees, bring the hallux into a corrected position while manually pushing the first metatarsal as far laterally as possible. Evaluate the alignment, keeping the metatarsal and hallux straight.
- Grasp the hallux in one hand and displace the proximal remnant medially so that, under direct vision, two longitudinal 0.062-inch Kirschner wires can be inserted.
- Hold the interphalangeal joint straight while drilling the wires from proximal to distal, emerging a few millimeters plantar to the nail plate.

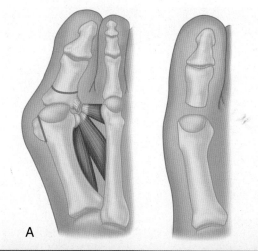

A

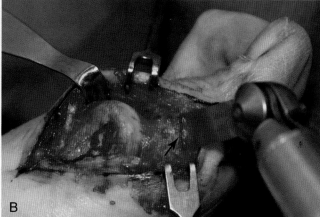

B

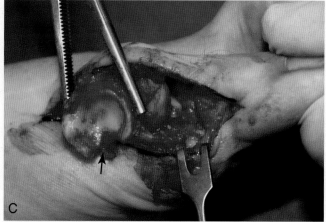

C

FIGURE 2.28   Keller technique. **A,** Resection of proximal phalanx, release of adductor tendon, and resection of medial eminence. **B,** Metaphyseal-diaphyseal junction of proximal phalanx *(arrow)*. **C,** Note concave plantar aspect of proximal phalanx for course of flexor hallucis longus tendon *(arrow)*. **SEE TECHNIQUE 2.2.**

- Return the foot to the corrected position and drill the wires into the metatarsal head.
- While holding the metatarsal as far laterally as possible, cross the joint and drive the wires out the plantar cortex just proximal to the head, while holding the hallux in 10 to 15 degrees of extension, neutral abduction, adduction, and rotation and with no translation dorsally or plantarward on the metatarsal head. The wires should penetrate

only 2 to 3 mm past the cortex to avoid tenderness over the wires with weight bearing.

- If the Kirschner wires tend to "walk" on the rounded articular surface of the metatarsal head, use a small hemostat snugged up against the wire while it is being drilled to allow accurate placement. Proper placement of the wires and the desired position of the hallux on the metatarsal may require several attempts. The medial aspect of the proximal phalanx should not rest medial to the medial aspect of the metatarsal head.

- Place the hallux in the neutral mediolateral plane and in 10 degrees of extension.

- Before the second wire is driven into the first metatarsal head, place the hallux in proper rotation, using the plane of the nail as a guide. The initial length of the hallux is maintained by the wires. Later, collapse occurs when the wires are removed, but improved encapsulation of the hemiarthroplasty, by maintaining length for the first few weeks, may help maintain a more desirable position long term.

- Cut the wires 2 to 3 mm distal to the skin edge.

- Remove the tourniquet and secure hemostasis.

- Close the capsule with interrupted 2-0 or 3-0 absorbable sutures. A firm, complete capsular closure is imperative. A box stitch is recommended. Increasing the curve of the needle manually is helpful.

- Starting proximal and plantarward, pass the suture through the capsule from the outside in.

- The second pass of the suture is from the inside out through substantial soft tissue on the plantar-medial aspect of the phalangeal base.

- Reenter the soft tissue at the base of the proximal phalangeal remnant dorsomedially for the third pass. Move the suture back and forth to ensure uninhibited excursion.

- Make the fourth pass from inside out through the dorsal capsule in line with the initial plantar capsular suture. Have an assistant grasp the ends of the capsule, pulling them together, while the tie is completed. This is basically a four-corner box stitch, which may leave a small area of capsule in the middle that cannot be approximated, but this is of no consequence.

- Intersperse interrupted sutures as needed to complete a firm closure.

- Release the tourniquet and close the skin with nonabsorbable 4-0 sutures.

- Apply a compression forefoot dressing extending just distal to the tarsonavicular tuberosity so that only the toenails are exposed and no loose edges of gauze are raised above the dressing. A snug but nonconstricting, layered, contoured forefoot dressing is vital to reduce edema.

- Cover the tips of the wires with circular adhesive bandages or commercially available "pin balls."

Several modifications of the Keller technique can expand the indications for its use with more severe deformities.

REMOVAL OF THE FIBULAR SESAMOID

- When the medial eminence and phalangeal base have been excised, remove the fibular sesamoid.

- Place a sturdy two-toothed retractor beneath the metatarsal head and have an assistant lift it dorsally.

- Using a Freer elevator or a small osteotome for its strength, mobilize the fibular sesamoid (Fig. 2.29A-C). This may be difficult in elderly patients with significant deformity and adherence of the sesamoid to the metatarsal head. Lift the metatarsal dorsally for exposure (Fig. 2.29D,E).

- When the sesamoid is mobile, identify the flexor hallucis longus tendon by placing traction on the hallux and flexing and extending the interphalangeal joint of the hallux. The tendon is visible just distal to and in alignment with the sesamoids, which straddle it.

- Identify and expose the lateral neurovascular bundle just lateral to the tendon by blunt dissection.

- Pull the plantar-medial capsule medially. This requires a firm grasp on the capsule. The medial traction brings the intersesamoid "ligament" into better view.

- Incise the intersesamoid ligament longitudinally with a No. 67 Beaver or No. 15 Bard-Parker blade. If tenotomy scissors are used, place one arm of the scissors under the ligament (this arm rests on the dorsal side of the flexor hallucis longus) and the other arm dorsal to the ligament.

- When the intersesamoid ligament is incised, grasp the sesamoid firmly with forceps or a small Kocher clamp, flex the toe at the interphalangeal and metatarsophalangeal joints to relax the flexor hallucis longus tendon, and pull the fibular sesamoid distally and medially.

- With release of the intersesamoid ligament, the medial surface of the fibular sesamoid is free from soft tissue. Distally, the sesamoid is free because of resection of the base of the proximal phalanx. This leaves two sides of the sesamoid, distal and medial, free of soft tissue.

- While pulling the sesamoid distally and medially, use a small blade to incise along the lateral margin of the sesamoid under direct vision. Keep pulling the head of the metatarsal dorsally and holding the hallux distracted and in flexion. This greatly aids in identification of the margins of the fibular sesamoid, particularly laterally and proximally.

- The most difficult part of the sesamoidectomy and that which should be done last is release of the proximal lateral corner of the sesamoid where the flexor hallucis brevis lateral head inserts. While incising the lateral capsular attachments to the sesamoid, do not bury the blade of the knife because the neurovascular bundle to the lateral side of the hallux is just lateral to the capsule.

- Now all attachments to the fibular sesamoid have been removed except the lateral head of the flexor hallucis brevis, which inserts on the proximal lateral margin of the sesamoid. This is a difficult section to remove; however, this section can be released under direct vision by pulling the sesamoid distally and medially and lifting the metatarsal head dorsally with a strong two-toothed retractor.

- When the sesamoid has been removed, insert two 0.062-inch Kirschner wires retrograde from the tip of the toe 2 to 3 mm plantar to the nail bed, leaving about 5 to 7 mm of the pins exposed at the base of the phalangeal remnant to help align the phalanx on the metatarsal before antegrade passage of the pins into the metatarsal (Fig. 2.29F).

LATERAL DISPLACEMENT OF THE FIRST METATARSAL

- Push the metatarsal laterally several times. Occasionally, this does not move the metatarsal, but some lateral mobility usually is present.

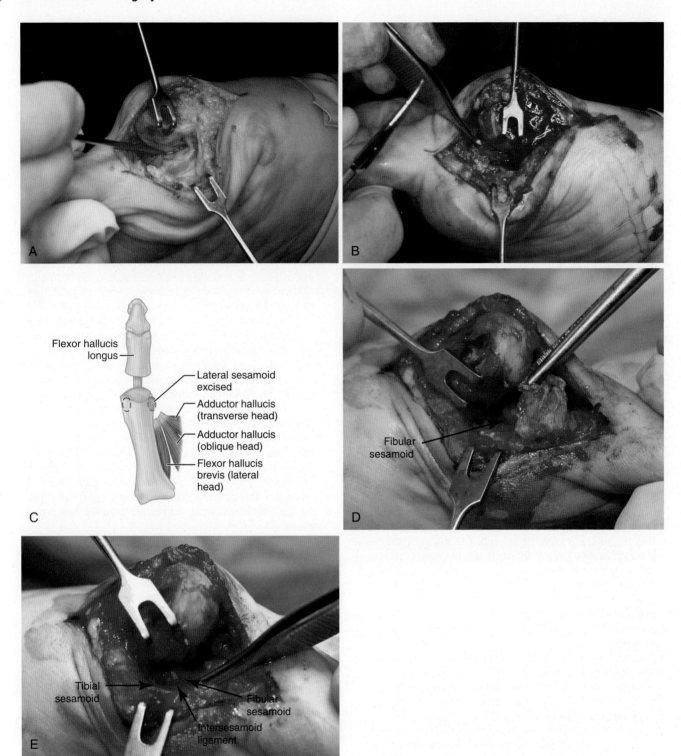

FIGURE 2.29 Excision of fibular sesamoid in modified Keller procedure. With base of proximal phalanx removed and medial eminence excision, exposure of fibular sesamoid is not as difficult from medial incision. **A,** Operative photograph showing elevation of first metatarsal with strong two-tooth retractor and use of small osteotome to mobilize fibular sesamoid and lateral capsuloligamentous (frequently contracted) structures. Osteotome is between metatarsal head and lateral sesamoid. When mobilization of fibular sesamoid is complete, entire sesamoid is visible for excision. Note chondromalacia of tibial sesamoid articular surface medial to osteotome. **B,** Fibular sesamoid has been excised, and lateral capsular structures and conjoined tendon (in forceps) have been released. Neurovascular bundle to lateral side of hallux is adjacent to these structures. **C,** Diagrammatic representation of modified Keller procedure. By excising fibular sesamoid, valgus moment of conjoined tendon of flexor hallucis brevis and adductor hallucis no longer pulls flexor hallucis longus tendon laterally (carrying hallux with it) through capsulosesamoid plantar plate and pulley system. **D,** Metatarsal head must be lifted dorsally to excise fibular sesamoid under direct vision. **E,** Note exposure of fibular sesamoid after mobilization of metatarsal head.

Continued

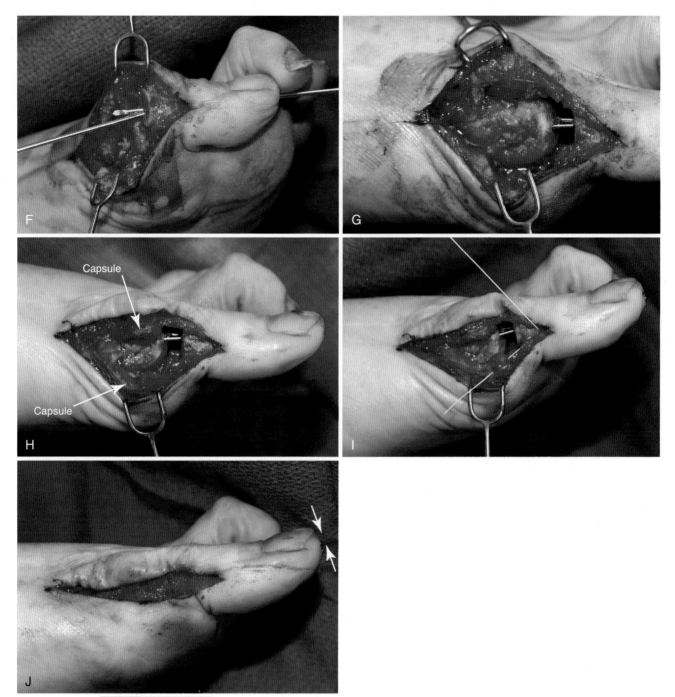

FIGURE 2.29, Cont'd **F,** Two 0.062-inch Kirschner wires are drilled distally. **G,** First metatarsal head is manually displaced laterally, and hallux is placed end-on the first metatarsal. Kirschner wires are drilled proximally across joint. **H,** Capsule is mobilized dorsally and plantarward. **I,** 2-0 or 3-0 absorbable sutures placed in purse-string fashion are used for capsular closure. **J,** Capsule must be closed over joint. Note pins cut off at skin level; they also can be bent at skin level. **SEE TECHNIQUE 2.2.**

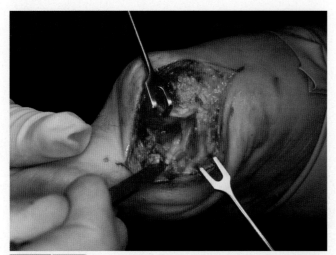

FIGURE 2.30 Firm fibrous band connects fibular sesamoid to base of proximal phalanx. Traction on band pulled hallux into valgus. Removing fibular sesamoid and holding hallux straight for 4 weeks improved results. **SEE TECHNIQUE 2.2.**

- While standing next to the patient looking distally at the dorsum of the foot, dorsiflex the ankle to neutral.
- Viewing the foot as the patient would, hold the first metatarsal firmly and move its distal end laterally. Hold this position with one hand and use the other hand to place the hallux on the metatarsal head and out to length.
- While holding the first ray straight with the foot vertical, have an assistant insert the wires from distal to proximal (Fig. 2.29G). Often these wires, which run through the first metatarsal and hallux, hold the first ray straight, and most of this correction is maintained after the wires have been removed.
- Close the capsule with a purse-string suture as previously described in the original technique (Fig. 2.29H-J).
- Presumably, the laterally displaced fibular sesamoid, when pulled proximally by the lateral head of the relaxed flexor hallucis brevis, pulls the flexor hallucis longus laterally through the sesamoid apparatus, which encases it and contributes to recurrent hallux valgus. In addition, while reoperating after a failed Keller procedure, we observed a strong, linear, fibrous attachment of the fibular sesamoid to the proximal phalangeal remnant (Fig. 2.30), which pulled the hallux into valgus when tension was applied to it. For these reasons, when the deformity is severe, the hallux and first metatarsal maintain better alignment if excision of the fibular sesamoid and lateral displacement of the metatarsal are added to the procedure.

  See also Video 2.1.

POSTOPERATIVE CARE A firm-soled, postoperative shoe is worn, and weight bearing is allowed to tolerance with or without the assistance of crutches or a walker. Bathroom privileges only are allowed for the first 72 hours. The foot is elevated except during meals and bathroom visits. After this period, the patient may be up and about as symptoms allow. Taking more pain medication to allow increased activity is discouraged. For 7 to 10 days after surgery, the foot should be elevated when the patient is sitting.

The dressing is changed at 19 to 23 days, and the wires remain in place for 21 to 28 days. If the hallux migrates proximally on the wires and the wires protrude too far before time to remove them, the tips are cut 1 to 2 mm distal to the skin edge. The Kirschner wires are removed in the office by placing a large or medium-sized needle holder longitudinally over the tip of the wire, rotating it back and forth gently, and pulling with gentle traction. To prevent excessive bleeding, the foot is elevated for 5 minutes after the wires have been removed. A good method of elevation is to place the patient supine with the unoperated knee flexed 90 degrees and the foot flat on the table and then to place the ankle of the operated foot on the flexed knee. A small plastic strip bandage is placed over the holes when the bleeding has stopped.

A small or medium-sized toe spacer (commercially available) is worn in the first web for an additional 4 to 6 weeks; this spacer is removed only for bathing. A wide, soft shoe is allowed after the pins have been removed. Dress shoes are allowed only after most of the edema has resolved, which may take 3 to 4 months. The expected results are a satisfactorily well-aligned hallux with 40 to 50 degrees of motion at the metatarsophalangeal joint, relief of pain, and some improvement in the variety of shoes that can be worn.

OSTEOTOMY OF THE DISTAL FIRST METATARSAL

Although distal metatarsal osteotomies were described by a number of authors, including Reverdin, Hohmann, Trethowan, and Truslow, a report by Mitchell of 100 osteotomies gave the procedure his name. The Mitchell osteotomy procedure consists of (1) removal of the medial eminence, (2) an osteotomy of the distal portion of the first metatarsal shaft, (3) lateral displacement and angulation of the capital fragment, and (4) medial capsulorrhaphy. Several large retrospective reviews of the Mitchell operation reported satisfactory results ranging from 74% to 94%, with a negligible nonunion rate and infrequent recurrence. However, the procedure is not without complications, the most troublesome being metatarsalgia, attributable to dorsiflexion malunion of the distal fragment or excessive shortening of the metatarsal, or both (Fig. 2.31). Metatarsalgia also has been reported after the peg-in-hole procedure. The Mitchell osteotomy, described in previous editions, is now rarely used.

A closing wedge osteotomy at the subcapital level of the first metatarsal to correct valgus of the hallux has its proponents. Although some emphasize that metatarsus primus varus is worsened, and recurrence of the valgus deformity of the great toe is likely, published series have not confirmed this. The issue of when a lateral release is indicated in the setting of a distal osteotomy remains. Schneider et al. evaluated three techniques of lateral release in 15 cadaver feet and found that release of the deep transverse metatarsal ligament and the adductor hallucis muscle did not contribute to correction of the valgus deformity. Transection of the lateral metatarsosesamoid suspensory ligament, however, led to successful release in this study. Much has been written in recent years about transarticular release with distal metatarsal osteotomy. The studies found that limited transarticular release provides comparable outcomes to a classic lateral release, with the advantage that it is a simple technique, patients can ambulate early, and there is no dorsal scarring. Ahn et al. emphasized that different precautions need to be taken for each procedure to avoid complications. As a general guide, we use the following procedures.

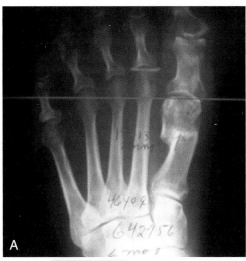 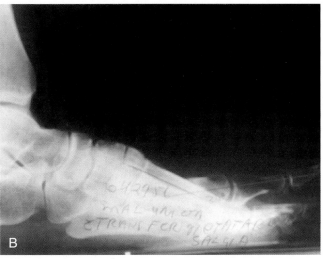

FIGURE 2.31 **A** and **B,** Anteroposterior and lateral weight-bearing radiographs of Mitchell procedure that, through excessive shortening and dorsally angulated malunion, has resulted in transfer metatarsalgia. This biplanar deformity is most difficult to correct.

Open dorsal release (adductor hallucis, lateral metatarsal sesamoid ligament, transverse metatarsal ligament, and lateral collateral ligament):
1. The toe is pronated in the resting position
2. Worsening pronation of the toe as it is extended
3. Sesamoid view indicates the tibial sesamoid is lateral to the crista; the crista is completely eroded
4. Sesamoid view indicates the fibular sesamoid is located in the first web space and likely will block any attempted lateral translation of the metatarsal head

Transarticular release of the lateral structures (lateral metatarsal sesamoid ligament and lateral collateral ligament):
1. Minimal resting position of the toe in pronation
2. Mild pronation of the toe as it is extended
3. Tibial sesamoid position at or medial to the crista on the sesamoid view

Open dorsal release with removal of fibular sesamoid:
1. Keller procedure (see Technique 2.2)
2. Severe recurrent deformity with persistent intrinsic malalignment (increases risk of subsequent varus)

DISTAL CHEVRON METATARSAL OSTEOTOMY

A popular osteotomy of the distal metatarsal is the chevron intracapsular osteotomy, which was described by Corless in 1976 as a modification of the Mitchell procedure to correct the bunion associated with mild-to-moderate metatarsus primus varus. The procedure consists of two parts: (1) correction of metatarsus primus varus by a V-shaped osteotomy in the sagittal plane through the metatarsal head and neck, followed by lateral shifting of the metatarsal head and trimming of the proximal fragment without internal fixation (because of the inherent stability of the osteotomy) and (2) correction of the hallux valgus by suturing a previously raised flap of joint capsule into the abductor hallucis tendon.

Several series of this osteotomy with adequate clinical follow-up have been published, with most reporting good results in 85% to 95% of patients, regardless of age. Modi-fications of the chevron osteotomy have included placing the arms of the V-shaped osteotomy at a 90-degree angle (instead of a 45- to 60-degree angle) and using a 2-mm drill hole as a marker at the apex of the intended V-shaped osteotomy (Horne et al.); placing the bone wedge taken from the exostosis into the dorsal limb of the osteotomy to supinate, plantarflex, and distract the metatarsal (Borton and Stephens); increasing the lateral displacement of the osteotomy to more than 50% of the width of the metatarsal head to expand its use to deformities with an intermetatarsal angle of up to 18 degrees (Murawski and Beskin; see Technique 2.6); and inclusion of an intracapsular-to-extracapsular extension of the osteotomy cuts, with the apex of the osteotomy at or slightly proximal to the center of the metatarsal head. The angle of the osteotomy is about the same (50 to 70 degrees), but the length of the two cuts can be modified to accommodate the small amounts of bone removal needed to correct metatarsals with excessive valgus position of the articular surface of the metatarsal head. Some stability is sacrificed at the osteotomy site, however, and internal fixation is recommended. Shifting the capital fragment laterally more than 5 to 6 mm is not recommended because of the loss of bone apposition. The primary advantage of the slightly more proximal placement of the osteotomy cuts is the correction of a wider range of deformities. Improved fixation techniques, however, may allow larger translation.

Prado et al. proposed a modification of the biplanar chevron osteotomy to treat internal rotation of the first metatarsal bone. After displacement of the distal metatarsal fragment laterally as in the conventional chevron procedures, the metatarsal rotational deformity is corrected by removing a medial wedge from the plantar fragment of the osteotomy. This allows the metatarsal head to be rotated, facilitating correction of pronation (Fig. 2.32).

The chevron osteotomy generally is recommended for patients younger than 50 years old with a hallux valgus angle of less than 40 degrees and an intermetatarsal angle of less than 15 degrees. Advantages of the chevron osteotomy over metatarsal neck osteotomy (the Mitchell procedure and its modifications) include its

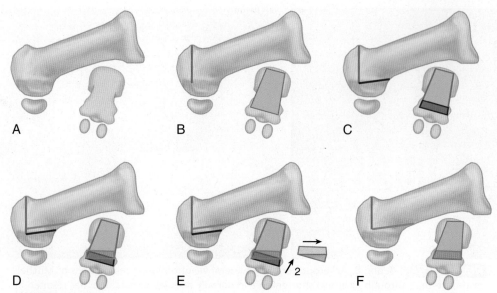

FIGURE 2.32 Rotational biplanar chevron osteotomy. **A,** Lateral and axial view of first metatarsal. **B,** Dorsal cut. **C,** First plantar cut. **D,** Second plantar cut. **E,** Removal of wedge. **F,** Rotation of fragments and correction of pronation. (From Prado M, Baumfeld T, Nery C, Mendes A, Baumfeld D: Rotational biplanar chevron osteotomy, *Foot Ankle Surg* May 21, 2019 [Epub ahead of print].)

location through cancellous bone, less shortening of the metatarsal, and its inherent stability. If the hallux valgus angle is more than 35 degrees, however, the hallux frequently is pronated and cannot be corrected by medial capsulorrhaphy alone or at the osteotomy. A hallux valgus angle of more than 30 degrees is not consistently correctable to a cosmetically acceptable angle (10 to 20 degrees), especially if the intermetatarsal angle is more than 12 degrees.

This procedure is most useful for younger patients (adolescence through the 30s) with a hallux valgus angle of 30 degrees or less and an intermetatarsal angle of less than 13 degrees; however, successful outcomes also have been reported in patients 50 years old or older. It narrows the forefoot, brings the hallux into cosmetically acceptable valgus (when combined with a medial capsulorrhaphy), and maintains adequate dorsiflexion of the first metatarsophalangeal joint to allow some variety in footwear.

The procedure consists of (1) medial eminence removal, (2) a V-shaped intracapsular osteotomy through the first metatarsal head, (3) lateral displacement of the capital fragment, (4) removal of the resulting projection of the first metatarsal, and (5) medial capsulorrhaphy. Fixation of the osteotomy with one or two Kirschner wires, a cortical screw, or a biodegradable pin adds stability to the osteotomy.

Although the intracapsular chevron procedure is included because of its longevity and results, in practice this osteotomy is rarely used at our institution. The modified extracapsular chevron is the workhorse distal osteotomy for mild to moderate deformity. It is most useful in the patient with a wide metatarsal and an intermetatarsal angle of less than 16 degrees, and can be used with or without a lateral release as long as care is taken not to overly strip the dorsal capsule from the head of the metatarsal (see Technique 2.4).

See also Video 2.2.

TECHNIQUE 2.3

(JOHNSON; CORLESS)

SKIN INCISION

- For tourniquet use and anesthesia, see Technique 2.1. Begin a dorsomedial incision at the midportion of the proximal phalanx and gently curve it dorsally and proximally over the medial eminence so that, coursing plantarward, it ends 2 cm proximal to the medial eminence along the medial subcutaneous surface of the first metatarsal shaft. Currently, we use a straight midline medial incision.
- Raise the skin flap gently, being careful to preserve the sensory nerve (the terminal branch of the medial division of the superficial peroneal nerve) to the dorsomedial aspect of the hallux. Protect as many branches of the superficial venous system as possible to decrease postoperative edema.
- Make a longitudinal capsular incision in the midline (medial) of the medial eminence and extend it distally along the shaft of the proximal phalanx and proximally along the metatarsal shaft until the medial eminence is exposed.
- Be careful not to loosen all the proximal attachments of the capsule on the metatarsal neck (an alternative capsular incision is the Y-shaped capsular incision).
- In addition, to preserve vascularity to the capital fragment, do not strip the capsule from the dorsolateral and lateral aspects of the metatarsal head and neck.

MEDIAL EMINENCE REMOVAL

- Begin the osteotomy dorsomedially at the parasagittal groove and direct the blade (9 mm wide) proximally and medially, angled toward the junction of the medial eminence with the metatarsal shaft.

- If using a power saw with a small blade (4 mm wide), take care not to scoop out a portion of the cancellous bone in the metatarsal head because this decreases the surface contact of the osteotomy and can delay union.

V-SHAPED OSTEOTOMY IN TRANSVERSE PLANE

- Using a power saw with a 9-mm-wide blade, begin the dorsal arm of the osteotomy in the metatarsal head near the subchondral bone. This usually is 3 to 4 mm proximal to the medial edge of the articular surface of the head of the first metatarsal. Angle the blade dorsally about 30 degrees from the longitudinal plane of the metatarsal.
- In a similar manner, angle the plantar arm of the osteotomy 30 degrees from the longitudinal plane of the metatarsal, making the angle between the two limbs 60 to 70 degrees. This angle is suggested to maximize metaphyseal cancellous bone contact while maintaining stability of the osteotomy when it is displaced. The stability decreases as the angle increases. An angle of less than 50 to 60 degrees places the proximal ends of the osteotomy limbs in the cortical bone of the metatarsal neck instead of in the cancellous bone of the metatarsal head.
- When making the second limb of the osteotomy, avoid diverging the blade from or converging it toward the first cut because this makes displacement of the capital fragment difficult.
- The arms of the V usually are 10 to 12 mm long. Do not overpenetrate the bone with the blade to avoid placing the blood supply to the head of the metatarsal further at risk.

LATERAL SHIFT OF THE CAPITAL FRAGMENT

- Stabilize the metatarsal shaft manually or with a towel clip while shifting the capital fragment laterally by thumb pressure. This lateral displacement should be 4 to 5 mm and no more than 40% to 50% of the width of the metatarsal.
- Care should be taken to avoid making the osteotomy unstable, which may occur if an instrument is used to lever the osteotomy open to facilitate displacement.

REMOVAL OF THE METATARSAL PROJECTION

- After displacement of the capital fragment laterally, a medial projection of the metatarsal on the proximal side of the osteotomy remains. Shape this projection into the contour of the metatarsal neck and distal shaft by beginning a saw cut dorsomedially and directing it medially and proximally.
- A small rongeur can be used, taking small bites with its beveled side, to smooth the medial surface of the two fragments further.

MEDIAL CAPSULORRHAPHY

- Bring the hallux into 5 degrees of valgus and inspect the osteotomy.
- If it is stable, proceed with the capsulorrhaphy; if not, internally fix the osteotomy and perform the capsulorrhaphy, which holds the hallux in 5 to 10 degrees of valgus.
- We prefer the pants-over-vest technique because of its strength, but excising a portion of the capsule dorsally and closing the capsule side-to-side also is appropriate. Pulling the plantar flap of the capsule dorsally (instead of vice versa) repositions the sesamoids if no contracture exists.

- Release of the adductor through the joint before the osteotomy is suggested if the hallux valgus angle is 30 degrees or more.

POSTOPERATIVE CARE Three days after surgery, the bulky soft dressing is removed, a small dressing and a short leg walking cast with dorsal and plantar toe plates are applied, and touch-down weight bearing is allowed with crutches until the osteotomy has healed (6 to 8 weeks).

MODIFIED CHEVRON DISTAL METATARSAL OSTEOTOMY

The modified chevron osteotomy is simply a more proximal placement of the apex of the osteotomy in the metatarsal head. Potential problems of this modification of the chevron osteotomy are instability of the osteotomy and insufficient metaphyseal bony contact. Proper placement of the osteotomy cuts is mandatory. The metatarsal osteotomy must be internally fixed. With some modifications, however, the chevron osteotomy can be used for more severe deformities (up to 35 degrees of hallux valgus and up to 15 degrees of first to second intermetatarsal diversion) (Fig. 2.33). As an alternative, the valgus appearance of the hallux can be corrected by an additional few degrees with an additional osteotomy of the proximal phalanx (see Akin procedure). This phalangeal osteotomy augments cosmetic correction only if the metatarsophalangeal joint has been rendered congruent in the corrected position. Also, a basal osteotomy of the proximal phalanx adjacent to the distal metatarsal osteotomy may cause more limitation of motion of the first metatarsophalangeal joint than a single osteotomy. The patient should be informed of this possibility.

In patients with mild to moderate deformity in whom a wide metatarsal is present, an absorbable pin is used for fixation (Fig. 2.34). For more severe deformity or in patients in whom there is a narrow metatarsal, fixation with Kirschner wires or screws is recommended as described below. Recent reports, as well as our experience, indicate significant patient satisfaction with this procedure even in more severe deformity. A more precise determination of the upper limits of deformity that can be treated with this procedure remains to be defined. Park et al. compared clinical and radiographic results of proximal and distal chevron osteotomies (both with soft-tissue release) in 110 patients with severe hallux valgus. They noted comparable results, with both methods resulting in significant improvement. Kim et al. also obtained good results in 56 patients with moderate or severe deformity. They noted that distal chevron osteotomy with lateral soft-tissue release can be useful in severe deformity if the lateral soft-tissue contracture is not severe and if the metatarsocuneiform joint is adequately flexible. Song et al. reported good results in 82.6% of 46 feet with moderate hallux valgus and in 82% of 42 feet with severe hallux valgus using an extended distal chevron osteotomy with a distal soft-tissue release. Seven complications were reported in each group.

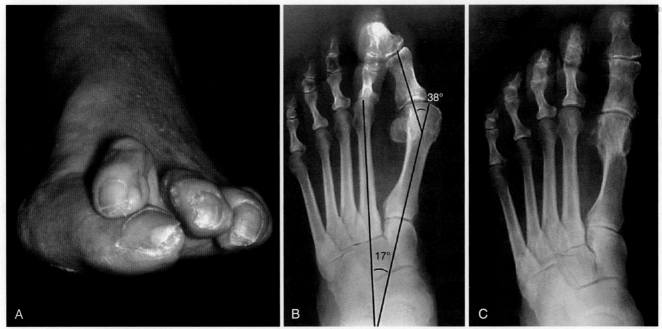

FIGURE 2.33   **A,** This degree of deformity (left foot) is difficult to correct with standard chevron osteotomy when apex is at subchondral bone of capital fragment. **B,** Standing radiograph of left foot before correction. **C,** Standing radiograph 1 year after chevron osteotomy, release of adductor hallucis, Akin osteotomy, and correction of hammer toe.

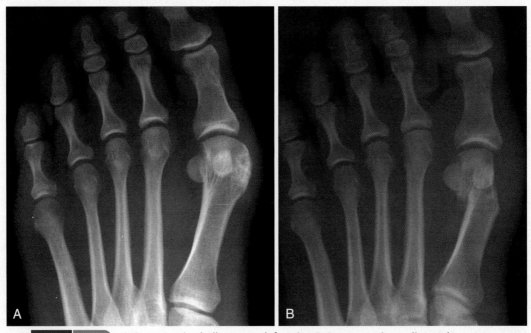

FIGURE 2.34   **A,** Preoperative hallux varus deformity. **B,** Postoperative radiograph.

TECHNIQUE 2.4

- See Technique 2.1 for use of the tourniquet and anesthesia. Make a medial midline incision as described in Technique 2.3, protecting the dorsal veins and dorsal and plantar sensory nerves to the medial side of the hallux (Fig. 2.35A).
- When the capsule is exposed, make a longitudinal incision along the dorsomedial aspect of the first metatarsal.

- Begin the second limb of the capsulotomy 1 to 2 mm proximal to the base of the proximal phalanx and in a coronal plane at right angles to the first limb of the capsulotomy (Fig. 2.35B).
- Extend the coronal incision plantarward 1 to 2 mm proximal to the junction with the tibial sesamoid (Fig. 2.35C).
- Raise the capsule, beginning medially and plantarward, by sharply dissecting it from the inside out and off the

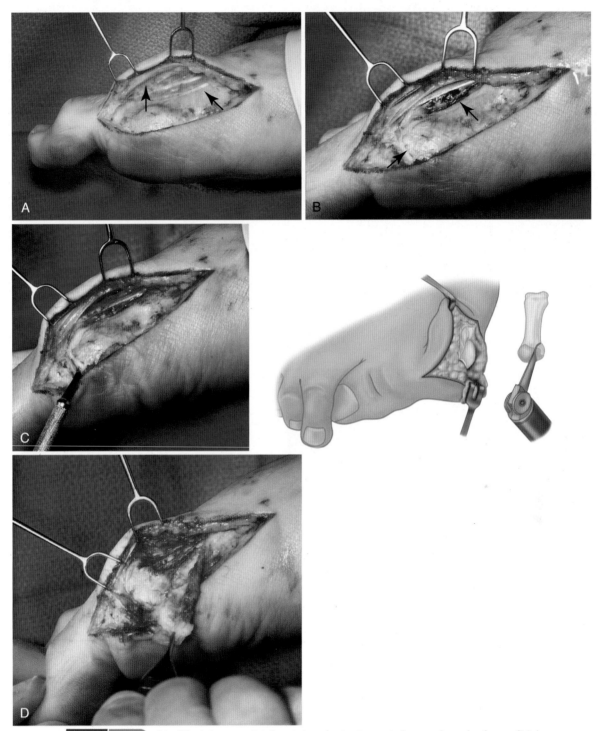

FIGURE 2.35 Modified chevron distal metatarsal osteotomy. **A,** Sensory branch of superficial peroneal nerve *(left arrow)* and accessory extensor hallucis longus *(right arrow)*. **B,** Inverted L-shaped capsulotomy. **C,** Transverse limb of L-capsulotomy. **D,** Reflection of capsule.

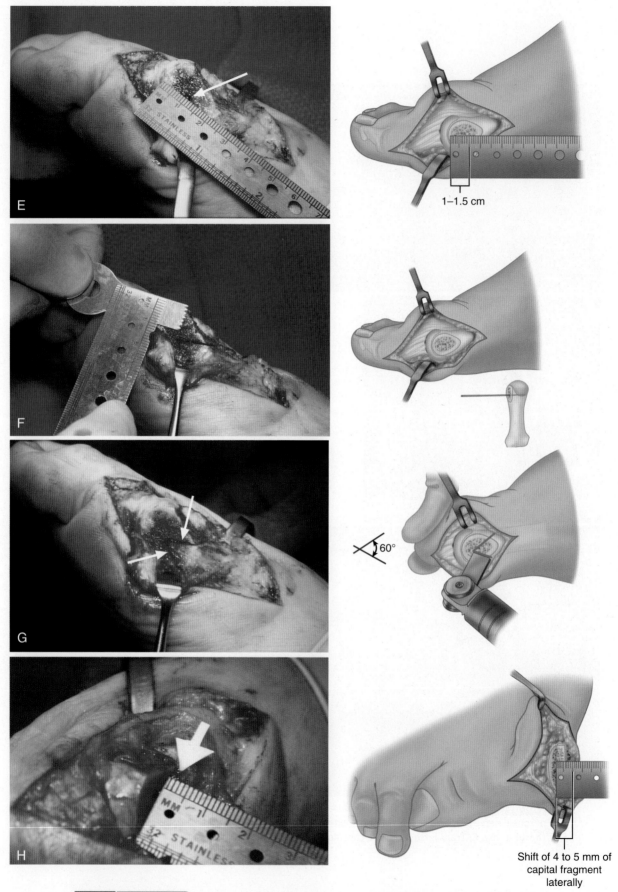

60°

Shift of 4 to 5 mm of
capital fragment
laterally

FIGURE 2.35, Cont'd   **E,** Apex of osteotomy is 1 to 1.3 cm proximal to articular surface,
depending on size of metatarsal head. **F,** Dorsal limb of osteotomy and width of saw blade. **G,**
Completion of osteotomy. **H,** Lateral translation of capital fragment. Note overhang of proximal
metatarsal *(arrow)*.

Continued

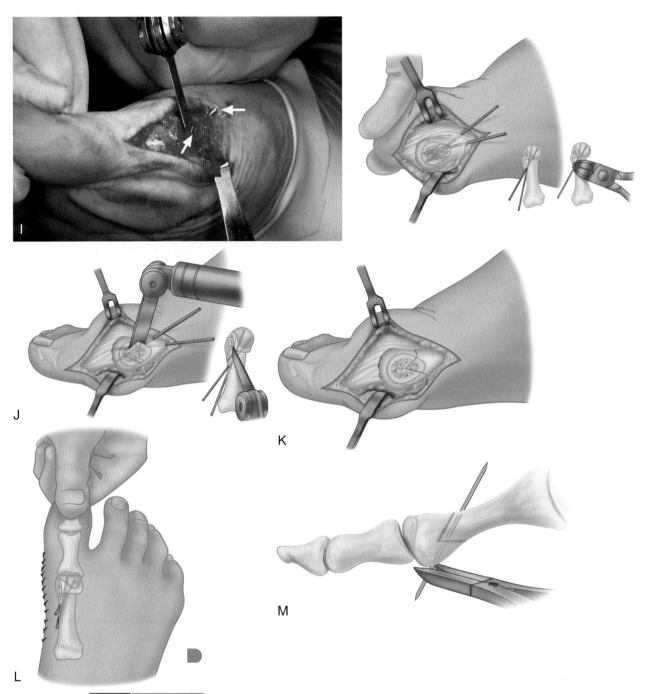

FIGURE 2.35, Cont'd **I** and **J,** Kirschner wire in place *(top arrow)*; resection of overhang of proximal metatarsal *(bottom arrow)*. **K,** Completed osteotomy. **L,** Hallux is placed in corrected position while dressing is applied. **M,** Absorbable pins that can be trimmed may be used as alternative. SEE TECHNIQUE 2.4.

- most prominent part of the medial eminence until its dorsal aspect is reached (Fig. 2.35D).
- Maintain the incision close to bone, curving over the medial eminence as the contour demands, and take a full-thickness piece of capsule from the medial eminence and proximally along the metatarsal shaft for 3 to 4 cm. This should leave the fascial attachment of the abductor hallucis in continuity with the periosteum and fascial covering of the first metatarsal shaft.
- Ensure that the plantar aspect of the metatarsal head where it meets with the shaft is adequately exposed so that the plantar osteotomy cut can be made under direct vision. Remove the medial eminence.
- Using a 0.062-inch Kirschner wire, and starting 1 to 1.3 cm proximal to the subchondral bone and in the center of the first metatarsal head, drill a hole from medial to lateral marking the apex of the intended osteotomy (Fig. 2.35E,F).
- Mark the limbs of the osteotomy with a sharp osteotome or a marking pen and begin the osteotomy with the dorsal cut. Avoid pushing the saw blade in and out of the bone; slowly glide the blade across the head-neck fragment with gentle back-and-forth rather than in-and-out movements.
- When there is no further resistance to the blade laterally, extract it and return to the centering hole. Ensure that the dorsal and lateral aspects of the cortical bone have been incised.
- Begin the plantar limb of the osteotomy at a point approximately 30 degrees from the midline or 60 degrees from the original dorsal osteotomy. Make this cut slowly and deliberately at right angles to the bone, exiting plantarward 2 to 3 mm proximal to where the articular surface of the metatarsal head meets the shaft (Fig. 2.35G). A small, right-angle retractor pulling the capsule plantarward increases exposure.
- If the osteotomy cuts have been made appropriately, the capital fragment usually displaces laterally with minimal lateral pressure; if this is not the case, either the osteotomy cuts are not parallel, or the plantar cortex or dorsal cortex, or both, has not been penetrated laterally.
- If gentle pressure on the head fragment does not displace it laterally while the shaft fragment is held stable, reposition the saw blade, being careful not to start the saw until the blade is in the depths of the osteotomy cut.
- When the capital fragment has been freed from the proximal fragment, shift it laterally 4 to 5 mm (Fig. 2.35H).
- Impact the head fragment on the shaft by applying gentle pressure to the hallux.
- While holding the capital fragment straight on the metatarsal shaft, internally fix the osteotomy. Insert one or two 0.062-inch Kirschner wires obliquely across the osteotomy site (Fig. 2.35I).
- Begin inserting the first wire dorsomedially and far enough proximally in the shaft to leave cortical bone between the pin and the cancellous portion of the distal-medial shaft when the overhanging ridge of bone is made flush with the capital fragment. Direct the wire so that it reaches the lateral aspect of the capital fragment.
- Insert the second wire into the metatarsal head at a point 3 to 4 mm plantar and parallel to the first.
- Test the osteotomy for stability and gently open the metatarsophalangeal joint by pushing the toe laterally.

- Examine the entire surface of the metatarsal head with a small Freer elevator to locate any Kirschner wire points. If the joint has been entered, retract the wire slightly so that it rests in subchondral bone. Because the entrance of the wire into subchondral bone and its exit through the cartilage of the head usually can be felt while drilling, withdrawing the wire about 2 mm usually places it in the proper position.
- Circumduct the hallux on the first metatarsal head; if any catching occurs, reinspect the joint for wire points. If there is any doubt, obtain radiographs.
- Incise the overhanging segment on the medial side of the proximal fragment and with a rasp smooth it flush with the capital fragment (Fig. 2.35J,K).
- Place the hallux on the metatarsal head in a congruous position, which can be determined by flexing, extending, abducting, adducting, and rotating the hallux on the first metatarsal head and observing the foot from the top (Fig. 2.35L).
- While an assistant holds the toe reduced, close the capsular incision by first closing its proximal part with two or three interrupted 2-0 or 3-0 absorbable sutures.
- Dorsally, pass the needle through the periosteum and deep fascia, over the metatarsal shaft, and through the accessory extensor hallucis longus tendon.
- Plantarward, the strong tissue is the deep, investing fascia over the abductor hallucis and the tendinous edge of this muscle; anchoring the capsular repair proximally before beginning the distal repair is important. Close the plantar-medial corner of the capsule with one or two interrupted sutures.
- The most important sutures, which hold the hallux congruously on the metatarsal head, form a pants-over-vest closure as follows. Enter the transverse limb of the capsular incision 2 to 3 mm plantar to the apex of the incision from the outside in; turn the needle 180 degrees, and reenter the corner of the capsule from the outside in. Reverse the needle 180 degrees and reenter it from the inside out, still on the proximal part of the capsule. Place the final pass of the stitch through the distal capsule on the dorsal side of the apex of the incision. Pull the capsule into the corner in a pants-over-vest manner and suture it. During capsular closure, observe the dorsal aspect of the foot while an assistant externally rotates the foot slightly to judge the proper alignment of the hallux.
- To obtain more correction of the valgus deformity, carefully imbricate the transverse or coronal limb of the capsulotomy. Do not attempt to correct hallux valgus interphalangeus by pulling the hallux into a more varus position at the metatarsophalangeal joint with imbricating sutures during capsular repair because hallux varus can develop if the imbrication is too tight. In most instances, close the transverse limb by approximating the edges, unless the capsule is so redundant that it requires partial excision. Finish closing the capsule at any weak points.
- The hallux should be in neutral to 5 degrees of valgus at completion of the capsulorrhaphy. Correct any varus by removing capsular sutures one at a time and observing the position of the hallux. Begin by removing one or more transverse limb sutures. If necessary, remove all of the distal capsular repair and start over.

- Secure hemostasis and close the wound in layers. Apply a forefoot dressing with the hallux taped in the proper position.
- Alternatively, an absorbable pin that can be trimmed may be used for fixation (Fig. 2.35M).

POSTOPERATIVE CARE The dressing and sutures are removed at 19 to 23 days, and a toe spacer is worn to hold the hallux in the proper position. A wooden-soled shoe is worn for 4 weeks, and then a deep, wide jogging shoe with a toe spacer is worn for the next 6 to 8 weeks. Usually by the third or fourth month a reasonably attractive shoe can be worn, but this varies. A short leg walking cast worn for 4 weeks after surgery is an alternative, but it is not routinely recommended except in adolescents. The Kirschner wires can be removed at 3 months or earlier if they cause symptoms, or they may be left if the patient is asymptomatic.

JOHNSON MODIFIED CHEVRON OSTEOTOMY

Johnson, who popularized the chevron osteotomy, also modified it by changing the length and position of the limbs of the osteotomy in the metatarsal head, which extended the indications for the osteotomy to severe deformities with intermetatarsal angles of 15 or 16 degrees. Also, in the modified procedure, a 2.7-mm screw is used for internal fixation. Johnson did not recommend this osteotomy for patients older than 60 years or for patients who had previous hallux valgus surgery or diminished joint mobility with crepitance.

TECHNIQUE 2.5

(JOHNSON)
- See Technique 2.1 for tourniquet use and anesthesia. Make a midline, longitudinal, medial capsular incision and expose the medial eminence.
- Expose the metatarsal head dorsally and plantarward just enough to see the dorsal and plantar limbs of the osteotomy, laterally enough to place a 2.7-mm screw. Avoid excessive stripping of the capsule.
- Using a power saw with a 9-mm blade, remove the medial eminence at an angle that is parallel to the medial border of the foot as opposed to the medial border of the cortical shaft or metatarsal.
- Begin the inferior or plantar limb of the osteotomy 5 or 6 mm proximal to the medial articular surface of the first metatarsal and midway between the superior and inferior margins of the metatarsal head in its center portion. This plantar extension of the osteotomy exits extracapsularly at the inferior aspect of the metatarsal head and neck junction or just proximal to that.
- The lateral portion of this osteotomy cut can be difficult, so ensure that it is completely through the bone before attempting to shift the metatarsal head laterally.

- Make the second limb of the osteotomy from the apex or distal extension of the first osteotomy and direct it dorsally at an approximate angle of 70 degrees to the first limb of the osteotomy. Exit this limb of the osteotomy dorsally just proximal to the dorsal border of the articular surface of the head of the metatarsal.
- Stabilize the metatarsal shaft proximally with a manual grip or a towel clip while the capital fragment is displaced laterally 4 to 6 mm without any tilting or opening of the osteotomy site medially, laterally, superiorly, or inferiorly.
- Compress the great toe longitudinally on the head of the metatarsal shaft fragment to impact the osteotomy site.
- For insertion of a 2.7-mm screw, use a 2-mm bit to drill a hole in the dorsal surface of the distal shaft of the metatarsal just proximal to the dorsal limb of the osteotomy. Leave an approximately 3-mm ledge of bone between the drill hole and the superior arm of the osteotomy.
- Direct the drill bit from proximal to distal at about a 10-degree angle and 10 to 15 degrees lateralward to place the screw in the substance of the transposed capital fragment.
- Pass the 2-mm drill bit through the dorsal cortex of the distal shaft of the metatarsal and then through the cancellous bone of the capital fragment into subchondral bone of the fragment.
- Ream the proximal aspect of the hole with a 2.7-mm drill bit to create a lag effect at the osteotomy and then measure the screw length (usually 16 to 18 mm) with a depth gauge.
- Tap the drill hole with a 2.7-mm tap. Insert the 2.7-mm screw and tighten it to close the osteotomy. Do not allow the screw to exit through the articular surface of the metatarsal head because it may impair sesamoid glide.
- Use a power saw to contour the overhang of the medial aspect of the distal metatarsal that resulted from lateral shift of the capital fragment with the medial aspect of the first metatarsal shaft. Do not skive laterally into the center of the shaft of the metatarsal. Use a small rongeur to smooth the dorsomedial aspect of the metatarsal head.
- Overlap the capsule while holding the hallux in neutral flexion and extension and about 10 degrees of varus and excise any excess capsule (usually 3 to 5 mm). Close the capsule with multiple 2-0 or 3-0 nonabsorbable sutures.
- After capsular closure is completed, the hallux should rest in a straight position with the medial aspect of the proximal phalanx resting against the medial aspect of the displaced capital fragment.
- Apply the dressing in such a way as to hold the hallux in proper position and to take some of the pressure off the medial capsular repair (see Fig. 2.35L).

POSTOPERATIVE CARE The patient is allowed partial weight bearing with crutches for the first 3 to 4 days; then the dressing is changed, and a short leg walking cast is applied. The cast, which should extend distal to the great toe for gentle support, is primarily for comfort and patient mobility, allowing ambulation without crutches or a walker. It is removed approximately 1 week later, and gentle exercises of the great toe are begun. A hallux valgus night splint is applied to protect the medial capsular repair, and a stiff-soled postoperative shoe is worn for approximately 3 weeks; after this a deep, wide, soft shoe can be worn.

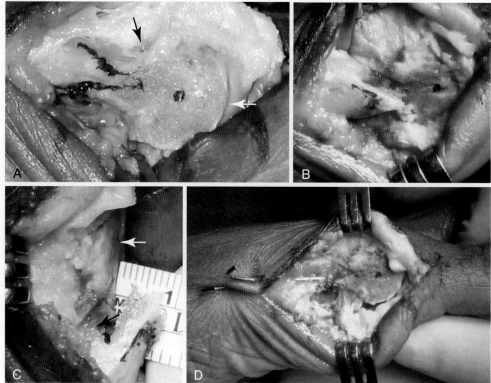

FIGURE 2.36   Increased displacement distal chevron osteotomy. **A,** Exposure and marking for osteotomy cuts. **B,** Sagittal view showing lateral translation of distal fragment. **C,** Dorsal view showing lateral translation of approximately 9 mm. *White arrow* points to the mark on center of metatarsal head; *black arrow* denotes lateral spike on which head fragment is perched. **D,** After placement of Kirschner wires and resection of residual medial bone flush with metatarsal head. (From Murawski DE, Beskin JL: Increased displacement maximizes the utility of the distal chevron osteotomy for hallux valgus deformity correction, *Foot Ankle Int* 29:156, 2008.) **SEE TECHNIQUE 2.6.**

INCREASED DISPLACEMENT, DISTAL CHEVRON OSTEOTOMY

The correction obtained by distal osteotomies is limited by the fact that approximately 1 mm of lateral translation corresponds to 1 degree of intermetatarsal angle correction. Murawski and Beskin described increasing the amount of displacement at the osteotomy more than 6 mm or the 50% maximum generally recommended in the literature for correction of severe deformities. Their indications for this procedure were symptomatic moderate-to-severe hallux valgus with an intermetatarsal angle of 18 degrees or less. They reported correction similar to that obtained with proximal crescentic osteotomy and chevron osteotomy with lateral soft-tissue release; however, the risk of hallux varus appears to be increased with their technique. A "medial diaphyseal bump" also was present in five of their 33 patients and was symptomatic in three. This procedure is technically difficult, and meticulous surgical technique is required.

TECHNIQUE 2.6

(MURAWSKI AND BESKIN)

- See Technique 2.1 for tourniquet use and anesthesia. If a lateral soft-tissue release is required for marked sesamoid

subluxation, expose the lateral capsule through a dorsal first web space incision and use a Freer elevator to identify the dorsal margin of the subluxed lateral sesamoid. Incise the capsule longitudinally from the phalanx to well proximal to the lateral sesamoid, which will allow medialization of the sesamoid complex during medial capsular repair at the end of the procedure.
- Make a standard medial incision centered over the metatarsophalangeal joint, followed by a longitudinal capsulotomy slightly plantar to the midaxis of the metatarsal.
- Reflect the capsule and remove the medial eminence with a sagittal saw, 1 to 2 mm medial to the articular margin or sagittal groove.
- Mark the apex and the limbs of the osteotomy with a surgical pen. The apex is 15 to 20 mm proximal to the joint, and the limbs are made with an angle of 35 to 45 degrees, exiting the diaphysis of the metatarsal (Fig. 2.36A). The position of the limbs is important: if they are too short, instability may be excessive, and if they are too long, translation or rotation of the distal head portion is difficult.
- Use a Freer elevator to gently strip the periosteum and soft tissue over the anticipated osteotomy cuts. To minimize vascular compromise, leave intact tissues distal to the osteotomies on the metatarsal head.
- Complete the osteotomy with a sagittal saw and gently translate the distal head fragment laterally while applying

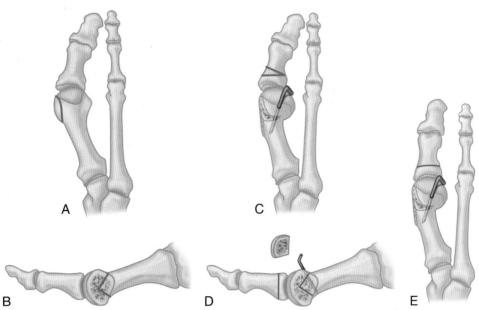

FIGURE 2.37　　Chevron-Akin double osteotomy. **A,** Resection of medial eminence parallel to medial border of foot. **B,** Chevron osteotomy cut is made, and metatarsal head is shifted laterally 2.5 to 3.0 mm. **C,** Osteotomy is fixed with 0.045-inch smooth pin, and protruding medial border of metatarsal is osteotomized flush with metatarsal head. **D,** Akin cut parallels concavity at base of proximal phalanx, and 1-mm wedge of bone is removed. **E,** Suture closure of Akin osteotomy corrects residual valgus of hallux. (From Mitchell LA, Baxter DE: A chevron-Akin double osteotomy for correction of hallux valgus, *Foot Ankle* 12:7, 1991.) **SEE TECHNIQUE 2.7.**

traction to the toe (Fig. 2.36B). Position the head fragment on the lateral spike of the proximal fragment (Fig. 2.36C). Up to 90% translation is possible and can be satisfactorily stabilized by two 0.054-inch smooth Kirschner wires.

- Insert the Kirschner wires percutaneously from the medial aspect of the proximal fragment, across the osteotomy site, and into the head fragment. Bend the pins and leave them percutaneous for ease in later removal.
- Cut and contour the large bony prominence on the proximal-medial metatarsal so that it is in line with the distal head at the medial margin (Fig. 2.36D).
- During closure of the medial capsule, remove a U-shaped wedge of tissue from the plantar portion near the level of the medial sesamoid. Close this defect with figure-of-eight sutures to correct the hallux valgus.
- Use a pants-over-vest suture configuration to close the plantar capsule to the dorsal capsule to improve sesamoid position.
- After closure, apply a standard soft dressing that gently supports the hallux in the corrected position.

POSTOPERATIVE CARE Patients are allowed to bear weight immediately on their heels with a stiff-soled postoperative shoe and crutches as needed. At 2 weeks, the sutures are removed and another bunion dressing is applied. Pins are removed 5 to 6 weeks after surgery, at which time the dressing and stiff shoe are discontinued. With larger osteotomy correction, radiographic healing can take 3 months or more, but the osteotomy usually is stable enough for normal activities of daily living within 2

months. Sports and strenuous activities should be delayed until 3 to 5 months after surgery.

CHEVRON-AKIN DOUBLE OSTEOTOMY

Mitchell and Baxter described a combination of the chevron and Akin osteotomies to gain greater correction of mild-to-moderate hallux valgus deformities. They reported satisfactory results in 95% of 24 feet in 16 patients using this combined procedure. They cautioned, however, that this procedure should not be used in feet that have advanced sesamoid subluxation with wide intermetatarsal angles.

TECHNIQUE 2.7

(MITCHELL AND BAXTER)
- See Technique 2.1 for tourniquet use and anesthesia. Make a longitudinal medial skin and capsular incision to expose both osteotomies, and make the distal metatarsal osteotomy first (Fig. 2.37A).
- Perform the chevron osteotomy as described in Technique 2.3 except place a single 0.045-inch smooth pin percutaneously dorsal to plantar and in a slightly more proximal position to secure the distal metatarsal osteotomy (Fig. 2.37B,C).
- The lateral displacement of the metatarsal head is approximately 3 mm.

- Do not perform an adductor tenotomy.
- Expose the proximal phalanx subperiosteally and perform a phalangeal closing wedge osteotomy as described in Technique 2.12. Direct the cut away from the articular surface so as to parallel the concavity of the base of the proximal phalanx, and remove a 1-mm wedge of bone (Fig. 2.37D). Do not attempt to remove the contiguous lip of the proximal phalanx.
- Place a 3-0 polyglactin 910 (Vicryl) suture from the periosteum on the distal side of the cut through the proximal undisturbed capsular tissues to maintain the osteotomy closure (Fig. 2.37E).
- Carefully imbricate the capsular incision with absorbable sutures to hold the toe in the corrected position.
- Close the skin with interrupted silk sutures and apply a bulky compressive dressing.

POSTOPERATIVE CARE Ambulation is allowed in a postoperative sandal the day of surgery as tolerated by the patient. The gauze wrap dressing is changed weekly for 2 weeks. The pin is removed, and an elastic bandage is used to hold the corrected toe position. Passive and active plantarflexion and dorsiflexion exercises of the great toe are encouraged at 2 weeks after surgery. At 4 weeks, the wearing of shoes is gradually resumed.

CHEVRON BUNIONECTOMY

Bennett and Sabetta reported a distal chevron metatarsal osteotomy bunionectomy using an intramedullary plate system in 63 feet with mild to moderate hallux valgus. Without fixation these osteotomies can displace, causing recurrence of the deformity; implants should therefore be strong and low-profile to avoid implant prominence. The implant they used allows for more translation of the capital fragment due to its intramedullary placement. All of their osteotomies healed, with no implant problems. They had seven minor complications; two patients complained of stiffness with no loss of motion, one patient developed a bursa over the area of the plate, and two patients had recurrence of the deformity.

TECHNIQUE 2.8

(BENNETT AND SABETTA)
- After a tourniquet is applied mid-calf, make a longitudinal incision on the medial side, centered over the first metatarsophalangeal joint. Make a longitudinal capsulotomy to expose the medial eminence.
- Resect the medial eminence with a sagittal saw in a line perpendicular to the sole of the foot, remaining medial to the sagittal sulcus.
- Make a chevron osteotomy 1 cm proximal to the metatarsophalangeal joint, perpendicular to the cut surface of the medial eminence at a 60-degree angle.
- Laterally translate the metatarsal head and impact onto the metatarsal shaft.

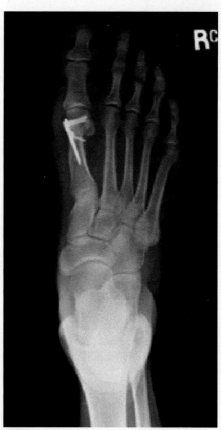

FIGURE 2.38   Chevron bunionectomy using Tornier Mini Maxlock extreme ISO plate system. (From Bennett GL, Sabetta JA: Evaluation of an innovative fixation system for chevron bunionectomy, *Foot Ankle Int* 37:205, 2016.) **SEE TECHNIQUE 2.8.**

- Stabilize the osteotomy site with the Tornier Mini Maxlock Extreme ISO plate system (Tornier, Wright Medical, Memphis, TN), placing the implant down the canal and securing it to the metatarsal head with two 2.4-mm locking screws placed medial to lateral. Insert the oblique nonlocking 2.4-mm screw to secure the implant to the metatarsal shaft (Fig. 2.38).
- Verify deformity correction and position of the implant with fluoroscopy.
- Close the skin in the usual fashion and apply a bulky dressing to the foot.

POSTOPERATIVE CARE Patients are kept minimally weight bearing for 1 week, then placed in a short boot and allowed heel weight bearing for a total of 5 weeks. Patients are weaned from the boot to an accommodative shoe, increasing activities as tolerated.

MINIMALLY INVASIVE OSTEOTOMY

There has been a growing interest in minimally invasive techniques for hallux valgus surgery, including large patient series. Although some authors have reported mixed or less than favorable results in the past, most now report satisfactory results with the percutaneous Akin or chevron-Akin osteotomies in patients with mild to moderate hallux valgus, especially with third-generation techniques. Magnan

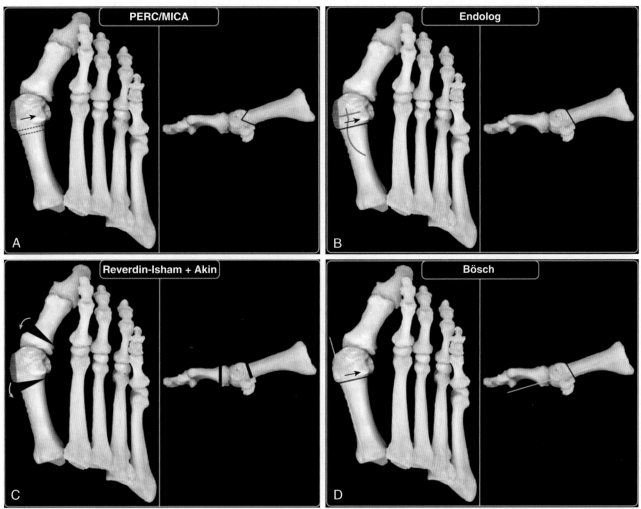

FIGURE 2.39 **A,** Minimally invasive chevron-Akin osteotomy and percutaneous extraarticular reverse-L chevron osteotomy. **B,** Endolog osteotomy technique. **C,** Reverdin-Isham technique. **D,** Bösch technique. (From Malagelada F, Sahirad C, Dalmau-Pastor M, et al: Minimally invasive surgery for hallux valgus: a systematic review of current surgical techniques, *Int Orthop* 43:625, 2019.)

et al. noted that they may even have utility in cases of recurrence. Comparison studies of open versus percutaneous techniques have shown comparable radiographic and clinical outcomes, with minimal soft-tissue dissection, avoidance of capsular disruption and lateral cortex penetration with the saw, decreased risk of vascular disruption, less perioperative pain, reduced operating time, use of distal ankle-blocks, high union rate, early weight bearing, and less risk of wound complications with the percutaneous techniques. Herrera-Perez et al. did note, however, that delayed union was common in their patients after the percutaneous Akin procedure.

A recent systematic review of four minimally invasive techniques (Bösch, MIS chevron-Akin, Reverdin-Isham, and Endolog) showed an overall complication rate of 13% among 23 studies (2279 procedures). Determining which procedure was the most effective could not be elucidated because there were too few studies on each surgical technique. However, the hallux valgus angle improved most with the chevron-Akin technique and the intermetatarsal angle with the Endolog technique (Fig. 2.39A,B). Another study of 80 patients found the combined Reverdin-Isham and Akin (Fig. 2.39C)

percutaneous osteotomy to be a reliable procedure for mild to moderate hallux valgus at 48-month follow-up, but the procedure had a steep learning curve, and results were less encouraging in patients with severe deformity. Complications of this technique included lack of joint congruency, stiffness, and recurrence (6% to 60%). The complication rates after the Bösch technique (SERI: simple, effective, rapid, inexpensive; Fig. 2.39D) have been reported to be between 0% and 22%, with reduced range of motion and dorsal or plantar malalignment of the metatarsal head being the most frequently reported. An anatomical study suggested intensive training for surgeons using the Bösch technique because the dorsal cutaneous nerve is at risk during this procedure.

Fernandez performed double (or triple when necessary) percutaneous osteotomies in 52 feet, reporting results comparable to other, more established techniques. He recommended this technique for intermetatarsal angles over 15 degrees and increased distal metatarsal articular angles in congruent joints. Lucattelli et al. obtained satisfactory preliminary results with a percutaneous procedure without using internal fixation in 195 patients. Overall, good results are being reported from centers that have developed these techniques, but longer-term follow-up and comparative trials are still needed.

MINIMALLY INVASIVE CHEVRON-AKIN OSTEOTOMY

Holme et al. and Lee et al. followed patients who had a third-generation minimally invasive chevron-Akin osteotomy and compared this new technique with older minimally invasive and open procedures, respectively. Their findings support the safety and success of this technique for hallux valgus correction. Lee et al. in a prospective randomized trial comparing 25 minimally invasive chevron-Akin procedures with 25 open surgeries obtained excellent results in 84% of patients and good results in 16%, with a complication rate of 24% (minimally invasive group) mainly due to

prominent screws. Holme et al. used headless screw fixation with excellent results in 40 consecutive patients at 12 months, and with a 10% complication rate.

TECHNIQUE 2.9

(LEE ET AL. AND HOLME ET AL.)
- With the patient supine and the feet over the end of the operating table, draw the dorsal and plantar outline of the first metatarsal.
- Make 3-mm incisions over the medial aspect of the first metatarsophalangeal joint and at the base of the flare of the medial eminence. Make a 5-mm incision at the medial aspect of the first tarsometatarsal joint (Fig. 2.40A).
- Introducing a 2 × 20-mm Shannon burr through the incision over the flare of the medial eminence, create a chevron osteotomy, removing 2 to 3 mm of bone. Direct the burr perpendicular to the axis of the second metatarsal (Fig. 2.40B). As the metatarsal head displaces laterally,

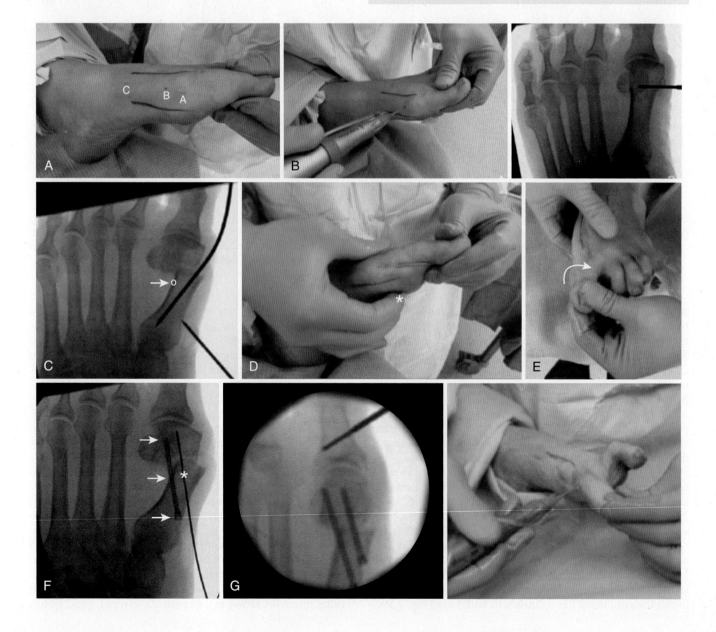

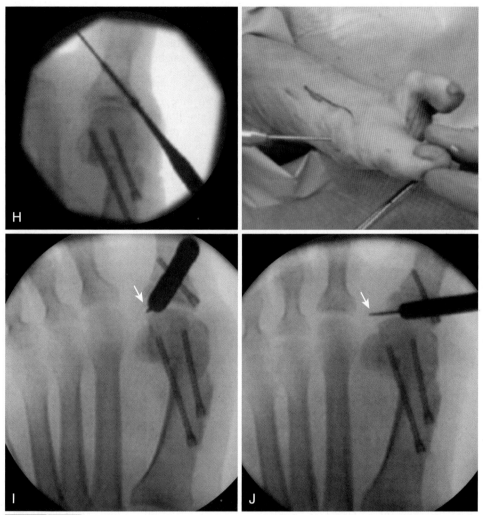

FIGURE 2.40 Minimally invasive chevron-Akin osteotomy. **A,** Initial stab incisions. **B,** Dorsal and plantar cuts of chevron osteotomy using a Shannon burr. **C,** Varus force applied with 2-mm Kirschner wire from translation of distal fragment (arrow shows targeted far cortex for initial guide pin, which enables three-point screw fixation). **D,** Clinical photo. Index finger supports metatarsal head to maintain alignment (*asterisk*). **E,** Correction maneuver for pronation. Supination force is applied as demonstrated by arrow. **F,** Three-point fixation of first proximal screw (*arrows*) and guide pin for second screw (*asterisk*). **G,** Initial placement of Shannon burr for apex of Akin osteotomy. **H,** Placement of screw after Akin osteotomy. **I,** For distal soft-tissue procedure, beaver blade is introduced from dorsum of first metatarsophalangeal joint lateral to extensor hallucis longus tendon. **J,** As varus force is applied to great toe, blade divides lateral plantar plate and lateral sesamoid phalangeal ligament. (From Lee M, Walsh J, Smith MM et al: Hallux valgus correction comparing percutaneous chevron/Akin (PECA) and open scarf/Akin osteotomies, *Foot Ankle Int* 38:838, 2017.) **SEE TECHNIQUE 2.9.**

the head fragment displaces distally by approximately 3 mm, counteracting shortening of the burr and ultimately the first metatarsal. The burr is also directed plantarly. In patients with a long first metatarsal, the burr can be directed more proximally to allow shortening of the first metatarsal.

- Perform the dorsal limb of the osteotomy vertically. For the plantar cut, direct the burr toward the skin of the heel to provide a short plantar limb.
- After the osteotomy is complete, introduce a 1.6-mm Kirschner wire from the medial base of the first metatarsal proximally, into the midaxis of the metatarsal bone,

perforating the far cortex of the distal first metatarsal so that the wire exits the bone approximately 1 cm proximal to the osteotomy (Fig. 2.40C-E). Withdraw the Kirschner wire and insert a 1-mm guidewire through the holes. This aids in placement of the proximal screw with three-point fixation.

- For screw insertion insert a 2-mm-diameter guidewire through the incision in the medial aspect of the first metatarsophalangeal joint and through the osteotomy into the shaft of the first metatarsal to allow displacement of the metatarsal head. This reduction maneuver is important. Use the right hand to ensure the head is in alignment in the lateral plane (see Fig. 2.40D); this prevents plantar and dorsal displacement of the first metatarsal head. Use the left hand and the 2-mm wire to displace the head laterally (see Fig. 2.40C-E), then correct pronation of the metatarsal head.

- Once alignment is corrected, advance the 1-mm guide-wire into the displaced first metatarsal head, then insert the 3.0-mm headless cannulated screw. To provide rotational stability and strength to the construct, insert a second screw (Fig. 2.40F).
- Obtain internal oblique views of the foot to confirm that the head of the screws are engaged in bone, as they may appear to be engaged on the anteroposterior view but are actually not.
- Perform an Akin osteotomy with a 2 × 12-mm Shannon burr and use a headless, cannulated 3.0-mm screw introduced from the medial base of the distal phalanx for fixation (Fig. 2.40G,H).
- For the soft-tissue release, insert a beaver blade from the dorsum of the first metatarsophalangeal joint just lateral to the extensor hallucis longus tendon (Fig. 2.40I,J). The blade divides the lateral plantar plate and the lateral sesamoid phalangeal ligament when varus force is applied to the big toe.
- Through the flare of the medial eminence, puncture the medial capsule just distal to the capsular attachment on the medial prominence using a periosteal elevator. Remove the medial eminence with a 3.1-mm-wedge burr and remove any medial prominence of the proximal first metatarsal at the site of the osteotomy. Confirm adequate removal on image intensification.
- Apply a nonadherent dressing, dry gauze, soft band, and crepe bandage.

POSTOPERATIVE CARE Patients are allowed full weight bearing as tolerated with the aid of crutches and a flat postoperative shoe for 2 weeks. To reduce swelling, the foot should be elevated for the first 10 days after surgery. Gentle plantar flexion stretching exercises of the first metatarsophalangeal joint are started after 2 weeks and scar massage is performed. Patients are allowed to wear sneakers with a straight medial last after 2 weeks.

OSTEOTOMY OF THE PROXIMAL FIRST METATARSAL

If varus of the first metatarsal, whether primary or secondary, contributes to the hallux valgus complex, correction near the origin of the deformity is reasonable, combined with a soft-tissue procedure at the first metatarsophalangeal joint to correct the valgus of the hallux. In addition, a few degrees' shift of the metatarsal at its base causes marked improvement at the distal end of the metatarsal; the forefoot is narrowed, and the chance of pressure symptoms over the former bunion is reduced. A patient without significant degenerative arthritis in the first metatarsophalangeal joint and with hallux valgus of more than 35 degrees and an intermetatarsal angle of more than 10 degrees (or a first to fifth intermetatarsal angle of ≥30 degrees with a hallux valgus of ≥35 degrees) may benefit from a proximal metatarsal osteotomy and a distal soft-tissue procedure at the metatarsophalangeal joint. Deformities with intermetatarsal angles of 13 degrees or less and hallux valgus angles of 30 degrees or less can be corrected by a less technically demanding procedure.

An osteotomy at the base of the metatarsal has the following advantages:
- Cancellous bone and broad contact surfaces of the fragments promote early stability (3 to 5 weeks) and union (6 to 8 weeks).
- Small changes in position at the osteotomy produce excellent correction at the distal end of the metatarsal where symptoms are most often located.
- The metatarsal is shortened minimally, if at all, unless the surgeon chooses a technique that intentionally shortens it (the width of the osteotomy cut itself is more than compensated for by the "straightening of the bone").
- Large angles between the first and second metatarsals can be corrected.
- Slightly tilting the distal fragment plantarward reduces load bearing by the second metatarsal, decreasing the chance of transfer metatarsalgia.
- Narrowing of the forefoot improves the variety of footwear possible and gives an excellent cosmetic result.

This type of osteotomy has the following disadvantages:
- Extensive soft-tissue dissection is required.
- The distal fragment tends to displace dorsally or migrate medially to its original position unless securely fixed internally.
- The second ray may be overloaded if the fragment displaces or migrates.
- Three incisions are required if the basilar osteotomy is performed dorsally.
- The procedure is more difficult to perform with regional block anesthesia.
- The immediate convalescence usually is characterized by more pain, swelling, and immobility than the convalescence that follows a distally placed osteotomy.
- Cast immobilization is more frequently needed.

Currently, the most frequently used proximal metatarsal osteotomies are the crescentic, chevron, Ludloff, and scarf osteotomies (Fig. 2.41). The specific technique of a proximal osteotomy probably is not as important as is meticulous attention to detail. Any proximal osteotomy that allows the first metatarsal to deviate laterally and remain stable in that position with no dorsal tilt to the distal fragment should accomplish the goal of narrowing the intermetatarsal angle. Overcorrection of this angle is possible, but this should not occur with careful attention to detail. If, however, the hallucal sesamoids are not reduced into their respective facets on the metatarsal head, recurrent metatarsus primus varus and hallux valgus may occur regardless of the degree of bony correction. Wagner et al. proposed a new proximal rotational metatarsal osteotomy to correct axial malrotation that may coexist with hallux valgus. It is performed through a single metatarsal oblique osteotomy and achieves correction through rotation only, with no second cut for wedge removal necessary. The procedure is indicated in moderate to severe deformities in patients younger than 50 years and only when there is axial malrotation present (Fig. 2.42).

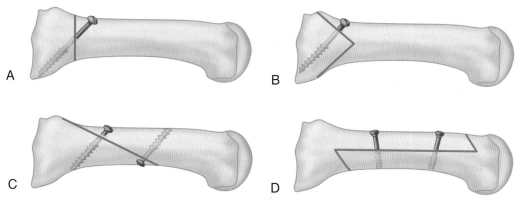

FIGURE 2.41 Four commonly used metatarsal shaft osteotomies. **A,** Proximal crescentic osteotomy. **B,** Proximal chevron osteotomy. **C,** Ludloff osteotomy. **D,** Scarf osteotomy. (From Trnka HG, Parks BG, Ivanic G, et al: Six first metatarsal shaft osteotomies: mechanical and immobilization comparisons, *Clin Orthop Relat Res* 381:256, 2000.)

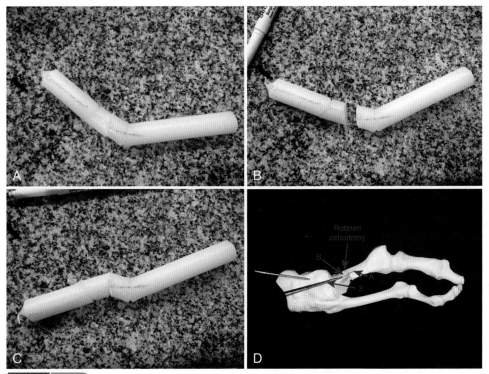

FIGURE 2.42 Rotational osteotomy for hallux valgus. **A,** Candlewax model showing deformity before osteotomy. **B,** Model showing osteotomy cut. **C,** Model after rotating the distal part. **D,** Bone model after correction through metatarsal external rotation. Note how lines *A* and *B* match on dorsum of metatarsal. *3,* Kirschner wire, which is used for osteotomy fixation. (From Wagner P, Ortiz C, Wagner E: Rotational osteotomy for hallux valgus. A new technique for primary and revision cases, *Tech Foot Ankle Surg* 16:3, 2017.)

PROXIMAL CRESCENTIC OSTEOTOMY WITH A DISTAL SOFT-TISSUE PROCEDURE

Mann, Rudicel, and Graves popularized the proximal crescentic osteotomy with a distal soft-tissue repair and documented their results in 109 feet. Of their patients, 93% had satisfactory results; only 7% were dissatisfied and continued to have pain or recurrence of the deformity. Although this procedure is technically demanding, it corrects intermetatarsal angles of 20 to 25 degrees and hallux valgus angles of 40 to 50 degrees. For patients with mild-to-moderate deformity, however, a simpler procedure may provide similar good results.

Most hallux valgus deformities that require a distal soft-tissue procedure also require a proximal osteotomy. This procedure is not recommended if excessive valgus posturing (>15 degrees) of the distal metatarsal articular angle

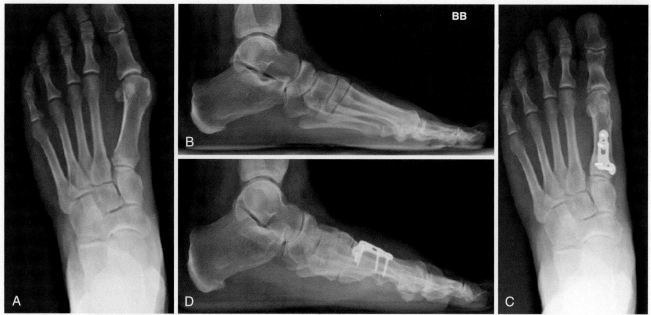

FIGURE 2.43   **A** and **B,** Anteroposterior and lateral views of severe hallux valgus. **C** and **D,** Post-operative anteroposterior and lateral radiographs 1 year after first metatarsal proximal crescentic and Akin osteotomies, showing maintained deformity correction. (From Stith A, Dang D, Griffin M, et al: Rigid internal fixation of proximal crescentic metatarsal osteotomy in hallux valgus correction, *Foot Ankle Int* 40:778, 2019.)

is present on the weight-bearing radiograph or in patients with moderate-to-severe degenerative arthritic changes of the metatarsophalangeal joint (Fig. 2.43). The decision to perform an osteotomy should be made at the time of surgery by passively reducing the intermetatarsal angle. If the first metatarsal does not move laterally, or if it springs back quickly into varus after the laterally directed pressure is released, a basilar osteotomy should be done.

TECHNIQUE 2.10

(MANN AND COUGHLIN)
- For tourniquet use and anesthesia, see Technique 2.1. This procedure is performed through three incisions. The first incision is made dorsally in the intermetatarsal space to release the adductor hallucis, the deep transverse intermetatarsal ligament, and the lateral capsule of the first metatarsophalangeal joint. The second incision is made midline-medial over the medial eminence to remove the medial eminence and perform a capsulorrhaphy. The third incision is made dorsally over the proximal end of the first metatarsal and extends a few millimeters over the medial cuneiform.
- Make the first incision in the first intermetatarsal space beginning at the proximal end of the web space and extending proximally 3 to 4 cm.
- Dissect the soft tissue with scissors to identify the branches of the deep peroneal nerve and be sure to protect them.
- Place a Weitlaner retractor in the first intermetatarsal space and widen this space to expose the adductor hallucis.
- Use a sponge to clear away the soft tissue in the first web space.

- The adductor hallucis approaches the base of the proximal phalanx in an oblique direction. When it has been identified, release it completely from the base of the proximal phalanx and from the lateral edge of the fibular sesamoid (Fig. 2.44A).
- Release the deep transverse intermetatarsal ligament that is plantar to this tendon (Fig. 2.44B). Because the neurovascular bundle to the first web space is immediately plantar to the transverse intermetatarsal ligament, use just the tip of the blade to release this. Placing a small Freer elevator on the plantar surface of this ligament helps avoid the neurovascular bundle as the incision is made.
- Make multiple small stab wounds in the lateral capsule.
- Complete the capsular release by manually forcing the hallux into 25 to 30 degrees of varus and pushing the first metatarsal lateralward.
- When the lateral release has been completed, release the deep transverse intermetatarsal ligament that attaches to the fibular sesamoid. Releasing the deep transverse intermetatarsal ligament prevents its deforming force on the fibulosesamoid from pulling the sesamoid apparatus laterally from under the metatarsal head.
- Push the first metatarsal head laterally. If it tends to rest in that position, an osteotomy is not necessary; however, if it springs back to the varus position, an osteotomy should be performed (Fig. 2.44C).
- Return to the adductor hallucis, which is completely freed, and lift it up into the wound from the bottom of the foot.
- Pass three absorbable 2-0 sutures first through the lateral capsule on the first metatarsal head just proximal to the lateral capsular release. Make a second throw of the suture through the adductor hallucis tendon and a third throw through the capsuloligamentous intrinsic tendinous

tissue on the medial side of the second metatarsal head. Do not tie these sutures, but hold them with hemostats and allow them to fall into the first web space.

- Make a second midline incision (Fig. 2.44D), avoiding the dorsal sensory branch of the superficial peroneal nerve dorsalward and the proper branch of the medial plantar nerve to the medial side of the hallux plantarward. Continue this incision down to the capsule and raise the dorsal flap deep to the dorsal sensory nerve.

- Raise the plantar flap on the capsule until the plantar aspect of the abductor hallucis muscle is reached, which is just a few millimeters from the tibial sesamoid. This is best done with the hallux in about 30 degrees of flexion, which relaxes the digital nerve just plantar to the dissection.

- Make a vertical incision in the capsule 2 to 3 mm proximal to the base of the proximal phalanx extending from a few millimeters medial to the extensor hallucis longus tendon in a plantar direction through the medial capsule and through the thickened portion of the capsule plantarward, which is actually the abductor hallucis tendon capsule junction. This vertical limb ends 2 mm medial to the tibial sesamoid. The most inferior portion of this vertical limb is best made from plantar to dorsal to avoid the digital nerve.

- Depending on the enlargement of the medial eminence and the subsequent redundancy and stretching of the medial capsule, remove an elliptical wedge of the capsule, measuring 4 to 8 mm wide at its widest section. Dorsally and plantarward, taper this incision into a V shape and excise the elliptical wedge of the capsule.

- Extend the capsular incision proximally, beginning at the dorsal edge of the vertical limb. This limb of the incision (an inverted L) should end 2 to 3 mm proximal to the junction of the medial eminence with the metatarsal shaft.

- Raise this capsular flap from dorsal distal to plantar proximal to expose the entire medial eminence.

- Remove the medial eminence. Do this in a plane parallel to the shaft of the first metatarsal and begin just medial to the sagittal groove (Fig. 2.44E).

- Begin a third incision on the dorsal aspect of the proximal third of the metatarsal. Extend this incision proximally over the dorsal surface of the medial cuneiform. Avoid the superficial peroneal nerve sensory branch to the hallux. Retract or ligate the dorsal venous arch.

- Identify the metatarsocuneiform joint and incise the periosteum of the first metatarsal and medial cuneiform longitudinally medial to the extensor hallucis longus tendon.

- Score the dorsal aspect of the metatarsal transversely at 1- and 2-cm levels distal to the metatarsocuneiform

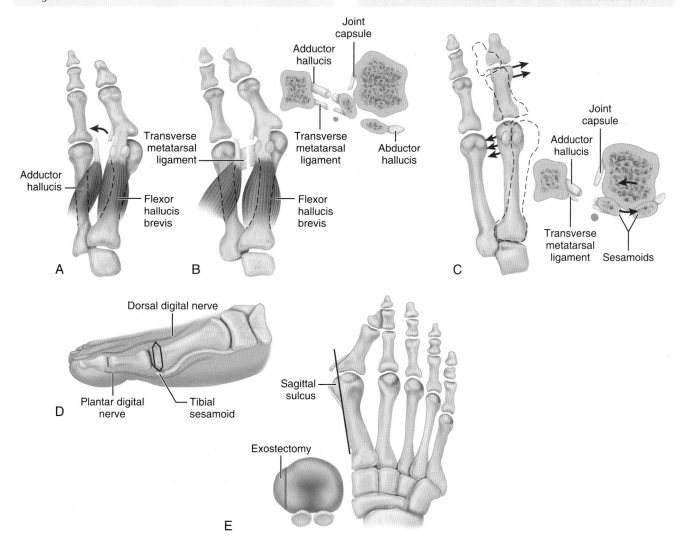

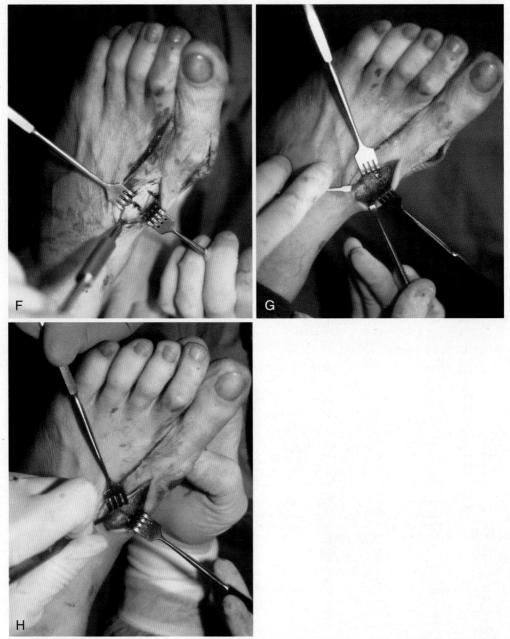

FIGURE 2.44 **A,** Adductor tendon released from insertion into lateral aspect of fibular sesamoid and base of proximal phalanx. **B,** Transverse metatarsal ligament has been transected. *Inset* shows that at this point, contracted lateral joint capsule, adductor hallucis, and transverse intermetatarsal ligament have been released. **C,** If metatarsal head springs back medially when pushed laterally, osteotomy should be considered. **D,** Medial capsular incision, beginning 2 to 3 mm proximal to base of proximal phalanx. Second incision is made 3 to 8 mm more proximal, removing flap of tissue. Size of flap is determined by severity of deformity. Wedge of tissue approximately 6 mm is removed. Capsular cut is V-shaped through abductor hallucis tendon with apex at tibial sesamoid. Medial eminence is exposed by making incision along dorsomedial aspect of capsule and peeling it off medial eminence with sharp dissection. **E,** Removal of medial eminence is done on line projected along medial aspect of the first metatarsal shaft, and exostectomy should be done 1 to 2 mm medial to sagittal sulcus. **F,** Knife blade is in metatarsocuneiform joint, and two lines marked on metatarsal represent osteotomy site *(proximal line)* and location of screw for fixation *(distal line)*. **G,** Final position of screw and position of metatarsal after correction of first metatarsal. **H,** Note Freer elevator is displacing or rotating proximal fragment medially whereas first metatarsal head and distal fragment are being angulated laterally by manual pressure. (**A-D** from Mann RA, Coughlin MJ: *The video textbook of foot and ankle surgery*, St. Louis, 1991, Medical Video Productions; **E** from Mann RA, Coughlin MJ, editors: *Surgery of the foot and ankle*, ed 6, St. Louis, 1993, Mosby.) **SEE TECHNIQUE 2.10.**

articulation. The first scored mark represents the osteotomy site, and the second represents the area for placement of the screw for internal fixation of the osteotomy (Fig. 2.44F).

- Release the soft tissue dorsally, medially, and laterally, being careful to avoid the penetrating branch of the dorsalis pedis artery in the proximal part of the first intermetatarsal space.
- If a screw is to be used for fixation, make a glide hole. This is much easier to do at this point than when the metatarsal becomes less stable after the osteotomy.
- Drill a 3.5-mm hole 1 cm distal to the osteotomy site in the center of the metatarsal shaft and direct it proximally 45 degrees to the metatarsal shaft, penetrating only the dorsal cortex.
- Use a countersink to enlarge the entrance hole. It is important to enlarge this at its most distal extension rather than at the proximal edge of the drill hole because it gives the screw head a place to sit and does not permit it to rise dorsally, which might crack the cortical bridge into the osteotomy site as the screw is tightened.
- If a 5/16-inch smooth Steinmann pin is to be placed in an oblique direction from distal medial to proximal lateral, drill the hole in the medial aspect of the metatarsal before the osteotomy.
- Using a 1/16-inch drill bit, drill a hole in the medial aspect of the metatarsal in an oblique direction, crossing the osteotomy site.
- After the osteotomy is complete and the intermetatarsal angle has been corrected, the pin is placed through the drill hole into the proximal fragment and into the tarsus if necessary (Fig. 2.44G).
- Using an oscillating saw with a crescent-shaped saw blade (Fig. 2.45) placed convex distally, begin the osteotomy on the most proximal scored mark.
- The initial cut should just be a deeper scoring. Place the saw blade gently into the first metatarsal base without oscillation or manual turning of the blade.
- When this superficial scoring has been performed with the crescentic blade, evaluate the angle of the osteotomy carefully. It should not be perpendicular to the first metatarsal shaft, and it should not be perpendicular to the sole of the foot but should bisect that angle.
- Drop the handle of the saw 10 to 15 degrees proximally to direct the osteotomy correctly.
- When the dorsal cortex has been scored, complete the osteotomy by gently rocking the blade medially and laterally. Mann emphasized that the lateral aspect of the blade must exit the lateral side of the metatarsal shaft. It is not as important that the blade exit the medial side because a small osteotome can be used to complete that part of the osteotomy.
- When the osteotomy is completed, use a Freer elevator to ensure that there are no periosteal attachments medially or laterally that would prevent displacement of the osteotomy (see Fig. 2.44H).

The following steps are crucial:

- Displace the proximal fragment medially and hold with a Freer elevator or some other instrument.
- While holding the proximal fragment medially displaced, rotate the distal fragment around the osteotomy site (usually 2 to 4 mm of lateral displacement or rotation of the distal fragment).

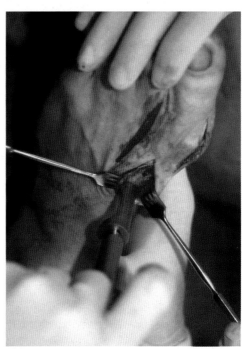

FIGURE **2.45** Curved saw blade is held firmly with one hand and stabilized with opposite hand. **SEE TECHNIQUE 2.10.**

- Do not let the distal fragment slide dorsally or plantarward.
- Have an assistant complete the drilling, tapping, and placing of the screw while the surgeon holds the osteotomy in the corrected position.
- With the osteotomy held reduced, enter the initial hole with a centering device, sometimes referred to as a "golf tee" or "mushroom," which guides the 2- or 2.5-mm drill bit into the basilar fragment.
- Use a 4-mm tap and insert a 4-mm fully threaded cancellous screw (usually 26 mm long).
- Be careful on the last few turns of the screw that the head of the screw does not rise dorsally on the cortex, because this would fracture the intervening cortical bridge. If this appears to be happening, remove the screw and countersink deeper so that part of the head of the screw would rest just plantar to the cortex.
- According to Mann, making the osteotomy convex distally should prevent overcorrection of the intermetatarsal angle.
- A useful technical tip is to use the countersink in the drill hole before placing the screw. This gently removes bone from the distal part of the screw hole, allowing the screw to sit firmly in the metatarsal (Fig. 2.46A). If this is not done, as the screw is placed the screw head abuts this bone distally and the screw displaces dorsally. This causes the fragile dorsal lip of bone between the screw hole and the osteotomy to break and lose the ability to achieve stable fixation with a screw. Because the screw is placed at an angle to the cortex, a true countersinking is not actually done but a pathway for the screw head to travel is created (Fig. 2.46B); a small burr can be used for this.
- After completing screw or pin fixation of the osteotomy, return to the dorsal wound in the first intermetatarsal space and tie the three sutures to bind the adductor hal-

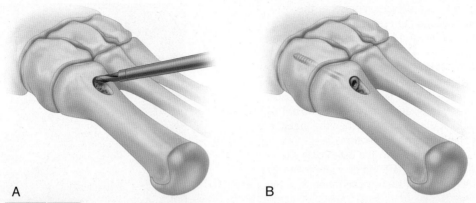

A   B

FIGURE 2.46 Screw hole preparation. **A,** Notch is made for passage of screw head. Drilling should begin near surface of bone, not in depths of notch. **B,** Screw head sits in untapered end of notch after passing through it. Joint or fusion surfaces remain well reduced. (From Manoli A, Hansen S: Screw hole preparation in foot surgery, *Foot Ankle* 11:105, 1990.) **SEE TECHNIQUE 2.10.**

lucis and the first and second metatarsal heads together. The first ray should rest in a corrected position. An X-plate also has been described for fixation of this osteotomy (Fig. 2.47).

- Close the medial capsule to hold it in place. Excise only the capsular overlap. Mann emphasized the importance of passing the sutures through the abductor hallucis tendon and capsule toward the plantar aspect of the vertical limb of the capsulotomy. Place the hallux in about 5 degrees of varus while the sutures are tied. It is unnecessary to close the dorsal proximal limb of the inverted-L capsulotomy.
- Apply a bulky compression dressing and remove the tourniquet.

POSTOPERATIVE CARE It is our practice after a proximal procedure to place the patient in a bulky bandage and a short leg walking cast and allow weight bearing, changing the cast at 2 weeks and allowing a postoperative shoe at 4 weeks. No benefit has been found to using postoperative taping after surgery.

The major complications of this procedure have been hallux varus, dorsiflexion malunion of the osteotomy site with transfer metatarsalgia, and limitation of motion of the first metatarsophalangeal joint; however, these complications are infrequent, and most patients are satisfied with their outcomes.

SCARF OSTEOTOMY

The scarf osteotomy is a horizontally directed displacement Z-osteotomy made at the diaphyseal level (Fig. 2.48). In architectural and carpentry terminology, "scarf" refers to a joint made by notching, grooving, or otherwise cutting the ends of two pieces and fastening them together so that they overlap and join to form one continuous piece. This configuration has a high level of intrinsic stability, particularly in the sagittal plane, and provides a broad surface area for bony healing. Cadaver studies confirmed that under

loaded conditions the scarf osteotomy has double the stability of a distal chevron or proximal crescentic osteotomy. Another reason for the popularity of the scarf osteotomy is its versatility. It allows lateral displacement of the plantar bone fragment to reduce the intermetatarsal angle, medial displacement of the capital fragment to correct hallux varus, plantar displacement to increase the load of the first ray, and elongation or shortening of the first metatarsal. The stability of the osteotomy allows early weight bearing and return to activities. The scarf osteotomy usually is combined with a lateral soft-tissue release, excision of the medial bony eminence, and medial capsulorrhaphy, and occasionally with a proximal phalangeal osteotomy.

Reported patient satisfaction with the outcomes of the scarf osteotomy is approximately 90%; however, a frequently reported complication has been "troughing" of the metatarsal with loss of height resulting in functional malunion with elevation of the first ray, occurring in as many as a third of patients. Other reported complications include delayed union, rotational malunion, proximal fracture, infection, early deformity recurrence, transfer metatarsalgia, osteonecrosis of the first metatarsal head, prominent screw causing irritation, screw back-out, neuralgia, and complex regional pain syndrome (CRPS). In a more recent report of 150 patients followed for at least 2 years, 91% were satisfied with their results; only 14 patients had "significant" complications, which included severe undercorrection or overcorrection, pain, osteoarthritis, metatarsal head osteonecrosis, troughing, and recurrence of the deformity. Choi et al. evaluated the clinical and radiographic results in 51 patients after the scarf osteotomy of the first metatarsal with soft-tissue realignment, noting that it was a reliable procedure with a low rate of complications and recurrence. American Orthopaedic Foot and Ankle Society (AOFAS) hallux score, SF-36 score, and visual analog scores improved postoperatively, reaching statistical significance. In addition, statistically significant improvement was noted in all radiographic measures, including hallux valgus angle, intermetatarsal angle, and medial sesamoid position. The complication rate was 15% and included symptomatic hardware for which four patients required reoperation, hallux varus, and progression of first metatarsophalangeal joint arthritis.

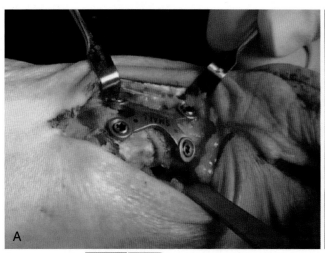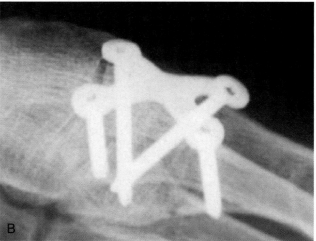

FIGURE 2.47 Clinical photo and radiograph of X-plate. (From Pauli W, Koch A, Testa E, et al: Fixation of the proximal metatarsal crescentic osteotomy using a head locking X-plate, *Foot Ankle Int* 37:218, 2016.) **SEE TECHNIQUE 2.10.**

Current indications for the scarf osteotomy are mild-to-moderate deformities (intermetatarsal angle of 11 to 18 degrees and hallux valgus angle of 20 to 40 degrees). Because the scarf osteotomy is an "overlapping" osteotomy, the limit of correction is not primarily the intermetatarsal angle but the width of the first metatarsal (the wider the metatarsal, the more correction possible). The minimal overlapping between the two fragments that still allows sufficient stability is one third of the metatarsal width, although very experienced surgeons might push this to one-fourth overlap. First ray instability caused by ligamentous laxity around the first Lisfranc joint rather than failure of the windlass mechanism secondary to hallux valgus deformity is a contraindication to the scarf osteotomy, but this is rare. Other contraindications are osteoarthritis of the metatarsophalangeal joint and severe osteoporosis. This procedure is technically demanding, and there is a steep learning curve. Suggested methods for preventing "troughing" include avoiding the cancellous bone with the step-cuts, using a noncompressing screw, making the long limb of the osteotomy from the first metatarsal head to its base parallel to the inferior metatarsal shaft, and making the short limbs of the osteotomy 45 degrees to the long limb.

TECHNIQUE 2.11

(COETZEE AND RIPPSTEIN)

- With the patient supine, administer general or regional anesthesia and apply a thigh tourniquet (see Technique 2.1).
- Make a skin incision that runs medially and longitudinally over the first metatarsophalangeal joint, extending from about the proximal half of the proximal phalanx to the middle part of the first metatarsal.
- Subperiosteally free the dorsal aspects of the proximal phalanx and first metatarsal from the overlying soft tissues. To preserve the blood supply to the distal fragment, do not detach the soft tissues on the plantar aspect of the first metatarsal.

- With the medial aspect of the first metatarsal exposed, make a three-cut Z-shaped osteotomy.
- Begin the longitudinal cut at the level of the metatarsal head, 5 mm from the joint at the junction between the dorsal third and the plantar two thirds of the metatarsal. Depending on the severity of the deformity to be corrected, make this cut longer or shorter, but generally reaching the proximal part of the diaphysis. In the frontal plane, this cut is parallel to the weight-bearing plane or slightly oblique from dorsomedial to plantar-lateral to bring the metatarsal head more plantar if required.
- Make the first transverse cut distally and dorsally, perpendicular to the long axis of the second metatarsal if the length of the first metatarsal has to remain equal. The transverse cut usually runs parallel to the cartilage line of the metatarsal head. To lengthen the metatarsal, orient the transverse (short) cut in the horizontal plane from medial-proximal to distal-lateral at an angle that will allow distal translation. If shortening of the first metatarsal is desired, orient the transverse cut from medial-distal to lateral-proximal in the horizontal plane; the more oblique the cut and the larger the lateral shift, the more shortening will occur.
- Alternatively, shorten the metatarsal by removing a segment of bone of the amount of desired shortening by making a second cut just proximal to the first one. This is a more predictable method of obtaining shortening.
- Make the second transverse cut strictly parallel to the first transverse cut, plantar at the proximal end of the longitudinal cut (Fig. 2.49A). Take care to avoid making this cut convergent to the first one because this would prevent the shifting of the head fragment (locking effect) (Fig. 2.49B).
- Translate the plantar-distal portion laterally to close the intermetatarsal gap (Fig. 2.49C). If necessary, rotation can be done to correct any pathologic distal metatarsal angle.
- If the required distal metatarsal articular angle correction is important, the proximal-lateral corner of the head fragment can impinge on the second metatarsal, preventing full correction; in this situation, resect this corner.

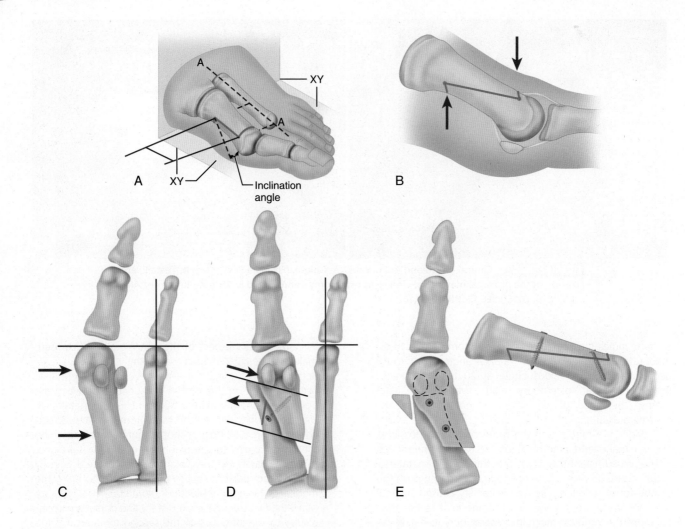

FIGURE 2.48 Scarf osteotomy. **A,** Placement of Kirschner wires at corner point of planned osteotomy. Standard orientation for lateral translation is 90 degrees to longitudinal axis of second metatarsal (A) and in approximately 20 degrees horizontal inclination to plantar surface (XY). **B,** Osteotomy cuts. **C,** Lateral displacement is obtained if short osteotomy cuts are perpendicular to longitudinal axis of foot. **D,** Proximally oriented inclination of short osteotomy cuts caused shortening depending on angle of inclination and amount of translation. **E,** After lateral displacement, osteotomy is fixed with two minifragment screws. (**A-D** redrawn from Kristen KH, Berger C, Stelzig S, et al: The scarf osteotomy for the correction of hallux valgus deformities, *Foot Ankle Int* 23:221, 2002; **E** redrawn from Jones S, Al Hussainy HA, Ali F, et al: Scarf osteotomy for hallux valgus: a prospective clinical and pedobarographic study, *J Bone Joint Surg* 86B:830, 2004. Copyright British Editorial Society of Bone and Joint Surgery.) **SEE TECHNIQUE 2.11.**

- Insert a Kirschner wire from the proximal fragment distally into the distal fragment, taking care to not place it where the distal screw will be placed for definitive fixation. The use of a wire instead of a clamp prevents stripping of the soft tissues beneath the distal fragment, better preserving its vascularity (Fig. 2.50A,B).
- Perform a simulated loading test on the forefoot. The hallux should be reduced or nearly reduced on the metatarsal head, and the metatarsal head should be reduced over the sesamoids. If this is not the case, either an Akin osteotomy or an additional lateral soft-tissue release with tenotomy of the adductor tendon is done, depending on the cause

of the residual subluxation. Check the sesamoid reduction either clinically or radiographically with a mini C-arm.
- Use two minifragment screws (2 or 2.7 mm) to secure the osteotomy.
- Remove the exposed medial eminence and dorsal-medial metatarsal shaft.
- If any hallux valgus deformity remains, the cause of this residual deformity should be treated before closing the capsule medially, because the capsule will not be able to hold the correction over time if the hallux valgus deformity is not adequately corrected by osteotomy and soft-tissue release (Fig. 2.51).

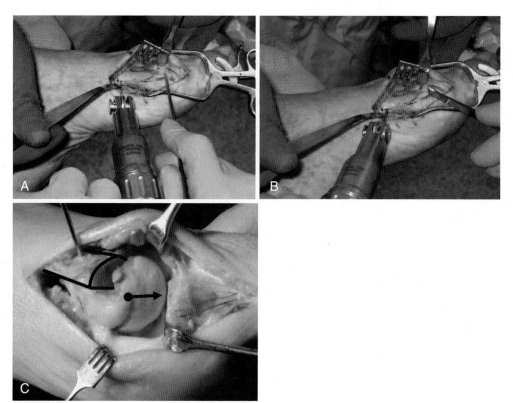

FIGURE 2.49 Scarf osteotomy. **A,** Two short arms of Z-cut should be perfectly parallel to allow capital fragment to displace laterally. To lengthen metatarsal, both short arms should project from medioproximal to laterodistal and remain parallel. **B,** If short arms converge, osteotomy is impossible to displace laterally. **C,** With short arms of Z parallel, capital fragment is easily displaced laterally. (From Coetzee JC, Rippstein P: Surgical strategies: scarf osteotomy for hallux valgus, *Foot Ankle Int* 28:529, 2007.) **SEE TECHNIQUE 2.11.**

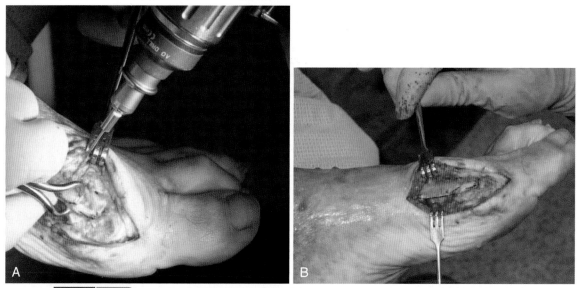

FIGURE 2.50 Scarf osteotomy. **A,** Capital fragment is displaced laterally while proximal fragment is held with clamp. Osteotomy is temporarily stabilized with Kirschner wire. **B,** Two screws are used to securely stabilize osteotomy. (From Coetzee JC, Rippstein P: Surgical strategies: scarf osteotomy for hallux valgus, *Foot Ankle Int* 28:529, 2007.) **SEE TECHNIQUE 2.11.**

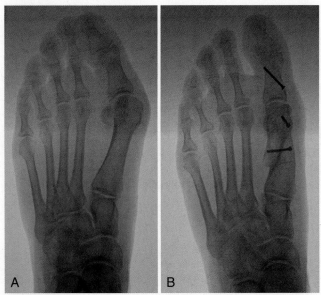

FIGURE 2.51   **A,** Patient with moderate metatarsus primus varus and hallux valgus deformity. **B,** Both intermetatarsal angle and hallux valgus are corrected; Akin osteotomy also was done to obtain complete correction of hallux valgus. (From Coetzee JC, Rippstein P: Surgical strategies: scarf osteotomy for hallux valgus, *Foot Ankle Int* 28:529, 2007.) **SEE TECHNIQUE 2.11.**

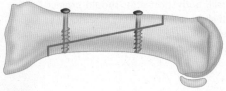

FIGURE 2.52   Shortening depth of short arms of Z osteotomy limits amount of metatarsal collapse, avoiding "troughing." (From Coetzee JC, Rippstein P: Surgical strategies: scarf osteotomy for hallux valgus, *Foot Ankle Int* 28:529, 2007.) **SEE TECHNIQUE 2.11.**

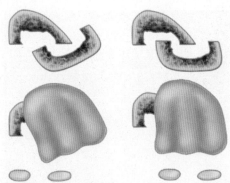

FIGURE 2.53   Troughing can lead to functional elevation of the first ray or rotational malunion. (From Coetzee JC, Rippstein P: Surgical strategies: scarf osteotomy for hallux valgus, *Foot Ankle Int* 28:529, 2007.) **SEE TECHNIQUE 2.11.**

- Repair the medial joint capsule, deflate the tourniquet, obtain hemostasis, and close the incisions in routine fashion.

POSTOPERATIVE CARE Patients are allowed heel-touch weight bearing for 2 weeks in a postoperative shoe

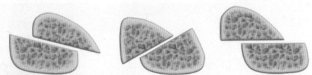

FIGURE 2.54   Depending on the direction of long arm of the Z osteotomy, capital fragment of first metatarsal can be displaced plantar, dorsal, or neutral. (From Coetzee JC, Rippstein P: Surgical strategies: scarf osteotomy for hallux valgus, *Foot Ankle Int* 28:529, 2007.) **SEE TECHNIQUE 2.11.**

followed by 4 weeks of partial weight bearing before starting a rehabilitation program.

After many years of experience with the scarf osteotomy, Coetzee et al. made several recommendations for changes to the technique.

The distal and proximal arms of the Z should be limited to 2 to 3 mm in depth. Although this theoretically reduces the stability of the osteotomy, this has not been observed clinically, and the short cuts avoid the cancellous portion of the metatarsal, thus reducing the risk of troughing (Fig. 2.52), which is the most frequent problem with this osteotomy. Troughing occurs when the cortices wedge into the softer cancellous bone of the metatarsal shaft, causing a functional elevation or dorsiflexion of the first ray that can lead to a pronated first metatarsal and lesser metatarsal overload (Fig. 2.53). Shortening the short arms of the osteotomy either eliminates the problem or allows only 2 mm of subsidence. Another way to limit troughing is to keep the long arm of the Z as long as possible, which allows the short arms to be in the metaphysis that has a less dense cortex.

The procedure should be limited to younger people with strong healthy bone that prevents troughing. In elderly patients, the cancellous bone may be very soft and unable to support the cortical overlay.

Multiple adjustments should be made as needed. Depending on the direction of the long arm of the Z, the distal (capital) fragment can be displaced in a plantar or dorsal direction. Angling the long arm from dorsomedial to plantar lateral displaces the capital fragment plantarly by 1 to 2 mm, increasing the weight bearing under the first metatarsal (Fig. 2.54). Plantarflexing or dorsiflexing the first metatarsal or adding a rotational component to the osteotomy increases its stability and versatility. The metatarsal can be lengthened a few millimeters without compromising the stability of the osteotomy by cutting the short arms of the Z parallel from proximal-medial to distal-lateral. Although seldom necessary, the metatarsal can be shortened by removing equal segments on the short arms of the Z.

LUDLOFF OSTEOTOMY

In 1918, Ludloff described an oblique osteotomy of the first metatarsal oriented from dorsal-proximal to distal-plantar. He originally shortened the metatarsal without using internal fixation; this technique was abandoned for many years because of its inherent instability. With the development of newer fixation methods that added stability, the technique has gained popularity. Biomechanical studies have shown that the Ludloff osteotomy fixed with lag screw compression is more rigid than proximal crescentic and other proximal first metatarsal osteotomies and that it provides lateral and angular correction similar to those of crescentic and closing wedge osteotomies with less elevation and shortening. In addition to mechanical stability that allows early ambulation, suggested advantages of the Ludloff osteotomy include simplicity (involving only a single cut in the bone), angular correction through bony rotation that allows the surgeon to "dial in" the precise amount of correction desired, and slight supination of the cut (8 degrees) that allows plantarflexion of the first metatarsal, theoretically minimizing the risk of transfer metatarsalgia further. Reported complications include prominent hardware requiring removal, hallux varus, delayed union, superficial infection, and neuralgia.

TECHNIQUE 2.12

(CHIODO, SCHON, AND MYERSON)
- For tourniquet use and anesthesia, see Technique 2.1. Separate dorsal and medial incisions are used.
- First make the dorsal incision aligned over the first web space and then release the transverse metatarsal ligament, adductor hallucis tendon, and lateral capsule.
- Make an 8-cm medial longitudinal incision next, extending from the metatarsocuneiform joint to the base of the proximal phalanx, to expose the medial aspect of the first metatarsal and metatarsophalangeal joint.
- Make a cruciate or L-shaped medial capsulotomy.
- Begin the oblique osteotomy approximately 2 mm distal to the metatarsocuneiform joint and extend it from dorsal-proximal to plantar-distal; the plane of the osteotomy should be oriented at an angle approximately 30 degrees from the long axis of the first metatarsal so that it exits the plantar-distal metatarsal a few millimeters proximal to the sesamoids.
- When the proximal three fourths of the osteotomy has been completed, loosely fix it with a cannulated lag screw (3 or 3.5 mm) placed perpendicular to the plane of the cut (Fig. 2.55A). Position this screw within the proximal rather than the middle portion of the osteotomy to bring the center of correction proximally toward the apex of the deformity to increase the correction and minimize shortening of the first metatarsal.
- Complete the osteotomy and rotate the distal fragment around the axis of the screw until the desired correction of the intermetatarsal angle is obtained (Fig. 2.55B).
- When the desired correction is obtained, tighten the screw.
- Insert a second, more distal screw perpendicularly across the osteotomy (Fig. 2.55C).
- If there is space, a third screw can be added. If screw purchase is poor for the second screw, two supplemental axial Kirschner wires can be used without significant loss of fixation strength. Fixation with threaded Kirschner wires alone provides adequate strength when screw fixation is impossible because of a short osteotomy or an intraoperative metatarsal fracture.

POSTOPERATIVE CARE Patients are allowed to bear weight as tolerated immediately on the heel and lateral forefoot in an open, hard-soled surgical shoe, followed by gradual resumption of full weight bearing on the flat foot as tolerated. Dressing changes are done at 7 to 10 days, and the postoperative shoe is discontinued at 4 to 6 weeks when evidence of bone healing and stability of the osteotomy are noted radiographically.

PROXIMAL OPENING WEDGE OSTEOTOMY AND DISTAL CHEVRON OSTEOTOMY

Braito et al. described the results of combining a proximal opening wedge osteotomy with a distal chevron osteotomy in 36 feet with severe hallux valgus (hallux valgus angle ≥20 degrees and an intermetatarsal angle ≥13 degrees). Although they obtained favorable outcomes radiographically and clinically in most patients, seven minor complications were reported, and there were three severe complications that were related to the technique and required revision surgery. They noted that this double osteotomy allows for correction of each component of the deformity in patients with an abnormal distal metatarsal articular angle, but it has substantial complications, including loss of fixation, wound infection, nonunion, overcorrection, and undercorrection.

TECHNIQUE 2.13

(BRAITO ET AL.)
- Under tourniquet control perform a lateral soft-tissue release, including incision of the lateral metatarsosesamoidal ligament, release of the adductor hallucis tendon at its attachment to the fibular sesamoid, and a longitudinal incision of the lateral metatarsophalangeal joint capsule through a separate distal dorsomedial approach.
- Through a proximal dorsomedial approach, perform a horizontal osteotomy of the first metatarsal, completing the opening wedge maneuver to the required correction.
- Accomplish fixation using an open-wedge locking plate.
- Through the dorsomedial incision of the lateral release, perform a distal chevron osteotomy, with the apex in the center of the first metatarsal head.
- Shift the metatarsal head laterally (or medially in patients with an increased distal metatarsal articular angle) by either impacting the metatarsal head onto the shaft or by excising a medial wedge from the distal dorsal cut.
- Confirm sesamoid position fluoroscopically and insert one or two 1.2- to 1.4-mm antegrade Kirschner wires for fixation of the first metatarsal head.
- If there is concomitant hallux valgus interphalangeus, an Akin osteotomy can be performed.

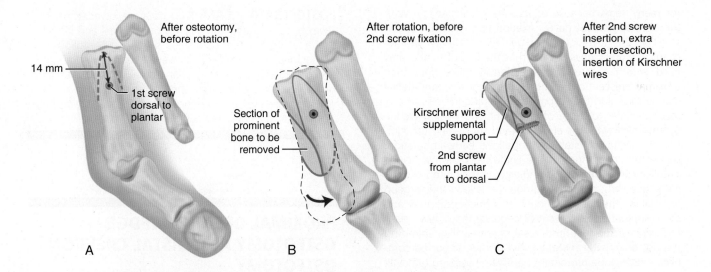

FIGURE 2.55 Ludloff osteotomy. **A,** Placement of first screw after osteotomy and before rotation of distal fragment. **B,** Rotation of distal fragment. **C,** Placement of supplementary Kirschner wires after placement of second screw and resection of bone. (From Schon LC, Dorn KJ, Jung HG: Clinical tip: stabilization of the proximal Ludloff osteotomy, *Foot Ankle Int* 26:579, 2005.) **SEE TECHNIQUE 2.12.**

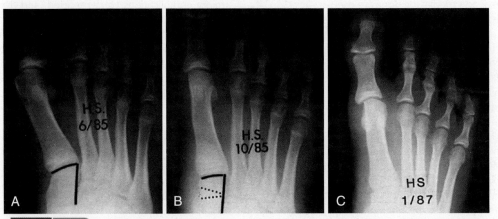

FIGURE 2.56 **A,** Metatarsus primus varus and open physis in an adolescent. **B,** After opening wedge cuneiform osteotomy and distal soft-tissue realignment. **C,** At 18-month follow-up visit. Note incongruous metatarsophalangeal joint. (From Coughlin MJ: Juvenile bunions. In Mann RA, Coughlin MJ, editors: *Surgery of the foot and ankle*, ed 6, St. Louis, 1993, Mosby.)

POSTOPERATIVE CARE A corrective soft dressing is to be worn for 2 weeks and the patient mobilized immediately in a custom shoe, which is to be worn for 6 weeks. Partial weight bearing is recommended at 2 weeks with progressive weight bearing over the next 4 to 6 weeks.

MEDIAL CUNEIFORM OSTEOTOMY

Medial cuneiform osteotomy, first described by Riedl, was originally used for the correction of primus varus but subsequently has been used to treat hallux valgus deformity in adolescents with open proximal metatarsal physes, especially patients with an abnormally wide intermetatarsal angle (Fig. 2.56). The osteotomy is combined with removal of the medial eminence and imbrication of the medial capsule. This procedure is particularly useful in combination with a closing wedge distal metatarsal osteotomy and proximal phalangeal osteotomy for more severe deformities, especially those with a congruent metatarsophalangeal joint.

TECHNIQUE 2.14

(RIEDL; COUGHLIN)

- For tourniquet use and anesthesia, see Technique 2.1. Center a medial longitudinal incision over the first cuneiform.

The medial cuneiform is approximately 2 cm long, and the osteotomy should be centered in the middle of the bone.

- Identify the navicular-cuneiform and the metatarsocuneiform joints.
- Direct the osteotomy in a mediolateral plane and carry it to a depth of 1.5 cm (Fig. 2.57A,B), ensuring that the dorsal and plantar cortices are transected.
- The medial eminence of the metatarsal head can be used as an interposition graft, or, in adolescents with little medial eminence, a wedge-shaped piece of bone from the iliac crest or lyophilized, freeze-dried iliac bicortical graft can be used. A 3-cm-long graft is required because of the height of the first cuneiform. The base of the graft should be 1 cm or less and should taper to a fine point at the apex. Remove all cortical bone.
- Distract the osteotomy site with a lamina spreader and impact the bone graft (Fig. 2.57C).
- Fix the osteotomy with crossed 0.062-inch Kirschner wires (or a 3.5 to 4.5 mm fully threaded cortical or cancellous screw) and close the wound in the routine manner.

POSTOPERATIVE CARE A short leg, well-padded, nonwalking cast is worn for 6 weeks, followed by a removable walking boot until both ends of the graft are incorporated. This may take 4 to 6 months.

PROXIMAL PHALANGEAL OSTEOTOMY

In 1925, Truslow popularized the term *metatarsus primus varus*, or varus of the first metatarsal, and recommended correcting this component to treat hallux valgus. In the same year, Akin suggested a medially based closing wedge osteotomy at the base of the proximal phalanx, combined with medial eminence removal to correct the deformity of the hallux. He also suggested removal of the medial condylar flare of the base of the proximal phalanx. With minor modifications, this procedure has proved helpful in correcting hallux

valgus in selected patients, mostly as an adjunctive procedure to the primary bunion repair; it rarely is indicated alone for correction of hallux valgus deformity, and in most patients this procedure should be performed along with some other procedure to correct all components of the hallux valgus.

The degree of deformity should be measured on weight-bearing anteroposterior radiographs. The intermetatarsal angle, the metatarsophalangeal angle, and the interphalangeal joint angle all are measured to determine the degree of metatarsus primus varus, hallux valgus, and hallux valgus interphalangeus. Persistent lateral displacement of the sesamoids after completion of the bunion procedure predisposes to recurrence of the valgus deformity. The Akin procedure is of limited value if the sesamoid apparatus is subluxed. The phalangeal articular angle and degree of hallux valgus interphalangeus can be determined by measuring on the weight-bearing anteroposterior radiograph the degrees of difference between a perpendicular line drawn among lines parallel to the phalangeal articular surfaces (Fig. 2.58). The Akin osteotomy corrects approximately 8 degrees of valgus for each 2.5 to 3 mm of wedge removal at the base of the proximal phalanx. Measurement of the distal metatarsal articular angle also is recommended in determining if the Akin osteotomy is indicated. If this is more than 10 to 15 degrees and a basilar osteotomy has been used to correct the excessive intermetatarsal angle, the Akin procedure may gain an additional correction of the valgus of the hallux without disrupting joint congruity. This procedure was not originally combined with adductor tenotomy or lateral capsulotomy, but this modification is attractive for elderly patients who primarily desire that the hallux and second toe do not impinge on each other.

In two radiograph studies, Dixon et al. and Park et al. found an increased incidence of hallux valgus interphalangeus after hallux valgus correction on postoperative radiographs. These studies underscore the need for attention to detail in the preoperative assessment of this component of the deformity and perhaps the more aggressive use of the Akin osteotomy.

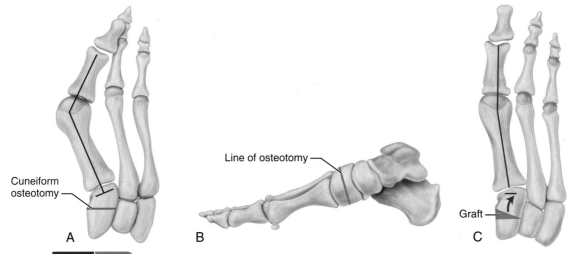

Cuneiform osteotomy

A

Line of osteotomy

B

Graft

C

FIGURE 2.57 **A,** Anteroposterior projection of medial cuneiform osteotomy before distraction. **B,** Lateral view of cuneiform osteotomy. **C,** Osteotomy site distracted, and bone graft impacted. (From Coughlin MJ: Juvenile bunions. In Mann RA, Coughlin MJ, editors: Surgery of the foot and ankle, ed 6, St. Louis, 1993, Mosby.) **SEE TECHNIQUE 2.14.**

The patient profile for the procedure if used *alone* is as follows:

- Patient older than 55 years
- Excessive hallux valgus interphalangeus (in patient of any age)
- Hallux valgus of no more than 25 degrees
- Intermetatarsal angle of less than 13 degrees
- Good metatarsophalangeal joint motion without localized joint pain

Contraindications for the procedure are the following:

- Rheumatoid arthritis
- Moderate-to-severe osteoarthritis at the metatarsophalangeal joint
- Intermetatarsal angle more than 13 degrees
- Hallux valgus angle more than 30 degrees
- Subluxation laterally of the tibial sesamoid more than 50% of its width
- Open physis of the proximal phalanx

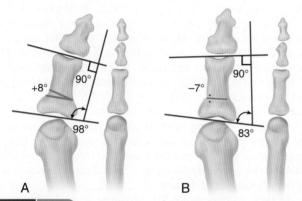

A and **B**, Measurement of phalangeal articular angle to assess hallux valgus interphalangeus and amount of correction postoperatively. (From Beskin JL: Akin's phalangeal osteotomy for bunion repair. In Myerson M, editor: *Current therapy in foot and ankle surgery*, St. Louis, 1993, Mosby.)

Although the originally described osteotomy at the base of the phalanx is contraindicated if the physis is open, an osteotomy at the neck of the phalanx can be performed to correct hallux valgus interphalangeus even in adolescents. Combining this procedure with another bunion procedure, if the primary one does not correct the deformity sufficiently or if a patient has severe hallux valgus interphalangeus, is reasonable (Fig. 2.59).

The Akin procedure is most useful to correct hallux valgus interphalangeus or to add 5 to 10 degrees of additional correction if the primary procedure has not satisfactorily corrected the deformity and if the aforementioned criteria regarding correction of the intermetatarsal angle and sesamoid position have been achieved. The procedure often is appropriate in elderly patients with moderate deformities when combined with adductor release and medial eminence removal and with medial capsular imbrication if the capsule is strong enough to suture. It must be emphasized to the patient, however, that the cosmetic appearance of the toe would not be appreciably changed, although the hallux should fit in a shoe better and should not cause symptomatic impingement of the second toe.

Numerous fixation methods, such as screws, staples, and sutures, can be used for the Akin procedure. Liszka et al. noted comparable fixation among these, but suture fixation is more economical and avoids hardware-related complications.

AKIN PROCEDURE

TECHNIQUE 2.15

- For tourniquet use and anesthesia, see Technique 2.1. This procedure can be done with ankle-block anesthesia. Make a longitudinal medial incision along the proximal

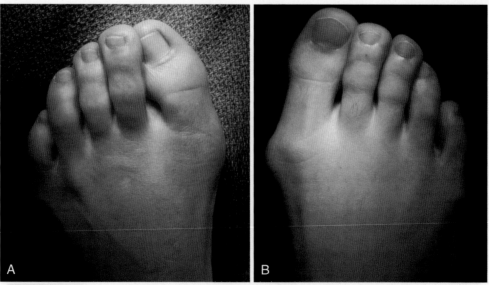

A, Mild hallux valgus and significant hallux valgus interphalangeus is a deformity that can be corrected with an Akin osteotomy. **B,** Deformity that is *not* appropriate for Akin osteotomy.

two thirds of the phalanx and extend it over the medial eminence to expose the distal metatarsal shaft capsule 2 to 3 mm proximal to its attachment on the metatarsal neck.

- Expose the proximal phalanx by sharp dissection (not with a periosteal elevator) just enough to make the osteotomy cuts. Avoid stripping the periosteum any more than is necessary because delayed union or nonunion may result. Also, raise the capsule surrounding the exostosis by sharp dissection and expose the medial eminence, but preserve as much of the proximal capsular attachment to the metatarsal neck as possible.
- Remove the medial eminence as previously described, using the parasagittal groove as a starting mark. Smooth the rough margins of the cancellous bone remaining after exostectomy with a rongeur or rasp (Fig. 2.60A).
- Make a midline incision as a continuation of the medial incision from the bunionectomy, extending to the interphalangeal joint. Protect the plantar and dorsal cutaneous nerves to the hallux.
- Elevate the periosteum medially as much as necessary to expose the flexor hallucis longus and extensor hallucis longus so that they can be protected with a small Hohmann retractor.
- Make the first osteotomy cut parallel to the Kirschner wire from medial to lateral, not penetrating the far cortex. A medium-sized blade should be used because a fine blade may burn the bone and cause delayed union (Fig. 2.60B).
- Make a second osteotomy cut 2 to 5 mm from the first (depending on the deformity that requires correction) and angle the cut toward the same point on the lateral cortex as the first. Ideally, do not penetrate the lateral cortex but just weaken it so that only minimal force is necessary to close the osteotomy medially. Passing the saw blade along the two cuts will accomplish this. Correct residual pronation of the hallux by rotating the distal part of the proximal phalanx.
- If an ankle tourniquet was placed, remove it at this point to assess the alignment of the toe. Also remove the Kirschner wire used to determine alignment of the osteotomy. If an adequate bone bridge is present, the hole left by Kirschner wire removal can be used for suture fixation.
- Determine rotation of the toe and use a Kirschner wire to make a corresponding hole opposite the first hole. Pass a 2-0 braided nonabsorbable suture through the holes.
- Close the osteotomy and advance a 0.045-inch Kirschner wire from proximal to distal, plantar to the midline of the phalanx (Fig. 2.60C).
- Confirm the position of the wire, bend it at bone level, and cut and bury it. Tie the suture securely (Fig. 2.61).
- Close the periosteum with 2-0 braided absorbable suture to cover the knot of bone fixation suture and close the skin with 5-9 nylon sutures. Apply a forefoot bandage, incorporating the interphalangeal joint of the hallux.

POSTOPERATIVE CARE The patient is instructed to rest and elevate the extremity for 72 hours, with bathroom privileges only, but weight bearing to tolerance is allowed. Generally, no cast is needed. In adolescent patients with excessive hallux valgus interphalangeus, however, it is best to use a short leg walking cast that extends past the toes for the first month. The sutures and pins are removed at 3 to 4 weeks, and a deep, wide, soft shoe can be worn. After the pins have been removed, gentle active and passive ranges of motion are begun. The osteotomy usually is clinically stable at 4 to 6 weeks, but radiographic healing may take 3 to 6 months or longer. Nonunion is uncommon, occurring in only 1% of patients.

Recently, a distal Akin osteotomy has been described for operative correction of symptomatic hallux valgus interphalangeus deformity. Usually intervention for this deformity is not required unless symptomatic. However, the degree of the hallux valgus interphalangeus angle does not necessarily correlate with symptoms, and clinical findings are better indicators for operative intervention. The traditional Akin osteotomy is done at the base of the proximal phalanx, but in hallux valgus interphalangeus the deformity is at the other end. Vander Griend moved the osteotomy to the distal end because the apex of the deformity in his series was at the interphalangeal joint, with an increase in both the hallux valgus interphalangeus angle and distal phalangeal articular angle. He noted that the site of osteotomy should be modified to be closer to the center of rotation angle. Good results were obtained by his patients (Fig. 2.62), with no infection, pain, stiffness, swelling, or sensitivity with wearing shoes at follow-up. There was one intraoperative complication (a fracture extending into the interphalangeus joint), but this was not symptomatic at 1 year.

TRIPLE OSTEOTOMY

Operative correction of mild hallux valgus has traditionally been obtained with the chevron osteotomy. For moderate to severe deformities, the scarf or opening wedge osteotomies are used as well as the Lapidus procedure. Double and triple osteotomies can be performed in severe deformity, and among these is a double first metatarsal osteotomy combined with a proximal phalangeal osteotomy and lateral release to provide adequate correction of incongruent deformities. Good bony correction can be obtained initially without the lateral release; however, Booth et al. noted an 8-degree mean loss of correction of the hallux valgus angle without it. Their decision to not include a lateral release was based on concerns of soft-tissue stripping of the metatarsal head and the extensive medial incision required. Preserving the soft tissues lateral to the first metatarsal head theoretically may preserve the blood supply to the metatarsal head. Two particular disadvantages of this technique were persistent postoperative swelling and the possibility of requiring implant removal. Their suggestion was to include lateral release in this triple osteotomy to prevent early recurrence.

ARTHRODESIS OF THE FIRST METATARSOPHALANGEAL JOINT

In properly selected patients, arthrodesis of the first metatarsophalangeal joint for hallux valgus is the most appropriate operation (Figs. 2.63 and 2.64). Mann and Katchurian reported a 4- to 5-degree average reduction in the intermetatarsal angle after arthrodesis alone, suggesting that proximal metatarsal osteotomy combined with arthrodesis is not indicated except for the most severe deformities. Most recently, a study by McKean et al. concurred with this conclusion, demonstrating that the hallux valgus angle and first-second

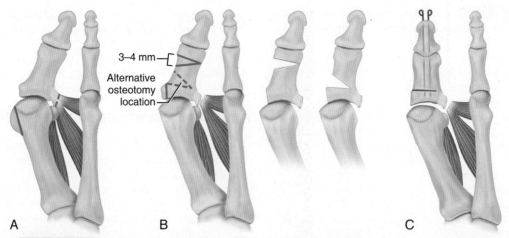

FIGURE 2.60 Akin procedure. **A,** Medial eminence removal and adductor tenotomy. **B,** Basilar osteotomy and removal of medial condyle. *Shaded area* shows alternative location of phalangeal closing wedge osteotomy. **C,** Final position of hallux. **SEE TECHNIQUE 2.15.**

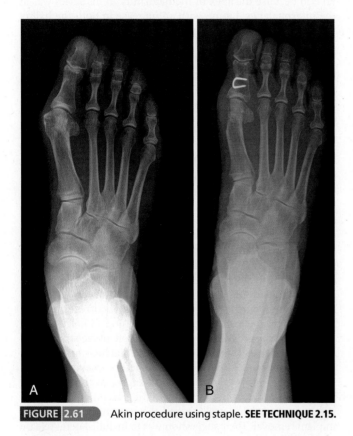

FIGURE 2.61 Akin procedure using staple. **SEE TECHNIQUE 2.15.**

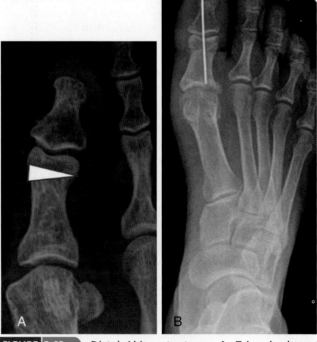

FIGURE 2.62 Distal Akin osteotomy. **A,** Triangle-shaped wedge is amount of bone to be removed. **B,** Postoperative view. (From Vander Griend R: Correction of hallux valgus interphalangeus with an osteotomy of the distal end of the proximal phalanx (distal Akin osteotomy), *Foot Ankle Int* 38:153, 2017.)

intermetatarsal angle were acceptably corrected in 17 patients with arthrodesis without a proximal first metatarsal osteotomy. Grimes and Coughlin reported excellent or good outcomes in 24 (72%) of 33 feet an average of 8 years after arthrodesis for treatment of a variety of failed hallux valgus procedures, including the proximal and distal osteotomies, McBride procedure, exostectomy, and resection arthroplasty. The use of arthrodesis in young, active patients or those who participate in sports has been questioned because there is loss of motion of the first metatarsophalangeal joint. Da Cunha et al. attempted to answer this question in a study of 50 patients who were involved in sports (golfing, walking, biking, running, swimming) using a sports-specific,

patient-administered questionnaire. They found that 96% of patients were satisfied after surgery with regard to return to sports and physical activities even though 21% found their activity to be more difficult. Forty-five percent of patients returned to their preoperative level of activity in less than 6 months and were able to return to 89% of their preoperative physical activities. As in all foot and ankle arthrodesis procedures, care should be taken in patients who smoke because of the increased risk of nonunion. All patients undergoing bony procedures, especially arthrodesis, are advised to take vitamin D supplements unless they are medically contraindicated.

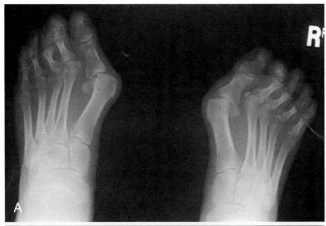

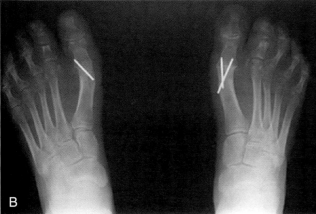

FIGURE 2.63 **A,** Hallux valgus in 46-year-old woman. **B,** One year after arthrodesis.

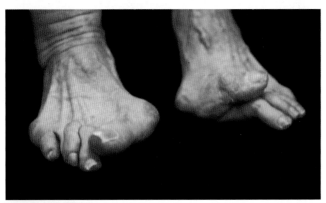

FIGURE 2.64 Severe hallux valgus is good indication for arthrodesis of first metatarsophalangeal joint, particularly in recurrent hallux valgus after previous attempt at correction (left foot).

Arthrodesis of the first metatarsophalangeal joint for hallux valgus is indicated in the following circumstances:

- Severe deformity (an intermetatarsal angle > 20 to 22 degrees, a hallux valgus angle > 45 degrees, and severe pronation of the hallux) (Fig. 2.65), especially when painful callosities are present beneath the second and third metatarsal heads with an atrophic forefoot pad
- Degenerative arthritis with hallux valgus. Although uncommon, erosion along the lateral aspect of the sagittal

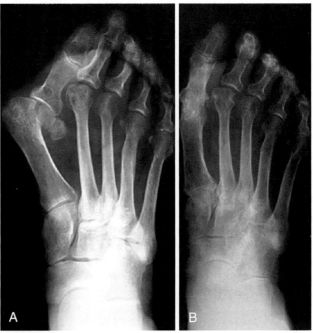

FIGURE 2.65 **A,** Severe hallux valgus with severe metatarsus primus varus. **B,** After proximal metatarsal osteotomy and arthrodesis of first metatarsophalangeal joint.

groove with loss of articular cartilage occasionally is seen in patients older than 60 years.
- Possibly for mild-to-moderate deformity when motion of the metatarsophalangeal joint is limited and painful. Resection arthroplasty is a reasonable alternative.
- Recurrent hallux valgus. The McBride procedure, a metatarsal osteotomy, or a Keller procedure may be used instead.
- Hallux valgus caused by muscle imbalance in patients with neuromuscular disorders, such as cerebral palsy, to prevent recurrence
- Posttraumatic hallux valgus with severe disruption of all medial capsular structures that cannot be adequately reconstructed
- Hallux valgus in patients with rheumatoid arthritis. Arthrodesis of the first metatarsophalangeal joint is preferred to resection arthroplasty, particularly in patients younger than 55 to 60 years.

The surgical technique for arthrodesis of the first metatarsophalangeal joint may vary according to the type of osteotomy and the kind of fixation used. Joint surfaces may be cut flat or tapered, or reamers may be used to create a "cup-and-cone" configuration. Fixation may include Kirschner wires, cortical or lag (compression) screws, or dorsal plates. Biomechanical assessment of five commonly used arthrodesis techniques determined that the most stable construct was obtained with an oblique lag screw and a dorsal plate. Various arthrodesis plates are now manufactured with contoured dorsiflexion angles of 9 to 10 degrees. These low-profile plates in combination with a lag or compression screw provide strong fixation that allows immediate full weight bearing without a cast. Specially designed, precontoured plates are preferred to improvised plates because bending leads to poor control over dorsiflexion and may increase the incidence of plate failure. After preparation of the joint for arthrodesis, a crossed screw configuration is used, either a variable pitch headless compression screw or a partially threaded compression screw followed by a crossing fully threaded screw for increased stability and thread purchase. Ideally, one screw passes plantar to the axis of motion of the metatarsophalangeal joint (on the tension side of the construct). This procedure avoids potential hardware prominence dorsally but is not indicated in osteoporotic bone. It is easier to perform with a straight medial approach as opposed to a dorsal or dorsomedial approach (Fig. 2.66). A biomechanical comparison study was conducted to determine load to failure and stiffness of fully threaded screws and locking plates. Fully threaded compression screws had similar load to failure as low-profile plates; however, screws had significantly greater stiffness.

ARTHRODESIS OF THE FIRST METATARSOPHALANGEAL JOINT WITH SMALL PLATE FIXATION

TECHNIQUE 2.16

(MANKEY AND MANN)

- For tourniquet use and anesthesia, see Technique 2.1. Begin a dorsal incision on the medial edge of the extensor hallucis longus tendon a few millimeters proximal to the interphalangeal joint of the hallux, and extend it proximally 5 to 6 cm (Fig. 2.67A). Incise the skin and subcutaneous tissue and the extensor mechanism. Identify and preserve the proper branch of the superficial peroneal nerve to the dorsomedial aspect of the hallux. Carry the incision through the extensor mechanism at the base of the proximal phalanx and through the periosteum over the first metatarsal.
- With sharp dissection, expose the first metatarsophalangeal joint dorsally, medially, and laterally.
- Uncover the medial eminence, using small, right-angle retractors to expose fully three sides of the metatarsophalangeal joint.
- Remove any dorsal osteophytes at the base of the proximal phalanx or over the metatarsal head with a rongeur.
- Using a 9-mm-wide blade in a power saw, remove the distal surface of the first metatarsal 3 to 4 mm proximal to the articular cartilage, making the cut perpendicular to the shaft of the first metatarsal (Fig. 2.67B).
- Align the hallux with the first metatarsal in 15 degrees of dorsiflexion to the plantar surface of the foot or 25 to 30 degrees of dorsiflexion to the inclination angle of the first metatarsal and approximately 15 degrees of valgus and neutral rotation (Fig. 2.67C, D).
- With the hallux in this position, remove the base of the proximal phalanx parallel to the previous cut in the first

metatarsal. Leave as much metaphyseal flare of the base as possible for later screw fixation.
- In severely eburnated bone, drill multiple small holes in the base of the proximal phalanx and in the head of the first metatarsal with a 0.062-inch Kirschner wire; if cancellous bone is reached after making the osteotomy cuts, this step is unnecessary.
- When the hallux is aligned properly, fix it temporarily with one or two 0.045-inch Kirschner wires placed from dorsal distal to proximal medial. These wires must be placed in the upper quarter of the phalanx and metatarsal head to leave room for the interfragmentary screw to be placed just plantar to the midline of the proximal phalanx (Fig. 2.67E).
- Ensure that all soft tissue has been excised around the base of the proximal phalanx, with no soft tissues invaginated in the arthrodesis site, and that the flexor hallucis longus tendon has been preserved.
- Place an interfragmentary 4-mm cancellous screw through the plantar-medial aspect of the base of the proximal phalanx directed laterally into the metatarsal head. Using a drill guide, drill a glide hole with a 3.5-mm bit and then drill the hole with a 2-mm bit. This should be placed at the flare of the base of the proximal phalanx where there is good bone stock. Measure the length of the screw, tap the hole, and insert the screw. A countersink usually is not required for the screw head but can be used if there is concern that the head of the screw would lever in a dorsal direction and crack through the cortical bridge. Just before final tightening of the screw, remove the Kirschner wires to maximize compression.
- Remove the medial eminence and ensure that no osteophytes remain on the lateral side.
- Mann emphasized that in rheumatoid feet the bone stock may be so poor that interfragmentary screw fixation is impossible. In that case, use a dorsal plate or intramedullary Steinmann pins.
- When limited fixation with the interfragmentary screw is achieved, place a one-quarter tubular AO plate or its equivalent dorsally. Usually, three holes are made in the metatarsal and two in the proximal phalanx, but in some patients the phalanx is long enough to place three screws on each side of the arthrodesis site. Secure the plate proximally with a 4-mm cancellous screw. No lag technique is needed, and no compression is gained with this type of plate. If the bones are quite small, use 2.7-mm screws designed for the one-quarter tubular plate. First secure the plate proximally through the screw hole closest to the arthrodesis site (Fig. 2.67F, G).
- Before the final seating of the screw, check the position of the arthrodesis and the plate. The plate should rest in the midline of the hallux and proximal phalanx, and the lateral edge of the proximal phalanx should line up with the lateral edge of the first metatarsal head.
- Place another screw in the metatarsal and two or three screws in the proximal phalanx. Measure the screw lengths accurately so that they do not impinge on the flexor hallucis longus. Place the final screw in the most proximal hole in the plate.

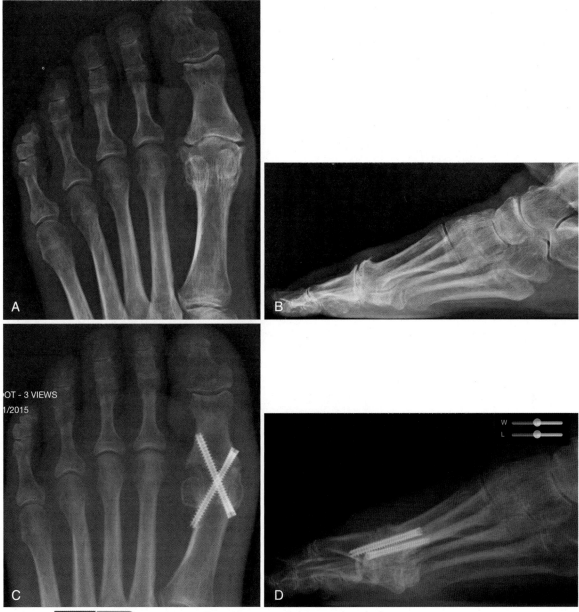

FIGURE 2.66 A and B, Hallux valgus. C and D, Crossed-screw fixation.

- If there are any small areas of unapposed bone, use the deep surface of the medial eminence for cancellous bone graft.
- Close the capsule with 2-0 absorbable suture, repositioning the extensor hallucis longus dorsally, and close the skin with nonabsorbable sutures.
- Apply a compression dressing to the foot and secure it around the ankle using multiple unfluffed fluffs and gauze wrap.

POSTOPERATIVE CARE The dressing is changed to a more snug-fitting dressing at the first postoperative visit, and the patient is allowed to bear weight to tolerance with a postoperative shoe. Assisted walking with crutches or a walker is optional. Fusion usually is complete by 12 weeks after surgery, and the patient is allowed to wear any shoes that accommodate the foot.

ARTHRODESIS OF THE FIRST METATARSOPHALANGEAL JOINT WITH LOW-PROFILE CONTOURED DORSAL PLATE AND COMPRESSION SCREW FIXATION

TECHNIQUE 2.17

(KUMAR, PRADHAN, AND ROSENFELD)

- For tourniquet use and anesthesia, see Technique 2.1. Through a dorsal approach (or through previous incision if a revision), expose the joint capsule and divide it longitudinally medial to the extensor hallucis longus; retract the tendon laterally.

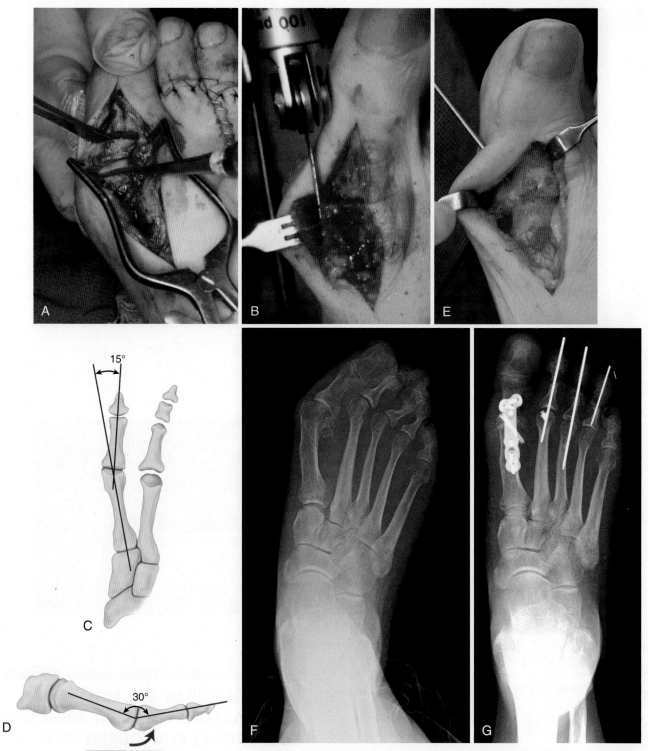

FIGURE 2.67 Technique for arthrodesis of first metatarsophalangeal joint. **A,** Dorsal skin incision. **B,** Excision of metatarsal head. **C,** Fusion site placed in 15 to 20 degrees of valgus. **D,** Approximately 30 degrees of dorsiflexion in relation to metatarsal shaft or 10 to 15 degrees of dorsiflexion in relation to floor. **E,** Kirschner wire placed. **F** and **G,** Radiographs before and after plating, respectively. (From Mann RA, Coughlin MJ, eds: *Surgery of the foot and ankle*, ed 7, St. Louis, 1999, Mosby; *C* and *D* from Mann RA, Coughlin MJ: *The video textbook of foot and ankle surgery*, St. Louis, 1991, Medical Video Productions.) **SEE TECHNIQUE 2.16.**

- Reflect the capsule and collateral ligaments from the metatarsal head and mobilize the flexor hallucis longus inferiorly.
- Prepare the joint surfaces using spherical reamers to create concentric concave-convex surfaces (see Technique 2.18).
- Appose the joint surfaces in optimal position and temporarily fix them with a Kirschner wire.
- Check sagittal alignment using a flat tray to simulate weight bearing. Position the metatarsophalangeal joint to allow a heel clearance of approximately 1 inch with simulated weight bearing.
- Remove any dorsal prominences.
- Determine valgus alignment by comparison to the opposite hallux; keep rotation to neutral using the nail plate as a guide.
- Confirm by direct observation that the dorsiflexion angle is 15 to 25 degrees and secure the reduction with an interfragmentary compression screw.
- Apply a precontoured titanium alloy low-profile plate dorsally and fix with standard screws.
- Fill any minor local defects or cysts with bone graft taken from the reamers, close the wound in layers, and apply a compression bandage.

POSTOPERATIVE CARE Patients are allowed full weight bearing immediately in a flat postoperative shoe, using crutches if needed. The compression bandage is removed at 2 weeks. At 6 weeks, wearing of normal shoes is permitted.

TRUNCATED CONE ARTHRODESIS OF THE FIRST METATARSOPHALANGEAL JOINT

Multiple manufacturers produce reaming systems designed for this procedure. Alternatively, this procedure may be performed by fashioning cup-and-cone surfaces by hand.

TECHNIQUE 2.18

(JOHNSON AND ALEXANDER)
- With the patient under regional or general anesthesia (see Technique 2.1 for tourniquet use and anesthesia), make a medial midline incision over the metatarsophalangeal joint between the branch of the superficial peroneal nerve dorsally and the proper branch of the medial plantar nerve plantarly. Begin the incision over the proximal half of the proximal phalanx and extend it proximally over the medial eminence and along the shaft of the first metatarsal.
- Do not raise any flaps until bone is reached. We recommend raising a small flap at this point to ensure that the superficial peroneal nerve, which is vulnerable at the level on the metatarsal where the medial eminence enters the shaft, is not tethered in the midline medially because the protruding medial eminence displaces the nerve dorsally at the site of the bunion.
- By sharp dissection, denude the base of the proximal phalanx and the metatarsal head of soft tissue, being careful to preserve the flexor hallucis longus tendon. The base of the proximal phalanx must be visible end on.

- Place a guidewire in the center of the base of the proximal phalanx and drill it into the subchondral bone of the head of the proximal phalanx.
- With a conical reamer, ream the proximal phalanx (Fig. 2.68A).
- Expose the metatarsal head and insert a guide pin into it. This guide pin must be placed at an appropriate angle in reference to the dorsal aspect of the first metatarsal. Use an angle guide to ensure dorsiflexion of the hallux 25 to 30 degrees to the inclination angle of the first metatarsal (Fig. 2.68B).
- When the guide pin has been properly positioned in the metatarsal head, place the truncated cone reamer system for the metatarsal head over the guide pin (Fig. 2.68C) and use it to produce a truncated cone configuration of the distal metatarsal for optimal cancellous bone contact (Fig. 2.68D).
- Impact the two prepared surfaces and place a fully threaded 4-mm cancellous screw from the medial base of the proximal phalanx laterally into the metatarsal head. Countersink the screw head and avoid fracture through the cortical bridge of the medial aspect of the base of the proximal phalanx. Use a lag technique by overreaming the phalangeal side of the arthrodesis.
- Before placement of the screw, temporary fixation with one or two 0.062- or 0.045-inch Kirschner wires may be needed. Occasionally, in osteoporotic bone, two crossed screws may be needed for secure fixation.

POSTOPERATIVE CARE The patient may walk flat-footed, bearing weight to tolerance, in a postoperative shoe with specific instructions not to load the hallux. The dressing is changed at 2-week intervals, and the arthrodesis is manually tested each time. If the fixation is not rigid, the patient wears a cast for 6 weeks. If an interposition graft was necessary, such as for marked bone loss at the first metatarsophalangeal joint from previous total joint replacement or hemiarthroplasty, the postoperative management is altered. No weight bearing is allowed for 3 months, during which time the patient wears a cast. A walking cast is applied until the arthrodesis is solid.

ARTHRODESIS OF THE FIRST METATARSOCUNEIFORM ARTICULATION (LAPIDUS PROCEDURE)

Arthrodesis of the first metatarsal cuneiform joint is included in the section on arthrodesis for convenience but could properly be listed as an option in patients in whom the deformity is enough to require a proximal metatarsal osteotomy. It provides powerful correction of varus of the first ray and allows improved stability of the medial column of the foot. It is often helpful in combined flatfoot deformity in the setting of posterior tibial tendon insufficiency, instability of the first ray, and corresponding moderate to

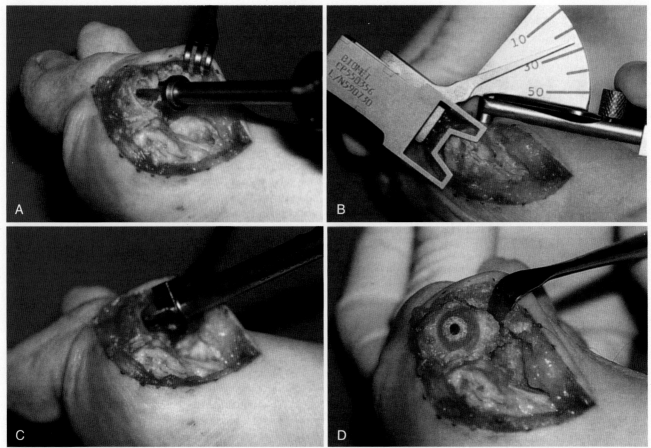

FIGURE 2.68   Truncated cone arthrodesis. **A,** Preparation of phalangeal base with end-cutting reamer. **B,** Metatarsal angle guide for reaming. **C,** Cutting truncated cone with side-cutting reamer. **D,** Base of proximal phalanx after reaming. (From Johnson KA, editor: Master techniques in orthopaedic surgery: the foot and ankle, New York, 1994, Raven.) **SEE TECHNIQUE 2.18.**

severe hallux valgus (Figs. 2.69 and 2.70). McAlister et al. evaluated the corrective ability of this arthrodesis in 99 patients based on the first intermetatarsal angle, hallux valgus angle, and tibial sesamoid position. They found a significant decrease in all three parameters from preoperative to all postoperative time periods. Faber et al. compared the Lapidus procedure with a simple Hohmann distal closing wedge metatarsal osteotomy in 101 feet. At a mean follow-up of 9.25 years, they found no difference in clinical or radiographic outcomes between the two procedures. Ellington et al. evaluated 32 feet with recurrent hallux valgus in which preoperative evaluation determined clinical hypermobility in 96% and radiographic signs of instability in 52%. The average preoperative hallux valgus angle, intermetatarsal angle, and distal metatarsal angle showed statistically significant correction postoperatively from preoperative values. Good to excellent results were reported by 87% of patients.

TECHNIQUE 2.19

(MYERSON ET AL.; SANGEORZAN AND HANSEN; MAULDIN ET AL.)

- For tourniquet use and anesthesia, see Technique 2.1. The procedure is performed through three incisions: over the medial eminence, dorsally in the first web space, and dorsally over the metatarsocuneiform articulation.
- Make the first incision medially over the medial eminence and incise the capsule in an inverted-L shape distally (Fig. 2.71A,B). Remove the medial eminence.
- Make a second incision dorsally in the first web space and release the adductor hallucis from its attachments at the base of the proximal phalanx and the lateral margin of the fibulosesamoid ligament. Incise the capsulosesamoid ligament in an axial plane, and mobilize the sesamoids beneath the metatarsal head. Do not resuture the adductor hallucis in the first intermetatarsal space.
- Make a third incision dorsally over the first metatarsocuneiform articulation. This should be long enough to expose adequately the dorsal venous arch and the most medial branch of the superficial peroneal nerve. To find the joint, make a longitudinal incision with a small blade over the base of the first metatarsal onto the medial cuneiform with gentle subperiosteal dissection medially and laterally. Avoid the penetrating branch of the dorsalis pedis artery during the lateral dissection.
- Remove the small wedge of bone from the articulation laterally and plantarward to ensure plantarflexion of the first metatarsal (Fig. 2.71C,D). Remove as little bone as possible. Myerson recommended removing only the articular cartilage laterally and plantarward,

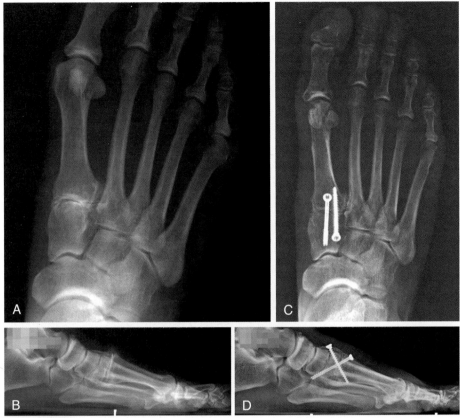

FIGURE 2.69 Arthrodesis of first metatarsal cuneiform articulation (Lapidus). **A** and **B**, Preoperatively. **C** and **D**, Postoperatively.

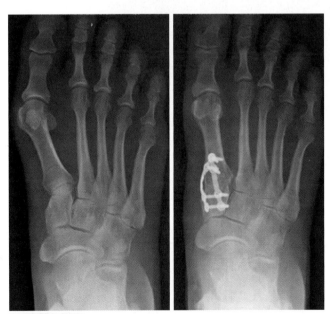

FIGURE 2.70 Preoperative and postoperative radiographs demonstrating tarsometatarsal arthrodesis with biplanar miniplate construct. (From Ray JJ, Koay J, Dayton PD, et al: Multicenter early radiographic outcomes of triplanar tarsometatarsal arthrodesis with early weightbearing, *Foot Ankle Int* 40:955, 2019.)

leaving the articular surface of the medial aspect of the joint intact.

- The first metatarsal should plantarflex and adduct, and the dorsal part of the arthrodesis site should never be

wider than the plantar part, which is difficult to achieve because of the deep plantar recession at the base of the first metatarsocuneiform articulation.

- Use a small, flexible, thin chisel blade or a long-handled, small rongeur to reach deep within the joint. Osteotomes, even thin ones, are not recommended because too much bone is removed dorsally.
- Hold the metatarsal in the corrected position with a 0.062-inch Kirschner wire and verify correct positioning of the metatarsal with radiographs or fluoroscopy.
- Insert two 3.5-mm cortical screws (if room allows) dorsal to plantar from the medial cuneiform proximally into the first metatarsal distally, using a lag screw technique by overdrilling the proximal cortex. Tighten the screws sequentially (Fig. 2.71E).
- Use a small burr to create two or three small troughs on the dorsal and medial sides of the arthrodesis site and fill them with autogenous bone graft. The small quantity of bone graft required can be obtained from one of the adjacent tarsal bones, the calcaneus, or the distal tibia.
- Move the first metatarsophalangeal joint through a range of motion to locate the exact position in which the joint is most congruent. This step is important because if the intermetatarsal angle is undercorrected, or if the hallux valgus angle is excessive, placing the hallux in a straight position may cause impingement or incongruency, resulting in loss of motion of the first metatarsophalangeal joint.
- When the position of first metatarsophalangeal joint congruency is located, repair the capsule in that position.
- If the hallux impinges on the second toe or is in unattractive valgus, perform an Akin basal phalangeal osteotomy,

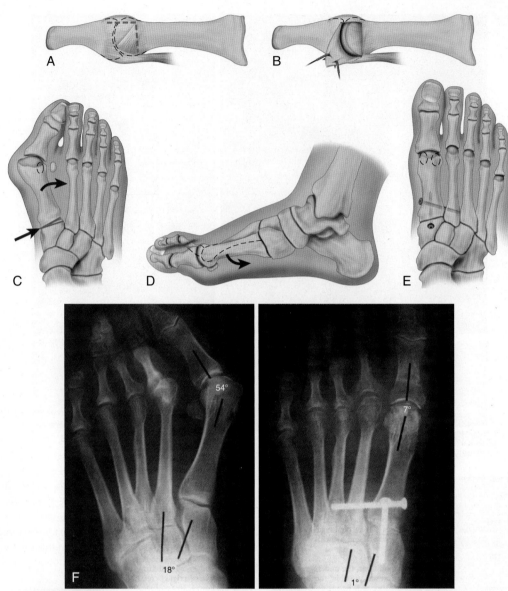

FIGURE 2.71   Lapidus procedure. **A,** Capsular flap is inverted-L with apex dorsal and proximal. **B,** Medial eminence exposed after peeling flap. Flap can be resutured or attached to neck of metatarsal through drill hole. **C** and **D,** Correction of metatarsus primus varus achieved by translation and slight rotation of metatarsal. **E,** Screw position. **F,** Correction obtained. (**A-D** from Myerson M, editor: *Current therapy in foot and ankle surgery,* St. Louis, 1993, Mosby.) **SEE TECHNIQUE 2.19.**

rather than force the hallux into a straight position, producing incongruency of the joint.
- If the corner of the L-shaped capsulotomy cannot be resutured because of a lack of soft tissue, use a Kirschner wire to drill a small hole in the metatarsal neck for attachment of the capsule.

POSTOPERATIVE CARE   Initially, a non–weight-bearing cast is used. When the patient can bear weight to comfort in the cast, a walking cast is applied and is worn until 6 weeks after surgery. A removable walking cast can be used for the next 3 to 6 weeks. Myerson et al. emphasized that swelling can be bothersome for 4 to 6 months, and the patient cannot expect to wear normal shoes until this period is over (Fig. 2.71F).

ARTHRODESIS OF THE FIRST METATARSOCUNEIFORM ARTICULATION (LAPIDUS PROCEDURE) WITH PLATE FIXATION

TECHNIQUE 2.20

(SORENSEN, HYER, BERLET)
- After administration of a popliteal block and induction of general anesthesia, prepare and drape the limb using standard sterile technique. Exsanguinate the operative

limb and apply and inflate a thigh tourniquet (300 mm Hg) (see Technique 2.1 for tourniquet use and anesthesia).

- For the sequential lateral release, make the first incision over the first intermetatarsal space to allow fibular sesamoid ligament recession, conjoined adductor tenotomy, deep transverse metatarsal ligament transection, and lateral capsular "pie crusting" with attenuation by putting the hallux into 45 degrees of varus stress.
- Make the second incision over the medial first metatarsophalangeal joint.
- Make an inverted-L medial capsular incision and resect any hypertrophic medial eminence.
- Make the third incision over the dorsomedial aspect of the first metatarsocuneiform joint.
- Expose the joint through a transverse capsulotomy and distract the joint with Steinmann pins and a Hintermann retractor to increase exposure.
- Use an osteotome and mallet to denude the corresponding surfaces of the joint of articular cartilage, taking care to maintain the subchondral plate. Make sure the joint is fully exposed, as deep as 3 cm, to ensure adequate removal of the entire cartilaginous surface.
- Scallop and fenestrate the subchondral plate to promote angiogenic and osseous growth.
- Preserve the peripheral rim of subchondral bone to retain as much length as possible and to provide added stability for internal fixation.
- If bone graft or bone marrow aspirate is used, place it within the fusion site.
- Manually reduce the first metatarsal in the transverse plane and attain sagittal position by engaging the windlass mechanism through dorsiflexion of the hallux. If necessary, use a large bone reduction clamp to hold the first metatarsal to the second in the transverse plane.
- With the metatarsal in the corrected position, place a guide pin across the joint for insertion of a partially threaded cannulated, titanium screw. Use fluoroscopy to ensure adequate correction and guide pin placement in all planes.
- Measure the guide pin and place the cannulated screw using standard AO technique.
- Apply a four-hole locking plate over the dorsomedial aspect of the joint, placing four corresponding locked screws of varying lengths according to standard AO technique (Figs. 2.72 and 2.73).
- Close the incisions in standard fashion and apply a modified Jones compression posterior splint.

POSTOPERATIVE CARE Patients remain strictly non–weight bearing for the first 10 to 14 days, followed by 4 weeks of protected weight bearing as tolerated in a cam-walker, with transition into regular shoes at about 6 weeks.

Because of the challenging technique and prolonged convalescence of this procedure, it is most beneficial for patients with recurrence of the metatarsus primus varus component of the hallux valgus complex after failed bunion surgery; for patients with marked ligamentous laxity; or for patients with cerebral palsy who have spastic equinovalgus, metatarsus primus varus, and hallux valgus. Because of improvements in surgical technique and

fixation methods, which have reduced the nonunion rate from as high as 20% in earlier series to less than 5% in more recent ones, the necessity for cast immobilization has been questioned, and immediate protected weight bearing in a postoperative shoe has been described after the Lapidus arthrodesis.

SPECIAL CIRCUMSTANCES
■ HALLUX VALGUS IN THE CASE OF METATARSUS ADDUCTUS

The association of metatarsus adductus with hallux valgus is relatively uncommon; however, when present, treatment of the hallux valgus deformity can be difficult because of the complex issues involved. Obtaining correct measurement of the first to second intermetatarsal angle is challenging, and it makes transposition of the first metatarsal head difficult. Also, patients may have additional associated problems from altered biomechanics of the foot and instability of the metatarsophalangeal joint, including metatarsalgia, pes planovalgus, and lesser toe deformities. There is a paucity of literature on the exact treatment and outcomes of hallux valgus with associated metatarsus adductus. Shibuya et al. noted no relationship between the metatarsus adductus deformity and the final outcome after hallux valgus correction in 154 patients. Loh et al. likewise concluded in their study of 206 patients who underwent a scarf procedure that metatarsus adductus did not predispose patients to poorer functional outcomes. However, Aiyer et al. found the rate of radiographic recurrence to be around 30% in 587 patients with underlying metatarsus adductus undergoing hallux valgus correction compared to 15% of patients without metatarsus adductus regardless of the type of procedure. Shima et al. reported 10-year follow-up results of 17 patients (21 feet) who had metatarsus adductus and underwent a proximal crescentic first metatarsal osteotomy and an abduction osteotomy of the proximal third of the second and third metatarsals. At most recent follow-up, 11 of the 21 feet were not painful, nine were mildly painful, and one was moderately painful. The mean hallux valgus, intermetatarsal, and metatarsus adductus angles significantly decreased postoperatively; however, recurrence was noted in four feet. Sharma and Aydogan have provided a comprehensive surgical algorithm that they used in four patients who had significant relief of pain (Box 2.2; Fig. 2.74).

■ HALLUX VALGUS IN MEN

It is well known that hallux valgus occurs more frequently in women than men at a ratio of 15:1, according to Nery et al. However, when it occurs in men, there are several notable differences. A family history of hallux valgus was noted by these researchers in 68% of men compared with 35% of women. Age at onset also was earlier in men, and they had a higher severity of deformity and increased radiographic angle measurements, especially the distal metatarsal articular angle. As opposed to women, no correlation with type of shoes worn was found among the men. In another study, the same authors also found that the scarf osteotomy produced inferior results in men.

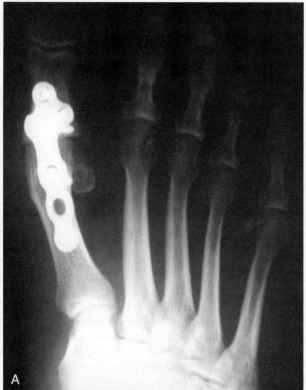

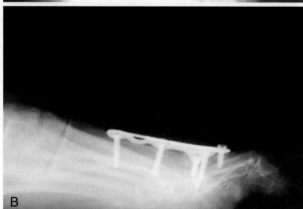

FIGURE 2.72   Anteroposterior **(A)** and lateral **(B)** radiographs of first metatarsophalangeal arthrodesis fixed with dorsal plate and screws. (From Berlet GC, Hyer CF, Glover JP: A retrospective review of immediate weightbearing after first metatarsophalangeal joint arthrodesis, *Foot Ankle Spec* 1:24, 2008.) **SEE TECHNIQUE 2.20.**

■ HALLUX VALGUS IN ATHLETES

Given the progressive nature, hallux valgus may eventually affect performance in athletes. To meet the demands of an athlete's sport, a functional metatarsophalangeal joint is necessary, especially considering that four times weightbearing force is generated during running or jumping. In addition, adequate range of motion is required for some sports. Symptoms in athletes can range from pain with footwear to loss of momentum, and even decreased athletic performance. When considering surgery, one must bear in mind that a less than perfect outcome in an athlete may be a career ender. Choosing the appropriate procedure is of paramount

importance. As with all patients, it is necessary to perform a thorough evaluation and assess the types of activities and goals of the patient. Also imperative is an effective postoperative rehabilitation program.

Traumatic hallux valgus is a common injury in athletes and is a variation of what is known as "turf toe." Covell et al. believe that this injury often is not recognized because athletes may not remember an inciting event. Nevertheless, failure to treat this injury can lead to progressive deformity, pain, and inability to continue the sport. However, even with treatment many athletes cannot return to play. Covell et al. reported good results in 14 of 19 patients 3.4 months after surgery, but one quarter of their patients were not able to resume their sporting activity.

■ HALLUX VALGUS IN CEREBRAL PALSY

Symptomatic hallux valgus in patients with cerebral palsy is uncommon. It occurs most commonly in spastic diplegic patients with equinovalgus deformity. Varus of the first metatarsal may contribute to the hallux valgus deformity. A symptomatic dorsal bunion also may occur if extension of the first metatarsal develops secondary to muscle imbalance. Indications for surgery include pain (usually at the first metatarsophalangeal joint), inability to find properly fitting shoes, interference with walking, and recurrent skin breakdown because of pressure from bony deformity.

Arthrodesis of the first metatarsophalangeal joint is most frequently recommended for this condition because it is the most reliable and enduring procedure for hallux valgus in patients with spastic cerebral palsy. Good results have been reported at 3 to 5 years after arthrodesis; Bishay et al. reported excellent or good results in all 24 feet treated with arthrodesis in adolescents with spastic cerebral palsy. A combination of proximal osteotomies of the first metatarsal and proximal phalanx, with appropriate tendon transfers, also has been beneficial.

If the hindfoot is not in marked valgus, a proximal osteotomy of the first metatarsal or an arthrodesis of the first metatarsocuneiform joint to correct metatarsus varus combined with an Akin osteotomy of the proximal phalanx, transfer of the adductor hallucis to the first metatarsal, and lateral capsular release to correct the hallux valgus deformity may result in permanent correction. If a first metatarsal extension posture causes a dorsal bunion, the distal fragment can be plantarflexed at the same time the varus is corrected. If arthrodesis of the first metatarsophalangeal joint is performed, the recommended position is 15 to 20 degrees of valgus and 10 to 15 degrees of extension, as measured by the plantar surface of the foot and hallux. The operative techniques for the metatarsal and phalangeal osteotomies are described earlier in this chapter, as is the technique for arthrodesis of the first metatarsophalangeal joint. When an osteotomy is combined with a soft-tissue procedure, the latter should be performed before the metatarsal is inclined laterally.

JUVENILE AND ADOLESCENT HALLUX VALGUS (10 TO 19 YEARS OLD)

It is helpful for the surgeon to consider adolescents with hallux valgus separately from adults with the deformity for the following reasons:

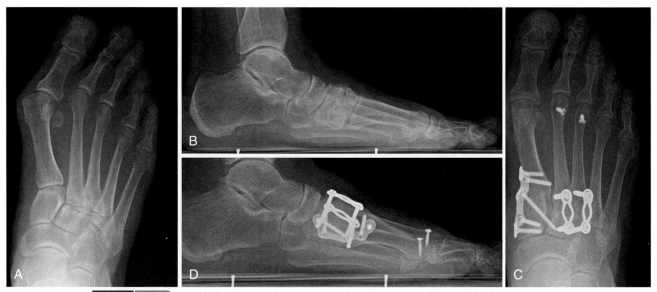

FIGURE 2.73   Lapidus procedure. **A,** Preoperative radiograph with severe valgus deformity. **B,** Lateral view demonstrating instability of first tarsometatarsal joint. **C,** Postoperative anteroposterior correction of deformity. **D,** Postoperative lateral view. **SEE TECHNIQUE 2.20.**

BOX 2.2

Algorithm for Severe Hallux Valgus Associated With Metatarsus Adductus (Sharma and Aydogan)

Reconstruction is done in the following order:
1. If pes planovalgus deformity is present, perform a medial sliding calcaneal osteotomy.
2. Perform distal soft-tissue release of the first metatarsophalangeal joint.
3. Perform a bunionectomy.
4. Prepare the tarsometatarsal joint surface for arthrodesis.
5. For metatarsus adductus correction, perform second and third metatarsal base oblique rotational osteotomies.
6. For hallux valgus correction, reduce the first tarsometatarsal joint and perform arthrodesis.
7. Fix the second and third metatarsal base oblique rotational osteotomy.
8. For correction of coronal metatarsophalangeal joint subluxation, perform Weil shortening osteotomies with lateral collateral ligament release.
9. If hallux valgus interphalangeus correction is necessary, perform an Akin closing wedge osteotomy of the proximal phalanx.

From Sharma J, Aydogan U: Algorithm for severe hallux valgus associated with metatarsus adductus, *Foot Ankle Int* 36(12):1499, 2015.

- Pain, either at the metatarsophalangeal joint or beneath the lesser metatarsal heads, may not be the primary complaint in many instances.
- A bunion secondary to the medial eminence and bursal hypertrophy may be a minor part of the deformity.
- Varus of the first metatarsal with a widened intermetatarsal angle is almost always present.
- Hypermobile flatfoot with pronation of the foot during weight bearing frequently is associated with the deformity.

- Recurrence of the deformity is more frequent, especially in the presence of flatfoot deformity.
- Hallux valgus interphalangeus may be prominent, yet easily overlooked, and may cause unsatisfactory correction of the deformity.
- The family history frequently is positive for hallux valgus.
- Soft-tissue procedures alone are unlikely to result in permanent correction.
- Osteotomy, single or double, of the first metatarsal is almost always necessary to obtain and maintain correction of the deformity.

The indications for surgical correction of a hallux valgus deformity in an adolescent are neither rigid nor clearly defined, and the timing of the procedure during adolescence is not agreed on. Debate continues over whether the procedure should be postponed until the physes of the phalanx and metatarsal are closed, whether radiographic confirmation of progression should be documented before recommending surgery, and whether pain should be a primary indication for operative treatment, as in adults. Several well-documented series recommend operative correction only for adolescents with painful, progressive deformity after the physes have closed. Other well-documented, retrospective studies indicate that surgery before 15 years of age, with or without open physes, yields the best long-term results, especially if preservation of normal metatarsophalangeal motion is considered an essential element of acceptable results.

Any adolescent 12 to 18 years old with cosmetically unattractive hallux valgus deformity that the patient and family report to be progressive and whose family history is positive for hallux valgus is considered a candidate for surgery. Pain and shoe-fitting problems are even stronger indications for operative correction of the deformity. The patient and family must be informed of the chance of recurrence of the deformity and, if the patient is free of pain before surgery, that no guarantee can be made that pain will not develop after surgery.

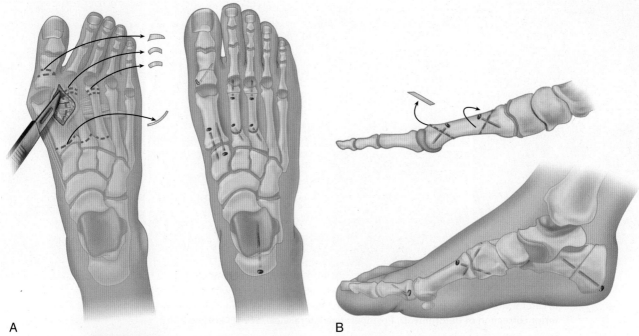

A   B

FIGURE 2.74   Sharma operative technique. **A,** Medial sliding calcaneal osteotomy, distal soft-tissue release of first metatarsophalangeal joint, first tarsometatarsal joint arthrodesis, second and third metatarsal base oblique rotational osteotomy with fixation and metatarsal neck Weil shortening osteotomy with lateral collateral ligament release, and Akin closing wedge osteotomy of proximal phalanx. Overall improvement in physical appearance of foot, including overall width. Arrows indicate Weil shortening osteotomies and metatarsal base oblique rotational osteotomies with fixation. **B,** Lateral view of operative technique. Arrows indicate medial sliding calcaneal osteotomy, first tarsometatarsal joint arthrodesis, and Akin closing wedge osteotomy of proximal phalanx of hallux.   (From Sharma J, Aydogan U: Algorithm for severe hallux valgus associated with metatarsus adductus, *Foot Ankle Int* 36:1499, 2015.)

Valgus angulation of the metatarsophalangeal joint can be caused not only by displacement of the hallux in a lateral direction on the metatarsal head but also by tilting of the articular surfaces of the respective sides of the joint in relation to the long axis of the metatarsal or phalanx, and an increased distal metatarsal articular angle may be the defining characteristic of juvenile hallux valgus. Recognition of this distinction is important to avoid excessive lateral tilt of the distal articular surface of the metatarsal after correction of the hallux valgus angle. An abnormal obliquity to the metatarsocuneiform articulation, allowing the first metatarsal to slide into varus, also has been implicated as a primary deforming factor in adolescent hallux valgus.

The medial eminence may or may not require excision, depending on its size. Any intermetatarsal angle of 10 degrees or more requires a metatarsal osteotomy. If the intermetatarsal angle is corrected to 6 degrees or less, and the hallux valgus angle is corrected to 15 degrees or less, the likelihood of unattractive, symptomatic recurrence is rare. Pronation of the great toe in juvenile and adolescent patients is uncommon but may result from pronation of the first ray and not simply of the hallux. If this is true, derotation to the neutral position should be performed at the time the varus inclination of the metatarsal is corrected. In addition, an osteotomy of the proximal phalanx may be required to correct residual hallux valgus not corrected by the primary procedure.

The most difficult combination of deformities to correct is hypermobile flatfoot, metatarsus primus varus, and hallux valgus; recurrence is common. Often, proximal metatarsal osteotomy or distal metatarsal osteotomy, or both, is required. The patient and parents should be fully advised that no operative procedure always prevents recurrence of the deformity in this particular anatomic configuration.

Any procedure that relieves discomfort, retains a functional range of motion of the metatarsophalangeal joint, corrects the excessive valgus posture of the hallux, and narrows the forefoot probably would please the patient and the family. Considering these criteria, the following procedures are useful, alone or in combination, for correcting hallux valgus in juveniles and adolescents. Adductor tenotomy, lateral capsulotomy, medial eminence removal, and medial capsulorrhaphy are recommended in patients with lesser deformity and lower intermetatarsal angle, hallux valgus angle, and distal metatarsal articular angle.

If the first metatarsal physis is fully open in an immature foot, a medial opening wedge osteotomy distal to it, with use of the resected medial eminence for a graft, is recommended. If the metatarsal physis is closed or near closure, a proximal crescentic osteotomy is recommended because it changes the metatarsal length little if at all. Internal fixation is used (Fig. 2.75; see Technique 2.10). Proximal crescentic osteotomy and a distal soft-tissue procedure can be used for older adolescent patients with moderate-to-severe deformities, but

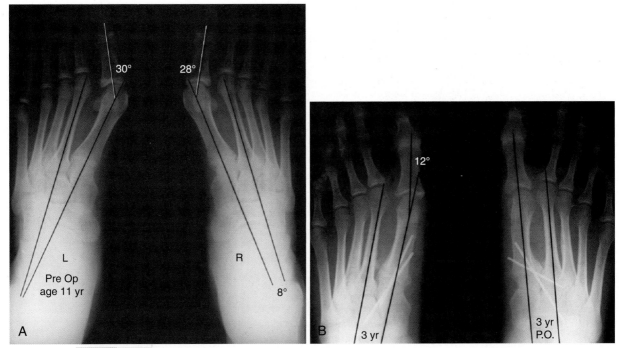

FIGURE 2.75 Adolescent hallux valgus treated by proximal osteotomy, adductor tendon release, medial capsular imbrication, and medial eminence removal. **A,** Preoperative standing radiographs. **B,** Postoperative standing radiographs. Note incongruous metatarsophalangeal joint on right probably from overcorrection of intermetatarsal angle.

this procedure is contraindicated in juvenile and adolescent patients who have increased distal metatarsal articular angles. This procedure is recommended for older adolescent patients who are near the end of foot growth and who have moderate-to-severe deformities.

The chevron osteotomy (see Technique 2.4) has been recommended for deformities with a hallux valgus angle of 30 degrees and an intermetatarsal angle of 15 degrees. The modified chevron osteotomy may be helpful in moderate deformity (Fig. 2.76). If the physis is open, this location for the osteotomy is even more advantageous. Most published series do not recommend the chevron osteotomy for hallux valgus with intermetatarsal angles of more than 12 degrees.

The scarf osteotomy (see Technique 2.11) also has been used for correction of moderate to severe adolescent hallux valgus, with contradictory outcomes reported. Some authors recommend the scarf osteotomy because of its stability and low recurrence rate and others urge caution in the use of this technique because of the high rate of recurrence. Suggested advantages of the scarf osteotomy include its stability (which allows unlimited weight bearing at 1 week after surgery) and its versatility (which obviates the need for a second osteotomy). Currently, reports in the literature provide little guidance about its usefulness in adolescents with hallux valgus because the numbers are too small and follow-up too short.

Mild-to-moderate deformities in adolescents can be corrected by proximal or distal metatarsal osteotomy combined with soft-tissue realignment, but care must be taken not to disturb the physis of the first metatarsal. In more severe deformities (hallux valgus angle > 30 degrees and intermetatarsal angle > 13 degrees), the cosmetic correction using either one of those procedures has not been consistently satisfactory. Peterson and Newman described double first metatarsal osteotomies, an opening wedge proximally, and a closing wedge distally to correct the abnormal distal metatarsal articular angle and the abnormal intermetatarsal angle. The technique has been modified by using plate and screw fixation with an osteoperiosteal flap to decrease laxity in the medial capsular repair. The use of Steinmann pins distally ensures optimal alignment but also can result in first metatarsophalangeal joint stiffness, and longitudinal pin fixation is not recommended.

Lateral hemiepiphysiodesis has been described as an alternative to osteotomy for the treatment of symptomatic or progressive juvenile hallux valgus. The rationale for lateral hemiepiphysiodesis is that gradual correction of the more proximal metatarsal deformity will lead to improved forefoot loading during gait and result in correction of the more distal metatarsophalangeal deformity. Most reports of this procedure are anecdotal, with short follow-up times and no objective assessment of outcomes. The largest series to date is that of Davids et al., which included seven children (11 feet) with a 4-year follow-up. They concluded that this procedure is appropriate for symptomatic or progressive hallux valgus in children with 2 years or more of growth remaining in whom nonoperative methods have failed. In their patients, however, the average corrections of the hallux valgus and first-second intermetatarsal angles were small (2.3 degrees and 3.5 degrees, respectively), and a significant correction was obtained in only six of 11 feet.

For severe deformities in adolescents, a triple osteotomy may be necessary: a medial cuneiform opening wedge osteotomy, a distal metatarsal osteotomy to correct the abnormal distal metatarsal articular angle, and an Akin osteotomy. This

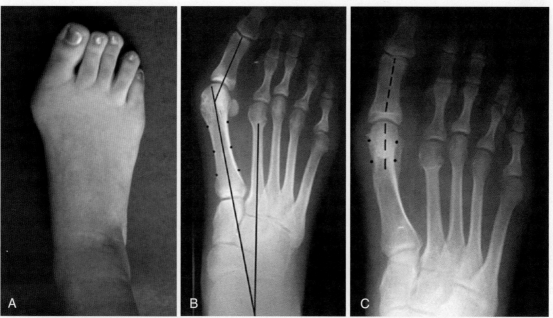

FIGURE 2.76   **A,** Moderately severe hallux valgus in 17-year-old patient. **B,** Note congenital shortening of second metatarsal on radiograph. **C,** After chevron osteotomy and adductor release.

procedure is recommended only for patients with markedly splayed forefeet and a widened first to fifth metatarsal angle of more than 30 degrees, an excessive first to second intermetatarsal angle of more than 15 degrees, a hallux valgus angle of more than 35 degrees, and a distal metatarsal articular angle of more than 15 degrees. The Akin osteotomy is described in Technique 2.15.

If the deformity at the interphalangeal joint is prominent when the metatarsus primus varus and hallux valgus have been corrected, a proximal phalangeal osteotomy may be needed. The osteotomy can be performed near the base of the proximal phalanx if the physis is closed or at the neck if the physis is open. If a phalangeal osteotomy is required, the pronation and the valgus at the distal hallux must be corrected. The patient and the family should be informed before surgery that two separate osteotomies may be needed to correct the deformity.

The original rationale for arthrodesis of the first metatarsocuneiform articulation was an assumed developmental varus posture of the first metatarsal as the prime offender in the hallux valgus complex; currently it generally is reserved for severe deformity. Although good or excellent results have been reported in about 75% of patients, primary complications include nonunion (approximately 10%), malunion with associated dorsal bunion of the first metatarsal and transfer metatarsalgia to the lesser metatarsals, hallux varus, and traumatic cutaneous neuromas. Dorsiflexion of the first metatarsal resulting from a malunion at the arthrodesis site can cause a dorsal bunion that severely limits first metatarsophalangeal motion, and transfer metatarsalgia may occur from decreased weight bearing on the first ray. Technical aspects reported to improve results include the use of bone grafts to preserve metatarsal length, rigid fixation with a two-screw technique, and avoidance of dorsiflexion at the arthrodesis site by placing the first metatarsal in approximately 5 degrees of plantarflexion compared with the preoperative weight-bearing angle of inclination of the first metatarsal.

DOUBLE FIRST METATARSAL OSTEOTOMIES

TECHNIQUE 2.21

(PETERSON AND NEWMAN)

- For tourniquet use and anesthesia, see Technique 2.1. Begin a longitudinal incision over the medial side of the first metatarsal, and curve it dorsally over the metatarsophalangeal joint onto the medial side of the base of the proximal phalanx.
- Incise the periosteum in the midline longitudinally and create a distally based, Y-shaped capsular flap, which is retracted distally.
- Expose the metatarsal diaphysis and both metaphyses subperiosteally on the dorsal, medial, and volar surfaces, leaving the periosteum intact laterally (i.e., three fourths of the circumference of the metatarsal is exposed).
- Excise the medial eminence and preserve the medial sulcus if present (Fig. 2.77A).
- Remove a wedge of bone with its base medial from the junction of the head and neck of the metatarsal to create a transverse closing wedge osteotomy (Fig. 2.77B). The width of the base of the wedge medially is 5 to 8 mm, depending on the size of the bone and the amount of correction desired. In adolescent patients, the size of the bone does not vary much, although that of boys usually is larger than that of girls. The angle of the apex differs with the degree of deformity, but usually it is approximately 20 degrees. The angle should be measured carefully with a sterile goniometer. This closing wedge allows the entire head of the metatarsal, the metatarsal and proximal phalangeal joint surfaces, and the great toe to angle medially

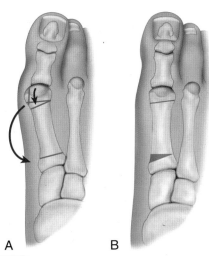

FIGURE 2.77 **A** and **B,** Double first metatarsal osteotomies (see text). **SEE TECHNIQUE 2.21.**

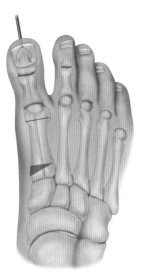

FIGURE 2.78 Intramedullary fixation with Steinmann pin secures longitudinal alignment of metatarsal and both phalanges. **SEE TECHNIQUE 2.21.**

to a neutral position, placing the phalanges in line with the first metatarsal shaft. This procedure corrects the hallux valgus deformity without disturbing the capsular or articular surface relationships of the metatarsophalangeal joint. At this point, any malrotation of the toe can be corrected.

- Leaving the distal osteotomy without fixation, hold the diaphysis of the metatarsal with a bone clamp and make a second transverse osteotomy perpendicular to the metatarsal about 1.5 cm distal to the proximal articular surface of the metatarsal.
- Insert the 20-degree wedge that was removed from the distal end of the bone into this proximal opening wedge osteotomy to correct the abnormally wide first to second intermetatarsal angle.
- Insert a 3/16-inch smooth Steinmann pin under direct vision, beginning at the tip of the great toe 2 or 3 mm below the end of the nail in its midpoint.
- Drive the pin through the distal phalanx, the proximal phalanx, and all four pieces of the metatarsal. When the pin gets to the metatarsal, its position in the closing wedge osteotomy can be seen. Close the osteotomy and drill the pin down the shaft of the metatarsal.
- Similarly, at the proximal osteotomy, the tip of the pin can be seen as it is carried into the proper position. Place the bone graft and drive the pin into the graft and into the proximal metatarsal fragment to provide firm fixation. This prevents malunion in the sagittal and axial planes. It does not control rotation in the frontal (coronal) plane (Fig. 2.78). Rotation of the fragment and the hallux is prevented by holding the hallux in neutral rotation while the Y capsular flap is resutured (into the bone if necessary). A well-applied forefoot dressing also helps to control rotation.
- Apply a bulky compression bandage, and a few days after surgery apply a short leg, non–weight-bearing cast.

POSTOPERATIVE CARE Six weeks after surgery, the cast and pin are removed (without anesthesia), and a short leg walking cast is applied, which is worn approximately 5 weeks.

MODIFIED PETERSON PROCEDURE

TECHNIQUE 2.22

(ARONSON, NGUYEN, AND ARONSON)

- For tourniquet use and anesthesia, see Technique 2.1. Make a straight medial incision from the palpable base of the first metatarsal to the midproximal phalanx. While retracting the veins and nerves dorsally and plantarly, use blunt dissection to expose the periosteum of the metatarsal. Raise flaps dorsal to the extensor hallucis longus tendon and plantar to the tibial sesamoid, exposing the plantarly subluxed abductor hallucis tendon.
- With a marking pen, identify the location of the medial periosteal incision. The incision extends from just distal to the physis to the base of the bunion and branches in a U-shaped fashion to include the bunion and the proximal phalanx (Fig. 2.79A). Sharply incise the periosteum from the physis to the U and incise the U dorsally and plantarward across the metatarsophalangeal joint to the base of the proximal phalanx.
- Use a beveled osteotome or oscillating saw to raise an osteoperiosteal distally based flap over the bunion (Fig. 2.79B). Raise the flap from distal to proximal with a 1-mm thickness of bone.
- Retract the flap distally and incise the residual capsular attachments to expose the metatarsal head (Fig. 2.79C).
- Add Hohmann retractors subperiosteally at the metatarsal neck and use an oscillating saw to remove the remaining bunion at the sulcus. Save the bone wafer for possible bone grafting.
- Calculate the size of the closing wedge using preoperative standing radiographs and intraoperative fluoroscopy. This calculation is based on exact measurement of the hallux

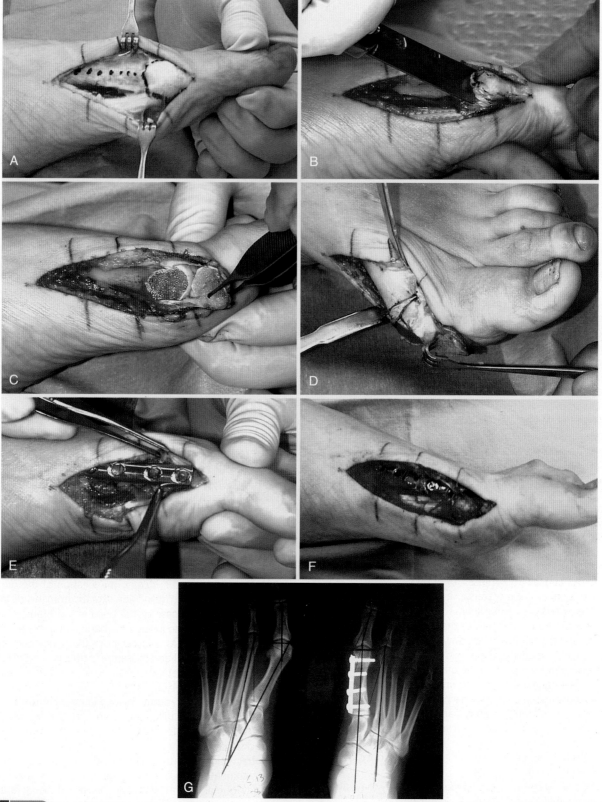

FIGURE 2.79 Modified Peterson bunion procedure. **A,** Medial longitudinal incision extends from base of first metatarsal to base of proximal phalanx with flaps from extensor hallucis longus tendon plantarward. **B,** Distally based osteoperiosteal flap is raised with 1-mm-thick bone cut after subperiosteal stripping of first metatarsal. **C,** Flap is retracted distally, exposing sulcus to remove remaining bunion. **D,** Distal closing wedge at base of bunion cut. Width of medial wedge equal to sine of hallux valgus angle multiplied by diameter of metatarsal. Attempt is made to greenstick osteotomy laterally. **E,** Proximal osteotomy made with saw and "greensticked" laterally allows space for one 3.5-mm screw. Plate is selected that fits adjusted length of metatarsal with proximal opening wedge graft inserted and distal osteotomy closed. Proximal screw is placed loosely into plate, allowing osteoperiosteal flap to be pulled under distal end of plate, while correcting great toe into supination. **F,** Periosteum closed over proximal plate and distally to osteoperiosteal flap. Abductor tendon is pulled up to its normal medial position. **G,** Appearance of foot after completed osteotomies and plate fixation. (**A-F** from Aronson J, Nguyen LL, Aronson EA: Early results of the modified Peterson bunion procedure for adolescent hallux valgus, *J Pediatr Orthop* 21:65, 2001; **G** courtesy Dr. James Aronson, Little Rock, AK.) **SEE TECHNIQUE 2.22.**

valgus angle, either on the preoperative radiograph (taking into account any magnification) or by determining the sine of the angle using the diameter of the metatarsal at the level of the cut as the hypotenuse.

- Make the distal cut at the base of the previous bunion cut and base the proximal cut on the previously calculated number of millimeters. For example, the width of the wedge is exactly half the diameter of the metatarsal for a 30-degree hallux valgus angle (sine 30 = 0.5). Leave enough distal metatarsal head to allow insertion of a single 3.5-mm screw (Fig. 2.79D). Make the osteotomy with an attempt to greenstick the lateral cortex. Save the wedge for later bone grafting.
- Make a second cut transversely in the proximal metatarsal, leaving enough space for another 3.5-mm screw between the cut and the physis. Lever open the proximal osteotomy with a straight osteotome, again attempting to greenstick the lateral cortex. The precalculated wedge (degrees to millimeters) is derived from the prior bone wedges to equal the intermetatarsal angle exactly. Insert this wedge into the proximal osteotomy, creating an opening wedge medially to reduce the intermetatarsal angle. Close the distal osteotomy manually.
- Stabilize the osteotomies with a four-hole small fragment tubular plate or a five- or six-hole mini tubular plate with three to five 3.5-mm screws (Fig. 2.79E). Plate size is determined by the space available between the physis and the metatarsal head. Insert the first screw into the proximal hole, loosely fixing the plate. The distal hole of the plate must fit exactly over the metatarsal head.
- Reduce the sesamoids indirectly by manually supinating the great toe.
- Pull the distally based osteoperiosteal flap under the plate to cover the distal osteotomy and pull it slightly dorsal to hold the supination correction. Be careful that the flap is not too tight, or it would decrease metatarsophalangeal motion.
- Place the distal screws across the osteoperiosteal flap into the metatarsal head.
- Place the remaining two or three central screws with inboard compression of each osteotomy.
- Close the periosteum over the plate up to the distal end, where it is approximated to the osteoperiosteal flap (Fig. 2.79F,G).
- Transfer the abductor hallucis tendon from the plantar to medial base of the proximal phalanx or to the extensor hallucis longus over the periosteal closure.
- It is imperative to confirm metatarsophalangeal motion before closing.
- Apply a short leg cast to the toes over loosely placed cotton gauze over the wound and in the first web space.

POSTOPERATIVE CARE The patient remains non–weight bearing in the short leg cast for 6 weeks, at which time radiographs are obtained. If healing is evident, weight bearing to tolerance is allowed in a hard-soled shoe or sandal, which is worn for 4 weeks. Active range of motion of the ankle, foot, and toes is begun when the cast is removed.

FIRST CUNEIFORM OSTEOTOMY

Coughlin recommended the first cuneiform osteotomy (Fig. 2.80) for severe deformities with a hypermobile first ray. It can be combined with a distal first metatarsal osteotomy and an Akin proximal phalangeal osteotomy (triple osteotomy).

TECHNIQUE 2.23

(COUGHLIN)

- For tourniquet use and anesthesia, see Technique 2.1. Make a medial longitudinal incision over the medial cuneiform.
- Dissect the tibialis anterior subperiosteally and lift it anteriorly, leaving its remaining portion intact on the base of the first metatarsal.
- Identify the cuneiform-navicular and cuneiform–first metatarsal articulations with a small knife blade. The medial cuneiform is 3 cm wide × 3 to 3.5 cm long.
- Use a 9-mm-wide saw blade on a power sagittal saw to make the osteotomy in the center of the cuneiform, parallel to the cuneiform-metatarsal joint, which would be at an angle of 10 to 15 degrees distal to the coronal plane. This angle of the osteotomy would give the least disruption of the intermediate cuneiform–second metatarsal and medial cuneiform articulations.
- Because the medial cuneiform is only about 1.5 cm deep, carry the saw blade through a little more than 1 cm and use a small blade (4 mm wide) to create perforations through the lateral cortex. This maintains some stability of the bony fragments and prevents them from shifting in a dorsoplantar direction.
- Open the plantar aspect of the osteotomy with a small, smooth-tipped lamina spreader or small osteotome.
- Using iliac crest allograft material, cut a 1-cm, wedge-shaped graft. (We have found these allografts to be useful in procedures around the foot.) Tap the graft in place, reducing the first metatarsal varus. Although this usually is stable, Coughlin recommended using crossed 0.062-inch Kirschner wires to ensure that the graft does not slip.
- If the distal metatarsal articular angle is excessive, perform a closing wedge osteotomy at the metatarsal head and neck junction.
- Make a medial incision over the medial eminence and remove any medial eminence present (usually there is little medial eminence in juvenile patients).
- Make a 5- to 8-mm-wide, laterally based wedge osteotomy in a transverse or axial direction. Ensure that the width of the blade (1 mm) is included in the measurements on each side of the wedge (the wedge itself should not be more than 4 to 7 mm wide).
- Remove the medially based wedge of bone. If needed, the wedge can be used as additional bone graft in the cuneiform osteotomy.
- Correct the distal metatarsal articular angle and fix the osteotomy with two 0.062-inch Kirschner wires inserted

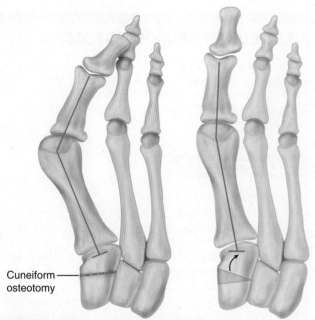

Cuneiform osteotomy

FIGURE 2.80   Opening wedge cuneiform osteotomy. (Redrawn from Coughlin MJ, Mann RA: Hallux valgus. In Mann RA, Coughlin MJ, editors: *Surgery of the foot and ankle*, ed 8, Philadelphia, Elsevier, 2007, p 319.) **SEE TECHNIQUE 2.23.**

from proximal to distal. If the wires penetrate the joint, they can be backed out into subchondral bone.
- If excessive hallux valgus interphalangeus remains, or if the double osteotomy at the cuneiform and distal first metatarsal does not adequately correct the deformity even with soft-tissue repair, perform a third osteotomy at the base of the proximal phalanx. The Akin osteotomy (see Technique 2.15) consists of a 3- to 4-mm wedge, based medially, just distal to the insertion of the extensor hallucis brevis and held with either sutures or crossed pins. We use pins placed longitudinally across the interphalangeal joint from distal to proximal, ending in the subchondral bone of the base of the proximal phalanx.

COMPLICATIONS AFTER SURGERY FOR HALLUX VALGUS

Complications after hallux valgus procedures can be discouraging for patients and physicians. Long-time practice experience, detailed physical and radiographic evaluations, excellent surgical technique, and careful postoperative care do not guarantee that a complication will not occur. Recurrence of the original hallux valgus deformity or development of the opposite deformity (hallux varus), malunion, clawed hallux, transfer keratotic lesions that cause intractable discomfort, and other complications all have been reported to occur after surgery. A systematic literature review of 229 patients found a pooled rate of postoperative dissatisfaction and first metatarsophalangeal joint pain of 10.6% and 1.5%, respectively, with an overall recurrence rate of 4.9%.

■ PREVENTING COMPLICATIONS

In the treatment of hallux valgus, preventing a complication begins at the time of initial evaluation of a patient. A careful physical examination can identify problems that ultimately may lead to failure in certain patients. Before any decision is made regarding treatment of hallucal disorders, the feet should be examined carefully with the patient sitting, standing, and lying supine and prone. As much or more time should be spent evaluating the deformity clinically as is spent reviewing the radiographs.

Although a bunion typically is present with hallux valgus deformity, this is not always the case. Also, first metatarsal varus is not always present. Rotation of the hallux is an important element of the deformity and may tell a great deal about the prospects for a successful outcome, as would the condition of the entire capsulosesamoid apparatus. Recurrence of hallux valgus deformity is more likely when subluxation or dislocation of the first metatarsophalangeal joint is present. Li et al. noted that excessive length of the first ray is a risk factor for recurrence, and they recommend taking this into consideration prior to surgery for improved outcomes.

Sensory nerve dysfunction has been noted in patients with hallux valgus both as a symptom of the deformity and after surgery. Jastifer et al. prospectively evaluated 57 feet undergoing surgery for hallux valgus deformity to determine if surgery and correction of the deformity had any effect on these symptoms. They found that sensory deficits can be caused by the deformity and can improve up to 24 months after correction. In a separate study, Jastifer et al. also found a high prevalence of osteochondral lesions in patients with hallux valgus, the significance of which was unknown. They did not see a correlation between these osteochondral lesions and the severity of the deformity or clinical outcome.

Pronation of the hallux (frequently an indication of severe deformity), dislocation of the sesamoids laterally, fixed deformity, pes planus, joint hypermobility, and a tight heel cord may increase the likelihood of recurrence of the deformity after hallux valgus repair. Pentikainen et al. found recurrence of hallux valgus deformity in 73% of patients (mild 14%, moderate 57%, and severe 1%). The preoperative congruence, distal metatarsal articular angle, sesamoid position, hallux valgus angle, and first to second intermetatarsal angle all had an effect on recurrence. Noting these clinical points may help to avoid failed hallux valgus surgery.

As in the physical examination, radiographic examination of the feet is incomplete without weight-bearing views (see Box 2.1, Boxes 2.3 to 2.5). The difference in the magnitude of the deformity on non–weight-bearing and weight-bearing views often is striking. A concise, detailed evaluation of weight-bearing radiographs is imperative before planning a procedure to correct hallux valgus deformity. Correction of each anatomic component contributing to the hallux valgus deformity is necessary to avoid or correct a complication.

Long-term assessment of radiographic outcomes of distal metatarsal osteotomies has revealed that the incidence of recurrent deformity may be considerably higher than previously thought but may actually be well tolerated by the patient.

Observations on Weight-Bearing Lateral Views

Observations on weight-bearing lateral views that help determine the degree of valgus thrust on hallux metatarsophalangeal joint during the stance phase of gait, which influences treatment decisions

Collapse deformity of metatarsocuneiform, cuneiform-navicular, or naviculotalar articulation

Increased talocalcaneal angle, suggesting valgus posture of hindfoot

Calcaneal inclination angle (≥10 degrees is normal; reduced angle indicates valgus hindfoot and possibly pes planus)

Dorsiflexion of first metatarsal, indicating incongruous reduction into concavity of base of proximal phalanx

Angle between diaphysis of proximal phalanx and diaphysis of first metatarsal (≥20 degrees is normal)

Delineation of cortical outlines of fifth, fourth, and third metatarsals even if overlapped (if fifth and fourth metatarsal cortical borders are not clearly outlined on weight-bearing lateral radiograph, pronation of foot should be suspected)

BOX 2.4

Observations on Non–Weight-Bearing Medial Oblique Views

Arthritic changes in first metatarsal–medial cuneiform articulation

Calcaneonavicular tarsal coalition not visible on other views

BOX 2.5

Observations on Weight-Bearing Sesamoid View

Observations on weight-bearing sesamoid view (especially useful in evaluation of recurrent hallux valgus deformity): Repositioning the intrinsic and extrinsic muscles and the capsulosesamoid apparatus into their anatomic positions is the key to correction, and the weight-bearing sesamoid view is helpful in planning the best means to accomplish this.

Location of sesamoid bones in relation to their facets on first metatarsal (often difficult on an anteroposterior view)

■ TRANSFER METATARSALGIA

Postoperative development of pain or a callus under the second metatarsal head is not common but may be more common than previously thought. Care in the preoperative assessment to take into consideration the presence of a short, hypoplastic metatarsal or the presence of a callosity under the adjacent metatarsal head may suggest a bunion correction that either lengthens, or at any rate, does not shorten, the metatarsal. Even with careful planning, a transfer callosity happens occasionally preoperatively.

The condition of the plantar skin and the presence and location of callosities provide clues as to the biomechanical cause of transfer metatarsalgia. It is important to observe the contact pattern and presence and location of keratoses during examination. Weight-bearing dorsoplantar, lateral, and oblique non–weight-bearing views should be obtained. MRI may help to determine if there is bone, cartilage, or soft-tissue damage and to rule out stress fracture of the lesser rays or Freiberg disease. CT is helpful in detecting subchondral cysts, osteophytes, loss of bone, nonunion or malunion, or alterations in the metatarsal heads.

Maceira et al. noted that nonoperative treatment should be attempted first, including analgesics, off-loading of the painful joint, padding, orthoses, shoe modifications (i.e., wider toe box, rocker-bottom), and stretching exercises. When these fail, surgery of the first toe or lesser toes may be necessary. The type of surgery will depend on the pathology (i.e., shortening lesser toe metatarsal osteotomies when there is only shortening of the first metatarsal, proximal gastrocnemius release for a second toe rocker metatarsalgia, combined procedures of the first metatarsal and lesser metatarsals). Rose et al. reported significant improvement both clinically and radiographically in 31 patients after a scarf procedure for recurrent hallux valgus secondary to iatrogenic first brachymetatarsia with resultant transfer metatarsalgia. They believe that the scarf osteotomy reduces the load transferred to the lesser metatarsal heads by restoring the length and alignment to a short metatarsal, allowing weight bearing under the first metatarsal head. Nakagawa et al. also stressed the importance of preserving the first metatarsal length during osteotomy to prevent metatarsalgia.

■ RECURRENT DEFORMITY AFTER SIMPLE BUNIONECTOMY

Recurrence of the deformity is a frequent complication after simple bunionectomy (medial eminence excision and capsular imbrication). Although it is tempting to do a minor procedure for a minor deformity, soft-tissue repair alone should not be done except in elderly patients with skin breakdown over the medial eminence even if the hallux is congruously reduced on the first metatarsal head and the hallux valgus and intermetatarsal angles are normal. A first web space dissection and lateral release always should be done with medial eminence removal and medial capsular imbrication.

If the hallux does not remain in the desired position at the conclusion of surgery, adduction of the hallux recurs. The adductor must be released not only from the proximal phalanx but also from its conjoined insertion with the lateral head of the flexor hallucis brevis on the fibular sesamoid. Whether reattaching the adductor to the capsule at the lateral side of the first metatarsal head (or through a tunnel in the metatarsal neck) is an improvement over adductor tenotomy alone in correcting the deformity and preventing recurrence is inconclusive. Tenotomy alone probably is effective, but the entire adductor insertion must be incised, and a section must be removed proximal to the metatarsophalangeal joint.

The capsular release and repair also are important factors that may contribute to recurrence. The lateral capsule is incised beginning at the lateral margin of the extensor hallucis longus tendon and progressing plantarward to the lateral edge of the fibular sesamoid, or multiple perforations are made in the lateral capsule and the capsulotomy is completed by manually placing the hallux in 20 to 25 degrees of varus before returning it to a normal position. Also, if the excessive medial capsule is not trimmed to hold the hallux in correct alignment, recurrence is likely.

Failure to reposition the articular surface of the metatarsal head to a normal 5- to 15-degree alignment with the metatarsal shaft (see Fig. 2.5) would compromise correction. If the metatarsophalangeal joint is congruent but is in a position of unacceptable valgus, correction can be obtained by a proximal phalangeal osteotomy or distal metatarsal osteotomy, or both if needed. The distal metatarsal osteotomy (chevron configuration) allows for a slight tilting of the metatarsal head to correct the valgus position of the articular surface if a medially based sliver of bone no wider than the saw blade is removed from the dorsal proximal side of the chevron cut. A phalangeal osteotomy corrects another 3 to 4 degrees of valgus of the hallux, but this is primarily for interphalangeal joint valgus and most often is used as supplemental correction with a soft-tissue procedure.

Failure to reduce the sesamoid sling allows the lateral head of the flexor hallucis brevis muscle to pull the hallux into valgus along with the extensor hallucis longus and flexor hallucis longus muscles (Fig. 2.81). These extrinsic muscles, particularly the flexor hallucis longus, bowstring laterally across the metatarsophalangeal joint, increase the valgus moment, and increase the chances of recurrence of the deformity. Releasing the capsulosesamoid ligament in an axial plane is integral to repositioning the sesamoid apparatus.

Postoperative care may be as crucial to success of hallux valgus surgery as the actual procedure, especially after soft-tissue repair. Adequate serial dressing changes and taping (with ½-inch adhesive tape) maintain the hallux in the desired position (0 to 5 degrees of valgus or 10 to 15 degrees of valgus if the fibular sesamoid has been excised). These dressing changes must continue until the hallux rests unattended in the proper alignment, which usually takes 4 to 8 weeks. A toe spacer is worn for another month. In addition, an abnormally long first ray, made even longer by straightening of the toe, can contribute to the recurrence of the deformity. Stockings and narrow shoes must be avoided for at least 12 weeks because of their deforming force.

RECURRENT HALLUX VALGUS WITH NORMAL DISTAL METATARSAL ANGLE AFTER BUNIONECTOMY

The magnitude and rigidity of the recurrent deformity should be used as guides to treatment. As a rule, a deformity that occurred after a soft-tissue procedure should not be treated with another soft-tissue procedure unless the deformity is completely flexible (the hallux can be easily reduced into varus, and the first metatarsal freely translates laterally by manual pressure). First web space dissection, lateral release, and repeat medial capsular imbrication with manual medial displacement of the first metatarsal are recommended in patients with mild, flexible deformity that is symptomatic despite appropriate shoes. For severe deformity, Kitaoka and Patzer recommended proximal first metatarsal osteotomy with distal soft-tissue reconstruction (see Technique 2.10). They emphasized, however, that although their results were satisfactory, they were not as successful as well-performed primary surgeries that appropriately corrected the valgus deformity. Indications for a soft-tissue repair are listed in Box 2.6.

FIRST WEB SPACE DISSECTION, LATERAL RELEASE, AND REPEAT CAPSULAR IMBRICATION (HALLUX VALGUS ANGLE LESS THAN 30 DEGREES AND FIRST-SECOND INTERMETATARSAL ANGLE LESS THAN 15 DEGREES)

TECHNIQUE 2.24

- Make a straight midline medial incision, extending from the middle of the proximal phalanx to 3 to 4 cm proximal to the first metatarsophalangeal joint. This incision is in the plane between the most medial branch of the superficial peroneal nerve and the dorsomedial aspect of the hallux and the proper branch of the medial plantar nerve to the medial side of the hallux. This nerve rests plantarmedially and blends with overlying superficial fascia so well that it is quite vulnerable to injury.

- Raise a dorsal flap the entire length of the incision until the extensor hallucis longus tendon and dorsal aspect of the first metatarsophalangeal joint are exposed proximally and the extensor hood is exposed distally. The plane of dissection of the dorsal flap is important. Do not enter the extensor mechanism, but raise the flap adjacent to it so that the flap would carry with it the dorsal veins and dorsal sensory nerve. Use blunt dissection proximally because the dorsal nerve frequently is in the center of the incision where the medial eminence joins the metatarsal shaft.

- Using an inverted-L configuration, extensively expose the area dorsally (relative to the initial procedure) to maximize the effectiveness of the capsular imbrication. Commonly, a thin slip of accessory extensor tendon is visible. This is a helpful landmark; however, if it is not present, locate the dorsal and medial juncture of the rounded distal first metatarsal head.

- Using either the medial aspect of the accessory tendon or the dorsomedial border of the first metatarsal as a starting point, complete a capsular-periosteal excision from the first metatarsophalangeal joint line to the junction of the middle and distal thirds of the metatarsal.

- Begin the transverse limb of this incision at the joint line. Traction on the hallux helps to identify the distal edge of the metatarsal head and avoid injury to the articular cartilage. The transverse limb extends from dorsal to plantar through the capsule and the conjoined capsular-abductor hallucis tendon insertion and terminates 2 to 3 mm medial to the tibial sesamoid.

- With a small, pointed blade, carefully raise the medial capsule from bone. Begin at the plantar aspect and develop the capsular flap until the junction of the inverted-L is reached. Dorsally, at the joint line, raise the flap by

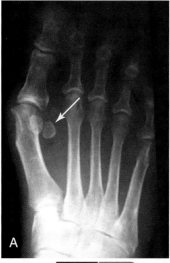
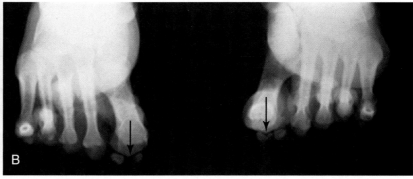

FIGURE 2.81 **A,** Failure to reduce sesamoid sling apparatus after soft-tissue procedure for hallux valgus. **B,** Recurrence of deformity caused pain beneath tibial sesamoid.

BOX 2.6

Indications for Soft-Tissue Repair for Recurrent Hallux Valgus

First-second intermetatarsal angle of ≤13 degrees

Hallux valgus angle of ≤30 degrees

Normal distal metatarsal articular angle (<10-15 degrees)

Minimal degenerative changes at first metatarsophalangeal joint

Fifty to 60 degrees of passive motion of first metatarsophalangeal joint

Subluxation but not complete dislocation of sesamoid bones

Ability to displace first metatarsal laterally at metatarsocuneiform joint from its abnormal varus inclination

Some degree of longitudinal arch present when weight bearing, determined clinically and radiographically

If arch is improved with passive dorsiflexion of hallux while standing, deformity is not fixed (structural pes planus) and a soft-tissue repair is likely to endure

---

sharp dissection with the point of the small bladed knife. Avoid penetrating or placing a buttonhole in the capsule because an intact flap results in stronger capsular repair.

■ When this capsular flap is elevated and the hallux is placed in marked valgus, almost the entire head of the metatarsal can be seen by distracting, dorsiflexing, and plantarflexing the hallux. Avoid the temptation to reach across the joint to release the lateral capsuloligamentous structures and continuous intrinsic tendon insertion through the medial incision. Although occasionally it may be successful, the predictability of permanent correction is improved with a formal web space dissection and direct exposure of the structure to be released. This surgery is for recurrence of valgus deformity, so every effort must be made to decrease the likelihood of a second failure. A second incision in the first web space into the first intermetatarsal space allows more complete lateral release.

■ Return the dorsal skin flap to its anatomic position.

■ Bring the hallux to neutral and begin an incision 2 to 3 mm proximal to the web space. With varus tension on the hallux, make an incision proximally 4 to 5 cm. Although this seems to be a lengthy incision just to release the lateral structures, exposure must be complete, and with a shorter incision the skin would be under constant tension. The deeper dissection is kept at or distal to the metatarsal head.

■ When the skin incision is complete, cauterize any dorsal veins inhibiting deeper dissection. Using blunt dissection, expose and retract the subcutaneous fat and deep peroneal nerve.

■ Clear the distal aspect of the web space of the transverse cutaneous ligaments (natatory ligaments) with blunt dissection to expose the first dorsal interosseous muscle and overlying fascia, the superficial transverse intermetatarsal ligaments, and the depth of the web space plantarward. In this space, the neurovascular bundle emerges from beneath the distal aspect of the intermetatarsal ligament.

■ The adductor hallucis tendon rests dorsal to the deep transverse intermetatarsal ligament. To expose the adductor muscle-tendon unit, place a small self-retaining retractor between the first and second metatarsals with the distal edge of the retractor proximal to the deep transverse intermetatarsal ligament and its lateral arm beneath or deep to the first dorsal interosseous muscle. Spread the first and second metatarsals and continue blunt dissection, exposing the adductor hallucis, the conjoined tendon and its muscle belly, the juncture of the adductor hallucis muscle with the lateral head of the flexor hallucis brevis, the adductor hallucis tendon with the lateral capsule of the first metatarsophalangeal joint, and the lateral border of the fibular sesamoid. It is difficult to distinguish the adductor tendon from the capsule and fibular sesamoid; the easiest way is to find the junction proximal to the joint where the adductor muscle becomes confluent with the muscle belly of the lateral head of the flexor hallucis brevis (Fig. 2.82).

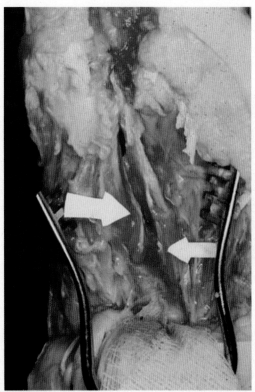

- With the adductor hallucis muscle-tendon unit clearly demarcated and retracted laterally, remove the tendon from the capsule and the capsulosesamoid ligament and the lateral border of the fibular sesamoid. This tendon's insertion is more plantar than anticipated. Ensure that all of it is resected, particularly from its fibular sesamoid attachment.
- Displace the tendon laterally and remove it by sharp dissection from its insertion into the base of the proximal phalanx. This is a wider insertion than anticipated.
- Bring the tendon proximally, dissecting on its deep or plantar surface.
- When proximal to the metatarsophalangeal joint, cut out a section of the tendon and place the muscle in the depths of the wound. Removing the adductor tendon without severing the deep transverse intermetatarsal ligament contiguous with its plantar surface is difficult. Section this ligament to allow medial mobility of the fibular sesamoid; remember that the neurovascular bundle to the first web space is immediately plantar to the ligament.
- With the fibular sesamoid visible in an axial plane, release it from the capsulosesamoid ligament, exposing the articular surface of the fibular sesamoid. This allows evaluation of the mobility of the sesamoid.
- If the fibular sesamoid cannot be placed into its facet on the inferior surface of the first metatarsal head or the hallux reduced on the first metatarsal head, section the lateral capsule from dorsal (at the level of the extensor hallucis brevis and extensor hallucis longus tendons) to the fibular sesamoid. This release is in the frontal or coronal plane.

- At this point, evaluate the mobility of the first metatarsal, the hallux, and the sesamoids. If all components contributing to the deformity can be corrected passively, most of the correction probably would be maintained. (This repair for recurrent hallux valgus does not consider the variant of excessive valgus posture of the articular surface of the first metatarsal head [distal metatarsal articular angle].) If the fibular sesamoid is excised, however, even more caution is required to avoid overtightening the medial capsule, which would cause a varus deformity.
- While an assistant displaces the first metatarsal laterally and places the hallux congruously reduced on the first metatarsal head under direct view, begin the capsular repair. Do not displace the first metatarsal too far laterally because this may lead to a hallux varus deformity. When the hallux is placed in a neutral position and held there with a capsular repair, the hallux rests in varus relative to the articular surface of the first metatarsal, even though it appears to be well aligned. Initially, displace the first metatarsal completely laterally, until it abuts the second metatarsal. This position of the first metatarsal produces a negative intermetatarsal angle. Allow the first metatarsal to spring back about one half of the total displacement and reduce the hallux on the first metatarsal head under direct observation. Close the capsule to maintain this position.
- Place two sutures proximally to anchor the capsule to the proximal confluence of the first metatarsal periosteum and the tendon of the abductor hallucis (Fig. 2.83A). This proximal anchoring would allow the transverse limb of the repair to have a stable base against which to pull, allowing the capsular repair to exert maximal restraints on the hallux and first metatarsal. Use 3-0 absorbable sutures on a small needle and increase the curve of the needle maximally to facilitate passage through cramped areas. Use the "two-bite" technique in suture passing; otherwise, the strength of repair may be compromised.
- To close the dorsal capsule, the corner of the raised capsular flap is tucked under the dorsal corner of the capsule. To accomplish this, start the dorsal capsule closure through the transverse limb, 3 to 4 mm from its junction with the longitudinal limb of the dorsal capsule. This is an outside-in stitch. Reverse the needle and enter the raised capsular flap on its transverse limb 3 to 4 mm from its junction with the longitudinal limb of the capsular flap. This also is an outside-in stitch. Reverse the needle again and reenter the capsular flap that was just exited; however, reenter it on the opposite side (its longitudinal limb), from inside out. At this point, ensure that the suture moves freely in the dorsal and the distal sides of the raised capsular flap. To lock this stitch at any passage would compromise not only the strength of the capsular repair but also the entire procedure.
- When it is known that the suture is freely movable, make the last stitch by reversing the needle for a final time and passing an inside-out suture through the stationary dorsal capsule, 3 to 4 mm proximal to the junction of the dorsal limb and stationary transverse limb. Pull on each end of the suture, in turn, ensuring that the suture

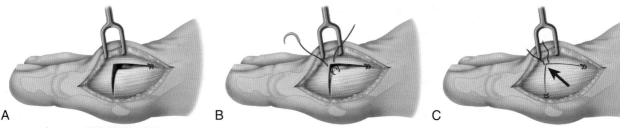

FIGURE 2.83 **A,** Two proximal sutures anchor capsule to proximal confluence of first metatarsal periosteum and tendon of abductor hallucis. **B,** Corner of raised capsular flap is sutured beneath corner of stationary dorsal capsule. **C,** Two or three sutures are placed in transverse limb of incision. **SEE TECHNIQUE 2.24.**

moves through the flaps freely. Maintaining the exact position of correction regarding the first metatarsal and hallux alignment, pull the corner of the raised capsular flap beneath the corner of the stationary dorsal capsule (Fig. 2.83B).

- Place two or three sutures in the transverse limb not more than 2 to 3 mm from the joint (Fig. 2.83C). Occasionally, 2 to 3 mm of excessive capsule must be excised from the transverse side of the raised capsular flap. Do not excise too much of the capsule or place the sutures in the transverse capsular limb too far from the joint. Overtightening of the transverse capsular repair can pull the hallux into varus, which may not be recognized until weight-bearing radiographs are obtained postoperatively.
- This repair should maintain acceptable alignment while allowing 40 to 50 degrees of passive motion. Do not try to move the joint passively through a greater arc of motion because the strength of capsular repair may be compromised.
- Dorsiflex the foot to neutral by pushing up on the arch, not the forefoot, and inspect the forefoot. Gently push the hallux medially and laterally to determine if the hallux stays in the corrected position.
- If the medial capsular repair is not tight enough and the hallux drifts laterally, add one transverse stitch at a time until this laxity is corrected. Remove a stitch and replace it if necessary until the tension is sufficient for the hallux to remain reduced on the first metatarsal head without drifting medially or laterally.
- If the hallux is pulled medially by the capsular repair, remove one suture from the transverse limb of the capsular repair. Continue to alter the tension on the capsular repair until the hallux remains in the correct position.
- Before skin closure, obtain a radiograph with the foot placed flat on a cassette or transparent image board to ensure the hallux is congruously reduced.
- As crucial to success as repair of the capsule is the meticulous application of a forefoot dressing holding the hallux in the corrected position. Use 4 × 4-inch gauze sponges, unfolded (some sectioned) for the interdigital spaces, and 2- and 3-inch rolling gauze, wrapped over the conforming dressing. Apply a 3- or 4-inch elastic gauze wrap, placed loosely on the forefoot with a dressing to avoid constriction but to allow gentle pressure as the edema resolves.

POSTOPERATIVE CARE The patient wears a rigid-soled, loosely applied shoe for 3 weeks. Weight bearing to tolerance is allowed immediately but limited to the bathroom. For 3 days after surgery, the patient should rest supine with the foot elevated 18 inches. After this, the patient can be up and about to tolerance. Driving is allowed when the patient can drive with confidence. The same dressing is kept dry and left in place for 19 to 23 days. The sutures are removed at 3 weeks, and a medium toe spacer is placed in the first metatarsal space for another 3 weeks. Shoes should not place pressure on the great toe. Wearing of dress shoes, even ones with a low heel and round toe box, is discouraged for at least 3 months. For postoperative management, a "rule of three" applies: 3 days of rest and elevation, 3 weeks in a postoperative shoe and dressing, and 3 months before the swelling is sufficiently reduced to attempt wearing a low-heeled, round toe box dress shoe with a soft, yielding material for the box.

RECURRENT VALGUS DEFORMITY WITH ABNORMAL DISTAL METATARSAL ARTICULAR ANGLE

When an increased distal metatarsal articular angle is present in recurrent hallux valgus, reducing the hallux would place the metatarsophalangeal joint incongruously on the metatarsal head (Fig. 2.84). The phalanx would rest in varus on the first metatarsal head and would leave the lateral aspect of the first metatarsal head uncovered. This deformity is corrected with medial capsulorrhaphy, distal metatarsal displacement osteotomy (chevron; see Technique 2.4), and first web space dissection with lateral soft-tissue release. Osteonecrosis of the first metatarsal head is a risk with distal metatarsal osteotomy and lateral release, but the extent of necrosis and its clinical significance are unknown. This complication probably is not to be feared as much as previously thought. Procedures that treat the coronal plane alignment may be particularly helpful in this circumstance (minimally invasive surgery with rotation or the Lapidus procedure).

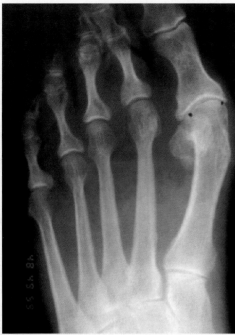

FIGURE 2.84 Anteroposterior weight-bearing radiograph in elderly woman, 20 years after McBride bunionectomy. In reality, this is congruous hallux valgus that assumed its normal position on first metatarsal head after soft-tissue realignment for hallux valgus. Biplanar correcting distal metatarsal osteotomy is needed.

CORRECTING DISTAL METATARSAL OSTEOTOMY

TECHNIQUE 2.25

■ The incision, inverted-L capsulotomy, elevation of the capsular flap, web space dissection, lateral release, partial adductor resection, and capsular flap closure are the same as in the soft-tissue repair technique previously described (see Technique 2.24). The web space dissection, lateral release, and adductor release and tendinous resection should be done before the osteotomy because the displaced metatarsal head after the osteotomy markedly limits exposure of the tissues to be released or resected. Keep the dissection distal to the neck of the first metatarsal when the soft-tissue release is performed. This preserves some perfusion to the first metatarsal head.

■ Perform a chevron osteotomy as described in Technique 2.4. One reason for recurrence is an unrecognized and uncorrected excessive distal metatarsal articular angle. The goal is to reduce the valgus tilt of the articular surface of the first metatarsal head to approximately 10 degrees and bring the hallux into a congruous position on the metatarsal head by a medial capsulorrhaphy with or without a first web space dissection and lateral soft-tissue release.

■ To reduce the distal metatarsal articular angle to an acceptable value, remove a 1- to 2-mm wedge-shaped sliver of bone from the medial aspect of the distal metatarsal (or from the capital fragment), a "closing wedge oste-

otomy." The size of the wedge is deliberately small because slight impaction occurs medially as the surfaces are manually pressed together.

■ Use small absorbable or nonabsorbable pins to secure the osteotomy.

■ Reduce the hallux congruously on the articular surface of the metatarsal head and maintain the position with capsulorrhaphy.

■ Evaluate the repair radiographically by imaging or plain films. Obtain an anteroposterior radiograph with the foot resting flat (flex the knee) on a cassette or radiolucent image board. Although this is not routinely necessary with an initial repair, it should always be done when surgically treating recurrence of a hallux valgus deformity.

RECURRENT DEFORMITY AFTER BASILAR METATARSAL OSTEOTOMY AND FIRST WEB SPACE DISSECTION OR RELEASE

Recurrent deformity after basilar metatarsal osteotomy and first web space dissection or release should be treated with a second basilar metatarsal osteotomy, medial capsular imbrication of the first metatarsophalangeal joint, and first web space dissection with release of the contracted lateral structures. Alternatively, in selected patients, particularly men, an arthrodesis of the first metatarsophalangeal joint is reasonable. Indications for this procedure include (1) an intermetatarsal angle of 14 degrees or more, (2) a hallux valgus angle of more than 30 degrees, (3) a normal distal metatarsal articular angle (10 to 15 degrees), (4) a splayed forefoot, (5) minimal-to-mild osteoarthritic changes at the first metatarsophalangeal joint (arthrodesis is indicated if the articular cartilage is damaged), (6) markedly subluxed or dislocated sesamoid bones, (7) 50 to 60 degrees of passive range of motion of the first metatarsophalangeal joint, and (8) arch structures that increase valgus stress on the metatarsophalangeal joint.

A combination of chevron and Akin osteotomies can be used for greater correction of valgus deformity, but this combined procedure should be used with caution if sesamoid subluxation and a wide intermetatarsal angle are present.

For severe recurrent deformity after basilar metatarsal osteotomy, arthrodesis of the first metatarsophalangeal joint often is the most appropriate operation. The surgical technique varies according to the type of osteotomy and the kind of fixation used. Nonunion, malunion, and degenerative arthritis of the interphalangeal joint of the hallux are the most frequent complications after arthrodesis of the first metatarsophalangeal joint. Accurate positioning of the hallux is essential during the procedure. Lapidus recommended combining arthrodesis of the first metatarsal-medial cuneiform joint with distal soft-tissue release for treating severe recurrent deformities.

RECURRENT DEFORMITY IN ELDERLY PATIENTS WITH OSTEOARTHRITIS

Resection and Arthrodesis or Replacement Arthroplasty of the First Metatarsophalangeal Joint. Resection (Keller) arthroplasty can be used for correction of recurrent deformity in elderly patients who have limited physical demands on their feet and have some degree of osteoarthritis at the first metatarsophalangeal joint. Its usefulness may be expanded if the hallux, after resection of its base, is secured to the first metatarsal with two longitudinal Kirschner wires (see Technique 2.2) after the metatarsal is manually displaced laterally as far as possible. Excision of the fibular sesamoid bone is recommended before the hallux is secured to the first metatarsal.

The results of replacement arthroplasty of the first metatarsophalangeal joint for correction of recurrent hallux valgus have varied. Replacement arthroplasty of the first metatarsophalangeal joint has been recommended for patients with rheumatoid arthritis and severe destruction of the metatarsophalangeal joints, but in most patients resection of the base of the proximal phalanx, lateral displacement of the first metatarsal, temporary internal fixation after fibular sesamoid excision, and medial capsular repair provide just as good results as replacement arthroplasty with less expense and fewer complications. Arthrodesis of the first metatarsophalangeal joint is a good choice for recurrent hallux valgus in elderly patients (see Fig. 2.64).

■ COMPLICATIONS AFTER CHEVRON OSTEOTOMY

Johnson described several complications of the chevron osteotomy and suggested the following ways to avoid them:

- Recurrent metatarsophalangeal joint valgus can be prevented by ensuring the medial capsular imbrication is firm and by maintaining the hallux in the proper position before skin closure.
- Insufficient narrowing of the forefoot, most often associated with preoperative metatarsus adductus and insufficient room to shift the metatarsal head laterally, can be avoided by paying careful attention to the preoperative radiographs.
- Osteonecrosis can be prevented by preserving the lateral blood supply to the capital fragment.
- Incongruity at the metatarsophalangeal joint results from failure to recognize a valgus posture of the articular surface before surgery or from closure of the osteotomy medially, placing the capital fragment in a straight or a varus position.
- Unfulfilled patient expectations can be minimized by providing a detailed explanation of the benefits and drawbacks of bunion surgery. A common mistake is trying to correct too much valgus deformity with this procedure; it is most useful in mild-to-moderate deformities.

If lateral capsular perforation distal to the metatarsal head and release of the adductor hallucis tendon across the joint are required, they should be done distal to the vascular supply of the metatarsal head; however, these seldom are necessary for the degree of deformity described for this procedure. Two technical errors can result in damage to the vessels that supply the metatarsal head: cutting of the first dorsal metatarsal artery by overpenetration of the saw blade and incorrect placement of the proximal arms of the osteotomy inside the joint capsule. A correctly performed chevron osteotomy, with or without a lateral capsular release, should not disrupt the vascular supply to the first metatarsal head, and a "safe zone" for performance of the chevron osteotomy and the lateral capsular release was identified by Jones et al. (Fig. 2.85). A cadaver study identified the plantar lateral corner of the metatarsal neck as the major site of vascular ingress into the first metatarsal head, suggesting that the long plantar limb of a chevron osteotomy should exit well proximal to the capsular attachment to decrease the risk of postoperative osteonecrosis.

Loss of correction after a chevron osteotomy is relatively common. Kaufman et al. examined preoperative radiographic measurements to determine correlations with recurrence and found that increased deformity (intermetatarsal angle, hallux valgus angle, distal metatarsal angle, and sesamoid position) preoperatively were statistically significantly correlated with loss of correction postoperatively.

Malunion after a chevron osteotomy is uncommon if three steps in operative technique are followed: (1) The osteotomy is internally fixed and manually tested, and fixation is augmented with additional fixation if any movement occurs; (2) the distal fragment is placed plantar or inferior to the proximal fragment and secured in that position with internal fixation; and (3) weight bearing is guarded if fixation is not rigid.

The difficulty in correcting a dorsal malunion after chevron osteotomy is preserving length. The initial chevron osteotomy often shortens the hallux 3 to 5 mm, and impaction and necrosis at the osteotomy site can decrease length another 3 to 5 mm, resulting in 6 to 10 mm of shortening that causes transfer metatarsalgia beneath the second metatarsal head or prevents relief of existing metatarsalgia. Although a second metatarsal transfer lesion was noted to occur in 2.7% of patients in one study after distal chevron metatarsal osteotomy, it did not appear to be correlated with the amount of first metatarsal shortening. Varus or valgus malunion can occur after a chevron osteotomy, but this is not as common as dorsal malunion. Varus or valgus malunion of a chevron osteotomy, even with mild-to-moderate incongruity of the first metatarsophalangeal joint, is tolerated better by the patient than a dorsal malunion with transfer metatarsalgia. Regardless of the plane of the malunion, the surgical technique to correct the deformity is basically the same.

To determine if generalized ligamentous laxity is a risk factor for recurrence of hallux valgus, Cho et al. compared recurrence rates in patients with and without ligamentous laxity who underwent a chevron osteotomy. Twenty-two of 23 patients with generalized ligamentous laxity had recurrence, and 17% of 175 patients without laxity had recurrence at a mean follow-up of 46.3 months. These authors noted no statistically significant differences in clinical or radiographic outcomes between those with and without laxity after the chevron osteotomy.

CORRECTION OF MALUNION OF THE CHEVRON OSTEOTOMY

TECHNIQUE 2.26

- Expose the distal metatarsal from the junction of the middle and distal thirds to the base of the proximal phalanx.
- Inspect the previous osteotomy, but do not allow its "limbs" to predetermine the plane of the corrective osteotomy.
- With a 2-mm drill bit (even smaller if available), make a semicircle of unicortical holes from dorsal to plantar adjacent to or within the previous osteotomy site (an arc of approximately 150 degrees).
- Connect these holes using only the corner of a 5- or 6-mm sharp, straight, thin osteotome as a cutting edge. Do not penetrate the lateral cortex with the osteotome.

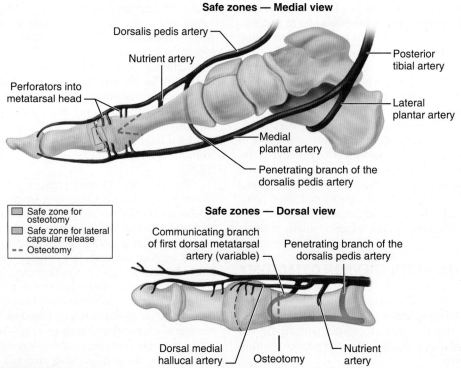

Safe zones — Medial view

Dorsalis pedis artery

Nutrient artery

Perforators into metatarsal head

Posterior tibial artery

Lateral plantar artery

Medial plantar artery

Penetrating branch of the dorsalis pedis artery

- Safe zone for osteotomy
- Safe zone for lateral capsular release
- -- Osteotomy

Safe zones — Dorsal view

Communicating branch of first dorsal metatarsal artery (variable)

Penetrating branch of the dorsalis pedis artery

Dorsal medial hallucal artery

Osteotomy

Nutrient artery

FIGURE 2.85 Safe zones for chevron osteotomy and lateral capsular release. Medial view shows that sites of cortical osteotomy must remain in interval between pericapsular perforators distally and nutrient artery proximally. Safe zone for lateral capsular release spares all perforators into metatarsal head proximally and all perforators into proximal phalanx distally, as long as capsulotomy is performed in line with metatarsophalangeal joint in coronal plane. Dorsal view shows relationship between osteotomy and nutrient artery and distal pericapsular perforators. First dorsal metatarsal artery and its branches are especially vulnerable to overpenetration of lateral cortex by oscillating saw. (From Jones KJ, Feiwell LA, Freedman EL, et al: The effects of chevron osteotomy with lateral capsular release on the blood supply to the first metatarsal head, *J Bone Joint Surg* 77A:197, 1995.)

- Using the 2-mm (or smaller) drill bit, make numerous holes in the lateral cortex through the unicortical osteotomized semicircle, and complete the osteotomy with a thin (4-mm-wide) blade on a small power saw. This technique reduces the amount of shortening.
- Manually rotate the head plantarward until the dorsal cortex of the capital (distal) fragment is inferior (plantar) to the dorsal cortex of the shaft (proximal) fragment. This slightly plantarflexes the first metatarsal head, allowing it to assume more of the weight-bearing load across the metatarsal heads.
- If the capital fragment has healed in varus or valgus, reverse the deformity until the capital fragment is reduced to normal anatomic alignment with the shaft. The malunion may be in two or more planes, but this "broomstick" osteotomy would allow correction of all planes of deformity.
- Internally fix the osteotomy with Kirschner wires, small screws, or absorbable pins. Interfragmentary wires are technically difficult to use in this location but are not contraindicated.

POSTOPERATIVE CARE Depending on the rigidity of fixation and body habitus of the patient and the anticipated compliance by the patient, protected weight bearing can begin immediately. A short leg cast that extends distal to the toes and crutches or a walker may be necessary. The patient should be told before surgery that permanent loss of some metatarsophalangeal joint motion is possible, but that function should not be compromised. Full, unprotected weight bearing is allowed when union of the osteotomy is apparent clinically and radiographically. Final range of motion often is not reached for 12 to 18 months postoperatively.

METATARSAL SHORTENING

Some shortening of the first metatarsal can occur with both proximal and distal chevron osteotomies, as well as with other types of osteotomy. The average shortening is reported to be 2 to 6 mm with distal osteotomies and nearly 3 mm with proximal osteotomies. Shortening of the first metatarsal may disrupt the normal weight-transfer mechanism, resulting in overload of the adjacent metatarsals with metatarsalgia and forefoot pain. Transfer metatarsalgia generally is treated conservatively with various orthoses, but when this treatment fails and symptoms are severe, operative treatment is indicated. Shortening or elevating osteotomies of the lesser metatarsals often are recommended. Although these osteotomies may be successful, the potential exists for several complications, including nonunion, floating-toe deformity, persistent metatarsalgia, and marked forefoot shortening. Rather than shortening the normal metatarsals and further altering the normal anatomy of the foot, distraction osteogenesis of the first metatarsal has been recommended to more closely restore normal foot anatomy and biomechanics. Hurst and Nunley described their technique using a unilateral, single-plane external fixator. There are few reports of the outcomes of this procedure, and we have no experience with it.

DISTRACTION OSTEOGENESIS FOR METATARSAL SHORTENING

TECHNIQUE 2.27

- After induction of anesthesia and sterile preparation of the foot, use fluoroscopic control and the fixator chosen for distraction to determine proper position of the holes for fixator placement.
- With a 1.5-mm Kirschner wire, drill the holes percutaneously along the medial side of the first metatarsal; insert four self-tapping pins with 2.5-mm tapered threads and 3-mm-diameter shafts into the holes. Place the distal two pins first and then the proximal pins.
- Orient the pins in the metatarsal so that the distraction force of the fixator will provide relative plantarflexion to the metatarsal head. To achieve this orientation, place the two distal pins in the plantar half of the distal metatarsal fragment, which will create a relatively plantarward distraction vector.
- Make a 2-cm incision along the medial border of the metatarsal between the second and third pins.
- Carry dissection down to the bone and sharply incise the periosteum longitudinally, leaving it intact laterally, anteriorly, and posteriorly.
- In the area of the proposed osteotomy, minimally strip the periosteum with a periosteal elevator and preserve it for later closure.
- Use a mini–sagittal saw to make a transverse osteotomy between the second and third pins, cooling the blade with normal saline irrigation.
- Confirm the adequacy and distractibility of the osteotomy by distracting the fixator 5 mm and obtaining a fluoroscopic image.
- Compress the distractor to achieve bone-on-bone contact and tighten it.
- Approximate the periosteum with 4-0 absorbable polyglactin suture and close the skin with simple sutures of 4-0 nylon; apply a soft dressing.

POSTOPERATIVE CARE The patient is discharged home on the day of surgery, with instructions to remain non–weight bearing on the operated foot. The dressing is removed at the first clinic visit 1 week after surgery, at which time the sutures are removed and radiographs are obtained. At this visit, patients are taught to distract the fixator at home by turning the external fixator key one-quarter turn four times a day to equal a distraction rate of 1 mm of lengthening per day. The goal is to obtain equal lengths of the first and second metatarsals to restore the normal "windlass" mechanism. Patients are kept non–weight bearing during the entire lengthening phase. When there is radiographic evidence of consolidation in the distracted segment, partial weight bearing is permitted. Daily passive range of motion of the metatarsophalangeal joint is encouraged during both the distraction and consolidation phases to prevent joint stiffness. The external fixator is kept in place until full consolidation is seen on multiple radiographic views. After removal of the fixator, full weight bearing and normal shoe wear are allowed as tolerated.

■ ACQUIRED HALLUX VARUS AND INTRINSIC MINUS HALLUX

Hallux varus (Figs. 2.86 and 2.87) is a complication of hallux valgus surgery that was not widely recognized until McBride in 1935 reported its occurrence in 5% of patients treated with his procedure (medial eminence removal, medial capsulorrhaphy, and fibular sesamoidectomy) (Fig. 2.88). Since then, many authors have reported this complication, with incidences ranging from 2% (Peterson et al.) to 17% (Trnka et al.) after almost all operations for hallux valgus, including distal and proximal metatarsal osteotomies. Few patients with hallux varus complain about appearance (only if varus is > 10 to 15 degrees) or discomfort (rare and usually associated with degenerative changes of the first metatarsophalangeal joint). The main causes for hallux varus after hallux valgus surgery are (1) complete release of the lateral structures of the metatarsophalangeal joint combined with excessive plication of the medial capsule, which pulls the sesamoids too far medially; (2) excessive resection of the medial eminence, leading to loss of medial bony buttress for the proximal phalanx; (3) excision of the fibular sesamoid; (4) release of the lateral head of the flexor hallucis brevis at its insertion into the fibular sesamoid; and (5) closure of the intermetatarsal angle to neutral or a negative value.

Hallux varus can be classified into two types: static (supple) and dynamic (fixed). There are two reasons to divide hallux varus deformities. The first is to place the focus on the intrinsic and extrinsic muscle imbalance, which explains the single and multiplanar types of deformity, and the second is to alert the surgeon that presurgical planning for correction would be different. Static hallux varus, which is supple, uniplanar, and passively correctable, usually is asymptomatic and mainly is a cosmetic complication. When the foot is viewed in a weight-bearing position, the hallux rests in varus, the metatarsophalangeal joint rests in a normal position in the sagittal plane (10 degrees to the plantar surface of the foot or 20 to 25 degrees to the first metatarsal), and the interphalangeal joint is in a normal position. Most often, the hallux is not rotated abnormally in an axial plane and does not assume a "snake-in-the-grass" appearance in the frontal plane. All the deformity occurs at the metatarsophalangeal joint, but only in the transverse or frontal plane. Dynamic hallux varus deformity is a multiplanar deformity that often is fixed, symptomatic, and difficult to correct surgically (Fig. 2.89). The term that best describes the deformity is *intrinsic minus deformity of the hallux with a varus component*. This

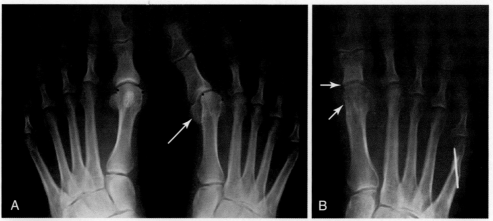

FIGURE 2.86 **A,** Hallux varus after McBride bunionectomy with subluxation of tibial sesamoid. **B,** Correction of hallux varus after Keller procedure.

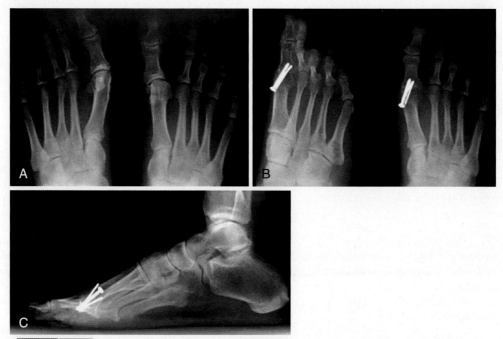

FIGURE 2.87 **A,** Relatively mild hallux varus with symptomatic degenerative arthritis of first metatarsophalangeal joint. **B** and **C,** Arthrodesis was chosen because of degenerative joint disease.

is a true intrinsic-extrinsic muscle imbalance. In dynamic hallux varus, the first metatarsophalangeal joint is hyperextended (usually with some degree of fixed soft-tissue contracture) and the interphalangeal joint is acutely flexed. The hallux is rotated, and its varus and extended posture makes shoe wear difficult. The most common complaint is that the toe box of the shoe rubs on the dorsomedial surface of the interphalangeal joint. A keratotic lesion may be present beneath the first metatarsal head, caused by the extended hallux pushing the first metatarsal head plantarward. The lesser toes may develop a hammer deformity and metatarsalgia as the hallux assists less and less in the stance phase of the gait cycle.

ANATOMY AND PATHOGENESIS

The intrinsic muscles balance the hallux on the first metatarsal head, whereas the extrinsic muscles add gross balance and

greatly increase the mobility of the hallux. The first metatarsophalangeal joint is a shallow, ball-and-socket joint with little stability from bony configurations. The tendon insertions of the abductor-adductor hallucis, the flexor hallucis brevis (both components), and the extensor hallucis brevis balance the hallux congruently on the first metatarsal head and act synchronously with the extrinsic muscle-tendon units of the extensor flexor hallucis longus. This balance is disrupted if the positions of these tendon insertions are altered relative to the axis of rotation in flexion or extension at the metatarsophalangeal joint.

The pathogenesis of hallux varus can best be explained after a McBride procedure with a fibular sesamoidectomy. Fibular sesamoidectomy and release of the adductor tendon can allow the tibial sesamoid (medial head flexor hallucis brevis) to drift medially, exerting a varus movement on the proximal phalanx (Fig. 2.90), and allow the

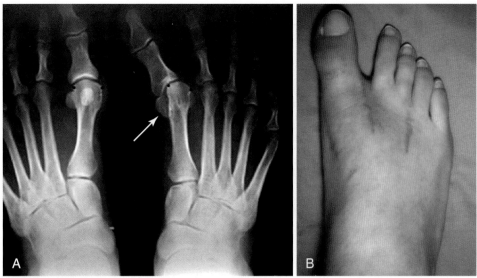

FIGURE 2.88 **A,** Fixed hallux varus after McBride bunionectomy. **B,** Hallux varus after McBride bunionectomy with fibular sesamoid excision. Removing fibular sesamoid removes valgus-producing moments of adductor hallucis and flexor hallucis brevis (lateral head) muscles.

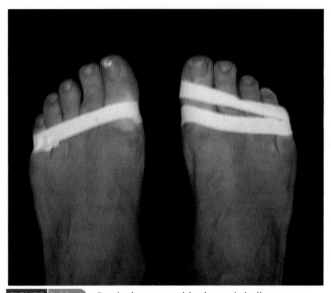

FIGURE 2.89 Passively correctable dynamic hallux varus.

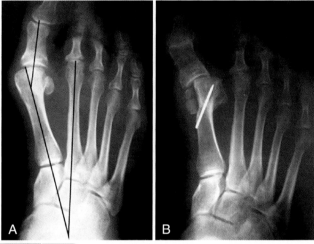

FIGURE 2.90 **A,** Hallux valgus deformity. **B,** Dislocation of tibial sesamoid after distal metatarsal osteotomy and fibular sesamoidectomy.

abductor tendon to overpower its antagonist, the released adductor tendon. With varus of the metatarsophalangeal joint, the extensor hallucis longus, the flexor hallucis longus, and the flexor hallucis brevis medial head are positioned medial to the midline in the axial plane, increasing the varus deformity. This is exactly the opposite of the mechanism of action in hallux valgus, in which the musculotendinous structures of the metatarsophalangeal joint accentuate the hallux valgus when they are positioned lateral to the axial midline of the metatarsophalangeal joint. After release of the lateral head of the flexor hallucis brevis from the fibular sesamoid (fibular sesamoidectomy) and medial subluxation of the medial head of the flexor hallucis brevis (tibial sesamoid), the medial head of the flexor hallucis brevis is no longer an efficient flexor of the metatarsophalangeal joint and is overpowered by the retained

extensors of the metatarsophalangeal joint, creating an extension deformity of the metatarsophalangeal joint. As extension of the metatarsophalangeal joint increases, the flexor hallucis longus tightens, and the extensor hallucis longus loosens, creating a flexion deformity of the interphalangeal joint (Fig. 2.91). This deformity may quickly become fixed and is described as *clawed hallux deformity* or *intrinsic minus hallucal deformity*.

Uniplanar deformity most commonly occurs when a mild-to-moderate hallux valgus deformity is treated with a lateral soft-tissue release combined with medial capsular imbrication and medial eminence excision. Excision of too much of the medial eminence (within or immediately lateral to the sagittal groove) has been cited as a major contributing factor to hallux varus. Excision of the fibular sesamoid and overcorrection of the first intermetatarsal angle to less than 5 degrees also can produce hallux varus

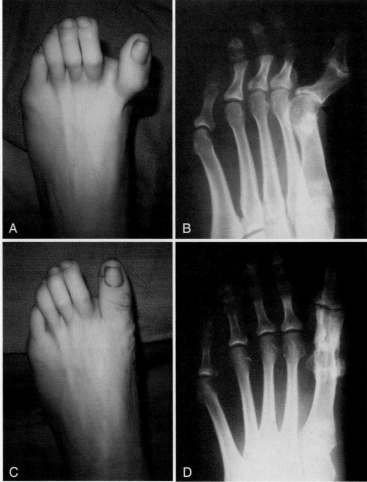

A and **B,** Hyperextension of metatarsophalangeal joint and hyperflexion of inter-phalangeal joint, in addition to varus and rotation of hallux. **C** and **D,** Dynamic (supple) deformity treated by arthrodesis of first metatarsophalangeal joint and plantar release of interphalangeal joint.

uniplanar deformity. Normally, the hallux rests on the first metatarsal head in about 10 degrees of valgus. If the inter-metatarsal angle is reduced to less than 5 degrees, and the hallux is reduced congruously on the metatarsal head, the necessary valgus angulation must be 15 degrees (5 degrees varus of the first metatarsal plus 10 degrees distal metatar-sal articular angle). Often the hallux is aligned parallel to the second toe if that toe is straight or to the medial border of the foot if it is not, but this clinically straight posture places the hallux into varus in relation to the articular sur-face of the first metatarsal head. When the lateral restrain-ing structures are released and the medial eminence is removed, the hallux is at risk of drifting further into varus. Overcorrection of the intermetatarsal angle and removal of the medial eminence at the sagittal groove instead of medial to it may contribute to the development of hallux varus deformity. Correction of the intermetatarsal angle to less than 5 degrees, excision of the fibular sesamoid, lat-eral capsulotomy, adductor release, and imbrication of the medial capsule, in combination or alone, may contribute to a hallux varus deformity. The powerful flexor hallucis bre-vis can be a significant valgus- or varus-deforming force if the sesamoid is not in its facet.

CORRECTION OF UNIPLANAR (STATIC) HALLUX VARUS DEFORMITY

Not all patients with acquired hallux varus require operative treatment. Varus deformity of 5 to 6 degrees is minimal and generally is only a radiographic finding, rather than a defor-mity that compromises the clinical result. In addition to an unsatisfactory appearance of the toe, some patients com-plain of difficulty wearing shoes, pain, instability, weakness with push-off, and metatarsalgia. A conservative program of modified shoe wear and taping of the hallux should be attempted in all patients before surgery is contemplated.

If uniplanar hallux varus develops after a soft-tissue proce-dure alone and is not fixed, weekly dressings and tapings of the hallux in a valgus posture of 10 to 15 degrees may correct the deformity if this treatment begins within the first 4 to 6 weeks, continues for 8 to 12 weeks, and is fol-lowed by treatment with a night splint that holds the hallux in slight valgus for an additional 3 months. If the deformity goes unnoticed for 2 months or longer after surgery and is symptomatic, however, surgical correction is required. This should be delayed until the soft tissue has no evidence of inflammation from the first procedure. A medial capsulotomy in the sagittal plane, placing the sesamoids in their proper location if subluxed medially, and holding the hallux in 10 to 15 degrees of valgus with a Kirschner wire for 6 weeks may be all that is necessary, especially if the deformity is passively correctable and 10 to 15 degrees of valgus is achievable. The success or failure rests almost entirely on the position and the moment of the flexor hallucis brevis. The surgical treatment of this deformity is straightforward, and results are predictable.

TECHNIQUE 2.28

SOFT-TISSUE CORRECTION

- Make an incision on the medial side of the hallux at the midline in the internervous plane, extending from the midportion of the diaphysis of the proximal phalanx to 4 to 5 cm proximal to the metatarsophalangeal joint. Raise a dorsal skin flap (on the capsule) 4 to 5 mm and a plantar flap 2 to 3 mm. Do not injure the dorsal sensory nerve near the junction of the (former) medial eminence and first metatarsal.
- Make a capsular incision in the midline medially.
- Elevate the dorsal and plantar capsular flaps until the dorsomedial corner of the first metatarsal and the tibial sesamoid plantarward are clearly exposed.
- After the hallux is adducted to the midline, flex and extend the first metatarsophalangeal joint. Carry the soft-tissue release dorsally and plantarward until the hallux can be placed into 10 to 15 degrees of valgus on the first metatarsal head. Flex and extend the hallux and passively dorsiflex it 40 to 50 degrees in this valgus position.
- Place a small osteotome or periosteal elevator between the articular surface of the tibial sesamoid and the first metatarsal head. If the tibial sesamoid slides back into its facet on the metatarsal head with passive valgus of the hallux or requires only gentle levering and pushing to reduce and maintain it in the facet, the correction will be long lasting. If the tibial sesamoid cannot be reduced and maintained in its facet, soft-tissue balance and realignment will fail, and an arthrodesis or hemiresection arthroplasty to loosen the soft tissue must be performed.
- With the hallux positioned in 15 degrees valgus, 10 degrees extension, and neutral rotation, place a 0.062-inch Kirschner wire obliquely from distal medial in the proximal phalanx to proximal lateral in the first metatarsal, starting at the metaphyseal-diaphyseal flair of the proximal phalanx.
- Cut the wire beneath the skin so that it can be removed in the office under local anesthesia. Leaving it external to the skin is more likely to cause premature removal from pin track soft-tissue irritation.
- Release the tourniquet and obtain hemostasis. *Do not close the capsule.* Close the skin with permanent 4-0 monofilament nylon sutures in one layer. Place simple stitches near the wound margins because the skin is under tension, and mattress sutures may compromise the blood supply to the skin margins further. Because neither capsular nor subcutaneous sutures are allowed, use more stitches than usual to avoid gaps between the stitches that could cause a synovial fistula or an infection.
- Apply a forefoot dressing. The dressing does not have to help maintain the reduced position of the hallux because

of the articular wire but should be gently conforming and snug to reduce edema.

- In the Hawkins technique, the lateral structures are released and the muscle-tendon unit of the abductor hallucis is transferred to the base of the proximal phalanx plantar to the transverse intermetatarsal ligament and through a long bone tunnel and sutured to the soft tissue medially. The adductor hallucis and flexor hallucis brevis conjoined tendon is moved proximally and sutured into the lateral aspect of the metatarsal head dorsal to the transferred abductor hallucis tendon (Fig. 2.92).

POSTOPERATIVE CARE The initial dressing is maintained for 10 to 14 days (19 to 21 days is permissible) to ensure skin healing without interruption of the dermal adhesion. A removable short leg walking boot is preferred to immobilize the ankle, but it is optional. The patient is allowed touch-down weight bearing with crutches for 3 weeks and then weight bearing to tolerance without crutches another 3 weeks in the removable walking boot. The boot can be removed only to bathe the first 3 weeks, after which it can be removed during bed and bath periods. The pin is removed in the office in 4 to 6 weeks. (If reduction was difficult, the pin should be left in for 6 weeks.) The pin should not be removed before 3 weeks unless pressing circumstances require it. If it is necessary to remove the pin earlier than planned, the hallux is taped to the second and third toes until the hallux has no tendency to drift medially from its valgus posture when the patient is standing.

DISTAL METATARSAL OSTEOTOMY, MEDIAL CAPSULAR RELEASE WITHOUT TENDON TRANSFER

Choi et al. described an alternative procedure for hallux varus after hallux valgus surgery in 19 patients (20 to 65 years of age). Thirteen patients had been treated by a scarf osteotomy, and six underwent a proximal chevron osteotomy initially. After their corrective surgery, 11 patients were very satisfied, seven were satisfied, and one was very dissatisfied. The mean hallux valgus angle, intermetatarsal angle, and distal metatarsal articular anlage improved significantly from preoperative to postoperative, and the mean relative length ratio of the metatarsus decreased significantly. Two patients had recurrences of the hallux varus deformity, one required no further procedures, and the other required repeat distal metatarsal osteotomy. No other complications were reported.

TECHNIQUE 2.29

- To expose the head of the first metatarsal, make a medial longitudinal incision through the previous scar. Make a T-shaped capsular incision, the horizontal one along the metatarsophalangeal joint line and the vertical one along the shaft of the first metatarsal.

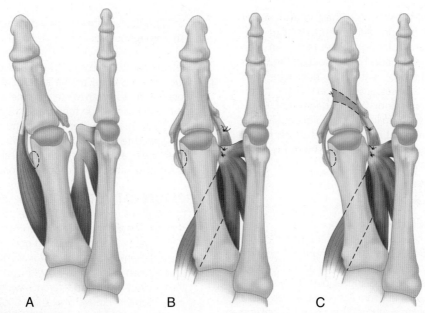

FIGURE 2.92 Hawkins technique for correction of hallux varus. **A,** Hallux varus secondary to muscle imbalance. **B,** Repositioning of abductor hallucis to remnant of adductor hallucis. **C,** Suturing of abductor hallucis lengthened by tendon graft into base of proximal phalanx and repositioning of conjoined tendon. (Redrawn from Hawkins FB: Acquired hallux varus: cause, prevention and correction, *Clin Orthop Relat Res* 76:169, 1971.) **SEE TECHNIQUE 2.28.**

- Perform a distal metatarsal chevron osteotomy at an angle of 60 degrees to the apex of the distal portion (Fig. 2.93A).
- Translate the distal fragment medially. Create a 1- to 3-mm medial biplanar closing wedge 8 to 10 mm proximal from the first metatarsophalangeal joint line. The degree of the medial closing wedge is based on the distal metatarsal articular angle.
- Fix the osteotomy with one or two Kirschner wires (Fig. 2.93B,C).
- Do not repair the medial capsules to allow for medial release.
- If severe varus instability remains, make a 2- to 3-mm transverse capsular excision through the previous scar over the dorsum of the first web. Tighten the lateral capsule.

POSTOPERATIVE CARE Immediate weight bearing is allowed in a wooden-soled rocker-bottom shoe for 6 to 8 weeks postoperatively. Passive exercises of the metatarsophalangeal joint are started at 2 weeks postoperatively.

TRANSFER OF EXTENSOR HALLUCIS LONGUS WITH ARTHRODESIS OF THE INTERPHALANGEAL JOINT OF THE HALLUX

Occasionally, an arthrodesis or tendon transfer may be required in a static, uniplanar deformity, but the patient must be informed preoperatively that one or the other may be required if the deformity cannot be corrected otherwise. When the metatarsophalangeal joint deformity is static, usually the interphalangeal joint deformity also is static. Extensor hallucis longus transfer usually is recommended for supple deformity of the metatarsophalangeal joint, combined with interphalangeal joint fusion whether the interphalangeal joint deformity is dynamic or static. For a combined supple interphalangeal and metatarsophalangeal joint deformity, transfer of only half of the extensor hallucis longus tendon without arthrodesis of the hallux interphalangeal joint is recommended to allow free interphalangeal joint motion; if the extensor hallucis longus transfer fails to correct the hallux varus and a subsequent metatarsophalangeal joint fusion is necessary, a better result will be obtained if the interphalangeal joint retains some motion. Fusion of the interphalangeal joint aids in the correction of the metatarsophalangeal joint extension by having the flexor hallucis longus flex the great toe at the metatarsophalangeal joint, rather than at the interphalangeal joint. Transfer of only half of the extensor hallucis longus is inappropriate, however, because it requires the extensor hallucis longus to perform two actions simultaneously: extension of the interphalangeal joint and adduction of the metatarsophalangeal joint. Both techniques correct the deformity, and both reduce motion at the metatarsophalangeal joint, occasionally severely. The patient must be informed that a correction of deformity may produce a reduction in motion.

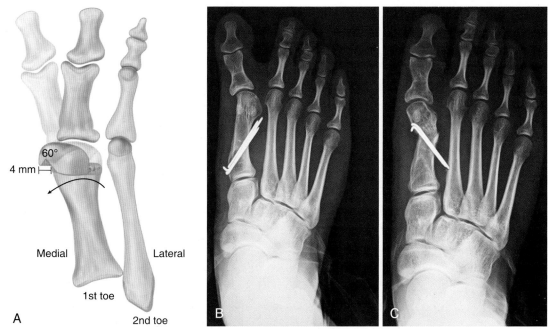

FIGURE 2.93 **A,** Distal chevron metatarsal osteotomy with medial translation of distal fragment. **B,** Hallux varus deformity with negative intermetatarsal angle that occurred after proximal chevron osteotomy. **C,** Twenty-four-month follow-up showing correction and congruent metatarsophalangeal joint. (From Choi KJ, Lee HS, Yoon YS, et al: Distal metatarsal osteotomy for hallux varus following surgery for hallux valgus, *J Bone Joint Surg* 93B:1079, 2011. Copyright British Editorial Society of Bone and Joint Surgery.) **SEE TECHNIQUE 2.29.**

TECHNIQUE 2.30

(JOHNSON AND SPIEGL)

- Begin an L-shaped incision between the midportions of the first and second metatarsals, extend it distally along the dorsolateral aspect of the great toe, and curve it medially near the insertion of the extensor hallucis longus tendon (Fig. 2.94A).
- Divide the extensor hallucis tendon at its insertion on the base of the distal phalanx. Avoid the dorsal sensory nerve and the nail bed.
- Perform an arthrodesis of the interphalangeal joint after removing the articular surfaces to permit a neutral position in the sagittal and coronal planes (Fig. 2.94B-D). The use of a 4-mm cancellous bone screw, advocated by Shives and Johnson, has proved beneficial.
- Drill a 2-mm-diameter hole longitudinally in a retrograde manner at the denuded articular surface of the distal phalanx (Fig. 2.94E). The drill should exit at a point 5 mm plantar to the tip of the nail in the midline of the toe.
- Appose the denuded articular surfaces, insert the drill bit distally at the tip of the phalanx, and, following the previously placed hole, drill into the base of the proximal phalanx and down the center of its medullary canal (Fig. 2.94F,G).
- Overdrill the distal phalanx with a 2.7-mm drill bit and tap the entire drill path with a 3.5-mm tap.
- Following the drill bit in a proximal direction, insert the 4-mm cancellous bone screw (Fig. 2.94H). The lag effect of this screw produces compression and firm fixation of the arthrodesis (Fig. 2.94I to M).
- When the arthrodesis is completed, dissect the extensor hallucis longus free from the extensor mechanism and proximal fascial attachments to 5 to 6 cm proximal to the metatarsophalangeal joint. The tendon should exhibit free excursion with gentle traction and relaxation (Fig. 2.95A).
- Pass a nonabsorbable suture back and forth through the distal 1.5 cm of tendon and lay it aside temporarily.
- Drill a 3.6-mm hole in the dorsoplantar direction in the lateral side of the proximal phalanx (Fig. 2.95B).
- With a hemostat, grasp the suture in the end of the tendon and pass it plantar to the deep transverse intermetatarsal ligament (see Fig. 2.95B). The transferred tendon cannot correct the hallux extensus or hallux varus if it is not passed plantar to a pulley that is plantar to the flexion-extension axis of the first metatarsophalangeal joint. Johnson and Spiegl stated that the earlier formed surgical scar in this region never interfered with use of the ligament as a suitable pulley.
- Pass the tendon through the hole in the phalanx from the plantar to the dorsal direction and place the hallux in the desired position (a medial capsulotomy and possibly a tibial sesamoidectomy may be required before the hallux can be positioned properly).
- Pull the extensor hallucis longus distally and suture it to itself (see Fig. 2.95C).
- Insert a 0.062-inch Kirschner wire obliquely across the joint, taking care not to impale the tendon and weaken it (see Fig. 2.95D).

POSTOPERATIVE CARE A compression dressing is worn for 2 days, followed by a short leg, non–weight-bearing cast, which is worn for 3 weeks. The cast is changed, and weight bearing is allowed in the new cast, which is worn for 3 more weeks. The Kirschner wire is removed, and

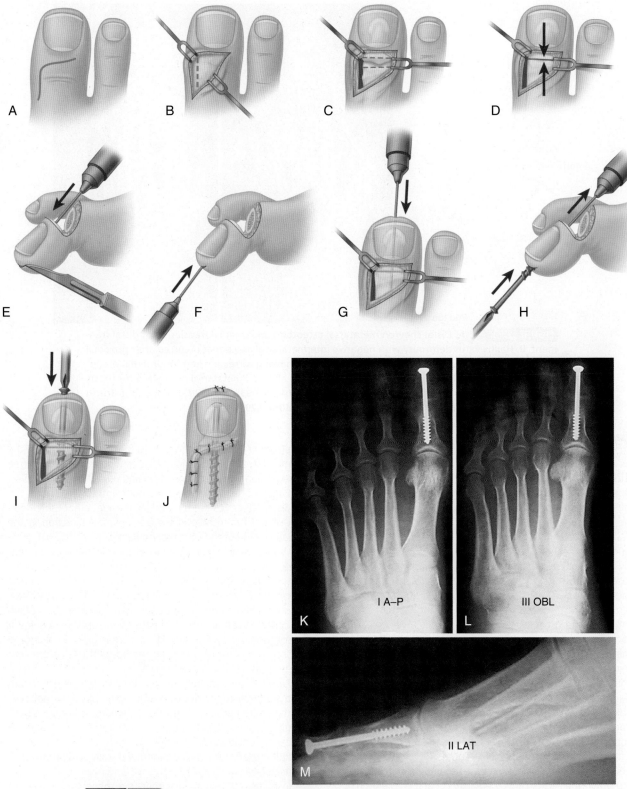

FIGURE 2.94 Johnson and Spiegl arthrodesis technique for correction of hallux varus. **A-C,** L-shaped skin incision, release of extensor hallucis longus, and preparation of joint for arthrodesis. **D-F,** Apposition of surfaces to confirm good bony apposition and retrograde drilling with 2-mm bit. **G,** Antegrade drilling of proximal phalanx. **H,** Insertion of 4-mm cancellous screw. **I,** Compression of arthrodesis site as lag effect is created. **J,** Closure. **K-M,** Radiographs of interphalangeal joint arthrodesis of great toe. (A-J redrawn from Shives TC, Johnson KA: Arthrodesis of the interphalangeal joint of the great toe: an improved technique, *Foot Ankle* 1:26, 1980.) **SEE TECHNIQUE 2.30.**

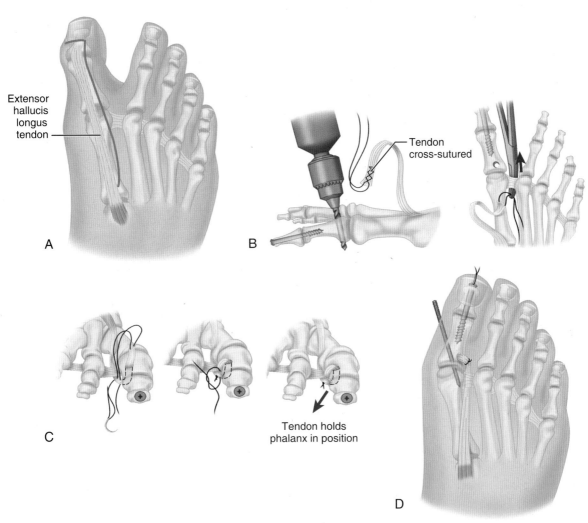

Extensor hallucis longus tendon

Tendon cross-sutured

A

B

Tendon holds phalanx in position

C

D

FIGURE 2.95 **A-D,** Transfer of extensor hallucis longus (Johnson and Spiegl technique) for correction of hallux varus (see text). (From Johnson KA, Spiegl P: Extensor hallucis longus transfer for hallux varus deformity, *J Bone Joint Surg* 66A:681, 1984.) **SEE TECHNIQUE 2.30.**

weight bearing is allowed without a cast (night splinting of the hallux in the desired position for another 10 to 12 weeks should be considered).

EXTENSOR HALLUCIS BREVIS TENODESIS

TECHNIQUE 2.31

(MYERSON AND KOMENDA; JULIANO ET AL.)
- Make a dorsal longitudinal incision in the first web space, extending proximally 2 inches.
- Retract the terminal branch of the deep peroneal nerve and transect the extensor hallucis brevis at the musculotendinous junction (Fig. 2.96A).

- Insert a 4-0 monofilament suture into the stump of the extensor hallucis brevis tendon and dissect it free of soft tissues to its distal attachment into the extensor hood. Do not interrupt this attachment.
- Free the proximal end of the extensor hallucis brevis from its attachment to the extensor hallucis longus tendon.
- Perform a dorsal and medial capsulotomy, or capsulectomy if required, to correct the extension deformity at the metatarsophalangeal joint.
- Release the abductor tendon with the medial capsulotomy. Before performing the extensor hallucis brevis tenodesis, completely release the dorsal and medial soft-tissue contractures, and assess the resting position of the hallux after this release. The deformity should now be passively correctable. If not, complete the capsulotomy or capsulectomy from sesamoid to sesamoid.
- Pass the stump of the extensor hallucis brevis tendon plantar to the deep transverse metatarsal ligament from distal to proximal (Fig. 2.96B).
- Apply tension to the extensor hallucis brevis tendon and assess alignment and rotation of the hallux. Because of the dorsal insertion of this tendon, there is a tendency to

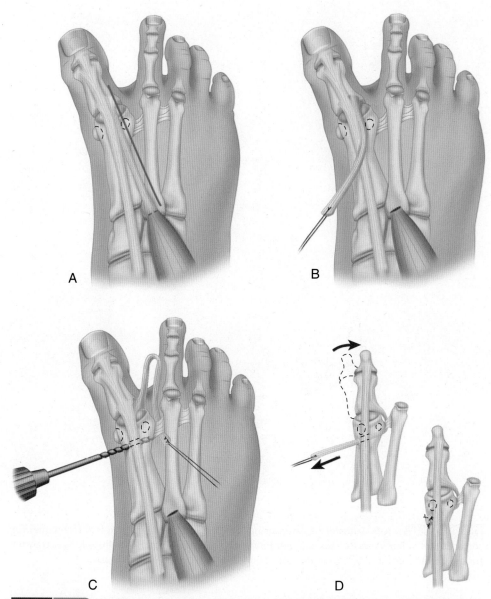

FIGURE **2.96** Hallux varus correction using extensor hallucis brevis tenodesis. **A,** Dorsal incision and transection of extensor hallucis brevis tendon. **B,** Transected tendon is passed deep to transverse metatarsal ligament from distal to proximal. **C,** Hole is drilled in dorsomedial first metatarsal. **D,** Extensor hallucis brevis tendon is pulled through drill hole and secured with sutures to periosteum or bone. (Redrawn from Juliano PJ, Meyerson MS, Cunningham BW: Biomechanical assessment of a new tenodesis for correction of hallux varus, *Foot Ankle Int* 17:17, 1996.) **SEE TECHNIQUE 2.31.**

supinate (internally rotate) the hallux as the extensor hallucis brevis tendon is proximally redirected. If this occurs, partially release the distal insertion of the tendon so that the attachment is not as dorsally located.

- Attach the extensor hallucis brevis tendon to the first metatarsal shaft under tension.
- With the tendon pulled in a proximal direction, assess the range of motion of the hallux metatarsophalangeal joint and compare with the motion with no tension on the tenodesis. Expect mild loss of passive flexion. The patient should be made aware of this preoperatively. Because the extensor hallucis brevis transfer is to function as a tenodesis and not as a dynamic tendon transfer, the goal is to apply the maximal tension on the tendon that would

interfere the least with range of motion at the metatarsophalangeal joint.

- The desired position of the hallux after correction is 5 degrees of valgus. Secure the extensor hallucis brevis tendon to the first metatarsal through a bone tunnel 1.5 cm proximal to the joint, or use a bone suture anchor (Fig. 2.96C,D). Use temporary pin fixation across the metatarsophalangeal joint for further stabilization if needed.

POSTOPERATIVE CARE Weight bearing is permitted in a wooden-soled surgical shoe immediately after surgery. The shoe is used for an additional 4 weeks, after which time a comfortable stiff-soled shoe is permitted. The hallux is taped into valgus for 2 months after surgery. At that time, the patient is permitted to pursue any desired activity. Range-of-motion exercises of the hallux metatarsophalangeal joint are encouraged as soon as the wound permits, unless a pin across the metatarsophalangeal joint was required for stability. If used, the pin should be removed in 7 to 10 days and motion begun.

CORRECTION OF DYNAMIC (MULTIPLANAR) HALLUX VARUS

Treatment of dynamic deformity of the metatarsophalangeal joint is most often either resection arthroplasty (resecting the proximal third of the phalanx) or arthrodesis of the metatarsophalangeal joint (Fig. 2.97). If all components in the axial, coronal, and sagittal planes are correctable passively, however, and passive motion at the metatarsophalangeal joint approaches normal in flexion and extension, soft-tissue repair of the deformity may be successful.

The "hanging toe" procedure (resection of all intrinsic muscle attachments to the base of the proximal phalanx when the proximal third is removed) should include the insertion of two longitudinal, parallel Kirschner wires to maintain the position in 5 to 10 degrees of valgus for 6 weeks. Before placing the Kirschner wires in a retrograde direction through the proximal and distal phalanges and then in an antegrade direction into the metatarsal head, tension on the extensor hallucis longus tendon should be evaluated by holding the foot and ankle in the neutral position and judging if this tendon is causing an extensor posture of the hallux. If so, the tendon should be lengthened no more than 1 cm before fixation. If a fixed flexion contracture of the interphalangeal joint has caused symptomatic dorsal calluses, one of two procedures is recommended: (1) an arthrodesis of the interphalangeal joint at the time of resection arthroplasty of the metatarsophalangeal joint or (2) a plantar plate release at the interphalangeal joint with pin fixation holding the joint in a neutral position (Fig. 2.98).

Techniques of arthrodesis of the metatarsophalangeal and interphalangeal joints are described in Techniques 2.17 to 2.20. The technique of resection arthroplasty is described in Technique 2.2.

CLAW TOE (INTRINSIC IMBALANCED HALLUX)

In claw toe, the metatarsophalangeal joint is hyperextended and the interphalangeal joint is flexed with or without a fixed contracture of either joint. Hallux extensus frequently is present, resulting in the inability of the patient to place the pulp of the great toe to the floor or to the sole of a shoe when standing; the pulp of the great toe misses the ground during the stance phase of gait. The crucial loss is the intrinsic muscle flexion moment at the metatarsophalangeal joint. This results in hyperextension of the metatarsophalangeal joint by the unopposed extensor hallucis longus and brevis tendons and in the inability of the extensor hallucis longus tendon to extend the interphalangeal joint because of loss of excursion (slackness), which is caused by hyperextension of the first metatarsophalangeal joint. The loss of intrinsic muscle control usually is secondary to bilateral sesamoidectomy or fibular sesamoidectomy and dorsomedial subluxation of the tibial sesamoid after medial capsular imbrication (Fig. 2.99).

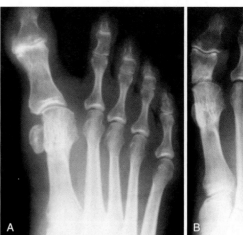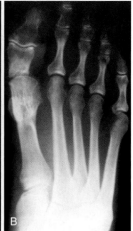

FIGURE 2.97   **A** and **B,** Preoperative and postoperative radiographs of middle-aged woman with multiplanar hallux varus deformity (clawed hallux) corrected by resection arthroplasty.

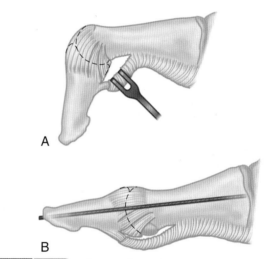

FIGURE 2.98   Plantar plate release. **A,** Exposure of plantar plate and partial release of flexor hallucis longus tendon. **B,** Excision of plantar plate from proximal phalanx. (Intramedullary Kirschner wire is recommended for 4 weeks.)

Arthrodesis of the interphalangeal joint, transfer of the extensor hallucis longus tendon into the neck of the metatarsal, and dorsal capsulotomy of the metatarsophalangeal joint constitute the treatment of choice to preserve metatarsophalangeal joint motion. Simple arthrodesis of the interphalangeal joint does not correct hyperextension of the metatarsophalangeal joint. In effect, the dorsal capsulotomy also lengthens the extensor hallucis brevis tendon when it heals with scar tissue in continuity. A Kirschner wire should be inserted to hold the metatarsophalangeal joint in the neutral position for 4 weeks. If degenerative articular changes are apparent radiographically, an arthrodesis of the first metatarsophalangeal joint is indicated.

LIMITATION OF METATARSOPHALANGEAL JOINT MOTION

An essential part of any soft-tissue procedure for hallux valgus is imbrication, or "reefing," of the medial capsule to

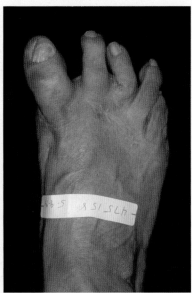

FIGURE 2.99 Dorsomedial subluxation of hallux after fibular sesamoidectomy, medial capsular imbrication, and displacement of tibial sesamoid medially.

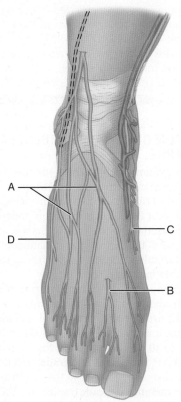

FIGURE 2.100 Two main branches of superficial peroneal nerve: medial (intermediate) branch to medial side of hallux and second and third dorsal web spaces and lateral branch to third and fourth dorsal web spaces (A). Deep peroneal nerve courses between first and second metatarsals to innervate skin of first web space dorsally (B). Saphenous nerve courses anterior to medial malleolus and innervates skin over dorsomedial aspect of hindfoot and midfoot (C). Sural nerve passes posterior to lateral malleolus and divides near calcaneocuboid joint into dorsal branch (which innervates fourth web space dorsally) and main trunk (which continues distally to supply skin of lateral side of fifth toe) (D). In practice, however, branch of superficial peroneal nerve to dorsomedial aspect of hallux is most vulnerable to injury.

correct the deformity without osteotomy or resection arthroplasty. Whether this capsulorrhaphy is performed coronally in the plane of the first metatarsophalangeal joint or longitudinally (sagittally) in the long axis of the first ray, the final outcome is soft-tissue plication around a mobile articulation. To maintain correction of the valgus, the capsulorrhaphy must be snug, which decreases metatarsophalangeal joint motion.

In our experience, even without intrinsic imbalance, loss of full flexion of the metatarsophalangeal joint is common after medial capsular plication but is seldom of clinical significance. Before any type of bunion surgery, patients should be informed that some loss of motion of the metatarsophalangeal joint may occur but that it should not decrease function or, in itself, produce symptoms. Wrapping the hallux during the postoperative period to hold the metatarsophalangeal joint in a neutral position or in 5 degrees of flexion is beneficial.

▌HALLUX EXTENSUS

Hallux extensus as an isolated deformity (i.e., without being a part of the hallux varus complex or a clawed hallux) is rare. One cause of such a deformity is laceration of the flexor hallucis longus tendon during sesamoidectomy or Keller resection arthroplasty. Consequently, the surgeon must ensure that the flexor hallucis longus tendon is intact by inspection and passive excursion after the sesamoid has been removed.

▌NEUROMA AND HEMATOMA

Neuroma and hematoma, inherent in any procedure on the foot, are largely avoidable with attention to anatomic detail and release of the tourniquet (if used), followed by meticulous hemostasis before wound closure. Because a neuroma of the foot may be a debilitating problem, illustrations of these cutaneous nerves are shown in Figure 2.100.

▌STRESS FRACTURES OF THE LESSER METATARSAL

Stress fractures occasionally occur in the second, third, or, in rare cases, fourth metatarsal, most often in postmenopausal women. Attempting to reduce weight on the first ray may overload the lesser metatarsals and cause a stress fracture. Protected weight bearing or use of a wooden-soled shoe usually relieves symptoms within 3 to 4 weeks. Occasionally, a stress fracture of the second or third metatarsal angulates apex plantar, however, resulting in dorsiflexion of the metatarsal head. This malunion shifts weight to the adjacent metatarsal heads, producing painful calluses. In osteoporotic patients when no callus is seen on radiographs, protection of a suspected fracture in a short leg walking boot or wooden (rigid) sole shoe is indicated to avoid this complication.

▇ COMPLICATIONS OF RESECTION ARTHROPLASTY OF THE FIRST METATARSOPHALANGEAL JOINT (KELLER PROCEDURE)

Resection arthroplasty continues to be recommended in certain patients with hallux valgus, especially elderly individuals with limited physical demands on their feet and some degree

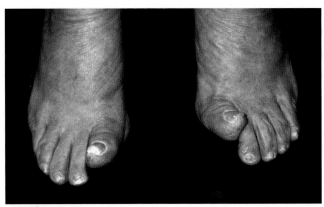

FIGURE 2.101 Hallux extensus on right foot and hallux extensus and recurrent valgus on left foot. These complications should be preventable when suggested techniques are used. (From Richardson EG, Graves SC: Keller bunionectomy. In Myerson M, editor: *Current therapy in foot and ankle surgery,* St. Louis, 1993, Mosby.)

of osteoarthritis of the first metatarsophalangeal joint. The procedure has not been embraced widely by orthopaedists, but it may have some merit in select patients, such as those with rheumatoid arthritis and severe destruction of the joints.

COCK-UP HALLUX

Complications of the Keller procedure are related to the intrinsic muscle attachments to the phalangeal base. Without the intrinsic muscles flexing the hallux, an extension deformity or contracture may develop at the first metatarsophalangeal joint with a concomitant flexion deformity at the interphalangeal joint. A callus that develops at the dorsum of the interphalangeal joint of the hallux is best treated by arthrodesis of the joint.

If the cock-up deformity of the hallux is severe and more than one third of the proximal phalanx has been excised (Fig. 2.101), an interposition corticocancellous bone graft may be necessary to correct the deformity at the metatarsophalangeal joint. This restores some length to the hallux and stabilizes the first metatarsophalangeal joint. This is a tedious procedure with a long recuperative period, however, and the arthrodesis commonly fails to unite. A simpler procedure should be chosen for patients with lesser degrees of bone shortening.

METATARSALGIA

Metatarsalgia present before surgery may be exacerbated by the Keller procedure. Because of unloading of the medial column by extreme varus of the first metatarsal, painful callosities often develop beneath one or more metatarsal heads. Realigning the first ray (bringing the first metatarsal closer to the second metatarsal) reduces the lesser metatarsal load and the likelihood of painful callosities beneath the second and third metatarsals. Patients should be instructed that the pain beneath the lesser metatarsal heads may not improve after the Keller procedure and possibly could worsen and require a pad relief inside the shoe.

■ COMPLICATIONS AFTER ARTHRODESIS OF THE FIRST METATARSOPHALANGEAL JOINT

The primary complications of arthrodesis of the first metatarsophalangeal joint are nonunion, malunion, and degenerative

arthritis of the interphalangeal joint of the hallux. Accurate positioning of the hallux at the time of surgery is essential, and repositioning may be necessary after temporary fixation. The plane of the nail of the hallux should be in the plane of the lesser toes. In reconstruction of a rheumatoid forefoot, the lesser metatarsophalangeal joints must be corrected before final positioning of the hallux. The proper position of the hallux is 15 degrees of dorsiflexion at the metatarsophalangeal joint relative to the plantar surface of the foot and 25 to 30 degrees of dorsiflexion relative to the inclination angle of the first metatarsal. In addition, 15 degrees of valgus is recommended to reduce the risk of degenerative changes in the interphalangeal joint and callus formation over the interphalangeal and metatarsophalangeal joints. Nonunion occurs in less than 10% of patients and usually is not painful.

HALLUX RIGIDUS

Hallux rigidus, a term coined by Cotterill in 1888, refers to limitation of motion of the metatarsophalangeal joint of the great toe. Although he did not call it *hallux rigidus,* in 1887 Davies-Colley reported the first resection of the base of the proximal phalanx for this disorder, which he called *hallux flexus* because of the flexion posture of the metatarsophalangeal joint with the foot plantigrade and the limited extension of the joint (Fig. 2.102). Although understanding of the condition has advanced through radiographic and histologic techniques, the pathogenesis of hallux rigidus is still not clearly defined, but its unrelenting destructive course is well appreciated. Cartilage damage is believed to initiate the synovitis, which leads to further cartilage destruction, osteophyte proliferation, and subchondral bone destruction.

The process may begin in adolescence when a single traumatic event at the metatarsophalangeal joint damages the dorsal articular surface of the metatarsal head. Repeated microtrauma also may cause articular cartilage damage. Other suggested causes include osteochondritis dissecans of the first metatarsal head secondary to an osteochondral fracture over the dorsal convexity of the joint surface, hyperextension of the first metatarsal, an abnormally long first metatarsal, and severe pronation of the foot. Adult hallux rigidus most often is caused by degenerative arthritis of the first metatarsophalangeal joint, whereas in adolescents, hallux rigidus usually results from localized cartilage damage to the first metatarsal head.

A system for grading the severity of hallux rigidus (Table 2.1) uses passive range-of-motion, clinical, and radiographic examinations to assign a grade from 0 to 4. Numerous grading systems have been used over the years, all with strengths and weaknesses. The classification system by Coughlin and Shurnas has been reported to reliably predict the outcome of operative treatment of hallux rigidus. Beeson et al. reported that the strengths to this classification system were that it includes best elements of prior systems, uses subjective and objective clinical examination and radiographic data to determine grade, includes a grade 0 for patients with no symptoms but loss of metatarsophalangeal joint motion, and includes joint pain during range of motion. The weakness of this classification system was that grades were applied retrospectively to the sample population at final follow-up.

Although metatarsus primus elevatus (dorsal position of the first metatarsal on a weight-bearing lateral radiograph) has been suggested as a primary causative factor in the pathogenesis

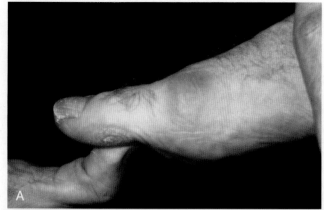

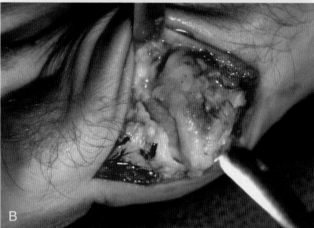

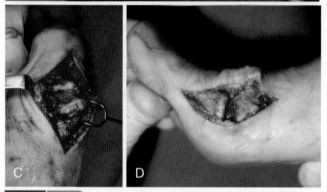

FIGURE **2.102**   Hallux rigidus. **A,** Marked limitation of metatarsophalangeal extension. **B** and **C,** Dorsal osteophyte and degenerative changes. **D,** Increased extension after joint debridement.

of hallux rigidus, this has not been clearly proven. No association has been identified between hallux rigidus and primus elevatus, first ray hypermobility, a long first metatarsal, Achilles or gastrocnemius tendon tightness, abnormal foot posture, symptomatic hallux valgus, adolescent onset, shoes, or occupation. Usuelli et al. reviewed clinical and radiographic data from 297 patients and found no etiologic correlation between primus elevatus and hallux rigidus. It is, however, associated with hallux valgus interphalangeus, bilateral involvement in patients with a familial history, unilateral involvement in patients with a history of trauma, and female sex.

McMaster reported that the most common microscopic finding in seven patients with hallux rigidus was a cleavage lesion in the articular cartilage of the first metatarsal head

without any detached subchondral bone and that the earliest radiographic finding was a small depression in the dome of the metatarsal head (Fig. 2.103). This finding is subtle and easily overlooked, however. The cleavage lesion on the metatarsal head is always between the apex of the dome and the dorsal margin of the articular surface. McMaster postulated that the characteristic tenderness over the dorsum of the first metatarsophalangeal joint and the limited dorsiflexion of the joint could be explained by the classic site of this lesion. When the hallux is extended, abutment of the proximal phalanx against the cleavage lesion in the articular cartilage produces pain and instinctive flexion of the joint, limiting extension. As the disease worsens, an osteophyte at the dorsal articular margin of the metatarsal head presents a mechanical abutment to extension. This is the usual condition of the patient at the initial presentation: degenerative arthritic changes in and around the first metatarsophalangeal joint. Often the first metatarsal is forced dorsally, decreasing its inclination angle on the weight-bearing lateral radiograph (primus elevatus). The elevation of the first metatarsal probably is secondary to the arthritic first metatarsophalangeal joint rather than causal.

NONOPERATIVE TREATMENT

In most patients, operative correction is required to relieve pain and improve function; however, Yee and Lau, in a review of the literature on hallux rigidus, determined that the evidence supports the use of nonoperative measures such as foot orthoses, shoe modifications, and injections of corticosteroid or sodium hyaluronate before surgery is considered (Fig. 2.104).

OPERATIVE TREATMENT

Although many operations have been recommended for the treatment of hallux rigidus, including dorsal wedge osteotomy at the base of the proximal phalanx or distal first metatarsal, the Keller procedure, and arthrodesis of the first metatarsophalangeal joint (Fig. 2.105), no one procedure has proved superior. Suggested indications for arthrodesis of the first metatarsophalangeal joint include loss of joint space evident not only on anteroposterior and lateral views but also on an oblique view of the first metatarsophalangeal joint, because the oblique view frequently shows remaining joint space not visible on the other two views and grade 4 or grade 3 hallux rigidus with more than half of the metatarsal head cartilage remaining (Fig. 2.106). Modern fixation techniques with interfragmentary compression screws or dorsal plates have produced high rates of fusion (94% to 98%) and patient satisfaction after arthrodesis for hallux rigidus. Gait studies have shown significant improvements in propulsive power, weight-bearing function of the foot, and stability during gait after arthrodesis for hallux rigidus.

The rationale for cheilectomy is relief of a painful mechanical impingement of the proximal phalanx on a dorsal osteophyte at the first metatarsal head. This is accomplished by removing the osteophyte and bony excrescences on each side of the articular margin and as much of the dorsal lip of articular cartilage as necessary to allow at least 70 degrees of dorsiflexion. Reported success rates of cheilectomy range from 56% to 92%, with better results in less severe grades of involvement (grade 1 or 2) and in patients older than 60 years. Nicolosi et al. evaluated the long-term efficacy of cheilectomy

TABLE 2.1

Grading of Severity of Hallux Rigidus (Coughlin and Shurnas)

GRADE	RADIOGRAPH	PAIN	MTP JOINT MOTION
0	Normal	None	Stiffness or slight loss
1	Minor narrowing of MTP joint space	Intermittent	Mild restriction
2	Moderate joint space narrowing, osteophyte formation	More constant	Moderate restriction
3	Severe joint space narrowing, extensive osteophyte formation	Constant (no pain at midrange of MTP joint motion)	Moderately severe restriction (<20 degrees total motion)
4	Same as grade 3	Pain at midrange of passive MTP joint motion	Same as grade 3

MTP, Metatarsophalangeal.

Modified from Coughlin MJ, Shurnas PS: Hallux valgus in men: II. First ray mobility after bunionectomy and factors associated with hallux valgus deformity, *Foot Ankle Int* 24:73, 2003.

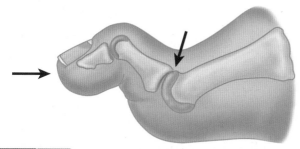

FIGURE 2.103 Location of chondral or osteochondral lesion produced by forceful extension and impaction of metatarsal head. (Redrawn from McMaster MJ: The pathogenesis of hallux rigidus, *J Bone Joint Surg* 60B:82, 1978.)

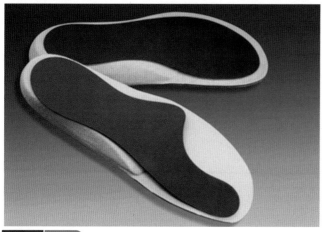

FIGURE 2.104 Spring Lite Plate.

for hallux rigidus in 58 patients. Results were good in 88%, with only 3% requiring subsequent arthrodesis. Sidon et al. reported long-term follow-up (average, 6.6 years) after cheilectomy in 169 feet with Coughlin grades 1-3 hallux rigidus. Twenty-eight of 169 feet had recurrence, and nine required a second procedure. Overall 69% of the patients were satisfied with the procedure. Gait analysis has shown that increased lateral metatarsal-head loading may occur after cheilectomy,

and these alterations in kinematics may result in further degenerative joint changes. However, Smith et al. reported their results of gait analysis in 17 patients 4 weeks before surgery and 1 year after surgery. They noted that cheilectomy resulted in significant increases in first metatarsophalangeal joint motion and AOFAS hallux scores. In addition, peak sagittal plane push-off power of the ankle improved.

Distal osteotomies of the metatarsals or phalanx with cheilectomy have been shown to be effective for mild to moderate hallux rigidus. Coutts and Kilmartin reported an 11-year follow-up of 27 dorsiflexion phalangeal osteotomies and found that 96% of patients with stage II hallux rigidus had pain relief, with 77% reporting complete pain relief. However, joint stiffness and footwear restrictions were ongoing issues in 35% of the women in their series. Results by Voegeli et al. in 31 patients showed satisfactory results in patients with stage II hallux rigidus; high patient satisfaction and improved range of motion were noted at 39-month follow-up. Cho et al. determined outcomes of the distal metatarsal dorsiflexion osteotomy using bioscrew fixation for advanced hallux rigidus in 42 patients. Although Foot and Ankle Ability Measure and AOFAS scores improved, dorsiflexion decreased over time, and there was a significant difference between patients with stage III and IV deformity. Based on the unfavorable results in stage IV hallux rigidus, these authors did not recommend this for patients with end-stage hallux rigidus. Viladot et al. reported clinical and radiographic outcomes after distal oblique osteotomy for stage II hallux rigidus at a mean follow-up of 40 months, noting that it was a viable alternative for moderate hallux rigidus with high patient satisfaction. They also compared the Youngswick-Austin osteotomy with distal oblique osteotomy and found comparable results. The Youngswick-Austin osteotomy has the benefit of being stable in three planes with only one screw for fixation, while distal oblique osteotomy requires two screws for stability. Distal oblique osteotomy, however, is a simpler technique because it requires only one cut instead of three.

A modification of the Keller procedure (resection arthroplasty) in which the extensor hallucis brevis and capsular tissue are used as interposition materials has been described for the treatment of severe hallux rigidus, but, as with cheilectomy, reported results vary. Sanhudo et al. reported good

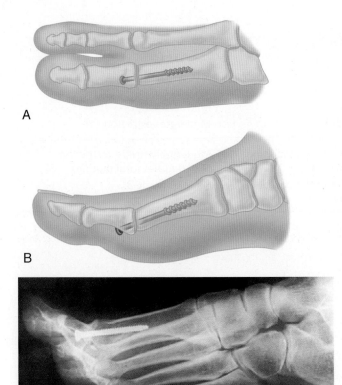

FIGURE 2.105 McKeever arthrodesis. **A** and **B,** Four-millimeter cancellous screw for internal fixation. **C,** Completed arthrodesis.

surgical outcomes in 75% of 25 feet. Schneider et al. reported a 23-year follow-up study on 87 Keller resection arthroplasties. The average AOFAS score was 83 points. SF-36 scores showed normal values, and pedobarographic assessment revealed only moderate alterations in weight bearing. Five feet required revision. Of those who did not require revision, 94% said they would have this procedure again. Johnson and McCormick reported a significantly higher postoperative AOFAS score after the modified oblique Keller capsular interposition arthroplasty compared with arthrodesis. Passive range of motion measured 54 degrees and active motion 30 degrees after the Keller arthroplasty, whereas after arthrodesis, range of motion was nonexistent. There was no difference between the two procedures in plantar pressure under the second metatarsal head, but the arthrodesis group had greater plantar pressure under the first metatarsal head.

Interposition arthroplasty has been modified by making an oblique proximal phalangeal resection that exits at the subchondral bone of the plantar aspect of the proximal phalanx in an attempt to preserve the attachment of the flexor hallucis brevis on the base of the proximal phalanx. Capsular interposition arthroplasty has been shown to be a safe, efficacious treatment in patients with advanced hallux rigidus, with high patient satisfaction.

Silicone-rubber, single-stem replacement arthroplasty components have been reported to produce satisfactory results, but the concern with this technique is silicone-rubber synovitis (Fig. 2.107). Outcomes after total joint arthroplasty of the first metatarsophalangeal joint have been compared

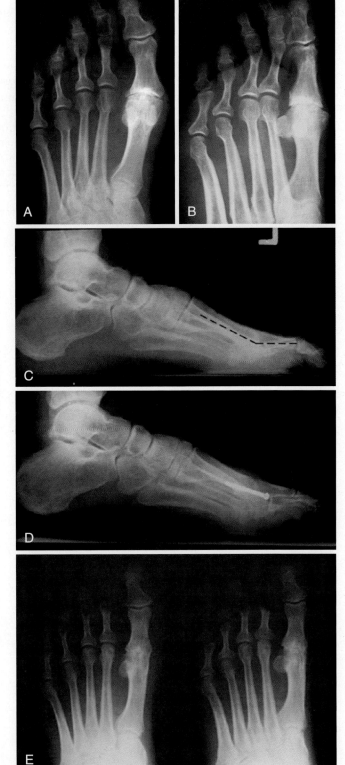

FIGURE 2.106 **A** and **B,** Anteroposterior and oblique views of severe hallux rigidus. **C-E,** Postoperative radiographs; note angle of arthrodesis.

with outcomes after arthrodesis. Arthrodesis was noted to be superior in pain reduction, outcomes, and patient satisfaction and had fewer complications and fewer revisions required

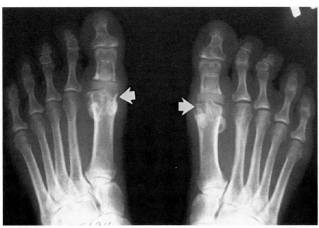

FIGURE 2.107 Hallux rigidus treated with silicone-rubber spacers; note erosion of bone at metatarsal head and thickening of soft tissue of hallux from silicone synovitis and edema. Prosthesis had to be removed.

(Stevens et al.; Stone et al.). Horisberger et al. reported outcomes of a new three-component metatarsophalangeal joint prosthesis (follow-up average of 50 months). Although this total joint arthroplasty provided significant pain relief at midterm follow-up, high variability was noted in component alignment, and range of motion deteriorated with time. Hemiarthroplasty of the proximal phalanx with a metallic resurfacing component also has been described, with high success rates reported, but large, controlled studies with long-term follow-up remain unavailable for evaluation of this procedure. One study of 23 hemiarthroplasties reported that 91% of patients were satisfied with their outcomes at 5.7-year follow-up and all had made significant gains in AOFAS scores. Despite continued interest in resurfacing procedures and total joint arthroplasty, there is a need for rigorous scientific study before implant arthroplasty can be recommended. Early results from metatarsal head resurfacing and ceramic total joint replacement seem encouraging, but more research is necessary.

A synthetic cartilage implant hemiarthroplasty procedure was developed in 2016. A hydrogel implant, approximately 8 to 10 mm, is implanted into the metatarsal head with resection of osteophytes at the dorsal first metatarsal and at the base of the proximal phalanx. The implant is left 1.5 mm proud to allow joint distraction. Outcome studies at 2 and 5 years have shown equivalent results to arthrodesis in terms of pain and function (90%). When stratified by hallux rigidus grade, success rates were almost identical between the synthetic implant and arthrodesis procedures. In a study by Baumhauer et al., less than 10% of the implant group required revision to arthrodesis. Cassinelli et al., however, reported that although 62% of patients were satisfied or neutral, 27% were very unsatisfied; 20% required reoperation, with 8% requiring conversion to an arthrodesis. A cost comparison study by Rothermel et al. revealed a higher direct aggregate cost for the hydrogel implant compared with arthrodesis. Regardless, this may be an option for patients who wish to retain motion of the metatarsophalangeal joint and obtain significant pain relief. This procedure is not indicated in patients with osteoporosis, bone defects, tumors, sesamoid arthritis, active infection, allergies to polyvinyl alcohol, or inflammatory arthropathies. Patients who have had other osteotomy procedures may have inadequate bone stock for implantation. Authors agree that patients should be counseled regarding pain and dysfunction in the early postoperative period, with pain improvement expected at 3 months. In our experience, radiographic parameters improve with this implant, but many patients have stiffness and low-grade pain. Procedures may best be used in advanced cases of hallux rigidus in patients who absolutely want to avoid arthrodesis.

CHEILECTOMY

The goal of this procedure is to remove the proliferative bone from around the metatarsal head so as to remove the buttress preventing dorsiflexion of the proximal phalanx on the metatarsal head (Figs. 2.108 and 2.109A).

TECHNIQUE 2.32

(MANN, CLANTON, AND THOMPSON)

- Make a dorsal skin incision about 1 cm proximal to the interphalangeal joint and continue it proximally about 5 cm across the metatarsophalangeal joint (Fig. 2.109B).
- Deepen the incision through the subcutaneous tissue and fat to expose the extensor tendon and hood (Fig. 2.109C).
- Lateral to the extensor hallucis longus, open the extensor hood and joint capsule to expose the dorsal, medial, and lateral aspects of the metatarsophalangeal joint (Fig. 2.109D).
- Remove any synovium and locate the dorsal and dorsolateral osteophytes on the metatarsal and the phalanx. Assess the degree of cartilage loss and remove any loose bodies (Fig. 2.109E).
- Plantarflex the metatarsophalangeal joint and remove 20% to 30% of the dorsal metatarsal head with a 6-mm osteotome (Fig. 2.109F). The amount of bone to be removed from the metatarsal head depends on the size of the dorsal exostosis and the severity of articular cartilage destruction. If the articular cartilage damage is minimal and the main problem is the dorsal exostosis, approximately 20% of the dorsal aspect of the metatarsal head is removed. If more articular damage is present, more of the metatarsal head should be removed. If articular damage is severe, one third of the dorsal aspect of the metatarsal head can be removed.
- Begin the resection just dorsal to the edge of what appears to be viable articular cartilage. Remove the osteophytes on the lateral aspect of the joint in line with the long axis of the metatarsal. This narrows the metatarsal head less medially than laterally than dorsally to plantarly.
- Correct any irregularities in the articular cartilage and remove remaining synovial tissue.
- Dorsiflexion of the metatarsophalangeal joint should now be possible to approximately 70 degrees (Fig. 2.109G). If this degree of dorsiflexion cannot be achieved, probably

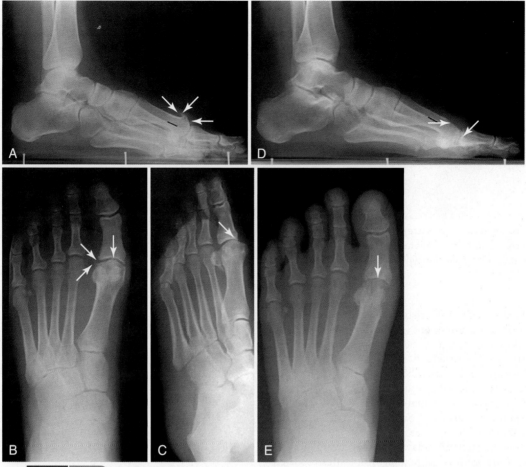

FIGURE 2.108 Hallux rigidus of left foot treated with cheilectomy. **A-C,** After surgery. **D** and **E,** One year after surgery.

more bone needs to be removed from the metatarsal head. Remove any dorsal osteophyte on the proximal phalanx.

- Sharply plantarflex the metatarsophalangeal joint and inspect the sesamoid area. If the sesamoid bones do not freely move distally as the hallux is extended, place a smooth instrument (Freer elevator) between the head of the metatarsal and sesamoids. Gently lever the instrument up and down until the contracted volar capsulosesamoid apparatus is more mobile. This usually allows a few degrees more dorsiflexion.

- Apply bone wax to the raw bone surfaces (if the patient is not allergic to bee venom) and close the joint capsule beneath the extensor tendon.

- Close the skin in a single layer. Apply a tight, well-padded compression dressing.

POSTOPERATIVE CARE After 12 to 18 hours, the compression dressing is removed and a smaller, snug dressing is applied. Patients are allowed to bear weight on the heel and as much of the foot as is comfortable. Crutches are not needed unless for patient comfort and are discontinued as soon as possible. At 10 to 14 days, the sutures are removed and active and gentle passive range-of-motion exercises are begun.

DISTAL OBLIQUE OSTEOTOMY FOR HALLUX RIGIDUS

Distal oblique osteotomy has several advantages: it only requires one cut, allows shortening, plantarflexion, and first metatarsal head translation as needed, and weight bearing is immediate. It is an effective surgical procedure for grade II hallux rigidus with a high patient satisfaction.

TECHNIQUE 2.33

(VOEGELI ET AL.)

- Place the patient supine and apply a pneumatic tourniquet after sedation and a local block are administered.
- Make a medial longitudinal incision over the first metatarsophalangeal joint and deepen the incision through the capsule.
- Resect the dorsal and medial first metatarsal head prominences and any periarticular osteophytes.
- Perform the osteotomy from dorsal-distal to plantar-proximal, with the angle ranging from 40 to 45 degrees in the sagittal plane and beginning immediately distal to the

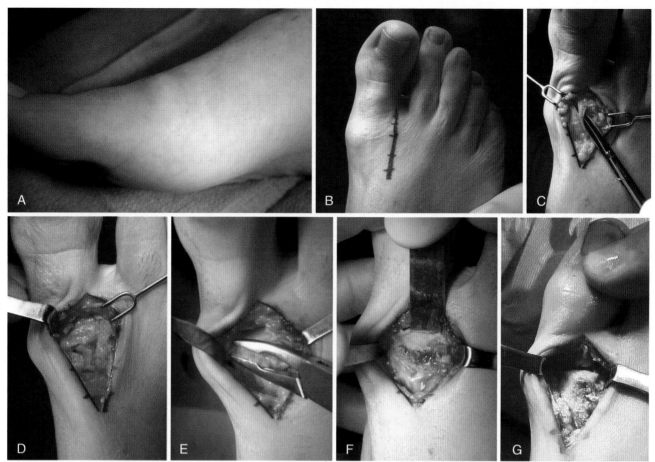

FIGURE 2.109 Cheilectomy. **A,** Patient with stage II (radiographically) hallux rigidus; note dorsal osteophyte over first metatarsal. **B,** Incision is placed at lateral border of extensor hallucis longus. **C,** Dorsal sensory nerve to hallux is protected. **D,** First metatarsophalangeal joint is exposed. **E,** Dorsal osteophytes are removed from metatarsal head and base of proximal phalanx. Dorsolateral osteophyte frequently is present and must be removed. **F,** Between 20 and 25% of metatarsal head is removed dorsally. **G,** Joint is distracted, any loose cartilage and bone are removed, and joint is moved through 60 to 70 degrees of motion. Palpation through skin is done to ensure that no abnormal bony prominences remain. Capsule is closed with two or three absorbable sutures, and skin is closed with nylon sutures. **SEE TECHNIQUE 2.32.**

proximal-most aspect of dorsal cartilaginous surface of the metatarsal head and ending plantar-proximal behind the vascular package, taking care not to violate vascularity of the metatarsal head.
- Transpose the capital fragment proximally and fix with two screws oriented from proximal-distal to dorsal-plantar.
- Repair the capsule with absorbable sutures and close the wound with simple sutures with no drainage. Apply a compressive dressing with the hallux splinted in neutral position.

POSTOPERATIVE CARE Immediate full weight bearing is permitted in a postoperative shoe for 6 weeks. Active and passive dorsiflexion and plantarflexion exercises of the first metatarsophalangeal joint are started on the first postoperative day.

"V" RESECTION OF THE FIRST METATARSOPHALANGEAL JOINT (VALENTI PROCEDURE)

Joint resection procedures generally have good clinical outcomes; however, young, active patients are a concern, especially those who are involved in sports and whose expectations and demands are higher than those of nonathletic patients. Foot surgery for athletes should decrease pain, increase joint motion, speed return to activity, and improve performance. In 1987 Valenti described a technique of an 80-degree sagittal plane "V" resection of the dorsal third or fourth of the metatarsal head and base of the proximal phalanx. In a study comparing the Valenti procedure with cheilectomy, dorsiflexion increased 27 degrees with the Valenti technique and only 13 degrees after cheilectomy. The Valenti procedure preserves length of the first ray, first metatarsal head plantarly, base of the proximal phalanx, flexor hallucis brevis, and sesamoid function. Joint-preserving procedures improve stability, motion, and function, but if revision becomes necessary, arthroplasty or arthrodesis may be the only options left; hence, Saxena et al. modified the technique to adequately decompress the joint with less bone resection, which allows for future arthrodesis or arthroplasty if necessary.

TECHNIQUE 2.34

(MODIFIED VALENTI, SAXENA ET AL.)

- Make a 4- to 6-cm dorsal linear incision over the first metatarsophalangeal joint, medial to the extensor hallucis longus tendon, and carry the dissection down to the joint capsule, taking care to avoid the medial dorsal cutaneous nerve branches. Cauterize minor vessels as necessary.
- Perform a dorsal capsulotomy, exposing the head of the metatarsal and base of the proximal phalanx, and sharply excise the hypertrophic synovium and bursal tissue.
- Evaluate the integrity of the articular cartilage, locating osteochondral defects or cystic lesions.
- Begin the metatarsal exostectomy below the degenerated articular cartilage (Fig. 2.110). Using a sagittal saw, excise the dorsal one fourth or one third of the osteochondral surface of the metatarsal head from distal-plantar to proximal-dorsal.
- Perform a proximal phalangeal exostectomy from dorsal-distal to proximal-plantar, removing only the exposed subchondral bone and preserving the entire flexor hallucis brevis tendon insertion. Avoid entering the medullary canals when performing these exostectomies.
- Remove any remaining hyperostosis on the metatarsal head and base of the proximal phalanx with a rongeur and round the edges with a burr. Confirm that there is no bony abutment and full range of motion in the sagittal plane. The lateral hyperostosis of the proximal phalangeal base should be removed with a rongeur and the hyperostosis of the metatarsal head may require a saw.
- Measure the amount of dorsiflexion to confirm it is 45 to 65 degrees, which may be necessary for normal gait and for the anticipated loss of some of the motion gained during healing. Using a Freer elevator release the plantar adhesions of the sesamoids if necessary.
- Close the capsule using the extensor hallucis brevis as an interpositional arthroplasty and drape it over the exposed metatarsal head but do not place plantarly.
- Perform skin closure in the standard fashion.

POSTOPERATIVE CARE Patients should remain non–weight bearing for 2 to 5 days until they no longer need pain medication. Sutures are removed 12 to 14 days after surgery. Formal physical therapy begins at approximately 3 to 4 weeks postoperatively. Patients are instructed on resuming normal walking and modalities to decrease swelling and pain. Sporting activity may begin when greater than 20 degrees of passive dorsiflexion is achieved. Patients are advised to continue ice application and first metatarsophalangeal joint range of motion exercises until they are at full recovery.

■ ARTHRODESIS OF THE FIRST METATARSOPHALANGEAL JOINT

The techniques of arthrodesis for hallux rigidus are the same as those described for hallux valgus.

■ RESECTION ARTHROPLASTY (KELLER PROCEDURE)

For resection arthroplasty, see Technique 2.2.

■ PROXIMAL PHALANGEAL EXTENSION OSTEOTOMIES

EXTENSION OSTEOTOMY OF THE PROXIMAL PHALANX

The purpose of this operation is to change unnecessary plantarflexion to needed dorsiflexion by a dorsal, closing wedge osteotomy of the proximal phalanx of the hallux. Combining cheilectomy with extension osteotomy of the proximal phalanx has been reported to improve patient satisfaction over that obtained with cheilectomy alone. O'Malley et al. reported their results with combined cheilectomy and osteotomy of the proximal phalanx in 81 patients at 4-year follow-up. Eighty-five percent of patients were satisfied with the result and only 5% required arthrodesis for persistent symptoms. Hunt and Anderson reported good or excellent results in 90% of 34 patients after a combined dorsal cheilectomy and a Moberg-Akin procedure. None of their patients required additional surgical procedures for ongoing symptoms. Perez-Aznar et al. reported a dorsal wedge phalangeal osteotomy in 42 feet (40 patients). Eighty-one percent had good or excellent results according to the AOFAS and visual analog scores. Two patients required revision for screw irritation.

TECHNIQUE 2.35

(THOMAS AND SMITH)

- Make a dorsomedial incision. Identify and protect the dorsomedial cutaneous nerve.
- Perform a metatarsophalangeal capsulotomy in line with the skin incision and reflect it dorsally and plantarly.
- Using a reciprocating saw, resect the medial eminence 1 to 2 mm to promote healing of capsule to bone after closure.
- To perform a limited dorsal cheilectomy, resect the dorsal portion of the distal first metatarsal with a power sagittal saw. This is less than the amount resected for traditional cheilectomy and is not based on the need for dorsiflexion to 60 degrees relative to the weight-bearing surface.
- Resect any osteophytes that may be present on the lateral aspects of the metatarsal head and the proximal phalanx.
- Identify and protect the flexor hallucis longus tendon.
- Place a 0.062-inch Kirschner wire transversely from medial to lateral, parallel to and as close to the articular surface of the proximal phalanx as possible without entering the joint or cartilaginous surface. This provides a marker to prevent penetration of the joint during the proximal phalangeal osteotomy (Fig. 2.111A).
- Make the proximal osteotomy immediately along the distal surface of the 0.062-inch Kirschner wire using an oscil-

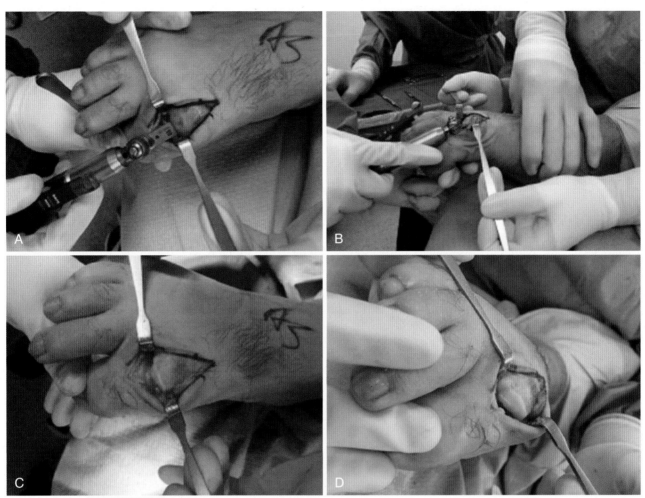

FIGURE 2.110   Modified Valenti arthroplasty. **A,** Starting point for first metatarsal osteotomy. **B,** Lateral view. **C** and **D,** After osteotomy. (From Saxena A, Valerio DL, Behan SA, Hofer D: Modified Valenti arthroplasty in running and jumping athletes with hallux limitus/rigidus: analysis of one hundred procedures, *J Foot Ankle Surg* 58:609, 2019.) **SEE TECHNIQUE 2.34.**

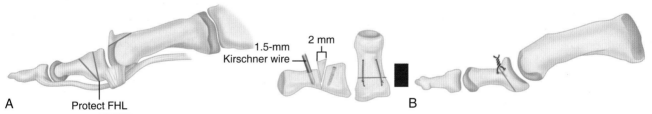

FIGURE 2.111   Thomas and Smith extension osteotomy of proximal phalanx. **A,** Amount of bone resected from first metatarsal. Bone is resected in line with dorsal metatarsal shaft. Dorsal width of proximal phalangeal osteotomy measures 6 mm. Care is taken to protect flexor hallucis longus (FHL) tendon. **B,** Lateral view of metatarsophalangeal joint after proximal phalangeal dorsal closing wedge osteotomy with 3-0 wire fixation in place. (From Thomas PJ, Smith RM: Proximal phalanx osteotomy for the surgical treatment of hallux rigidus, *Foot Ankle Int* 20:3, 1999.) **SEE TECHNIQUE 2.35.**

lating saw with a 0.5-mm blade width. To maintain stability of the osteotomy site, it is helpful if the first osteotomy is not completed until the second cut (more oblique and distal to the first) is made. The second, oblique cut allows removal of a measured 6-mm dorsal wedge of bone.
- Drill multiple 1.5-mm holes into the plantar cortex to weaken it and protect the flexor hallucis longus tendon.

- Close the osteotomy manually and secure it with a 3-0 wire placed through the 1.5-mm drill holes at the dorso-medial aspect of the osteotomy (Fig. 2.111B). Start the proximal drill hole just adjacent to the articular cartilage at the base of the proximal phalanx, 2 to 3 mm from the osteotomy. This avoids breaking the fragile suture tunnel.

- Pass the wire from proximal to distal, placing most of the tension on the distal side to prevent fracturing the delicate proximal hole.
- Close the capsule with interrupted nonabsorbable sutures. If possible, completely cover the osteotomy with soft tissue. Small staples or screws may be used as well.

POSTOPERATIVE CARE Patients are placed in a wooden-soled shoe for 6 weeks and are allowed to bear weight. At 1 to 2 weeks after surgery, passive dorsiflexion exercises are begun and plantarflexion is started at 3 to 4 weeks.

CONDITIONS OF THE SESAMOID

Because of increased awareness of pathologic conditions of the hallux sesamoids, injuries to the sesamoids during sports activities or falls from heights are recognized quickly, but more subtle pathologic conditions may escape diagnosis. Chronic inflammatory conditions of a traumatic, infectious, or arthritic origin are grouped under the diagnosis of sesamoiditis. Inflamed bursae, intractable plantar keratoses, or diffuse callus beneath the tibial sesamoid may herald underlying sesamoid pathologic conditions. In addition, chondromalacia, flexor hallucis brevis tendinitis, osteochondritis dissecans, and fracture all occur in the sesamoids.

The tibial sesamoid is the most commonly injured of the two because of its central location beneath the first metatarsal head. Hyperextension and axial loading are the most common mechanisms of injury resulting in fracture (or sprain of the capsuloligamentous complex). Repetitive stress through a syndesmotic union of a bipartite sesamoid can weaken the junction, however, and a displaced "fracture" can result. Favinger et al. noted a 14.3% prevalence of bipartite and multipartite hallux sesamoid in a series of 671 foot radiographs.

On physical examination, diffuse tenderness may be present around the metatarsophalangeal joint, but with careful palpation of each sesamoid, the tenderness becomes more localized. Any patient complaining of pain around the first metatarsophalangeal joint should have a thorough evaluation of the sesamoids.

Routine radiographs, including anteroposterior and oblique views, may be helpful (Fig. 2.112). The standard lateral view of the foot usually is not revealing. The medial oblique (sesamoid) view (Fig. 2.113) is helpful for evaluating a tibial sesamoid. The axial sesamoid view should always be obtained if a sesamoid pathologic condition is suspected (Fig. 2.114). The techniques for obtaining these views are shown in Figure 2.115.

If these radiographic views are normal but a sesamoid pathologic condition is suspected, a bone scan may be helpful. The nuclear medicine department should be informed that the sesamoids are under question so that they can modify the projections accordingly. A bone scan may be helpful, but the projections are important to rule out intraarticular metatarsophalangeal joint pathologic conditions.

A bipartite tibial sesamoid is present in about 10% of the population, and in 25% of these people the condition is bilateral. For this reason, the surgeon must be certain that a tender sesamoid with a division through it, as seen on the radiographs, is a fracture and not a bipartite sesamoid. The fibular sesamoid rarely is bipartite, and if clinical symptoms and routine radiographs suggest a fracture of this sesamoid, one is usually present. A bone scan is an excellent means of confirming this.

■ TREATMENT

The initial treatment depends on the severity of the clinical and radiographic findings (Fig. 2.116). Such diagnoses as sesamoiditis (the only positive finding being tenderness over the sesamoid), osteochondritis (Fig. 2.117), acute calcific tendinitis (usually of the lateral head of the flexor hallucis brevis), chronic tendinitis of the flexor hallucis brevis with occasional calcific tendinitis or a traction osteophyte in its insertion into the sesamoid, and bursitis can be treated with nonsteroidal antiinflammatory drugs, modification of activity, full-length shoe orthoses with a metatarsal pad and a relief beneath the first metatarsal head, a metatarsal bar on the sole of the shoe, or cast immobilization. This treatment is continued for several months. If no relief is obtained, excision of the sesamoid is indicated.

For fractures (Fig. 2.118), exostoses (Fig. 2.119), persistent bursitis, and painful keratoses (Figs. 2.120 and 2.121), excision of the involved sesamoid may be required. A lengthy (6 months) trial of nonoperative treatment may be tried first. Sesamoidectomy is most often done in athletically active patients who wish to return to their sports more rapidly; however, complications of surgery can delay return to activity. Bichara et al. demonstrated good results after sesamoidectomy for sesamoid fractures in 24 athletes at a follow-up of 35 months (range 8 to 70 months). Although they reported reliable pain relief and return to activity in patients, progressive hallux valgus occurred in one of 24 cases. Lee et al. reported their outcomes in 20 of 32 patients who had isolated tibial sesamoidectomies. Postoperative outcome measurements (visual analog scale, SF-36, and Foot Function Index) showed significant improvement in pain and function. Eighteen patients indicated that they could perform; six could not stand on their tiptoes, but this did not affect their activities of daily living or athletic pursuits; two patients developed transfer metatarsalgia, but only one had symptoms. No significant differences were noted between preoperative and postoperative radiographs in regard to the intermetatarsal angle, hallux valgus angle, distal metatarsal articular angle, or sesamoid alignment.

EXCISION OF THE SESAMOID

TECHNIQUE 2.36

- Make a 3-cm incision as shown in Figure 2.122A; alternatively, make an incision in the midline if the capsule is to be opened and turned plantarward and the sesamoid removed from inside out. The proper digital branch of the medial plantar nerve to the medial side of the pulp of the hallux is vulnerable with this incision, more so than with the straight medial incision in the midline, which is an internervous plane (Fig. 2.122B). With the incision more plantar, however, less capsular disruption is needed to remove the sesamoid.
- Locate the sesamoid by palpation to differentiate it from the metatarsal head.

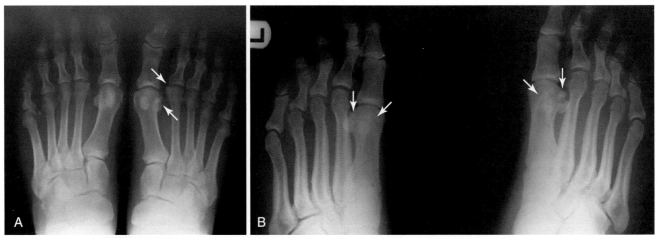

FIGURE 2.112 **A,** Standing anteroposterior view of both feet on same cassette allows comparison of sesamoids. This is especially helpful if fracture is suspected but bipartite sesamoid is present. Accessory sesamoids *(arrows)* are normal, although uncommon, findings. **B,** Oblique view profiles fibular sesamoid. Note cystic fibular sesamoid on right foot. This probably represents old fracture through syndesmotic union of bipartite sesamoid.

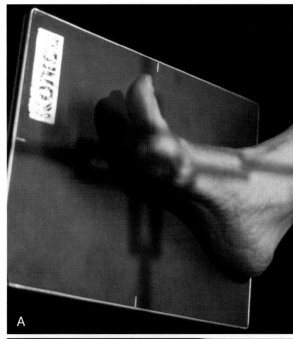

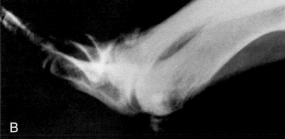

FIGURE 2.113 Tibial sesamoid is profiled on medial oblique view. **A,** Position of foot. **B,** Sesamoid in profile.

- "Shell" the sesamoid out of the capsule and plantar plate by incising across its plantar surface *and* articular surface, remaining ever aware of the flexor hallucis longus.

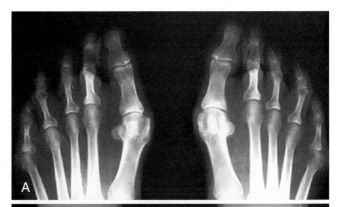

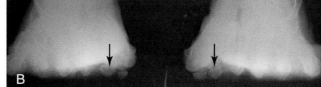

FIGURE 2.114 Hallux valgus **(A),** and, on axial sesamoid view **(B),** degenerative changes present with subluxation of sesamoids.

- When the flexor hallucis longus is identified, while keeping the great toe flexed 20 to 30 degrees, incise the intersesamoid ligament, grasp the tibial sesamoid and pull it medially, and complete the excision by releasing the flexor hallucis brevis medial head and its continuation distally to the base of the proximal phalanx of the hallux (Fig. 2.122C).
- Close the *medial* (not plantar) side of the capsule with absorbable sutures and close the skin with nonabsorbable sutures. A careful enucleation of the sesamoid can leave intact, small, thin slips of tendon of the flexor hallucis brevis, not losing all its flexion moment.

POSTOPERATIVE CARE A compressive forefoot dressing and postoperative rigid-soled shoe are worn for 12 to 16 days, and weight bearing to tolerance is permitted on the operated foot. The use of crutches or a walker is optional.

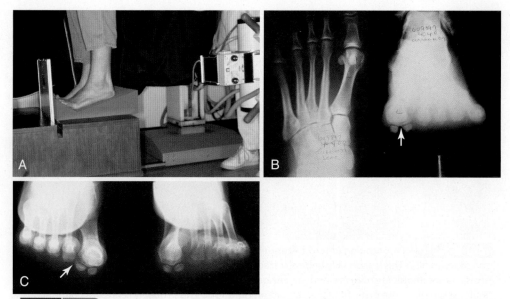

FIGURE 2.115   Techniques for obtaining axial sesamoid views. **A,** View may be taken with patient standing on inclined plane. **B** and **C,** Axial sesamoid view taken from front while patient stands on inclined plane.

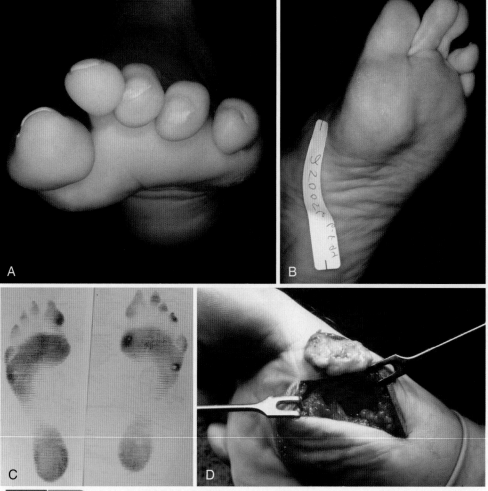

FIGURE 2.116   **A** and **B,** Plantarflexed first ray with callus beneath tibial sesamoid. **C,** On Harris pressure mat, note increased pressure beneath tibial sesamoid. **D,** Tibial sesamoid has been removed, and articular surface and corresponding facet of metatarsal head show degenerative changes.

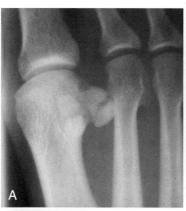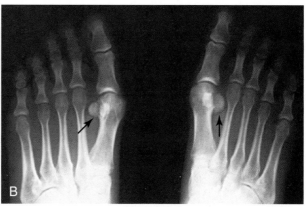

FIGURE 2.117 **A** and **B,** Oblique radiography is helpful for evaluating fibular sesamoid that rests between first and second metatarsals; note irregular lucency, indicating traumatic etiology.

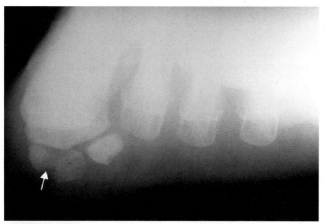

FIGURE 2.118 Axial sesamoid view showing fracture of tibial sesamoid.

The sutures are removed, and a wide, deep shoe of the patient's choice is allowed. Occasionally, a short leg walking cast is applied if the patient wants to be more active during the first 2 to 3 weeks. A metatarsal pad inside the shoe or metatarsal bar on the outside of the shoe is recommended for several months. These shoe modifications should have been used preoperatively so that the patient is not disturbed by their continual use until symptom free.

FIBULAR SESAMOIDECTOMY: PLANTAR APPROACH

TECHNIQUE 2.37

- If a plantar approach (Fig. 2.123A) is chosen for fibular sesamoidectomy, have an assistant hold the ankle dorsiflexed and use a headlight to see into the full depth of the wound. Avoid the flexor hallucis longus tendon and the neurovascular bundle to the first web space.

- Flex and extend the hallux and inspect the radiograph to locate the sesamoid. Beginning 1 to 1.5 cm distal to the metatarsophalangeal joint, make a longitudinal incision in the plantar surface of the foot, extending the incision proximally 3.5 to 4 cm between the first and second metatarsals.
- If the fibular sesamoid requires excision, it usually is subluxed.
- When the skin and fascial septa within the forefoot pad have been separated, insert a small self-retaining retractor.
- Using small, blunt-tip dissecting scissors, identify the neurovascular bundle to the first web space and retract it laterally or medially, depending on the position of the sesamoid (Fig. 2.123B).
- Palpate the sesamoids and flex and extend the hallux to locate the flexor hallucis longus tendon.
- Open the pulley over the flexor hallucis longus tendon and retract the tendon medially. This maneuver is made easier by having an assistant hold the foot in dorsiflexion at the arch with one hand and flexing the metatarsophalangeal joint to relax the flexor hallucis longus tendon with the opposite hand.
- At this point, the intersesamoid ligament should come into view; divide it completely (Fig. 2.123C). This may require moving the scalpel 1 or 2 mm laterally or medially to find the groove between the sesamoids.
- Incise the cleavage plane between the two sesamoids while retracting the flexor hallucis longus muscle medially and the neurovascular bundle laterally.
- Grasp the fibular sesamoid with a strong pick-up or small Kocher clamp and remove the lateral head insertion of the flexor hallucis brevis muscle on the proximal end of the sesamoid using direct vision (loupe magnification makes this easier but is not necessary).
- When the medial and proximal restraints of the sesamoid have been released, sever the attachment of the adductor hallucis muscle to its lateral distal edge close to the bone with a scalpel or scissors.
- Sever the last attachment of the sesamoid distally where the plantar plate continues its distal insertion into the proximal phalanx (Fig. 2.123D).
- When the sesamoid has been removed, inspect the wound carefully for any bleeding. Pressing on the edges of the wound helps identify any potential bleeding vessels, which should be cauterized.
- Excising the sesamoid does not release the adductor insertion on the base of the proximal phalanx. This can

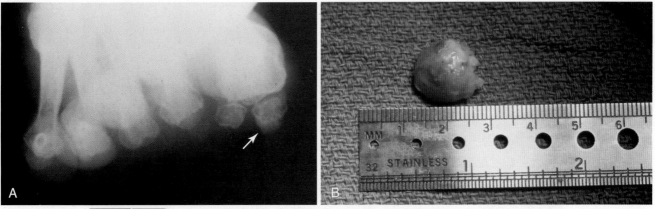

FIGURE 2.119   **A,** Exostosis on plantar surface of tibial sesamoid. **B,** Patient had keratotic lesion with intermittent ulceration. Excision of sesamoid is indicated.

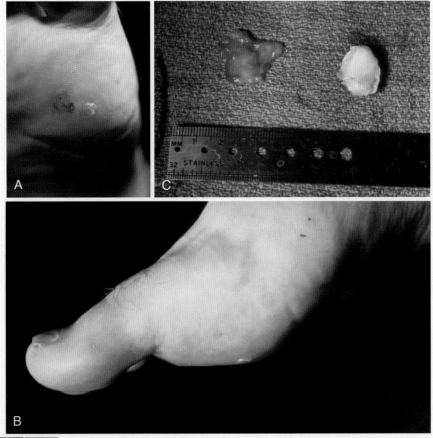

FIGURE 2.120   **A** and **B,** Persistent keratotic lesion and bursa beneath tibial sesamoid. **C,** Sesamoid and overlying bursa removed. Radiographs (not shown), including axial sesamoid view, were normal.

be released through the plantar incision. Continuing to retract the neurovascular bundle laterally and the flexor hallucis longus muscle medially, and adducting the hallux, while the opposite index finger palpates the adductor, helps identify the structure (Fig. 2.123E).

- Using right-angle retractors, expose the adductor, excise a small section of the tendon, and move the hallux medially.
- At the conclusion of this procedure, the surgeon should be unable to palpate any restraining structures on the fibular side of the metatarsophalangeal joint. The transverse

natatory fibers in the dorsal aspect of the web space should be released manually. All restraints pulling the hallux laterally (except the extrinsic tendons) must be removed.

- Inspect the neurovascular bundle and the flexor hallucis longus tendon.*

* McBride recommended an additional step: approximate the first and second metatarsal heads by passing a heavy suture either through the capsules of the adjacent first and second metatarsal heads or circumferentially around the metatarsal necks.

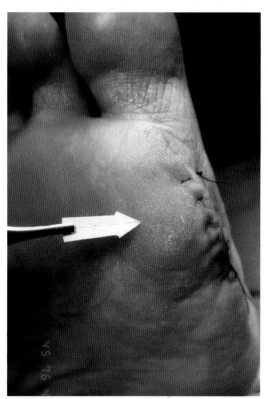

ARTHRITIS OF THE INTERPHALANGEAL JOINT

Arthritis of the interphalangeal joint, with or without flexion contracture, is common and often is preceded by trauma. It is occasionally well tolerated if a normally functioning first metatarsophalangeal joint is present, but pain and limitation of footwear often require an arthrodesis of the joint. A single headless compression screw has been quite satisfactory in our hands (Fig. 2.124). A supplemental 0.045-inch Kirschner wire may be used to control rotation (Fig. 2.125).

FIGURE 2.121 Diffuse keratosis that persisted over protracted period and was unresponsive to nonoperative management.

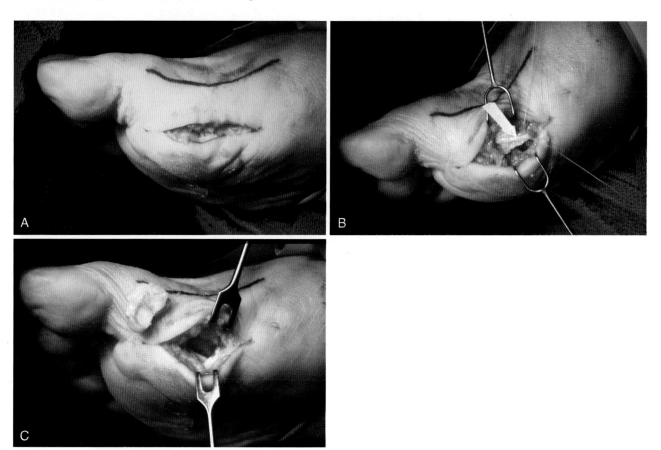

FIGURE 2.122 Removal of tibial sesamoid. **A,** Optional incision. **B,** *Arrow* and suture delineate proper digital nerve to medial side of hallux. Nerve blends with capsule and subcutaneous tissue, making it vulnerable by position and appearance. **C,** Excised sesamoid, tendon of flexor hallucis longus, and undersurface (tibial sesamoid facet) of metatarsal head. **SEE TECHNIQUE 2.36.**

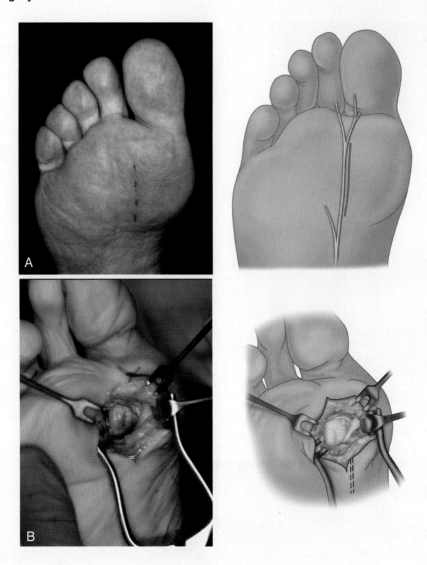

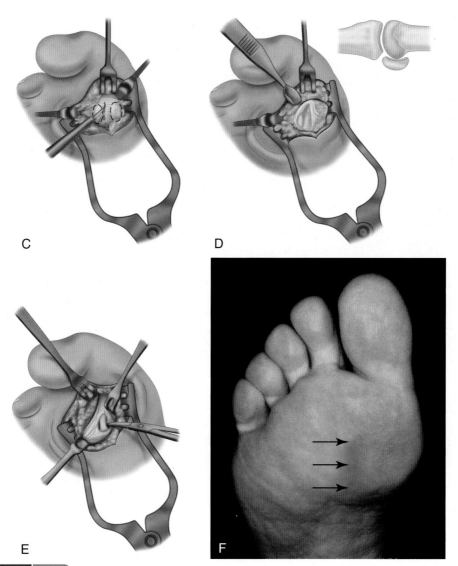

C

D

E

F

FIGURE 2.123 Fibular sesamoidectomy (plantar approach). **A,** Incision. **B,** Common digital nerve to first web space. **C,** Flexor hallucis longus tendon is retracted medially, and neurovascular bundle is retracted laterally; intersesamoid ligament is divided. **D,** Fibular sesamoid ligament is removed, and lateral border of tibial sesamoid is exposed. **E,** Tendon of oblique head of adductor hallucis. **F,** Healed plantar incision. **SEE TECHNIQUE 2.37.**

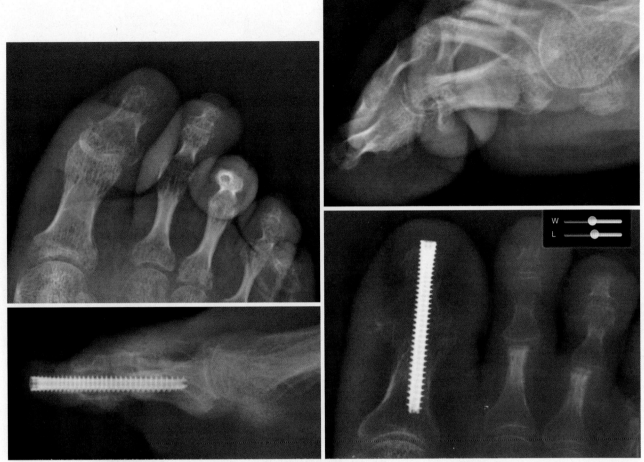

FIGURE 2.124   Headless compression screw in interphalangeal joint arthrodesis.

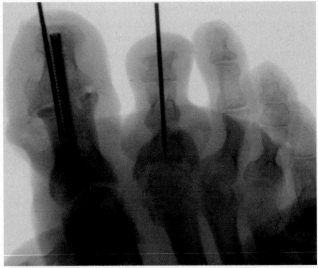

FIGURE 2.125   Interphalangeal joint fixed headless screw and additional Kirschner wires.

REFERENCES

HALLUX VALGUS

Ahn JY, Lee HS, Chun H, et al.: Comparison of open lateral release and transarticular lateral release in distal chevron metatarsal osteotomy for hallux valgus correction, *Int Orthop* 37(9):1781, 2013.

Ahn J, Lee HS, Seo JH, Kim JY: Second metatarsal transfer lesions due to first metatarsal shortening after distal chevron metatarsal osteotomy for hallux valgus, *Foot Ankle Int* 37(6):589, 2016.

Aiyer A, Shub J, Shariff R, Ying L, Myerson M: Radiographic recurrence of deformity after hallux valgus surgery in patients with metatarsus adductus, *Foot Ankle Int* 37(2):165, 2016.

Al Nammari SS, Christofi T, Clark C: Double first metatarsal and Akin osteotomy for severe hallux valgus, *Foot Ankle Int* 36(10):1215, 2015.

Angthong C, Yoshimura I, Kanazawa K, et al.: Minimally invasive distal linear metatarsal osteotomy for correction of hallux valgus: a preliminary study of clinical outcome and analytical radiographic results via a mapping system, *Arch Orthop Trauma Surg* 133(3):321, 2013.

Badekas A, Georgiannos D, Lampridis V, Bisbinas I: Proximal opening wedge metatarsal osteotomy for correction of moderate to severe hallux valgus deformity using a locking plate, *Int Orthop* 37(9):1765, 2013.

Bai LB, Lee KB, Seo CY, et al.: Distal chevron osteotomy with distal soft tissue procedure for moderate to severe hallux valgus deformity, *Foot Ankle Int* 31:683, 2010.

Barg A, Harmer JR, Presson AP, et al.: Unfavorable outcomes following surgical treatment of hallux valgus deformity: a systematic literature review, *J Bone Joint Surg Am* 100(18):1563, 2018.

Basile P, Cook EA, Cook JJ: Immediate weight bearing following modified Lapidus arthrodesis, *J Foot Ankle Surg* 49:459, 2010.

Bennett GL, Sabetta JA: Evaluation of an innovative fixation system for chevron bunionectomy, *Foot Ankle Int* 37(2):205, 2016.

Bhosale A, Munoruth A, Blundell C, et al.: Complex primary arthrodesis of the first metatarsophalangeal joint after bone loss, *Foot Ankle Int* 32(10):968, 2011.

Biz C, Fosser M, Dalmau-Pastor M, et al.: Functional and radiographic outcomes of hallux valgus correction by mini-invasive surgery with Reverdin-Isham and Akin percutaneous osteotomies: a longitudinal prospective study with a 48-month follow-up, *J Orthop Surg Res* 11:157, 2016.

Booth S, Bhosale A, Mustafa A, et al.: Triple osteotomy for the correction of severe hallux valgus deformity: patient reported outcomes and radiological evaluation, *Foot (Edinb)* 28:30, 2016.

Braito M, Dammerer D, Hofer-Picout P, Kaufmann G: Proximal opening wedge osteotomy with distal chevron osteotomy of the first metatarsal for the treatment of moderate to severe hallux valgus, *Foot Ankle Int* 40(1):89, 2019.

Brogan K, Lindisfarne E, Akehurst H, et al.: Minimally invasive and open distal chevron osteotomy for mild to moderate hallux valgus, *Foot Ankle Int* 37(11):1197, 2016.

Buciuto R: Prospective randomized study of chevron osteotomy versus Mitchell's osteotomy in hallux valgus, *Foot Ankle Int* 35(12):1268, 2014.

Campbell B, Miller MC, Williams L, Conti SF: Pilot study of a 3-dimensional method for analysis of pronation of the first metatarsal of hallux valgus patients, *Foot Ankle Int* 39(12):1449, 2018.

Cantanese D, Popowitz D, Gladstein AZ: Measuring sesamoid position in hallux valgus: when is the sesamoid axial view necessary? *Foot Ankle Spec* 7(6):457, 2014.

Chan CX, Gan JZ, Chong HC, et al.: Two year outcomes of minimally invasive hallux valgus surgery, *Foot Ankle Surg* 25(2):119, 2019.

Chen JY, Ang BF, Jiang L, et al.: Pain resolution after hallux valgus surgery, *Foot Ankle Int* 37(10):1071, 2016.

Chen JY, Lee MJ, Rikhraj K, et al.: Effect of obesity on outcome of hallux valgus surgery, *Foot Ankle Int* 36(9):1078, 2015.

Chiang CC, Lin CF, Tzeng YH, et al.: Distal linear osteotomy compared to oblique diaphyseal osteotomy in moderate to severe hallux valgus, *Foot Ankle Int* 33(6):479, 2012.

Cho BK, Park JK, Choi SM, SooHoo NF: Is generalized ligamentous laxity a prognostic factor for recurred hallux valgus deformity? *Foot Ankle Surg* 25(2):127, 2019.

Choi JH, Zide JR, Coleman SC, Brodsky JW: Prospective study of the treatment of adult primary hallux valgus with scarf osteotomy and soft-tissue realignment, *Foot Ankle Int* 34(5):684, 2013.

Choi KJ, Lee HS, Yoon YS, et al.: Distal metatarsal osteotomy for hallux varus following surgery for hallux valgus, *J Bone Joint Surg* 93B:1079, 2011.

Choi YR, Lee HS, Jeong JJ, et al.: Hallux valgus correction using transarticular lateral release with distal chevron osteotomy, *Foot Ankle Int* 33(10):838, 2012.

Covell DJ, Lareau CR, Anderson RB: Operative treatment of traumatic hallux valgus in elite athletes, *Foot Ankle Int* 38(6):590, 2017.

Day T, Charlton TP, Thordarson DB: First metatarsal length change after basilar closing wedge osteotomy for hallux valgus, *Foot Ankle Int* 32(5):S513, 2011.

Deenik A, Verburg A, Louwerens JW, et al.: Evidence of treatment algorithms for hallux valgus, *JSM Foot Ankle* 1(1):1003, 2016.

Dietze A, Bahlke U, Martin H, Mittlmeier T: First ray instability in hallux valgus deformity: radiokinematic and pedobarographic analysis, *Foot Ankle Int* 34(1):124, 2013.

Dixon AE, Lee LC, Charlton TP, Thordarson DB: Increased incidence and severity of postoperative radiographic hallux valgus interphalangeus with surgical correction of hallux valgus, *Foot Ankle Int* 36(8):961, 2015.

Edmonds EW, Ek D, Bomar JD, et al.: Preliminary radiographic outcomes of surgical correction in juvenile hallux valgus: single proximal, single distal versus double osteotomies, *J Pediatr Orthop* 35(3):307, 2015.

Ellington JK, Myerson MS, Coetzee JC, Stone RM: The use of the Lapidus procedure for recurrent hallux valgus, *Foot Ankle Int* 32(7):674, 2011.

Faber FW, van Kampen PM, Bloembergen MW: Long-term results of the Hohmann and Lapidus procedure for the correction of hallux valgus: a prospective, randomised trial with eight to 11-year follow-up involving 101 feet, *Bone Joint J* 95(B):1222, 2013.

Faldini C, Nanni M, Traina F, et al.: Surgical treatment of hallux valgus associated with flexible flatfoot during growing age, *Int Orthop* 40(4):737, 2016.

Farrar NG, Duncan N, Ahmed N, Rajan RA: Scarf osteotomy in the management of symptomatic adolescent hallux valgus, *J Child Orthop* 6(2):153, 2012.

Feilmeier M, Dayton P, Wienke JC: Reduction of intermetatarsal angle after first metatarsophalangeal joint arthrodesis in patients with hallux valgus, *J Foot Ankle Surg* 53(1):29, 2014.

Fernandez D: Percutaneous triple and double osteotomies for the treatment of hallux, *valgus* 38(2):159, 2017.

Feuerstein C, Weil Jr L, Weil Sr LS, et al.: Joint manipulation under anesthesia for arthrofibrosis after hallux valgus surgery, *J Foot Ankle Surg* 55(1):76, 2016.

Finney FT, Gossett TD, Hu HM, et al.: New persistent opioid use following common forefoot procedures for the treatment of hallux valgus, *J Bone Joint Surg Am* 101(8):722, 2019.

Fournier M, Saxena A, Maffulli N: Hallux valgus surgery in the athlete: current evidence, *J Foot Ankle Surg* 58(4):641, 2019.

Fraissler L, Konrads C, Hoberg M, et al.: Treatment of hallux valgus deformity, *EFFORT Open Rev* 1:295, 2016.

Giannini S, Cavallo M, Faldini C, et al.: The SERI distal metatarsal osteotomy and scarf osteotomy provide similar correction of hallux valgus, *Clin Orthop Relat Res* 471(7):2305, 2013.

Giannini S, Faldini C, Nanni M, et al.: A minimally invasive technique for surgical treatment of hallux valgus: simple, effective, rapid, inexpensive (SERI), *Int Orthop* 37(9):1805, 2013.

Gines-Cespedosa A, Alentorn-Geli E, Sanchez JF, et al.: Influence of common associated forefoot disorders on preoperative quality of life in patients with hallux valgus, *Foot Ankle Int* 34(12):1634, 2013.

Glazebrook M, Copithorne P, Boyd G, et al.: Proximal opening wedge osteotomy with wedge-plate fixation compared with proximal chevron osteotomy for the treatment of hallux valgus: a prospective, randomized study, *J Bone Joint Surg* 96A:1585, 2014.

Goldberg A, Singh D: Treatment of shortening following hallux valgus surgery, *Foot Ankle Clin* 19(2):309, 2014.

Gómez Galván M, Constantino JA, Bernáldez MJ, Quiles M: Hallux pronation in hallux valgus: experimental and radiographic study, *J Foot Ankle Surg* 38(5):886, 1996.

Harb Z, Kokkinakis M, Ismail H, Spence G: Adolescent hallux valgus: a systematic review of outcomes following surgery, *J Child Orthop* 9(2):105, 2015.

Hernandez LY, Goalnó P, Roshan-Zamir S, et al.: Treatment of moderate hallux valgus by percutaneous, extra-articular reverse-L chevron (PERC) osteotomy, *Bone Joint J* 98-B(3):365, 2016.

Herrera-Perez M, De Prado-Serrano M, Gutiérrez-Morales MJ, et al.: Increased rates of delayed union after percutaneous Akin osteotomy, *Foot Ankle Surg* 24(5):411, 2018.

Holme TJ, Sivaloganathan SS, Patel B, Kunasingam K: Third-generation minimally invasive chevron Akin osteotomy for hallux valgus, *Foot Ankle Int*, 2019, [Epub ahead of print].

Huang EH, Charlton TP, Ajayi S, Thordarson DB: Effect of various hallux valgus reconstruction on sesamoid location: a radiographic study, *Foot Ankle Int* 34(1):99, 2013.

Ianno B, Familiari F, De Gori M, et al.: Midterm results and complications after minimally invasive distal metatarsal osteotomy for treatment of hallux valgus, *Foot Ankle Int* 34(7):969, 2013.

Iyer S, Demetracopoulos CA, Sofka CM, Ellis SJ: High rate of recurrence following proximal medial opening wedge osteotomy for correction of moderate hallux valgus, *Foot Ankle Int* 36(7):756, 2015.

Jastifer JR, Coughlin MJ, Doty JF, et al.: Osteochondral lesions in surgically treated hallux valgus, *Foot Ankle Int* 35(7):643, 2014.

Jastifer JR, Coughlin MJ, Doty JF, et al.: Sensory nerve dysfunction and hallux valgus correction: a prospective study, *Foot Ankle Int* 35(8):757, 2014.

Kaipel M, Reissig L, Albrecht L, et al.: Risk of damaging anatomical structures during minimally invasive hallux valgus correction (Bösch technique): an anatomical study, *Foot Ankle Int* 39(11):1355, 2018.

Kaiser P, Livingston K, Miller PE, et al.: Radiographic evaluation of first metatarsal and medial cuneiform morphology in juvenile hallux valgus, *Foot Ankle Int* 39(10):1223, 2018.

Kaufmann G, Dammerer D, Heyenbrock F, et al.: Minimally invasive versus open chevron osteotomy for hallux valgus correction: a randomized controlled trial, *Int Orthop* 43(2):343, 2019.

Kaufmann G, Hofmann M, Brato M, et al.: Need for concomitant Akin osteotomy in patients undergoing Chevron osteotomy can be determined preoperatively: a retrospective comparative study of 859 cases, *J Orthop Surg Res* 14(1):277, 2019.

Kaufman G, Sinz S, Giesinger JM, et al.: Loss of correction after chevron osteotomy for hallux valgus as a function of preoperative deformity, *Foot Ankle Int* 40(3):287, 2019.

Khoury K, Staggers JR, Pinto MC, et al: Radiographic assessment of first tarsometatarsal joint shape and orientation, *Foot Ankle Int* 2019 [Epub ahead of print].

Kim YJ, Kim S, Young KW, et al.: A new measure of tibial sesamoid position in hallux valgus in relation to the coronal rotation of the first metatarsal in CT scans, *Foot Ankle Int* 36(8):944, 2015.

Kim HN, Park YJ, Kim GL, Park YW: Distal chevron osteotomy with lateral soft tissue release for moderate to severe hallux valgus decided using intraoperative varus stress radiographs, *J Foot Ankle Surg* 52(3):303, 2013.

Kimura T, Kubota M, Taguchi T, et al.: Evaluation of first-ray mobility in patients with hallux valgus using weight-bearing CT and a 3-D analysis system: a comparison with normal feet, *J Bone Joint Surg Am* 99(3):247, 2017.

Kraus T, Singer G, Svehlik M, et al.: Long-term outcome of chevron-osteotomy in juvenile hallux valgus, *Acta Orthop Belg* 79(5):552, 2013.

Kumar S, Pradhan R, Rosenfeld PF: First metatarsophalangeal arthrodesis using a dorsal plate and a compression screw, *Foot Ankle Int* 31:797, 2010.

Kuyucu E, Ceylan HH, Surucu S, et al.: The effect of incorrect foot placement on the accuracy of radiographic measurements of the hallux valgus and inter-metatarsal angles for treating hallux valgus, *Acta Chir Orthop Traumatol Cech* 84(3):196, 2017.

Lai MC, Rikhraj IS, Woo YL, et al.: Clinical and radiological outcomes comparing percutaneous chevron-Akin osteotomies vs open scarf-Akin osteotomies for hallux valgus, *Foot Ankle Int* 39(3):311, 2018.

Lai SWH, Tang CQY, Graetz AEK, Thevendran G: Preoperative mental health score and postoperative outcome after hallux valgus surgery, *Foot Ankle Int* 39(12):1403, 2018.

Lee HJ, Chung JW, Chu IT, Kim YC: Comparison of distal chevron osteotomy with and without lateral soft tissue release for the treatment of hallux valgus, *Foot Ankle Int* 31:291, 2010.

Lee M, Walsh J, Smith MM, et al.: Hallux valgus correction comparing percutaneous chevron/Akin (PECA) and open scarf/Akin osteotomies, *Foot Ankle Int* 38(8):838, 2017.

Li X, Guo M, Zhu Y, Xu X: The excessive length of the first ray as a risk factor for hallux valgus recurrence, *PloS One* 13(10):30205560, 2018.

Liszka H, Gądek A: Comparison of the type of fixation of Akin osteotomy, *Foot Ankle Int* 40(4):390, 2019.

Loh B, Chen JY, Yew AK, et al.: Prevalence of metatarsus adductus in symptomatic hallux valgus and its influence on functional outcome, *Foot Ankle Int* 36(11):1316, 2015.

Lucattelli G, Catani O, Sergio F, et al.: Preliminary experience with a minimally invasive technique for hallux valgus correction with no fixation, *Foot Ankle Int* 1071100719868725, 2019.

Maceira E, Monteagudo M: Transfer metatarsalgia post hallux valgus surgery, *Foot Ankle Clin* 19(2):285, 2014.

Magnan B, Negri S, Maluta T, et al.: Minimally invasive distal first metatarsal osteotomy can be an option for recurrent hallux valgus, *Foot Ankle Surg* 25(3):332, 2018.

Malagelada F, Sahirad C, Dalmau-Pastor M, et al.: Minimally invasive surgery for hallux valgus: a systematic review of current surgical techniques, *Int Orthop* 43:625, 2019.

Matthews M, Klein E, Youssef A, et al.: Correlation of radiographic measurements with patient-centered outcomes in hallux valgus surgery, *Foot Ankle Int* 39(12):1416, 2018.

McAlister JE, Peterson KS, Hyer CF: Corrective realignment arthrodesis of the first tarsometatarsal joint without wedge resection, *Foot Ankle Spec* 8(4):284, 2015.

Morandi A, Ungara E, Fraccia A, Sansone V: Chevron osteotomy of the first metatarsal stabilized with an absorbable pin: our 5-year experience, *Foot Ankle Int* 34(3):380, 2013.

McDonald E, Shakked R, Daniel J, et al.: Driving after hallux valgus surgery, *Foot Ankle Int* 38(9):982, 2017.

McKean RM, Bergin PF, Watson G, et al.: Radiographic evaluation of inter-metatarsal angle correction following first MTP joint arthrodesis for severe hallux varus, *Foot Ankle Int* 37(11):1183, 2016.

Nakagawa S, Fukushi J, Nakagawa T, et al.: Association of metatarsalgia after hallux valgus correction with relative first metatarsal length, 37(6):582, 2016.

Nery C, Coughlin MJ, Baumfeld D, et al.: Hallux valgus in males: Part 1: demographics, etiology, and comparative radiology, *Foot Ankle Int* 34(5):629, 2013.

Nery C, Coughlin MJ, Baumfeld D, et al.: Hallux valgus in males: Part 2: radiographic assessment of surgical treatment, *Foot Ankle Int* 34(5):636, 2013.

Neumann JA, Reay KD, Bradley KE, Parekh SG: Staple fixation for Akin proximal phalangeal osteotomy in the treatment of hallux valgus interphalangeus, *Foot Ankle Int* 36(4):457, 2015.

Nixon DC, McCormick JJ, Johnson JE, Klein SE: PROMIS pain interference and physical function screws correlated with the Foot and Ankle Ability Measure (FAAM) in patients with hallux valgus, *Clin Orthop Relat Res* 475(11):2775, 2017.

Ortiz C, Wagner P, Vela O, et al.: "Angle to be corrected" in preoperative evaluation for hallux valgus surgery: analysis of a new angular measurement, *Foot Ankle Int* 37(2):172, 2016.

Park CH, Lee WC: Recurrence of hallux valgus can be predicted from immediate postoperative non-weight-bearing radiographs, *J Bone Joint Surg Am* 99(14):1190, 2017.

Park HW, Lee KB, Chung JY, Kim MS: Comparison of outcomes between proximal and distal chevron osteotomy, both with supplementary lateral soft-tissue release, for severe hallux valgus deformity: a prospective randomized controlled trial, *Bone Joint J* 95(B):510, 2013.

Park JY, Jung HG, Kim TH, Kang MS: Intraoperative incidence of hallux valgus interphalangeus following basilar first metatarsal osteotomy and distal soft tissue realignment, *Foot Ankle Int* 32(11):1058, 2011.

Park JY, Jung HG, Kim TH, Kang MS: Intraoperative incidence of hallux valgus interphalangeus following basilar first metatarsal osteotomy and distal soft tissue realignment, *Foot Ankle Int* 32(10):962, 2011.

Park YB, Lee KB, Kim SK, et al.: Comparison of distal-soft-tissue procedures combined with a distal chevron osteotomy for moderate to severe hallux valgus: first web-space versus transarticular approach, *J Bone Joint Surg* 95A(21):e158, 2013.

Pauli W, Koch A, Testa E, et al.: Fixation of the proximal metatarsal crescentic osteotomy using a head locking X-plate, *Foot Ankle Int* 37:218, 2016.

Pentikainen I, Ojala R, Ohtonen P, et al.: Preoperative radiological factors correlated to long-term recurrence of hallux valgus following distal chevron osteotomy, *Foot Ankle Int* 35(12):1262, 2014.

Ponzio DY, Pedowitz DI, Verma K, et al.: Radiographic outcomes of postoperative taping following hallux valgus correction, *Foot Ankle Int* 36(7):820, 2015.

Prado M, Baumfeld T, Nery C, et al.: Rotational biplanar chevron osteotomy, *Foot Ankle Surg*, 2019, [Epub ahead of print].

Putti AB, Pande S, Adam RF, Abboud RJ: Keller's arthroplasty in adults with hallux valgus and hallux rigidus, *Foot Ankle Surg* 18(1):34, 2012.

Radwan YA, Mansour AM: Percutaneous distal metatarsal osteotomy versus distal chevron osteotomy for correction of mild-to-moderate hallux valgus deformity, *Arch Orthop Trauma Surg* 132(11):1539, 2012.

Ray JJ, Koay J, Dayton PD, et al.: Multicenter early radiographic outcomes of triplanar tarsometatarsal arthrodesis with early weightbearing, *Foot Ankle Int* 40:955, 2019.

Rippstein PF, Park YU, Naal FD: Combination of first metatarsophalangeal joint arthrodesis and proximal correction for severe hallux valgus deformity, *Foot Ankle Int* 33(5):400, 2012.

Rogero R, Fuchs D, Nicholson K, et al.: Postoperative opioid consumption in opioid-naïve patients undergoing hallux valgus correction, *Foot Ankle Int*, 2019, [Epub ahead of print].

Rose B, Bowman N, Edwards H, et al.: Lengthening scarf osteotomy for recurrent hallux valgus, *Foot Ankle Surg* 20(1):20, 2014.

Roukis TS: Nonunion after arthrodesis of the first metatarsal-phalangeal joint: a systematic review, *J Foot Ankle Surg* 50(6):710, 2011.

Santrock RD, Smith B: Hallux valgus deformity and treatment: a three-dimensional approach: modified technique for Lapidus procedure, *Foot Ankle Clin* 23(2):281, 2018.

Scala A, Vendettuoli D: Modified minimal incision subcapital osteotomy for hallux valgus correction, *Foot Ankle Spec* 6(1):65, 2013.

Schneider W: Influence of different anatomical structures on distal soft tissue procedure in hallux valgus surgery, *Foot Ankle Int* 33(11):991, 2012.

Shakked R, McDonald E, Sutton R, et al.: Influence of depressive symptoms on hallux valgus surgical outcomes, *Foot Ankle Int* 39(7):795, 2018.

Sharma J, Aydogan U: Algorithm for severe hallux valgus associated with metatarsus adductus, *Foot Ankle Int* 36(12):1499, 2015.

Shi GG, Henning P, Marks RM: Correlation of postoperative position of the sesamoids after chevron osteotomy with outcome, *Foot Ankle Int* 37(3):274, 2016.

Shibuya N, Jupiter DC, Plemmons BS, et al.: Correction of hallux valgus deformity in association with underlying metatarsus adductus deformity, *Foot Ankle Spec* 10(6):538, 2017.

Shima H, Okuda R, Yasuda T, et al.: Operative treatment for hallux valgus with moderate to severe metatarsus adductus, *Foot Ankle Int* 40(6):641, 2019.

Shine J, Weil Jr L, Weil Sr LS, Chase K: Scarf osteotomy for the correction of adolescent hallux valgus, *Foot Ankle Spec* 3(10), 2010.

Siekmann W, Watson TS, Roggelin M: Correction of moderate to severe hallux valgus with isometric first metatarsal double osteotomy, *Foot Ankle Int* 35(11):1122, 2014.

Song JH, Kang C, Hwang DS, et al.: Comparison of radiographic and clinical results after extended distal chevron osteotomy with distal soft tissue release with moderate versus severe hallux valgus, *Foot Ankle Int* 40(3):297, 2019.

Stith A, Dang D, Griffin M, et al.: Rigid internal fixation of proximal crescentic metatarsal osteotomy in hallux valgus correction, *Foot Ankle Int* 40:778, 2019.

Sutton RM, McDonald EL, Shakked RJ, et al.: Determination of minimum clinically important difference (MCID) in visual analog scale (VAS) pain and Foot and Ankle Ability Measure (FAAM) scores after hallux valgus surgery, *Foot Ankle Int* 40(6):687, 2019.

Tong CK, Ho YF: Use of minimally invasive distal metatarsal osteotomy for correction of hallux valgus, *J Orthop Trauma Rehabil* 16(16), 2012.

Usuelli F, Palmucci M, Montrasio UA, Malerba F: Radiographic considerations of hallux valgus versus hallux rigidus, *Foot Ankle Int* 32(8):782, 2011.

Vander Griend R: Correction of hallux valgus interphalangeus with an osteotomy of the distal end of the proximal phalanx (distal Akin osteotomy), *Foot Ankle Int* 38(2):153, 2017.

Wagner E, Ortiz C, Figueroa F, et al.: Role of a limited transarticular release in severe hallux valgus correction, *Foot Ankle Int* 36(11):1322, 2015.

Wagner E, Ortiz C, Gould JS, et al.: Proximal oblique sliding closing wedge osteotomy for hallux valgus, *Foot Ankle Int* 34(11):1493, 2013.

Wagner P, Ortiz C, Wagner E: Rotational osteotomy for hallux valgus. A new technique for primary and revision cases, *Tech Foot Ankle Surg* 16(3), 2017.

Wagner P, Wagner E: Is the rotational deformity important in our decision-making process for correction of hallux valgus deformity? *Foot Ankle Clin* 23(2):205, 2018.

Wülker N, Mittag F: The treatment of hallux valgus, *Dtsch Arztebl Int* 109(49), 2012.

Yamamoto Y, Yamaguchi S, Muramatsu Y, et al.: Quality of life in patients with untreated and symptomatic hallux valgus, *Foot Ankle Int* 37(11):1171, 2016.

Yanez Arauz JM, Del Vecchio JJ, Codesido M, Raimondi N: Minimally invasive Akin osteotomy and lateral release: anatomical structures at risk – a cadaveric study, *Foot (Edinb)* 27:32, 2016.

Young KW, Kim JS, Cho JW, et al.: Characteristics of male adolescent-onset hallux valgus, *Foot Ankle Int* 34(9):1111, 2013.

HALLUX RIGIDUS

Aynardi MC, Atwater L, Dein EJ, et al.: Outcomes after interpositional arthroplasty of the first metatarsophalangeal joint, *Foot Ankle Int* 38(5):514, 2017.

Baumhauer JF, Daniels T, Glazebrook M: New technology in the treatment of hallux rigidus with a synthetic cartilage implant hemiarthroplasty, *Orthop Clin North Am* 50(1):109, 2019.

Baumhauer JF, Singh D, Glazebrook M, et al.: Correlation of hallux rigidus grade with motion, VAS pain, intraoperative cartilage loss, and treatment success for first MTP joint arthrodesis and synthetic carilage implant, *Foot Ankle Int* 38(11):1175, 2017.

Baumhauer JF, Singh D, Glazebrook M, et al.: Prospective, randomized, multi-centered clinical trial assessing safety and efficacy of a synthetic cartilage implant versus first metatarsophalangeal arthrodesis in advanced hallux rigidus, *Foot Ankle Int* 37(5):457, 2016.

Cassinelli SJ, Chen S, Charlton TP, Thordarson DB: Early outcomes and complications of synthetic cartilage implant for treatment of hallux rigidus in the United States, *Foot Ankle Int*, 2019, [Epub ahead of print].

Cheung B, Myerson MS, Tracey J, Vulcano E: Weightbearing CT scan assessment of foot alignment in patients with hallux rigidus, *Foot Ankle Int* 39(1):67, 2018.

Cho BK, Park KJ, Park JK, SooHoo NF: Outcomes of the distal metatarsal dorsiflexion osteotomy for advanced hallux rigidus, *Foot Ankle Int* 38(5):541, 2017.

Chraim M, Bock P, Alrabai HM, Trnka HJ: Long-term outcome of first metatarsophalangeal joint fusion in the treatment of severe hallux rigidus, *Int Orthop* 40(11):2401, 2016.

Clement ND, MacDonald D, Dall GF, et al.: Metallic hemiarthroplasty for the treatment of end-stage hallux rigidus: mid-term implant survival, functional outcome and cost analysis, *Bone Joint J* 98-B(7):945, 2016.

Colò G, Alessio-Mazzola M, Dagnino G, Felli L: Long-term results of surgical treatment of Valenti procedures for hallux rigidus: a minimum ten-year follow-up retrospective study, *J Foot Ankle Surg* 38(2):291, 2019.

Coutts A, Kilmartin TE: Dorsiflexory phalangeal osteotomy for grade II hallux rigidus: patient-focused outcomes at eleven-year follow-up, *J Foot Ankle Surg* 58(1):17, 2019.

DaCunha RJ, MacMahon A, Jones MT, et al.: Return to sport and physical activities after first metatarsophalangeal joint arthrodesis in young patients, *Foot Ankle Int* 40(7):745, 2019.

Erkocak OF, Senaran H, Altan E, et al.: Short-term functional outcomes of first metatarsophalangeal total joint replacement for hallux rigidus, *Foot Ankle Int* 34(11):1569, 2013.

Fuld 3rd RS, Kumparatana P, Kelley J, et al.: Biomechanical comparison of low-profile contoured locking plate with single compression screw to fully threaded compression screws for first MTP fusion, *Foot Ankle Int* 40(7):836, 2019.

Glazebrook M, Blundell CM, O'Dowd D, et al.: Midterm outcomes of a synthetic cartilage implant for the first metatarsophalangeal joint in advanced hallux rigidus, *Foot Ankle Int* 40(4):374, 2019.

Goldberg A, Singh D, Glaebrook M, et al.: Association between patient factors and outcome of synthetic cartilage implant hemiarthroplasty vs first metatarsophalangeal joint arthrodesis in advanced hallux rigidus, *Foot Ankle Int* 38(11):1199, 2017.

Hogan MV, Mani SB, Chan JY, et al.: Validation of foot and ankle outcome score for hallux rigidus, *HSS J* 12(1):44, 2016.

Horisberger M, Haeni D, Henninger HB, et al.: Total arthroplasty of the metatarsophalangeal joint of the hallux, *Foot Ankle Int* 37(7):755, 2016.

Hunt KJ, Anderson RB: Biplanar proximal phalanx closing wedge osteotomy for hallux rigidus, *Foot Ankle Int* 33(12):1043, 2012.

Johnson JE, McCormick JJ: Modified oblique Keller capsular interposition arthroplasty (MOKCIA) for treatment of late-stage hallux rigidus, *Foot Ankle Int* 35(4):415, 2014.

Kline AJ, Hasselman CT: Metatarsal head resurfacing for advanced hallux rigidus, *Foot Ankle Int* 34(5):716, 2013.

Nagy MT, Walker CR, Sirikonda SP: Second-generation ceramic first metatarsophalangeal joint replacement for hallux rigidus, *Foot Ankle Int* 35(7):690, 2014.

Nicolosi N, Hehemann C, Connors J, Boike A: Long-term follow-up of the cheilectomy for degenerative joint disease of the first metatarsophalangeal joint, *J Foot Ankle Surg* 54(6):1010, 2015.

Nixon DC, Lorbeer KF, McCormick JJ, et al.: Hallux rigidus grade does not correlate with foot and ankle ability measure score, *J Am Acad Orthop Surg* 25(9):648, 2017.

O'Malley MJ, Basran HS, Gu Y, et al.: Treatment of advanced stages of hallux rigidus with cheilectomy and phalangeal osteotomy, *J Bone Joint Surg* 95A:606, 2013.

Perez-Aznar A, Lizaur-Utrilla A, Lopez-Prats FA, Gil-Guillen V: Dorsal wedge phalangeal osteotomy for grade II-III hallux rigidus in active adult patients, *Foot Ankle Int* 36(2):188, 2015.

Pinter Z, Hudson P, Cone B, et al.: Radiographic evaluation of first MTP joint arthrodesis for severe hallux valgus: does the introduction of a lag screw improve union rates and correction of the intermetatarsal angle? *Foot (Edinb)* 33:20, 2017.

Rothermel SD, King JL, Tupinio M, et al.: Cost comparison of synthetic hydrogel implant and first metatarsophalangeal joint arthrodesis, *Foot Ankle Spec*, 2019, [Epub ahead of print].

Sanhudo JA, Gomes JE, Rodrigo MK: Surgical treatment of advanced hallux rigidus by interpositional arthroplasty, *Foot Ankle Int* 32(4):400, 2011.

Saxena A, Valerio DL, Behan SA, Hofer D: Modified Valenti arthroplasty in running and jumping athletes with hallux limitus/rigidus: analysis of one hundred procedures, *J Foot Ankle Surg* 58(4):609, 2019.

Schneider W, Kadnar G, Kranzl A, Knahr K: Long-term results following Keller resection arthroplasty for hallux rigidus, *Foot Ankle Int* 32(10):933, 2011.

Sidon E, Rogero R, Bell T, et al.: Long-term follow-up of cheilectomy for treatment of hallux rigidus, *Foot Ankle Int*, 2019, [Epub ahead of print].

Smith SM, Coleman SC, Bacon SA, et al.: Improved ankle push-off power following cheilectomy for hallux rigidus: a prospective gait analysis study, *Foot Ankle Int* 33(6):457, 2012.

Stevens J, de Bot RTAL, Hermus JPS, et al.: Clinical outcome following total joint replacement and arthrodesis for hallux rigidus: a systematic review, *JBJS Rev* 5(11):e2, 2017.

Stone OD, Ray R, Thomson CE, Gibson JN: Long-term follow-up of arthrodesis vs total joint arthroplasty for hallux rigidus, *Foot Ankle Int* 38(4):375, 2017.

Taranow WS, Moor JR: Hallux rigidus: a treatment algorithm, *Tech Foot and Ankle Surg* 11(2):65, 2012.

Thomas D, Thordarson D: Rolled tendon allograft interposition arthroplasty for salvage surgery of the hallux metatarsophalangeal joint, *Foot Ankle Int* 39(4):458, 2018.

Viladot A, Sodano L, Marcellini L, et al.: Youngswick-Austin versus distal oblique osteotomy for the treatment of hallux rigidus, *Foot (Edinb)* 32:53, 2017.

Voegeli AV, Marcellini L, Sodano L, Perice RV: Clinical and radiological outcomes after distal oblique osteotomy for the treatment of stage II hallux rigidus: mid-term results, *Foot Ankle Surg* 23(1):21, 2017.

Vulcano E, Chang AL, Solomon D, Myerson M: Long-term follow-up of capsular interposition arthroplasty for hallux rigidus, *Foot Ankle Int* 39(1):1, 2018.

Wagner E, Wagner P, Ortiz C: Arthrodesis of the hallux metatarsophalangeal joint, *JBJS Essent Surg Tech* 5(4), 2015:e20.

SESAMOID INJURY

Bichara DA, Henn 3rd RF, Theodore GH: Sesamoidectomy for hallux sesamoid fractures, *Foot Ankle Int* 33(9):704, 2012.

Coughlin MJ, Kemp TJ, Hirose CB: Turf toe: soft tissue and osteocartilaginous injury to the first metatarsophalangeal joint, *Phys Sportsmed* 38:91, 2010.

Favinger JL, Porrino JA, Richardson ML, et al.: Epidemiology and imaging appearance of the normal bi-/multipartite hallux sesamoid bone, *Foot Ankle Int* 36(2):197, 2015.

Lee S, James WC, Cohen BE, et al.: Evaluation of hallux alignment and functional outcome after isolated tibial sesamoidectomy, *Foot Ankle Int* 26(10):803, 2005.

Rodrigues Pinto R, Muras J: Medial approach to the fibular sesamoid, *Foot Ankle Int* 31:916, 2010.

The complete list of references is available online at expertconsult.inkling.com.

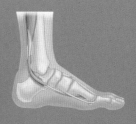

CHAPTER 3

DISORDERS OF TENDONS AND FASCIA AND ADOLESCENT AND ADULT PES PLANUS

Benjamin J. Grear

DISORDERS OF THE POSTERIOR TIBIAL TENDON

Chronic tenosynovitis (either traumatic, degenerative, or secondary to inflammatory arthritis), loss of continuity of the tendon (either complete or incomplete), and loss of the normal anatomic relationships of the tendon to its insertion or insertions (the accessory navicular) may render the posterior tibial tendon insufficient to perform its tasks of plantar-flexion, inversion, and stabilization of the medial longitudinal arch. For this reason, the term *insufficiency of the posterior tibial tendon* is descriptive. Further classification according to the just-mentioned etiologic factors is necessary for communicating the pathologic findings of this essential tendon of the foot. Other than the Achilles tendon, no other muscle-tendon unit distal to the knee can cause as many symptoms and functional deficits as loss of the posterior tibial tendon.

The etiology of progressive adult-acquired flatfoot deformity is multifactorial, and any pathologic condition that reduces the excursion of this tendon can produce the typical deformity of asymmetric flatfoot. It is important to note the difference between posterior tibial tendon insufficiency and flexible flatfoot deformity. With adult-acquired flatfoot deformity, the foot posture is acquired secondary to the insufficiency of the posterior tibial tendon, which leads to an asymmetric loss of arch. On the other hand, flexible pes planovalgus deformity (flexible flatfoot) is typically symmetric with a functioning posterior tibial tendon. This symmetric deformity is associated more with the patient's underlying anatomic morphology than with acquired tendon dysfunction. Nevertheless, patients with an underlying valgus foot posture can still develop tendon dysfunction and worsening deformity. Increased valgus orientation of the posterior facet

in the coronal plane and obesity have been associated with adult flatfoot deformity. In adult-acquired flatfoot deformity, the components of the deformity are hindfoot valgus, midfoot abduction at the midtarsal joint, and forefoot pronation, primarily at the midtarsal joint. This description applies best to the weight-bearing posture of the foot, and each component may vary in severity depending on the magnitude of posterior tibial dysfunction, the degree and location of the bony collapse of the medial longitudinal arch, the chronicity of the insufficiency, the rigidity of the deformity, and the configuration of the arch before the onset of posterior tibial tendon dysfunction.

The loss of the medial longitudinal arch can occur at the talonavicular, navicular-cuneiform, or cuneiform-metatarsal articulation or at more than one of these points. The weight-bearing lateral radiograph may show no collapse and may appear the same as the radiograph of the opposite, asymptomatic foot even with obvious clinical evidence of an asymmetric pes planus. To further complicate any discussion of posterior tibial tendon insufficiency, the nomenclature describing the components of the deformity is confusing. For example, it is obvious in the weight-bearing position that the heel is in valgus, the midfoot is in abduction, and the forefoot is in pronation. However, in reality, with the subtalar and midtarsal joints reduced anatomically (if the deformity is supple enough to allow it), the forefoot is not pronated but supinated, and in severe deformity this supination may be 60 to 70 degrees in the non–weight-bearing position. Restated in a different way, when examining the foot end-on with the hindfoot corrected to a neutral position, there is relative elevation of the first ray out of the neutral plane 60 to 70 degrees. Moreover, the terms *forefoot varus* and *supination* can be used interchangeably.

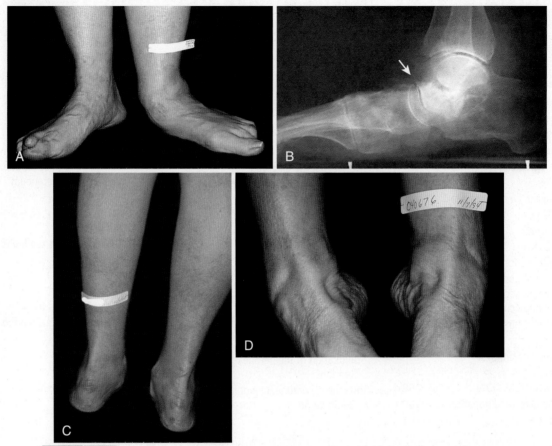

FIGURE 3.1   **A,** Patient with asymmetric pes planus. **B,** Talus slides distally, medially, and plantarward with loss of posterior tibial tendon and probable insufficiency of plantar calcaneonavicular ligament. **C,** Long-standing deformity. Achilles tendon contracture exacerbates heel valgus. **D,** In sitting position, when asked to hold foot in plantarflexion-inversion after being placed there passively by examiner, patient unconsciously used anterior tibial tendon. Also note increased supination (forefoot varus relative to longitudinal axis of calcaneus).

Recognition of secondary changes that occur in the hindfoot and forefoot with long-standing posterior tibial tendon insufficiency is important. As the hindfoot moves into valgus with midfoot pronation, changes occur in the ligamentous supporting structures of the medial arch, especially the spring ligament (calcaneonavicular ligament) in which significant stretching and elongation occur as it gradually loses support of the talar head. With increasing pressure and strain over the medial arch, the ligaments supporting the naviculocuneiform and cuneiform first metatarsal joints also may be elongated. In more severe cases, the deltoid ligament, especially the anterior or tibionavicular portion of the superficial deltoid ligament, may elongate, becoming a significant component of medial ankle instability. Deland et al. found that the most commonly involved ligament abnormality in this disease was the spring ligament but also demonstrated abnormalities in the anterior band of the superficial deltoid ligament, the plantar metatarsal ligaments, and the naviculocuneiform ligament.

CLASSIFICATION

Classification systems in general are useful only to the extent that they assist in planning treatment or in predicting the outcome of the condition. The classification system originally developed by Johnson and Strom in 1989 is useful in the management of posterior tibial tendon insufficiency. Stage I disease is characterized by swelling, pain, inflammation, and often effusion within the posterior tibial tendon sheath. Irritability is noted with passive eversion of the foot along the course of the posterior tibial tendon. Mild weakness to manual testing may be present; however, no deformity of the foot is demonstrated when compared with the opposite foot. The patient is able to invert the foot actively on a double-leg toe raise test and is able to perform a single-leg toe raise as described in the next section. Stage II disease is characterized by the loss of function of the posterior tibial tendon and inability to perform a single-leg toe raise. There is attempted compensation by use of the anterior tibial muscle and tendon unit as an accessory inverter of the hindfoot. In stage II disease the hindfoot remains flexible. With the hindfoot in neutral the forefoot can be brought into neutral. Generally, mild lateral or sinus tarsi impingement pain is present. Bluman et al. added two subcategories to Johnson and Strom's original classification: in stage IIA, less than 30% of the talar head is uncovered on standing anteroposterior radiographs and abduction deformity is minimal; in stage IIB, more than 30% of the talar head is uncovered and the abduction deformity is severe. In stage III disease, function of the posterior tibial tendon is lost, and a semirigid or rigid hindfoot deformity with valgus abduction occurs and degenerative changes may be apparent on radiographs. Significant lateral sinus tarsi pain is present. Stage IV disease was described by Myerson et al. and involves valgus positioning and incongruence of the ankle joint in addition to stage III findings.

The pertinent physical findings accompanying posterior tibial tendon insufficiency are illustrated in Figs 3.1 to 3.3.

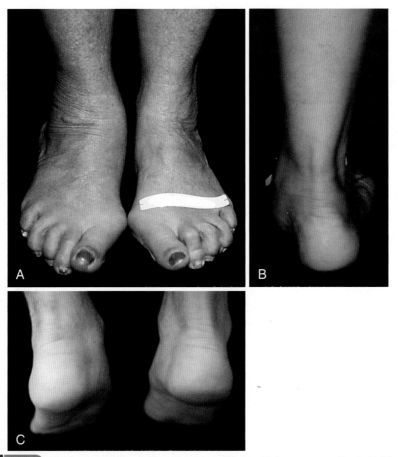

FIGURE 3.2   Patients with posterior tibial tendon insufficiency as result of attritional loss of continuity. Note that one or more of three major components of deformity may be excessive. **A,** Right heel is in some valgus and forefoot is pronated, but note marked midfoot abduction. This is important to note because not only would tendon transfer-substitute for posterior tibial tendon *not* correct this deformity, but also subtalar arthrodesis with heel in neutral would leave this component uncorrected. **B,** Standing position emphasizes multiple-plane deformity. **C,** Note convexity of medial side and concavity of lateral side on left foot.

DIAGNOSIS

A patient may have a variety of symptoms depending on the cause and chronicity of the insufficiency. If recurrent bouts of tenosynovitis are the cause, medial ankle and hindfoot pain may predominate. If the tenosynovitis goes unchecked, loss of excursion of the tendon may result either from mechanical blockage beneath the laciniate ligament that prevents the inflamed, edematous tendon and sheath from moving within the pulley system or from loss of voluntary contraction of the muscle-tendon unit because of pain. In other words, the patient "decommissions" the muscle-tendon unit because contraction is painful. With time, this becomes involuntary. The tendon can be palpated by the examiner at the medial malleolus by placing the foot in equinovarus and asking the patient to hold it there. Usually the deformity is not severe in tenosynovitis as long as continuity of the tendon is not lost (Fig. 3.4).

Patients may report foot and ankle fatigue after only limited activity, lack of support during ambulation, and limitation of footwear as a result of the foot "rolling out." However, pain is the most common primary complaint. This pain is medial at first, but with long-standing pronation it localizes laterally where the anterior surface of the lateral process of the talus impinges on the floor of the sinus tarsi (see Fig. 3.1B).

The deformity can become fixed, in which case lateral pain may become the presenting complaint. There may be a history of an acute injury with rapid collapse of the arch, but usually no traumatic event is noted by the patient, and gradual collapse of the arch is recalled.

Many authors have added to our understanding of the physical examination of the posterior tibial tendon–insufficient foot, but Mann, Specht, and Johnson emphasized that moving the heel into varus when raising the heel off the ground is difficult at best and virtually impossible if standing only on the affected foot. Therefore, in addition to examining the characteristic posture of the foot on weight bearing, the examiner should have the patient toe-stand while holding on to the examiner or the examining table for balance only and not support (single-limb heel rise). Some patients with supple deformities are able on toe-stand to "throw" the hindfoot-midfoot into a locked position, thereby inverting the heel even in the presence of complete loss of continuity of the tendon, but careful observation reveals the foot "jumping" into that position while gaining momentary support from the examiner or the examining table and using the gastrocsoleus muscle as the motor unit. Gradually rising on only the affected foot to the tip-toe position and inverting the heel at the end stage without concomitant external

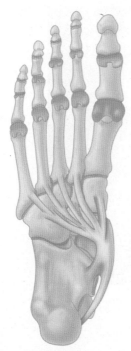

FIGURE 3.3   Posterior tibial tendon inserts into medial tuberosity of navicular (one main slip) and continues through second slip into plantar surface of foot, where it arborizes and inserts into all three cuneiforms, cuboid, and bases of second, third, fourth, and fifth metatarsals.

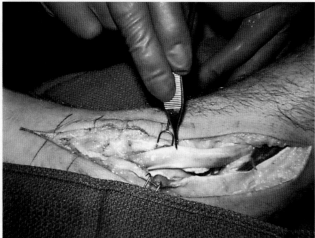

FIGURE 3.4   Patient with mild unilateral pes planus with tenosynovitis that was recalcitrant to all conservative treatment. Inflamed synovium is obvious along tendon, as is continuity of tendon. Loss of excursion and resultant deformity were caused by inflammatory synovial proliferation with its obstructive, painful sequelae at pulley. Radiographs were normal.

support is not possible for a patient with complete loss of continuity of the tendon.

DeOrio et al. described the "posterior tibial edema sign" in which the presence of subcutaneous pitting edema along the course of the posterior tibial tendon correlated with MRI findings of disease in 88% of patients. It is also important to evaluate the gait of patients with a suggested posterior tibial tendon pathologic process. In a normal, unaffected hindfoot

the stance phase of gait begins with the hindfoot in a neutral to slightly inverted position. Through midstance a valgus hindfoot position is obtained, and at terminal stance or toe-off position the hindfoot inverts, locking the midtarsal joint to produce a rigid lever for push-off. For the patient with posterior tibial tendon insufficiency, failure to invert the foot at the terminal stance position occurs. The inability to lock the hindfoot and produce a rigid lever during the point of gait at which most stress is placed through the arch of the foot creates a high strain level and ultimately pain through the arch.

Contracture of the gastrocnemius or gastrocsoleus complex frequently accompanies this condition early in the course of the disease. The hindfoot valgus position shortens the moment arm for the heel cord, leading to the contracture. By preventing dorsiflexion and inversion, the contracture further worsens the hindfoot valgus. The Silfverskiöld test is used to determine selective gastrocnemius muscle and gastrocsoleus (Achilles) contracture (Fig. 3.5). Treating the contracture conservatively or surgically is vital for successful treatment of posterior tibial tendon insufficiency.

Radiographic evaluation with standing anteroposterior and lateral views may or may not be helpful even with obvious clinical evidence of asymmetric pes planus. If the tendon is intact and the diagnosis is recurrent tenosynovitis, radiographs usually are normal even with some degree of flattening of the medial longitudinal arch clinically. More commonly, radiographs demonstrate changes as deformity occurs from tendon insufficiency. Radiographic parameters commonly used in the evaluation of posterior tibial tendon dysfunction include the lateral talus–first metatarsal angle, hindfoot alignment angle, hindfoot moment arm, calcaneal pitch, and talonavicular coverage angle.

In a normal foot, the talus–first metatarsal angle is 0 to 10 degrees on a standing lateral view. An increased angle indicates loss of the medial longitudinal arch. Overlapping metatarsals or loss of height of the medial cuneiform also indicates depression of the medial longitudinal arch. Loss of the calcaneal pitch angle may indicate both loss of the longitudinal arch and contracture of the gastrocsoleus complex. The standing lateral tibial-calcaneal angle (Fig. 3.6) has been found to be significantly increased in adults with flatfeet and Achilles tendon contracture, suggesting that this angle is a sensitive, reproducible, cost-effective method of identifying and quantifying Achilles tendon contracture in patients with adult-acquired flatfoot.

On the standing anteroposterior view, abduction of the forefoot through the midfoot may be characterized by an increase of the talus–first metatarsal angle, which normally should be 0. Additionally, a line drawn through the shaft of the second metatarsal should bisect the hindfoot angle that is formed by the intersection of lines along the longitudinal axis of the talus and calcaneus. Ellis et al. described two measurements for differentiating between mild (type IIa) and severe (type IIb) posterior tibial tendon insufficiency based on the degree of talonavicular abduction: lateral talonavicular incongruency angle and incongruency distance. The lateral talonavicular incongruency angle was significantly increased in those with type IIb insufficiency (Fig. 3.7), whereas the incongruency distance did not vary significantly between the two groups.

Saltzman et al. modified Cobey's method for radiographically imaging the coronal plane alignment of the hindfoot to quantify hindfoot valgus with the hindfoot moment arm

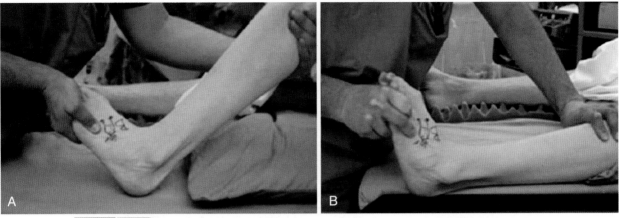

FIGURE 3.5 Silfverskiöld test to determine selective gastrocsoleus muscle tightness and contracture. Passive range of dorsiflexion of ankle is measured with knee flexed **(A)** and extended **(B)**. Significant reduction of dorsiflexion with knee extended may indicate need for gastrocnemius recession.

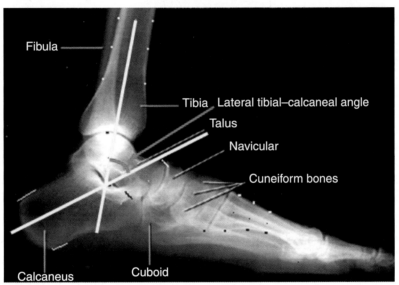

FIGURE 3.6 Measurement of standing lateral tibial-calcaneal angle (see text). (From Arangio GA, Wasser T, Rogman A: The use of standing lateral tibial-calcaneal angle as a quantitative measurement of Achilles tendon contracture in adult acquired flatfoot, *Foot Ankle Int* 27:685, 2006.)

measurement. More recently, Williamson et al. described the hindfoot alignment angle (Fig. 3.8), which correlated significantly with the hindfoot moment arm and was found to be a reliable measure of hindfoot valgus. Furthermore, hindfoot alignment radiographs demonstrate more pronounced valgus than clinical evaluation. In addition to standing foot radiographs, standing ankle radiographs are also useful in the diagnosis of tibiotalar joint valgus present in stage IV disease.

MRI has become a useful tool in evaluation of posterior tibial tendon insufficiency. Often it is helpful to know if a patient with a swollen, painful tendon and tendon sheath has degenerative changes within the tendon, tearing of the tendon, or simply peritendinitis with synovial effusion without tendon degeneration. MRI can aid in making the diagnosis. T2-weighted and fat-suppressed images are helpful in showing peritendinous effusions, as well as cystic degeneration within the tendon (Fig. 3.9). T1-weighted images are helpful in showing the anatomic contours of the tendon and whether

a disruption of the tendon has occurred. MRI also can aid in the diagnosis of spring ligament and tibionavicular ligament injury, two important medial arch stabilizers.

The advancement of weight-bearing CT scans with multiplanar images adds further insight for surgical planning. Because the deformity often is very dynamic, non–weight-bearing images may underestimate the amount of needed correction. On the other hand, weight-bearing CT scans provide multiplanar and three-dimensional reconstruction images that improve understanding of anatomic pathology.

If the weight-bearing films corroborate the clinical findings and locate the articular area of instability, preoperative counseling and surgical planning are facilitated if, indeed, surgical treatment is warranted (Figs. 3.10 and 3.11). However, the physician must be certain of the pathologic condition even if an expensive radiographic evaluation with MRI is necessary because other entities can mimic the posture of a foot with posterior tibial tendon insufficiency (Fig. 3.12). For example, degenerative arthritic deformities (Figs. 3.13

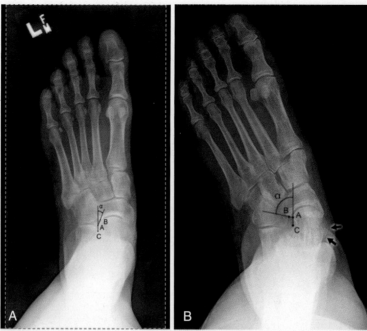

FIGURE 3.7   Incongruency angle is determined by drawing line joining lateral extent of talar articular surface *(point A)* and lateral extent of navicular surface *(point B)*. Second line is drawn between lateral aspect of talar neck at its narrowest segment *(point C)* and lateral extent of talar articular surface *(point A)*. Distal and lateral interval between these two lines forms incongruency angle. **A,** Incongruency angle in normal foot. **B,** Incongruency angle in type IIb flatfoot deformity. (From Ellis SJ, Yu JC, Williams BR, et al: New radiographic parameters assessing forefoot abduction in the adult acquired flatfoot deformity, *Foot Ankle Int* 30:1168, 2009.)

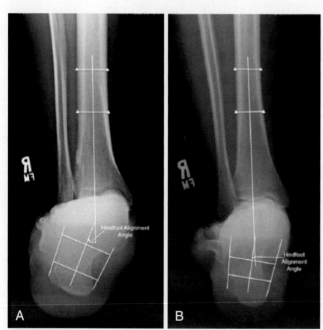

FIGURE 3.8   Depiction of hindfoot alignment angle measurements taken on a patient with flatfoot **(A)** and normal control patient **(B)**. (From Williamson ERC, Chan JY, Burket JC, et al: New radiographic parameter assessing hindfoot alignment in stage II adult-acquired flatfoot deformity, *Foot Ankle Int* 36:417, 2015.)

and 3.14), traumatic collapse distal to the midtarsal joint (Fig. 3.15), and tarsal coalitions, especially unilateral with a normal arch on the unaffected foot (Fig. 3.16), can cause such a deformity. Another entity that may confuse the examiner is the foot that has collapsed from neuropathic arthropathy (Fig. 3.17). Although the clinical examination may be strikingly similar, the radiographic examination should clarify the diagnosis (Fig. 3.18). Finally, idiopathic flexible pes planus must be excluded (Fig. 3.19). The association of the accessory navicular with posterior tibial tendon insufficiency is discussed in the following section on treatment.

TREATMENT

Although surgical management is highlighted in each section, conservative treatment often is successful in managing associated pain. Expectations of the patient regarding return to previous level of function should be ascertained before any treatment decisions are made.

■ STAGE I DISEASE (TENOSYNOVITIS)

Tenosynovitis is treated with rest, nonsteroidal antiinflammatory agents, and supportive modalities. Modalities may include walking boot with added medial longitudinal arch support, ankle corset, or short leg walking cast. After the acute inflammation of the tenosynovium subsides, rehabilitation of the calf and leg with physical therapy often is helpful. Success has been demonstrated with a comprehensive calf and leg

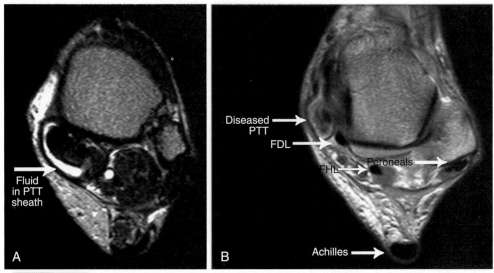

FIGURE 3.9 Magnetic resonance imaging is helpful to identify peritendinous effusion **(A)** and degeneration within the tendon **(B)**.

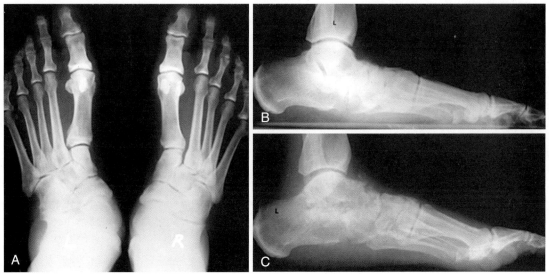

FIGURE 3.10 On anteroposterior view of both feet, note in symptomatic left foot uncovering of talar head as navicular and remaining part of foot move laterally into abduction. Intermetatarsal spaces at their base appear slightly widened; metatarsal-tarsal articulations appear in fact better than in right asymptomatic foot as result of pronation of forefoot. **A,** Divergence of anteroposterior talocalcaneal angle (Kite angle) is present. **B,** Standing lateral view shows plantarflexion of talus (head of talus moves plantarward, medially, and distally), loss of normal calcaneal pitch (and concomitant tightening of Achilles tendon), secondary collapse of navicular-cuneiform articular surfaces, and overlapping of medial four metatarsals from pronation of forefoot in weight-bearing position. This patient had traumatic rupture of posterior tibial tendon many years previously while engaging in sports. **C,** Traumatic arthritic changes followed, and eventually triple arthrodesis was required.

rehabilitation program that emphasizes graduated isometric strengthening exercises and gastrocsoleus complex stretching. Preventing recurrence of stage I disease can be assisted with the use of an orthotic device that incorporates a medial heel wedge and medial forefoot post to place the hindfoot in neutral, decreasing force requirements for the posterior tibial muscle and tendon unit. If conservative treatment fails, tenosynovectomy is indicated (Figs. 3.20 and 3.21). Open synovectomy remains our surgical treatment of choice for stage 1

disease, but tendoscopy has been reported to produce good results. Depending on the patient's underlying osseous morphology, adding adjuvant procedures to the synovectomy may be beneficial. Adding an osseous procedure such as a medializing calcaneal osteotomy or Cotton osteotomy to create a higher arch may also be warranted in patients with symmetrical pes planovalgus. These adjuvant procedures are further discussed in later sections of this chapter.

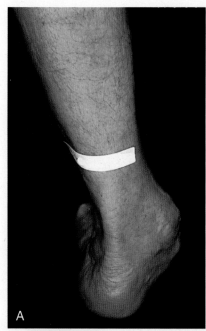
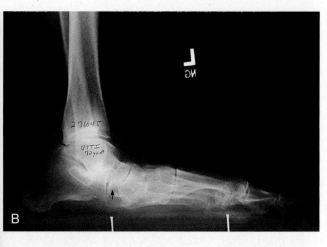

FIGURE 3.11 Attritional rupture of posterior tibial tendon at medial malleolus with arch collapse of unknown duration. **A,** Typical clinical findings of complete rupture of this tendon. **B,** Radiograph shows almost 90-degree rotation of talus.

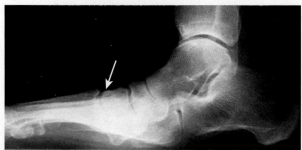

FIGURE 3.12 This foot mimicked arch collapse secondary to posterior tibial tendon disruption. Primary collapse was tarsometatarsal with secondary hindfoot collapse from osteoarthritis.

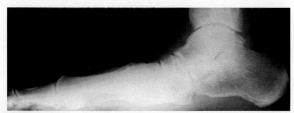

FIGURE 3.13 Collapse at navicular-cuneiform articulation on lateral view.

SYNOVECTOMY WITH REPAIR OF INCOMPLETE TEARS

TECHNIQUE 3.1

- Allow the foot to rest in gravity equinus.

- Starting at the inferior edge of the navicular tuberosity, carry a straight incision proximally 1 cm posterior to the prominence of the medial malleolus and continue it 3 to 4 cm proximal to the flexor retinaculum.
- Identify the tendon at the inferior margin of the wound and trace it proximally until the muscle is seen.
- Release the pulley behind the medial malleolus and the deep investing fascia of the distal leg (see Fig. 3.21).
- By sharp dissection remove all abnormal-appearing synovium.
- Inspect the tendon for longitudinal tears and intratendinous fibrosis.
- Trace the plantar slip of the tendon 1 cm distal to the tuberosity to be certain it is intact.
- If the tendon insertion into the navicular and the slip plantar to it appear intact, imbricate the tendon across the abnormal-appearing area. This imbrication is over a length of 1.0 to 1.5 cm.
- Leave the flexor retinaculum open and close the wound.

POSTOPERATIVE CARE The length of cast immobilization and protected weight-bearing varies depending on the appearance of the tendon at surgery, that is, the evaluation of its structural integrity and the extent of dissection necessary to rid the tendon of inflamed synovium. In most cases, weight bearing is delayed for 4 to 6 weeks and the leg is immobilized in a splint until the wound is healed (2 weeks). Mobilization of the tendon in the sheath is encouraged with minimal resistance exercises in a removable splint or boot to prevent intrasheath adhesions. In some markedly overweight patients with an abnormal-appearing tendon, after this extended period of support a double upright brace with a medial T-strap should be worn for 3 months.

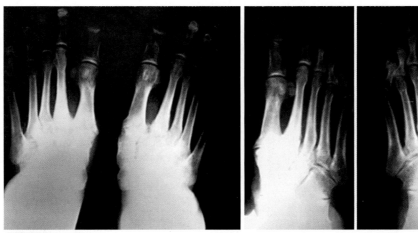

FIGURE 3.14 Anteroposterior and oblique radiographs showing degenerative arthritic changes at Lisfranc joints with resultant collapse deformity at these articulations. This probably represents erosive osteoarthritis with secondary enthesopathy and weakening of plantar metatarsal cuneiform, metatarsal cuboid, and intermetatarsal basilar ligaments. (Courtesy of W. Kenneth Bell, MD.)

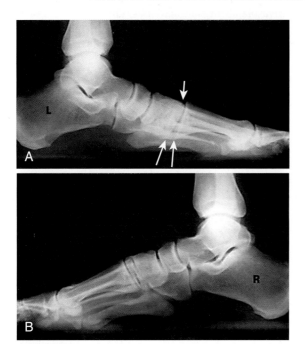

FIGURE 3.15 This 64-year-old carpenter felt pop in midfoot and noticed some time later flattened, pronated foot. Clinically, picture resembled posterior tibial tendon insufficiency, but tendon was intact. **A,** Radiographic weight-bearing view showed widening of metatarsal-cuneiform articulation plantarward and collapse at this articulation. **B,** Note also overlapping of metatarsals compared with uninjured right foot, indicating pronation of forefoot.

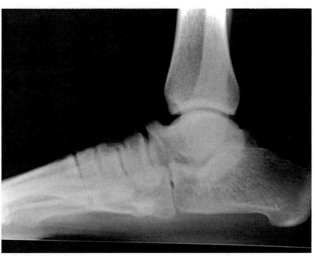

FIGURE 3.16 Middle facet tarsal coalition; note beaking of neck of talus and "C" sign.

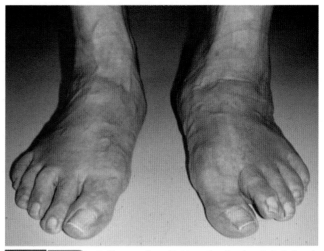

FIGURE 3.17 Collapse of medial longitudinal arch (left foot) resulting from diabetic neuropathy.

■ STAGE II DISEASE

Stage II disease, in which the hindfoot remains flexible and passively correctable, encompasses a wide spectrum of symptoms and varying physical and radiographic findings. Bluman et al. refined the classification system to reflect this spectrum in subtypes IIA and IIB. The principal difference between the subtypes is the amount of abduction of the midfoot through the talonavicular joint, with IIb being more severe (see Fig. 3.7). Conservative management of stage II disease often is successful, and most patients obtain pain relief with application of an orthotic device that has a medial post and an ankle-foot orthosis. A double-upright ankle-foot orthosis with a medial T-strap works well. The brace is configured to allow 20 to 30 degrees of plantarflexion and 10 degrees of ankle extension; however, despite its effectiveness, this large brace may not be acceptable

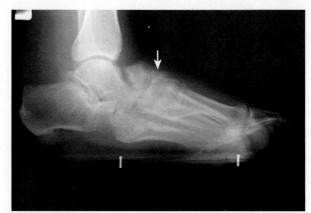

FIGURE 3.18 Standing lateral radiograph showing fracture and fragmentation of navicular with collapse of talus into resulting defect. Arrow points to attempted healing of fractures.

to patients. In these circumstances, a hinged polypropylene short leg ankle-foot orthosis (Richie brace) may be more acceptable. Although it is not as comfortable, it is lighter, can be used in a variety of shoes, and is more cosmetically acceptable. Patients who obtain significant relief with brace wear often find that after 9 to 12 months of routine brace use, they are able to wear regular shoes with insoles for longer periods of time without pain. At our institution, Lin et al. found that 70% of patients treated with double-upright ankle-foot orthoses (average duration of bracing, 15 months) were brace free and had not required surgery at 7-year follow-up; 61% of patients were "satisfied" with their outcomes, and 33% were "satisfied with minor reservations."

A patient who completes a structured physical therapy program also may avoid surgery. Alvarez et al. reported that after a median of 10 physical therapy visits over 4 months, 83% of patients had successful subjective and functional outcomes; 89% were satisfied with their outcomes. The rehabilitation protocol included the use of a short, articulated ankle-foot orthosis or foot orthosis, high-repetition exercises, aggressive plantarflexion activities, and an aggressive high-repetition home exercise program that included gastrocsoleus tendon stretching.

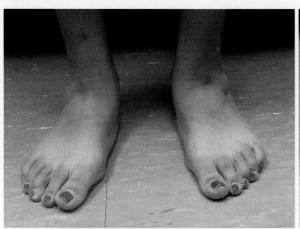
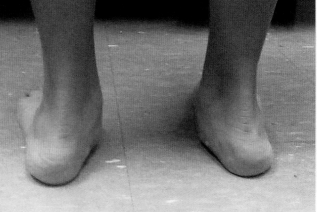

FIGURE 3.19 Idiopathic flexible flatfoot in adolescent patient.

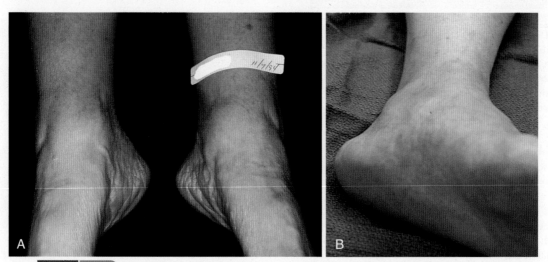

FIGURE 3.20 **A,** Persistent posterior tibial tenosynovitis on left was unresponsive to many weeks of casting and several months of double upright brace wear with medial T-strap. Note fullness behind medial malleolus on left not seen on right. **B,** Closer view of medial aspect of left ankle showing area of tenosynovitis.

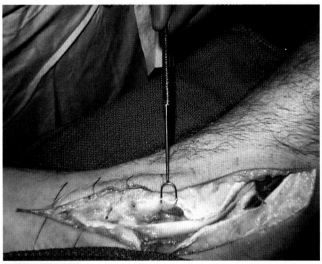

FIGURE 3.21 Abundant synovium surrounding posterior tibial tendon. This extended from inferior edge of flexor retinaculum to tuberosity of navicular. Evaluation for rheumatoid arthritis and seronegative spondyloarthropathy was negative. Patient was large-framed man who had mild unilateral pes planus and posterior tibial insufficiency secondary to tenosynovitis and loss of tendon excursion through pulley of flexor retinaculum (laciniate ligament). **SEE TECHNIQUE 3.1.**

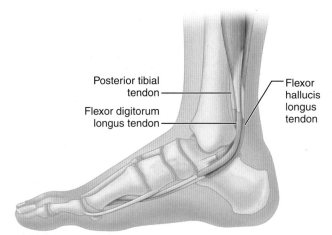

FIGURE 3.22 Technique for tendon transfer. Incision starts just behind musculotendinous border of posterior tibial tendon and courses behind medial malleolus to base of first metatarsal medially. **SEE TECHNIQUE 3.2.**

Surgical reconstruction is indicated for patients in whom conservative management is not acceptable or fails. Initial enthusiasm for *isolated* transfer of the flexor digitorum longus tendon to the navicular, with or without side-to-side augmentation using a remnant of the posterior tibial tendon, has waned because of a high incidence of failure. Therefore, in addition to reconstruction of the tendinous portion of the pathologic process, correction of the flatfoot deformity is indicated. Satisfactory results have been obtained with lengthening of the lateral column of the calcaneus (LCL), medial displacement of the tuberosity of the calcaneus (MDCO), a Z-shaped calcaneal osteotomy, or a combination of LCL and MDCO. Lateral column lengthening is achieved through an osteotomy of the body of the calcaneus between the anterior and middle facets of the subtalar joint, osteotomy between the posterior and middle facets, or a distraction arthrodesis at the calcaneocuboid joint. Malerba and De Marchi described a Z-shaped osteotomy that allows for rotation (lengthening) and translation. MDCO improves hindfoot alignment, but multiple authors have reported limitations of these osteotomies in stage IIB deformities. Iossi el al. proposed an algorithm to aid with surgical decision-making in which stage IIB deformities require the addition of a lateral column lengthening procedure; however, this algorithm is based on radiographic parameters and has not been validated with patient outcomes. Despite the power of LCL procedures to correct abduction deformities, they are associated with a higher rate of complications than MDCO and should be used judiciously; MDCO is a safe option for correction of mild abduction deformities. LCL through calcaneal cuboid arthrodesis is effective for correction, but it also has high complication rates. No one bony procedure is best, and surgeons should be familiar with both MDCO and LCL procedures.

Tendon transfer for reconstruction of the musculotendinous portion of the deformity is described first, followed by descriptions of each of the calcaneal osteotomies. Attention to the medial structures is important as well, with repair of the

spring ligament, arthrodesis of one or more midfoot joints, or cuneiform opening osteotomy (Cotton procedure) as adjunctive procedures to improve the integrity of the medial column. **Video 3.5** demonstrates posterior tibial tendon reconstruction with calcaneal osteotomy and flexor digitorum longus transfer.

TRANSFER OF FLEXOR DIGITORUM LONGUS OR FLEXOR HALLUCIS LONGUS TO TARSAL NAVICULAR

Although the flexor hallucis longus (FHL) has superior strength characteristics compared with the flexor digitorum longus, Wapner et al. demonstrated that the flexor digitorum longus may be more appropriate for reconstruction for posterior tibial tendon insufficiency because of its position. MRI has demonstrated adaptiveness of the flexor digitorum longus with muscle hypertrophy after transfer of the flexor digitorum longus tendon, and functional scores were significantly improved after this procedure.

We believe that it is important to evaluate the posterior tibial muscle belly when performing this transfer. With long-standing disease, the posterior tibial muscle becomes inelastic and fails to contract when touched with electrocautery and loses its normal color. In this case, it is inadvisable to supplement the flexor digitorum longus tendon with the remnant of the posterior tibial tendon. However, if the muscle appears normal, resection of the entire diseased segment of the posterior tibial muscle and side-to-side transfer using a Pulvertaft weave of the flexor digitorum longus and posterior tibial tendon are recommended.

TECHNIQUE 3.2

- Expose the posterior tibial tendon through an incision beginning 3 to 4 cm proximal to the tip of the medial malleolus. Curve it posterior to the malleolus and extend it to 3 to 4 cm distal to the navicular tuberosity (Fig. 3.22). This extensive incision is necessary to allow adequate evaluation of the condition of the posterior tibial muscle-tendon unit proximal to the flexor retinaculum. The incision

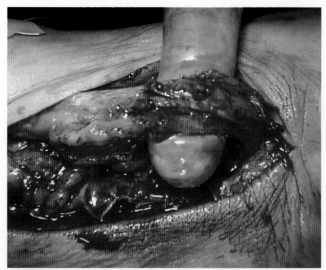

FIGURE 3.23 Complete rupture of posterior tibial tendon with proximal tendon ending within hypertrophied synovium. Once synovium was excised, complete rupture of posterior tibial tendon with healing by thin strand of scar in continuity was evident. Toes are to right. **SEE TECHNIQUE 3.2.**

should be distal enough not to compromise dissection around the medial plantar neurovascular bundle while reaching the Henry knot and exposing the crossover of the flexor digitorum longus and flexor hallucis longus.

- The posterior tibial tendon may be completely disrupted, with rounding of the proximal stump. The proximal stump may appear to end in hypertrophic synovial tissue (Fig. 3.23), but once the synovium is removed there may be a flimsy scar in continuity or a strong, dense, solid band of scar in continuity.
- If the tendon, once freed from its bed and with sustained slow tension, regains sufficient length, suture it with nonabsorbable suture to the undersurface of the navicular after the transfer is performed. Rarely can the tendon be advanced in this manner. Usually it is debrided and removed from its pulley proximal to the laciniate ligament and sutured to the adjacent tendon transfer under moderate tension.
- If the posterior tibial muscle-tendon unit has no excursion, which is uncommon even in long-standing deformity if dissected far enough proximally, then cut it short and discard it.
- Expose the flexor digitorum longus and FHL at the Henry knot lateral to the tuberosity of the navicular by dissecting along the superior border of the abductor hallucis muscle and retracting it plantarward. Branches of the medial plantar neurovascular bundle are along the path of dissection and about 2 cm lateral to the distal edge of the navicular. This dissection is tedious, and the distance to the tendons is surprisingly great.
- Using a right-angle smooth retractor to pull the intrinsic muscles plantarward, expose the tendons with blunt dissection. The FHL crosses dorsal to the flexor digitorum longus. Sever the tendon to be used at this point while flexing the toes. The strong tendinous cross ties will allow some active flexion by using the remaining intact muscle-

tendon unit. Rerouting the transferred tendon through the pulley of the posterior tibial tendon is unnecessary.

- Using successively larger drill bits (⅛ inch to ⁵⁄₁₆ inch), drill a hole perpendicular to the navicular in its midportion dorsal to plantar. Dissecting dorsally and plantarward to the midportion of the bone requires patience, but to stop short of this point may leave insufficient bony support medially to prevent the drill from cracking through the bone medially.
- Weave a 0 or 2-0 nonabsorbable suture through the distal 1.0 to 1.5 cm of the tendon and pass a straight hemostat or tendon passer with loop from dorsal to plantar.
- Holding to the suture ends, work the tendon up through the hole from plantar to dorsal until all slack is taken up. Then place the foot in equinovarus and further tighten the tendon.
- Using a small, free-cutting needle, suture the tendon to the adjacent periosteum. The foot should remain in this position when relaxed.
- Finally, if possible, advance the posterior tibial tendon and suture it to the adjacent periosteum and deep fascia. Wukich et al. described the use of a biotenodesis or interference screw to anchor the tendon in the tunnel.
- Holding the foot in equinovarus, apply a bulky dressing and a short leg splint.

POSTOPERATIVE CARE The splint is changed at 14 days after surgery, but the foot is maintained in equinovarus for 4 to 6 weeks. At 6 weeks a short leg walking cast or boot is applied and worn for an additional 3 to 4 weeks. Physical therapy is used to wean the patient from the boot and regain strength, balance, and range of motion. A molded arch support is encouraged after the cast is discontinued.

REPAIR OF SPRING LIGAMENT

Elongation and incompetence of the spring ligament from the loss of protective support of the posterior tibial tendon also contribute to the deformity. Many authors have suggested that the spring ligament should be routinely repaired as part of the medial soft-tissue procedure. Augmentation of the repair with nonabsorbable suture tape has become popular, but limited clinical evidence demonstrates its superiority over standard repair techniques.

TECHNIQUE 3.3

- After exposure and debridement of the posterior tibial tendon, locate the superomedial portion of the calcaneonavicular ligament just inferior to the head of the talus where it attaches to the plantar aspect and plantarmedial aspect of the tarsal navicular.
- Adduct the foot and forefoot into a neutral and slightly adducted position and excise a wedge of this ligament and plantar talonavicular capsule (Fig. 3.24A). The wedge should be 8 to 10 mm, depending on the magnitude of the deformity.
- Repair the spring ligament with multiple interrupted 2-0 braided, nonabsorbable sutures (Fig. 3.24B,C).

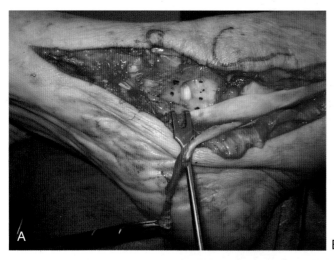
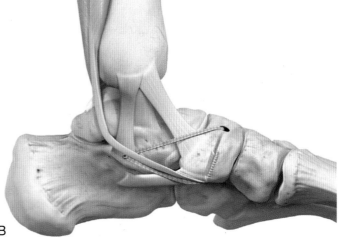
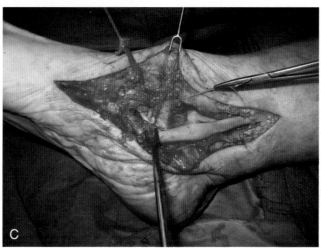

FIGURE 3.24 Repair of spring ligament. **A,** Portion of spring ligament to be excised. **B,** Nonabsorbable suture tape to augment primary repair or spring ligament. **C,** Repaired ligament. **SEE TECHNIQUE 3.3.**

If the spring ligament is so attenuated that it cannot be repaired, reconstruction of the ligament can be considered. Reconstruction may use an allograft or autograft tendon. Ryssman and Jeng described a reconstruction technique in which the posterior tibial tendon is used as an autograft. While leaving the posterior tibial tendon's native insertion on the navicular, the autograft tendon is secured proximally at the sustentaculum tali. Williams et al. described an autograft reconstruction technique using a peroneus longus transfer. Regardless of the spring ligament repair technique, a calcaneal osteotomy is almost always performed to support the soft-tissue repair.

RECONSTRUCTION OF THE SPRING LIGAMENT USING THE PERONEUS LONGUS

TECHNIQUE 3.4

(WILLIAMS ET AL.)

- Make a longitudinal incision over the fibula beginning 6 to 8 cm proximal to the tip of the lateral malleolus.
- Identify the peroneus longus and section it just proximal to the peroneal retinaculum. Tenodese the proximal end of the peroneus longus to the peroneus brevis.
- Make a 3-cm longitudinal incision along the plantarlateral aspect of the foot from the base of the fifth metatarsal proximally toward the cuboid tunnel.
- Release the attachments of the peroneus longus at the cuboid tunnel. Through the medial incision, use a right-angle clamp to hook around the peroneus longus tendon near its insertion site and deliver it gently through the medial incision. Leave the tendon attached to the base of the first metatarsal.
- Choose the location of the proximal tunnel according to the type of talonavicular deformity present. If significant plantar sag is present at the talonavicular joint, create a calcaneal tunnel (Fig. 3.25A); if only abduction is present through the talonavicular joint, create a tibial tunnel (Fig. 3.25B).
- For a calcaneal tunnel, place a Kirschner wire in the calcaneus immediately inferior to the sustentaculum tali, taking care not to damage the FHL tunnel. Advance the wire posteriorly and laterally across the calcaneus, exiting

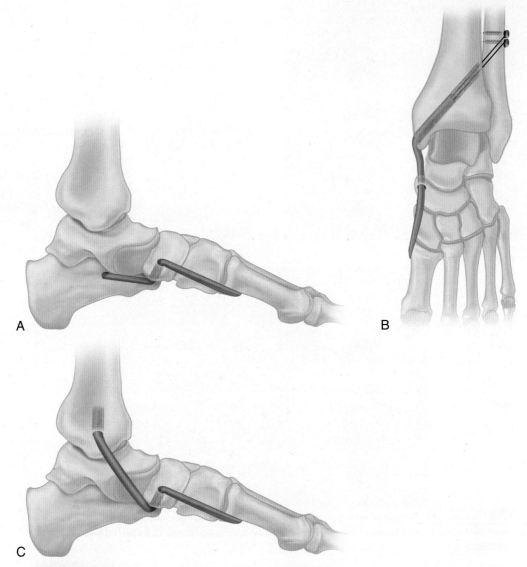

A

B

C

FIGURE 3.25   Reconstruction of spring ligament using peroneus longus autograft tendon transfer. **A,** Medial view showing calcaneal bone tunnel reconstruction. **B,** Anteroposterior view showing tibial bone tunnel reconstruction. **C,** Medial view of tibial bone tunnel reconstruction. (Redrawn from Williams BR, Ellis SJ, Deyer TW, et al: Reconstruction of the spring ligament using a peroneus longus autograft tendon transfer, *Foot Ankle Int* 31:567, 2010.) **SEE TECHNIQUE 3.4.**

above the medializing calcaneal osteotomy incision on the lateral side of the foot without violating the subtalar joint.

- For a tibial tunnel, identify a point between the anterior and posterior colliculi of the medial malleolus. Use a small Bennett retractor through the fibular incision to gain access to the lateral tibia just anterior to the fibula. Under fluoroscopic guidance, place a Kirschner wire from the medial malleolus directed proximally and laterally, taking care to avoid the ankle joint.

- For either tunnel placement, check the position with fluoroscopy, replace the Kirschner wire with a guidewire, and use a cannulated drill to create a tunnel 8 to 9 mm in diameter.

- Pass the graft from dorsal to plantar through the navicular tunnel and then through the calcaneal (Fig. 3.25A) or

tibial (Fig. 3.25B,C) tunnel. Tension the graft after fixation of the osteotomies.

- Place the foot in slight inversion and plantarflexion and in 5 to 10 degrees of adduction through the talonavicular joint as seen on a simulated weight-bearing view. Pretension the graft to remove creep before fixation.

- Place screws in the fibula or lateral calcaneus as posts to tie down the graft sutures. For a graft passed through a calcaneal tunnel, place a 3.5-mm screw anterior to the lateral exit of the tunnel. For a graft passed through a tibial tunnel, place the screw laterally on the fibula several centimeters proximal to the exit of the tibial tunnel.

- Use two sets of sutures to secure the graft while an assistant applies tension.

- Place bone graft from the medializing heel slide osteotomy in the tunnels.

POSTOPERATIVE CARE Non–weight bearing in a cast is continued for 12 weeks (cast changes at 6 and 10 weeks). If healing is evident on CT at 12 weeks, a removable boot is fitted, progressive weight bearing is allowed, and gentle stretching and strengthening are begun.

ANTERIOR CALCANEAL OSTEOTOMY (LATERAL COLUMN LENGTHENING)

Anterior calcaneal osteotomy has been studied extensively in the laboratory and has been shown to significantly improve the forefoot deformity, as well as the height of the arch. Although clinical studies could be characterized as intermediate at best, we have had significant success with this procedure. Variations of the calcaneal lengthening osteotomy exist. The traditional Evans lateral column lengthening calcaneal osteotomy (E-LLCOT) is created between the middle facet and anterior facets, and the Hintermann lateral column lengthening calcaneal osteotomy (H-LLCOT) is completed between the middle and posterior facets. Both have good clinical results. When compared directly, the H-LLCOT demonstrated less radiographic calcaneocuboid joint degenerative change, but this difference was not clinically relevant. In cadaver models, the H-LLCOT was associated with less injury to subtalar joint surfaces, but this finding may not be clinically relevant. Bolt et al. found that lateral column lengthening achieved greater realignment initially and maintained correction better over time while having a lower reoperation rate despite more frequent nonunion and radiographic progression of adjacent joint arthritis. In our experience, this procedure has been most helpful in patients who have a significant abduction deformity of the forefoot on standing anteroposterior radiographs. Complications such as graft collapse, nonunion, lateral column pain, development of arthritis at the calcaneocuboid joint, sural neuritis, and painful implants are relatively frequent and should be discussed with the patient. The use of tricortical allograft (Fig. 3.26) instead of autograft has been demonstrated by multiple authors to have equivalent healing and complication rates. Gross et al. reported good union rates (96%) and pain relief in patients treated with lateral column lengthening using a porous titanium wedge.

TECHNIQUE 3.5

- After preparation of the medial soft tissues and before final tensioning of the flexor digitorum longus tendon into the navicular, make a longitudinal incision over the lateral anterior process of the calcaneus. Take care to avoid injury to the sural nerve.
- Perform an osteotomy 1.0 to 1.5 cm proximal to the articular surface at the calcaneocuboid joint with a sagittal saw, taking care to aim the saw between the anterior facet and middle facet of the calcaneus. Avoid injuring the soft tissues just on the medial side of the calcaneus and the medial plantar nerve and artery.
- Distract the area using a combination of manual adduction of the forefoot and placement of 3/32-inch Steinmann

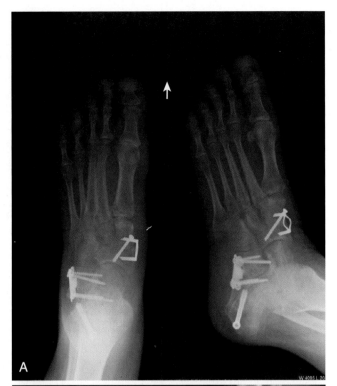

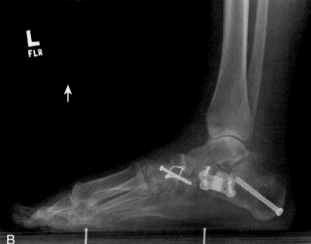

FIGURE 3.26 **A** and **B,** Lateral column lengthening with allograft in patient with severe decompensated flatfoot deformity; patient also had medial displacement calcaneal osteotomy and naviculocuneiform arthrodesis. **SEE TECHNIQUE 3.5.**

pins into the anterior process and the anterior body of the calcaneus. A hinged cervical lamina spreader, either smooth or with very small teeth, can be used to help distract the osteotomy.
- Harvest an appropriately sized graft from the iliac crest. Depending on the size of the patient, it should be 8 to 10 cm in width. Alternatively, a structural allograft can be used.
- Assess the foot for clinical and radiographic alignment before inserting the graft. Be certain that there is no overcorrection of the deformity.
- Fix the graft with a screw or plate. The subcutaneous nature of implants in this area often necessitates removal at a later date.

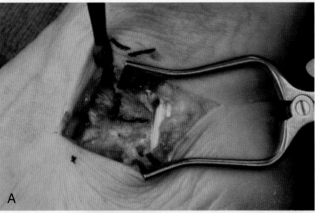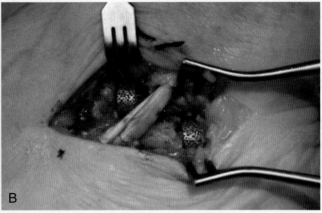

A   B

FIGURE 3.27 Scott and Berlet step-cut lengthening calcaneal osteotomy. (From Scott R, Berlet G: Calcaneal Z osteotomy for extra-articular correction of hindfoot valgus, *J Foot Ankle Surg* 52:406, 2013.) **SEE TECHNIQUE 3.6**.

- Sangeorzan et al. and others demonstrated success with lateral column lengthening through the calcaneocuboid joint. If this procedure is used, carry the incision more distally. Remove the opposing cartilaginous surface of the calcaneus and cuboid to cancellous bone and use a larger graft. In general, a 1.5-cm graft is routinely used in this situation. In our experience, it is more difficult to obtain union with this osteotomy.
- Tension the soft tissues, close the wound, and apply a short leg non–weight-bearing splint.

POSTOPERATIVE CARE Sutures are removed 2 weeks after surgery. Continued use of a non–weight–bearing cast is recommended for 8 to 10 weeks until evidence of bony union is present on anteroposterior and lateral radiographs. The patient then progresses to weight bearing.

STEP-CUT CALCANEAL LENGTHENING OSTEOTOMY (Z OSTEOTOMY)

Despite meticulous technique, the risks associated with lateral column lengthening have compelled surgeons to explore other techniques. Vander Griend described a lateral column lengthening technique through a "Z" cut osteotomy, and Scott and Berlet described a similar step-cut lengthening calcaneal osteotomy (SLCO). These techniques differ only slightly so they are described interchangeably. Similar to the more traditional lateral column lengthening, the SLCO allows for varus rotation through the calcaneus, but the horizontal limb improves osseous apposition, aiding with union rates. In 37 patients who underwent a SLCO for stage IIB posterior tibial tendon deficiency, Demetracopoulos et al. demonstrated excellent healing, good deformity correction, and improved clinical outcomes. When compared directly with traditional E-LLCOT, the SLCO had significantly increased healing times, fewer nonunions, less implant irritation, and small graft sizes while resulting in similar deformity correction and outcome scores.

TECHNIQUE 3.6

(SCOTT AND BERLET)
- Make a 5-cm linear incision over the peroneal tubercle.
- Carry dissection through the subcutaneous tissue with care to locate sural nerve branches.
- Incise the peroneal tendon sheath and mobilize the peroneal tendons.
- Mark the dorsal, vertical limb of the osteotomy site roughly 1.5 cm proximal to the calcaneocuboid joint.
- Moving proximally, mark the 2-cm horizontal limb and the proximal, plantar vertical limb. With the peroneus brevis reflected superiorly and the peroneus longus plantarly, make the horizontal osteotomy first.
- With the peroneals retracted plantarly, make the dorsal limb cut.
- With the peroneals retracted dorsally, create the plantar limb.
- Use a long arm distractor to rotate the osteotomy, and obtain an anteroposterior radiograph to determine the amount of talonavicular coverage needed.
- Use autograft, allograft, or porous titanium wedges to secure the osteotomy sites and maintain the correction (Fig. 3.27).

MEDIAL CALCANEAL DISPLACEMENT OSTEOTOMY

Medial calcaneal displacement osteotomy was popularized by Myerson as an alternative to lengthening of the lateral column. Myerson and Corrigan reviewed 32 patients treated with medial calcaneal displacement osteotomy and a medial soft-tissue procedure for stage II posterior tibial tendon dysfunction. At an average of 20 months after surgery, 30 of 32 patients were

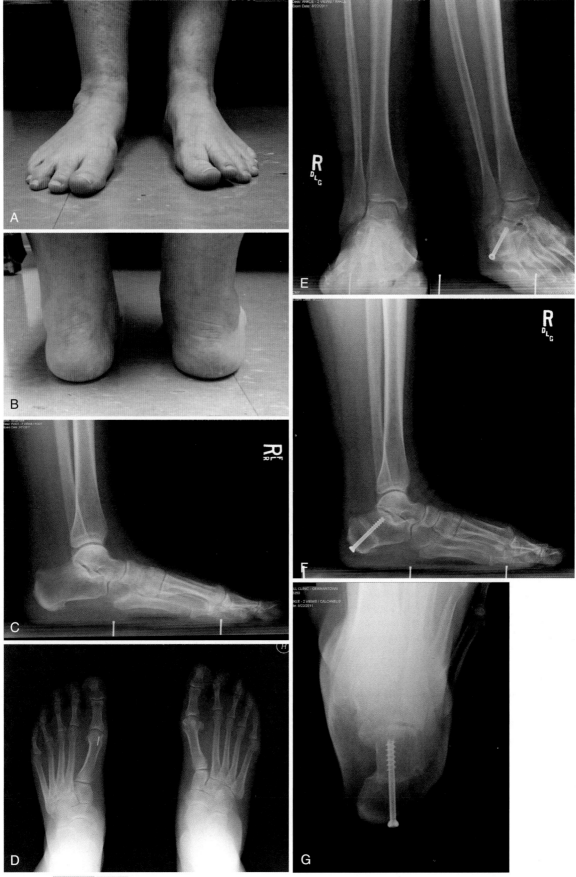

FIGURE 3.28 **A** and **B,** Clinical appearance of flatfoot deformity in 39-year-old man; note that midfoot abduction deformity is not severe. **C** and **D,** Preoperative radiographs. **E** to **G,** After medial calcaneal displacement osteotomy. **SEE TECHNIQUE 3.7.**

satisfied with the outcome of surgery, had improved function, and exhibited radiographic correction of the foot deformity. Ninety-four percent of the patients had pain relief and improvement in the arch of the foot and were able to wear regular shoes without orthotic support. Using three-dimensional gait analysis, Brodsky et al. determined that posterior tibial tendon reconstruction consisting of transfer of the flexor digitorum longus tendon to the navicular, reconstruction of the calcaneonavicular ligament, and medial displacement calcaneal osteotomy produced objective improvements in walking velocity, hindfoot motion, and power. The placement of the tuberosity of the calcaneus and the gastrocsoleus complex more medial to the axis of the subtalar joint improves the function of the gastrocsoleus complex as an inverter of the hindfoot, thereby assisting with the force necessary to invert the foot with less reliance on the transferred flexor digitorum longus tendon. We have found this procedure most useful in patients in whom standing anteroposterior radiographs do not demonstrate severe abduction deformity through the midfoot (Fig. 3.28). Advantages of this osteotomy include predictable healing of the osteotomy without the complication of increased calcaneocuboid joint pressure, which has been noted to occur with a lateral column lengthening.

With the increased popularity of minimally invasive surgery, a medializing displacement calcaneal osteotomy also has been described. In a comparative study, the minimally invasive osteotomy was found to be similarly effective with fewer wound and nerve complications than the more traditional open approach.

TECHNIQUE 3.7

- Position the patient supine with a large ipsilateral hip bump or a bean bag.
- Make an incision inferior and parallel to the peroneal tendons and posterior and inferior to the path of the sural nerve. Extend the excision from the upper border of the calcaneus anterior to the retrocalcaneal space to the inferior border of the calcaneus deep to the plantar fascia.
- Carry the dissection down to the periosteum and reflect the periosteum at the proposed osteotomy site.
- Make a transverse osteotomy in line with the skin incision using an oscillating saw blade (Fig. 3.29A). Make the cut at a right angle to the lateral border of the calcaneus and angle it posteriorly approximately 45 degrees to the plane of the foot.
- Place a toothless lamina spreader into the osteotomy site and spread it to mobilize the calcaneal soft-tissue attachments.
- Withdraw the lamina spreader, translate the posterior calcaneal tuberosity 10 mm medially (Fig. 3.29B), and secure it with an adequately sized cannulated screw (Fig. 3.29C). Take care to keep the posterior tuberosity from sliding proximally. Insert the screw from posteromedial and inferior to anterolateral and superior, that is, direct it toward the sinus tarsi.
- Close the lateral incision, and reposition the patient supine for the medial tendon transfer.

OPENING WEDGE MEDIAL CUNEIFORM (COTTON) OSTEOTOMY

With long-standing hindfoot valgus, the forefoot accommodates this deformity with increasing supination. This supination is accentuated after the hindfoot is corrected, creating an unbalanced foot. Thus, to balance the triangular support of the foot, the supination must be addressed through plantarflexing the medial column. An opening wedge medial cuneiform osteotomy (Cotton) plantarflexes the first metatarsal head, improving forefoot supination. Hirose and Johnson reported excellent results with no major complications in 16 patients treated with opening wedge osteotomy of the medial cuneiform as an adjunctive procedure in flatfoot correction (Fig. 3.30). However, Conti et al. warned that excessive plantarflexion of the medial cuneiform (cuneiform articular angle ≤ -2 degrees) correlates with worse outcomes than those with mild plantarflexion (cuneiform articular angle ≥ -2 degrees), so surgeons should avoid excessive plantarflexion. Suggested advantages of the Cotton osteotomy over first tarsometatarsal arthrodesis include predictable union, preservation of first ray mobility, and ability to vary the amount of correction.

TECHNIQUE 3.8

(HIROSE AND JOHNSON)
- Position the patient supine on the operating table with a pad under the ipsilateral buttock to internally rotate the affected leg.
- Prepare and drape the ipsilateral iliac crest donor site and the affected leg.
- Under tourniquet control, make a dorsal longitudinal incision over the medial cuneiform and the base of the first metatarsal and dissect through the skin and subcutaneous tissue.
- Retract the extensor hallucis longus medially to expose the dorsal portion of the medial cuneiform; identify the midportion of the bone with fluoroscopy.
- Use a microsagittal saw to make a transverse osteotomy from dorsal to plantar through the midportion of the medial cuneiform at the level of the second tarsometatarsal joint (Fig. 3.31A).
- Place an osteotome in the osteotomy and pull it distally to lever open the medial cuneiform osteotomy and plantarflex the first ray. Measure the amount of opening of the osteotomy to obtain the desired plantarflexion of the first ray; usually a 5- to 6-mm wedge of autograft bone is needed. The goal is plantarflexion of the first ray to the level of the fifth metatarsal to restore the normal "tripod" configuration (Fig. 3.32).
- Remove a tricortical iliac crest wedge of the measured width and denude it of soft tissue; trim the wedge with a microsagittal saw until it fits into the space created by opening the osteotomy (Fig. 3.31B).
- Place a small amount of cancellous bone graft into the most inferior aspects of the osteotomy.
- Use a bone tamp to impact the tricortical iliac crest graft from dorsal to plantar into the medial cuneiform osteotomy while the osteotomy is levered open with a narrow osteotome and a plantarflexion force is placed on the first metatarsal.

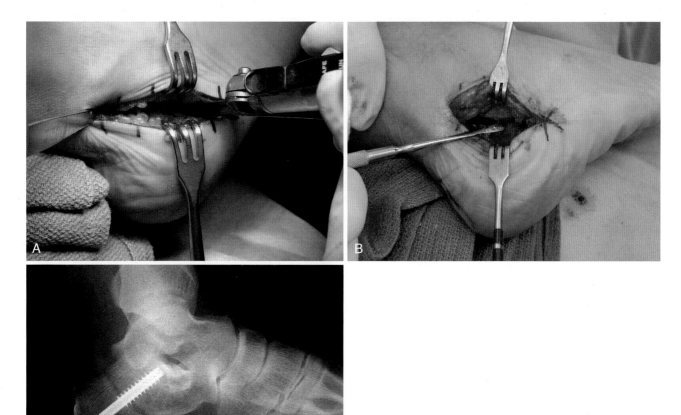

FIGURE 3.29 Medial displacement osteotomy. **A,** Transverse osteotomy made with oscillating saw. **B,** Posterior tuberosity displaced medially. **C,** Fixation with cannulated screw. (From Stephenson KA: Medial displacement calcaneal osteotomy, *Tech Foot Ankle Surg* 8:2, 2009.) **SEE TECHNIQUE 3.7.**

- Drive a guide pin for a 4.0- or 3.5-mm cannulated screw from the dorsal aspect of the distal portion of the cuneiform across the osteotomy and into the plantar aspect of the proximal fragment of the cuneiform. Insert a screw of the appropriate length and countersink it.
- Use the microsagittal saw to contour any portion of the iliac crest graft that protrudes outside the contours of the cuneiform.
- To avoid impingement against the second cuneiform, take care that the graft is not placed too far laterally.
- Close the incisions in routine fashion and apply a compressive dressing with plaster.

POSTOPERATIVE CARE At 7 to 14 days, the compressive dressing is changed for a non–weight-bearing cast. At 6 weeks, if fusion is evident on radiographs, weight bearing as tolerated is allowed.

SUBTALAR ARTHROEREISIS

The concept of arthroereisis probably dates to Grice's description of an extraarticular arthrodesis with insertion of bone graft into the sinus tarsi. To maintain the arch correction, the concept was to limit the ability of the calcaneus to externally rotate underneath the talus. Currently, this has evolved to the use of various sinus tarsi implants to block external rotation of the calcaneus relative to the talus or to prevent the anterior process of the calcaneus from abutting the lateral process of the talus as the foot pronates.

As described by Maxwell and Cerniglia, there are three biomechanical types of sinus tarsi implants. The first is a self-locking wedge, which is inserted in a screw fashion within the sinus tarsi between the lateral process of the talus and the anterior process of the calcaneus and prevents external rotation of the calcaneus on the talus (Fig. 3.33A). The second is described as an axis-altering device (Fig. 3.33B). This device is inserted intraarticularly under the lateral process of the talus, elevating the lateral aspect of the talus. The third type is an impact-blocking device, which is inserted extraarticularly in the floor of the sinus tarsi and acts to block external rotation of the calcaneus under the talus (Fig. 3.33C). Various plastic, metallic, and bioabsorbable materials are used for these implants. No studies compare the efficacies or safety of the differing available implants.

Multiple publications have demonstrated clinical and radiographic improvement with the use of subtalar arthroereisis in managing pes planus deformity in adults and children, but proper patient selection is crucial. Furthermore, this procedure is best utilized with other procedures (i.e., soft-tissue and osseous procedures) to maintain the correction

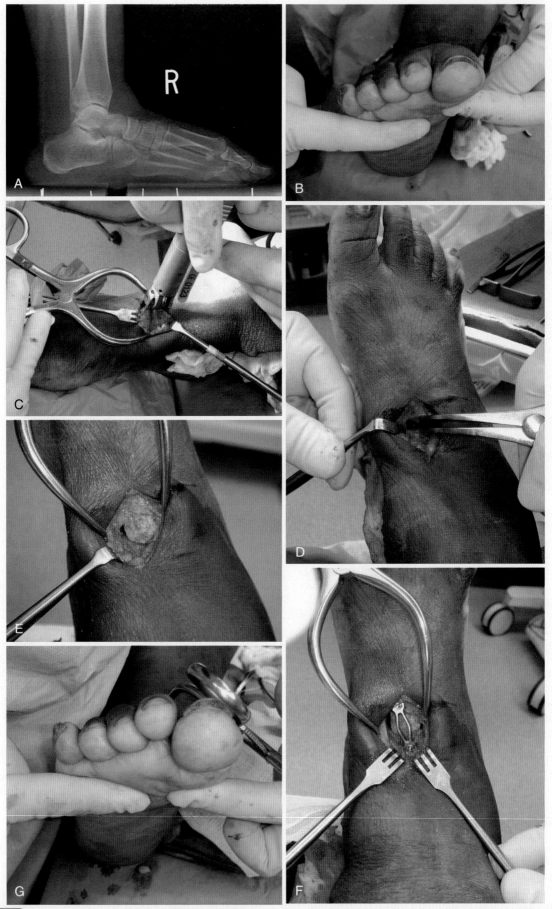

FIGURE 3.30   Opening-wedge medial cuneiform (Cotton) osteotomy. Preoperative radiographic **(A)** and clinical **(B)** appearance. **C,** Osteotomy made with microsagittal saw. **D,** Lamina spreaders used to open osteotomy. **E,** Graft in place in osteotomy. **F,** Fixation with "claw" plate and two cannulated screws. **G,** Postoperative appearance of foot. **SEE TECHNIQUE 3.8.**

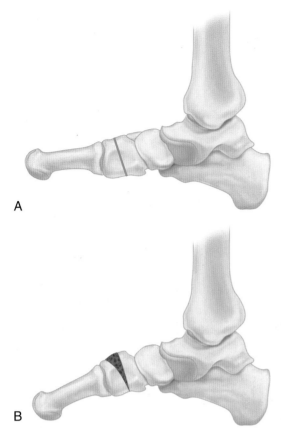

A

B

FIGURE 3.31   Opening wedge medial cuneiform osteotomy. **A,** Location of osteotomy. **B,** Insertion of bone wedge. (Re-drawn from Hirose CB, Johnson JE: Plantarflexion opening wedge medial cuneiform osteotomy for correction of fixed forefoot varus associated with flatfoot deformity, *Foot Ankle Int* 25:568, 2004.) **SEE TECHNIQUE 3.8.**

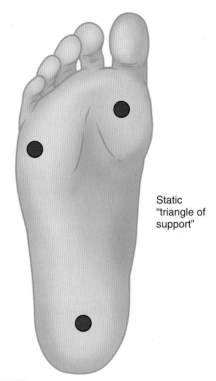

Static "triangle of support"

FIGURE 3.32   Triangle support of foot described by Cotton. **SEE TECHNIQUE 3.8.**

and should be limited to flexible pes planovalgus or early stage posterior tibial tendon deficiency (stage IIA) deformities. With a mean follow-up of 1 year, Chong et al. prospectively compared lateral column lengthening and arthroereisis in pediatric flexible flatfoot deformity. Both groups demonstrated clinical and radiographic improvement with minimal complications, and the authors recommended arthroereisis as a less-invasive alternative to lateral column lengthening. In a critical review of the literature, Metcalfe et al. found patient satisfaction rates of 79% to 100% in pediatric patients; however, arthroereisis was associated with a number of complications, including sinus tarsi pain, device extrusion, talar fracture, and undercorrection. Complication rates ranged from 5% to 18%. Similar positive results in adult populations have been reported in flexible posterior tibial tendon deficiency, but the need for implant removal remains high, ranging from 7% to 46%. Fortunately, no loss of correction has been reported once the implant is removed.

■ STAGE III DISEASE

In patients with stage III disease—rigid fixed deformity of the hindfoot and degenerative changes of the triple joint complex—arthrodesis is indicated if conservative measures have failed. Conservative measures include accommodative bracing such as a double upright ankle-foot orthosis. Multiple arthrodeses have been described for treatment of this deformity, including isolated talonavicular, isolated subtalar arthrodesis, talonavicular and calcaneocuboid arthrodesis, talonavicular

and subtalar arthrodesis, and triple arthrodesis. Historically, triple arthrodesis is the procedure of choice for this condition. However, Harper found that in elderly, low-demand patients, isolated talonavicular arthrodesis produced significant correction of the deformity with satisfactory pain relief. He reviewed the results in 29 patients treated with an isolated talonavicular arthrodesis with an average follow-up of 26 months; 25 of 29 patients (86%) were satisfied with no or minor reservations and achieved good or excellent results. Sammarco et al., in an effort to preserve the flexibility of the lateral column, corrected the deformity with subtalar and talonavicular arthrodesis without calcaneocuboid arthrodesis. They reported improvements in pain, function, cosmesis, and shoe wear, with only one nonunion in 16 feet, and recommended the procedure for patients whose calcaneocuboid joints are not involved in the primary disease. Denuding and compressing the talonavicular joint while preserving the calcaneocuboid joint was suggested to provide a relative lateral column lengthening, facilitating correction of forefoot abduction in flatfeet. Other authors have warned that the modified double arthrodesis has increased nonunion rates and worse outcomes than the standard triple arthrodesis. For mild stage III deformity, the "diple" (talonavicular and subtalar arthrodesis) is our procedure of choice, but including the calcaneocuboid joint is helpful for large corrections in severe deformity. The procedure for arthrodesis of the hindfoot is described in other chapter (Fig. 3.34).

▮ MEDIAL COLUMN STABILIZATION

As previously discussed, the deformity is not always the result of talonavicular joint subluxation, but instead the deformity may result from medial column instability (navicular-cuneiform or cuneiform-metatarsal instability). In reality, medial column instability often accompanies the hindfoot deformity, necessitating treatment of medial column stability in addition

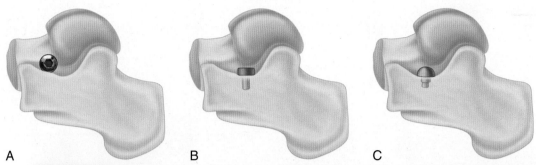

FIGURE 3.33 Maxwell and Cerniglia biomechanical classification of sinus tarsi implants. **A,** Self-locking wedge. **B,** Axis-altering device. **C,** Impact-blocking device.

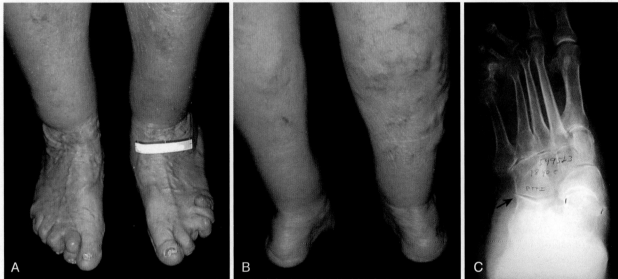

FIGURE 3.34 **A,** Patient with erosive osteoarthritis and posterior tibial tendon insufficiency. Note fixed hindfoot, midfoot, and forefoot deformities. Patient required triple arthrodesis. **B,** Posterior clinical view showing marked heel valgus bilaterally, worse on left. **C,** Weight-bearing anteroposterior view. With this degree of fixed deformity, "reconstructive" triple arthrodesis is required. Bone grafting is frequently needed.

to hindfoot procedures. Steiner et al. described correcting medial arch collapse at the level of the naviculocuneiform joint. In 34 feet treated with a subtalar and naviculocuneiform fusion, improved radiographic parameters and an excellent union rate (94%) were achieved. Stabilization of the medial column in flatfoot deformity, if not possible by soft-tissue procedures, may be achieved by either arthrodesis or osteotomy. Greisberg et al. described an isolated medial column arthrodesis to improve hindfoot alignment and reported improvement in all radiographic parameters in 19 patients.

ISOLATED MEDIAL COLUMN ARTHRODESIS

TECHNIQUE 3.9

(GREISBERG ET AL.)

- After induction of spinal or general anesthesia and application of a thigh tourniquet, assess the calf musculature

to determine if a gastrocnemius slide (Strayer) procedure is needed for contracture.
- Inflate the tourniquet and make a medial utility incision.
- If instability is present at the naviculocuneiform joint, use osteotomes to denude the medial and middle naviculocuneiform joints of cartilage and prepare them for fusion by perforating the subchondral bone with a small drill. The lateral naviculocuneiform joint usually is not included in the fusion. Reduce and stabilize the joints with multiple 3.5-mm lag screws passed from the navicular into the cuneiform.
- Treat any posterior tibial tendon degeneration as needed with tendon debridement or augmentation with the flexor digitorum longus.
- If the first tarsometatarsal joint is subluxed, approach it through a separate dorsal longitudinal incision to avoid injury to the anterior tibial tendon. Open the joint between the extensor hallucis longus and brevis tendons and prepare it for fusion with osteotomes and a small drill to perforate subchondral bone. Reduce and hold the joint with multiple 3.5-mm lag screws (Fig. 3.35). Typically, one screw is passed antegrade and the second ret-

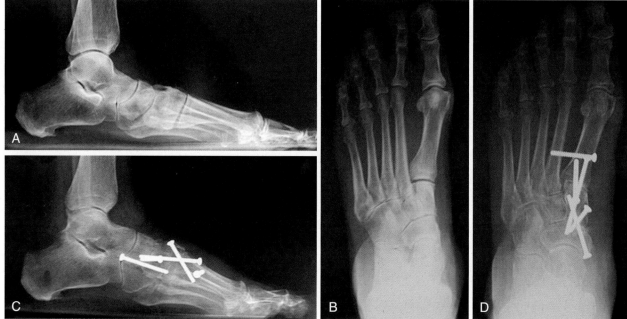

FIGURE 3.35 **A,** Patient with sag at naviculocuneiform and first tarsometatarsal joints; lateral process of talus is abutting anterior process of calcaneus. **B,** Varus of first metatarsal is consistent with instability of first tarsometatarsal joint; subluxation of talonavicular joint also is present. **C,** Lateral view 6 months after medial column arthrodesis shows improvement in talometatarsal angle and opening of sinus tarsi. **D,** Anteroposterior view shows improved talonavicular coverage. (From Greisberg J, Assal M, Hansen ST Jr, Sangeorzan BJ: Isolated medial column stabilization improves alignment in adult-acquired flatfoot, *Clin Orthop Relat Res* 435:197, 2005.) **SEE TECHNIQUE 3.9.**

rograde. A third screw is then used to hold the first metatarsal reduced to the second, especially when the area between the bases of the metatarsals is included in the fusion.

- Use a small burr to create small gaps for placement of cancellous bone graft, usually harvested from the proximal tibia.
- Deflate the tourniquet, close the wounds in routine fashion, and apply a cast.

POSTOPERATIVE CARE The patient is kept non–weight bearing in the cast for 6 weeks. If radiographs at that time show early consolidation of the fusions, weight bearing is advanced as tolerated. Patients usually can fully bear weight in regular shoes by 10 to 12 weeks after surgery.

◼ STAGE IV DISEASE

Chronic posterior tibial tendon deformity in which ankle joint incongruency in valgus is present is a most difficult problem. Although bracing is the mainstay of treatment, a subset of these patients will not have substantial pain relief and will require surgical repair and stabilization. For rigid deformities, the procedure of choice usually is arthrodesis of the ankle or tibiotalocalcaneal arthrodesis or, if the hindfoot deformity can be corrected, total ankle arthroplasty. In a select group of patients with flexible, reducible deformity, less than 10 degrees of tibiotalar tilt, and minimal lateral ankle joint arthrosis, consideration can be given to reconstruction of the deltoid ligament. Jeng et al. described a "minimally invasive" allograft

technique for deltoid ligament reconstruction for stage IV flatfoot deformity done in conjunction with triple arthrodesis.

MINIMALLY INVASIVE DELTOID LIGAMENT RECONSTRUCTION

TECHNIQUE 3.10

(JENG ET AL.)

ALLOGRAFT PREPARATION

- Before creation of the bone tunnels, prepare the allograft hamstring tendon.
- From a fully thawed allograft tendon, use about 20 cm for the reconstruction.
- Split the graft longitudinally, leaving approximately 6 cm intact. Place Krackow stitches of a no. 00 Orthocord (Ethicon, Somerville, NJ) nonabsorbable suture in all three limbs of the tendon graft and apply a preload to stretch the tendon and minimize creep after insertion.

DELTOID LIGAMENT RECONSTRUCTION

- Create a tibial tunnel by inserting a guidewire parallel to the joint surface at the level of the distal tibial physeal scar and centered in the sagittal plane within the tibia (Fig. 3.36).
- Confirm guidewire position with fluoroscopy, then drill a 6.5-mm tunnel 25 mm deep over the wire.

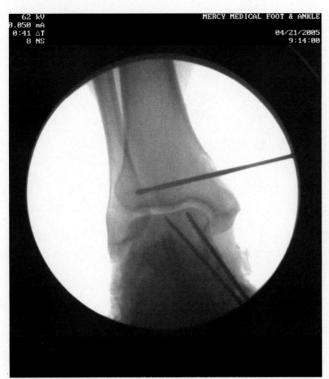

FIGURE 3.36 Reconstruction of deltoid ligament. Fluoroscopic view of guidewire for drilling of tibial tunnel for insertion of tibial limb of reconstruction. (From Jeng CL, Bluman EM, Myerson MS: Minimally invasive deltoid ligament reconstruction for stage IV flatfoot deformity, *Foot Ankle Int* 32:21, 2011.) **SEE TECHNIQUE 3.10.**

- Insert the nonsplit end of the tendon graft into this blind tunnel and fix it in place with a biotenodesis screw. Bioabsorbable polylactic acid interference screws of 6.25- to 8.0-mm diameter are used for tendon fixation depending on bone quality.
- With blunt dissection, create a subcutaneous tunnel from the insertion site inferiorly to the tip of the medial malleolus and pass the distal tendon limbs through this tunnel with a hemostat clamp.
- Make a longitudinal incision extending from the distal end of the medial malleolus to approximately 1 cm inferior to the sustentaculum tali.
- Excise the posterior tibial tendon and the remaining soft tissues (e.g., tendon sheaths and attenuated superficial deltoid fibers) as needed to gain access to the medial talar dome and sustentaculum. Take care not to damage the flexor digitorum longus or FHL tendons. The posteromedial neurovascular bundle of the ankle should remain posterior to all tunnels at the level of the ankle and posteroinferior to them at the level of the sustentaculum.
- Create a talar tunnel beginning at the medial center of tibiotalar rotation; approximate this position through the footprint of the previously transected deep deltoid fibers.
- Locate the junction of the lateral talar neck and body by palpation and make the lateral exit of the tunnel here (Fig. 3.37A).
- Taking care not to damage branches of the superficial peroneal nerve, use a small hemostat to bluntly dissect down to the most proximal portion of the lateral talar neck.

- Advance a guidewire along this axis and confirm its position with anteroposterior and lateral fluoroscopy.
- With a cannulated drill, drill a 5-mm tunnel over the guidewire in an anterograde direction.
- With a suture passer, pass the talar limb of the sutured tendon through the tunnel from medial to lateral.
- Hand-tension this limb of the tendon graft while holding the ankle and hindfoot in maximal inversion and place a 5.5-mm interference screw in the medial aspect of the tunnel to secure the graft.
- With digital palpation, locate the medial border of the sustentaculum tali. Advance a guidewire for a biotenodesis screw along an axis from the sustentaculum tali to a point approximately 1 cm superior to the peroneal tubercle on the lateral side of the calcaneus (Fig. 3.37B).
- Confirm position of the guidewire with fluoroscopy and create a 5-mm tunnel over the guidewire.
- Pass the free end of the remaining limb of the tendon graft through this calcaneal tunnel.
- Manually tension the graft to obtain congruent tibiotalar joint position on fluoroscopy and insert a 5.5-mm interference screw from medial to lateral into the calcaneal tunnel (Fig. 3.38).
- Close the incisions in routine fashion and apply a plaster splint.

POSTOPERATIVE CARE At 2 weeks after surgery, splint immobilization is removed and a cast boot is fitted. Weight bearing is begun 6 weeks after surgery, and immobilization is discontinued at 12 weeks.

POSTERIOR TIBIAL TENDON INSUFFICIENCY
■ INSUFFICIENCY OF POSTERIOR TIBIAL TENDON SECONDARY TO ACCESSORY NAVICULAR

Insufficiency of the posterior tibial tendon secondary to an accessory navicular presents unique problems. It would seem reasonable that if unilateral pes planus develops, excising the accessory navicular and advancing the posterior tibial tendon should suffice (provided the deformity is not severe and the opposite foot has an accessory navicular but no pes planus) (Fig. 3.39A,B); however, this most often is not the case. Whether excision of the accessory navicular and advancement of the posterior tibial tendon alters the medial longitudinal arch is doubtful.

Kidner believed that the support to the medial longitudinal arch offered by the posterior tibial tendon was compromised by its abnormal insertion into the accessory navicular, and he devised a procedure intended to correct this loss of suspension by the posterior tibial tendon. However, a cause-and-effect relationship between the accessory navicular and pes planus is uncertain. In a retrospective comparative radiographic series, the presence of an accessory navicular was associated with flatfoot radiographic parameters when compared to a control group, but many individuals with an accessory navicular had a normal medial longitudinal arch. Furthermore, the presence of an accessory navicular did not correspond with the severity or symptoms of the flat foot. Hence, any improvement in the medial longitudinal arch after a

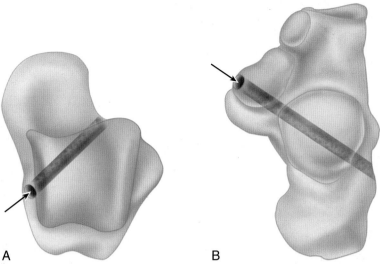

FIGURE 3.37 Reconstruction of deltoid ligament. Disarticulated superior views of talus **(A)** and calcaneus **(B)** show path of graft limbs. *Arrows* indicate entry points. Talar tunnel starts at footprint of deep deltoid ligament and exits at proximal lateral talar neck. Calcaneal tunnel starts at sustentaculum and exits 1 cm superior to peroneal tubercle. (From Jeng CL, Bluman EM, Myerson MS: Minimally invasive deltoid ligament reconstruction for stage IV flatfoot deformity, *Foot Ankle Int* 32:21, 2011.) **SEE TECHNIQUE 3.10.**

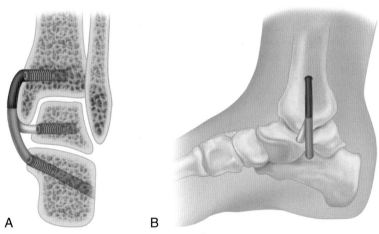

FIGURE 3.38 Coronal **(A)** and medial **(B)** views of completed reconstruction of deltoid ligament. (From Jeng CL, Bluman EM, Myerson MS: Minimally invasive deltoid ligament reconstruction for stage IV flatfoot deformity, *Foot Ankle Int* 32:21, 2011.) **SEE TECHNIQUE 3.10.**

Kidner procedure likely occurs only because of continued growth in the immature foot.

The accessory navicular bone has been classified by various authors into three primary types. Type I occurs primarily as a round sesamoid within the substance of the distal posterior tibial tendon. It rarely is associated with symptoms. Type II is associated with a synchondrosis within the body of the navicular at risk for disruption from traction injury or shear forces in the region. Type III, also known as a navicular beak or a cornuate navicular (Fig. 3.40), occurs with fusion of the accessory navicular bone to the body of the navicular. The presence of an accessory navicular bone likely is an autosomal dominant trait with incomplete penetrance. Recognition of the loss of structural integrity of the longitudinal arch is important because this component of the deformity would not be corrected by excising the accessory navicular and reinserting or even advancing

the posterior tibial tendon. In a skeletally mature foot, unilateral pes planus (see Fig. 3.39C,D) with a posterior tibial tendon insufficiency associated with an accessory navicular may require a combination of excision of the accessory navicular, advancement of the tendon, and lengthening of the lateral column (Evans procedure) (Fig. 3.41).

Generally speaking, the presence of an accessory navicular does not necessitate treatment unless symptomatic. Through a thorough history and examination, any foot pain must be correlated to the accessory ossicle because 10% to 14% of normal feet have an accessory navicular. With or without pes planus, an asymptomatic accessory navicular bone may become symptomatic after mild trauma, causing instability of the synchondrosis. Athletes may be less responsive to conservative treatment, suggesting that early operative treatment could be considered.

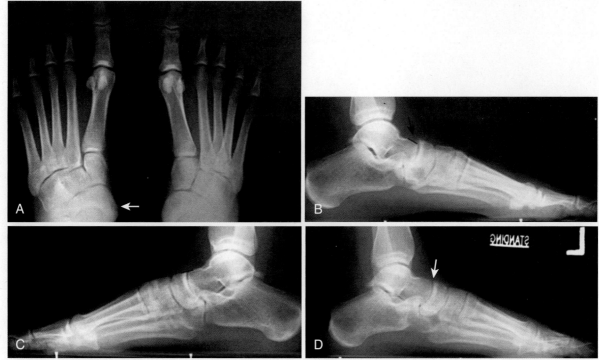

FIGURE 3.39   **A,** Bilateral cornuate navicular and, on left, accessory navicular *(white arrow)* in 19-year-old woman. Note on left pronation of forefoot (evidenced by opening up of metatarsal-tarsal joint spaces), apparent widening of intermetatarsal spaces, and uncovering of fibular sesamoid compared with right foot. On standing lateral views of left foot, which had unilateral pes planus, talus is plantarflexed **(B)** compared with asymptomatic right foot **(C). D,** After excision of navicular flush with medial cuneiform, advancement of posterior tibial tendon distally, and lengthening of lateral column of foot with calcaneal opening wedge osteotomy (Evans procedure). Talonavicular joint reduced congruously but not with just advancement of posterior tibial tendon.

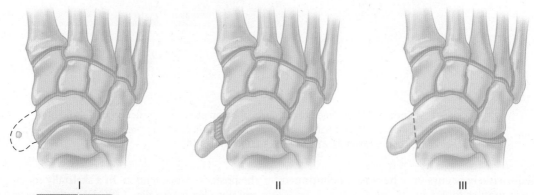

I   II   III

FIGURE 3.40   Classification of accessory navicular. Type I, small oval-to-round ossicle within the posterior tibial tendon; no bony or cartilaginous attachment to the navicular. Type II, larger lateral projection from the medial aspect of the navicular; fibrocartilaginous plate less than 2 mm wide and with an irregular outline separates tuberosity from body of the navicular. Type III, "horn"-shaped prominence connected to the navicular by a bony bridge. (Redrawn from Pretell-Mazzini J, Murphy RF, Sawyer JR, et al: Surgical treatment of symptomatic accessory navicular in children, *Am J Orthop (Belle Mead NJ)* 43:110, 2014.)

For painful synchondrosis with symmetric foot posture, excision and osseous union procedures have been successful. Cha et al., in a prospective study, compared two groups of patients (50 feet) with type 2 accessory navicular. Group 1 had simple excision of the accessory navicular, and group 2 had accessory navicular excision with advancement of the tendon. At a minimum of 3 years' follow-up, both groups showed pain improvement and no significant differences were present between the two groups.

Nakayama et al. described another technique in which percutaneous drilling to induce union of the synchondrosis produced excellent or good results in 30 of 31 feet.

Malicky et al. described accessory navicular fusion to the native navicular body as an alternative to excision. This

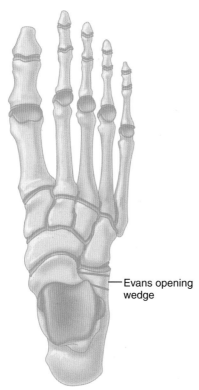

Evans opening wedge

FIGURE 3.41 Evans anterior calcaneal osteotomy helps restore and stabilize longitudinal arch by elongating lateral column of foot.

technique leaves the posterior tibial tendon attachment intact, removes the synchondrosis, and relies on bony union of the accessory navicular. Chung and Chu reported excellent or good results in 27 of 34 feet with fusion of the accessory navicular, but 6 feet developed a nonunion, resulting in a poor result.

KIDNER PROCEDURE

The Kidner procedure consists of excising the accessory navicular and rerouting the posterior tibial tendon into a more plantar position. The parents should be informed before surgery, however, that permanent correction of the arch sag cannot be certain. Relief of symptoms around the prominent tuberosity and reduction or elimination of fatigue from arch strain are predictable. Indications for the Kidner procedure include symptomatic accessory navicular bone with point tenderness in the region. In most patients with an acute injury to the synchondrosis, 6 to 8 weeks of cast or boot immobilization is recommended as a trial before surgical intervention.

LATERAL COLUMN LENGTHENING AND EXCISION OF ACCESSORY NAVICULAR

TECHNIQUE 3.11

INCISION AND REMOVAL OF ACCESSORY NAVICULAR

- Beginning 1.0 to 1.5 cm inferior and distal to the tip of the medial malleolus, arch the skin incision slightly dorsalward, peaking at the medial prominence of the accessory

navicular, and sloping distally to the base of the first metatarsal (Fig. 3.42A).
- After ligating the plantar communicating branches of the saphenous system, identify the posterior tibial tendon as it approaches the accessory navicular (Fig. 3.42B).
- Identify the dorsal and plantar margins of the tendon 2 cm proximal to the accessory navicular and expose the tendon distally, ending at the bone. By this means, the entire tendon can be exposed and the part extending plantarward toward its multiple insertions is not disturbed (Fig. 3.3).

TRANSPOSITION AND ADVANCEMENT OF THE SLIP OF THE POSTERIOR TIBIAL TENDON

- Using sharp dissection, shell the accessory navicular from the posterior tibial tendon, attempting to leave a small sliver of bone within the tendon if transposition of the tendon is planned (Fig. 3.42C).
- Resect the medial prominence of the main navicular flush with the medial border of the first cuneiform using a rongeur and rasp (Fig. 3.42D). Remove the portion of cuneiform using sharp dissection and shift it plantarward and laterally as far as possible.
- Suture the tendon to the apex of the medial longitudinal arch using periosteum and ligamentous tissue to secure the transposed tendon slip or by passing the sutures through holes drilled in the center of the navicular and tying them dorsally. Try to advance this slip of tendon while the talonavicular joint is reduced and the medial longitudinal arch is reestablished by holding the midfoot and forefoot in a cavovarus position.

EVANS LATERAL COLUMN LENGTHENING

This graft usually is 8 to 10 mm wide and is placed 1 cm proximal to the calcaneocuboid articulation. It is internally fixed with a single $\frac{3}{32}$-inch pin from the fourth intermetatarsal space, distal to proximal, crossing the calcaneocuboid articulation and cut beneath the skin. The pin is removed in 6 to 8 weeks using local anesthesia, and a short leg weight-bearing cast is worn for another 6 to 8 weeks. This should restore the arch (Fig. 3.39D).

SKIN CLOSURE AND CASTING

- Close the skin and subcutaneous tissue with absorbable sutures or adhesive skin strips so that the postoperative cast can remain in place for 4 weeks.
- Apply a long leg, bent-knee cast in two parts. The cast is well padded and gently molded into the longitudinal arch with the talonavicular joint reduced and the foot inverted. Extend the short leg cast above the knee with this joint flexed 45 degrees.
- If the patient is reliable and the parents are informed, a short leg cast with the foot in equinovarus is a reasonable alternative, but it must be a nonwalking cast.

POSTOPERATIVE CARE The cast applied in the operating suite is left on for 4 weeks unless neurovascular signs or evidence of infection demand its removal. At 4 weeks, a short leg cast, well molded into the arch with the foot plantigrade, is applied and partial weight

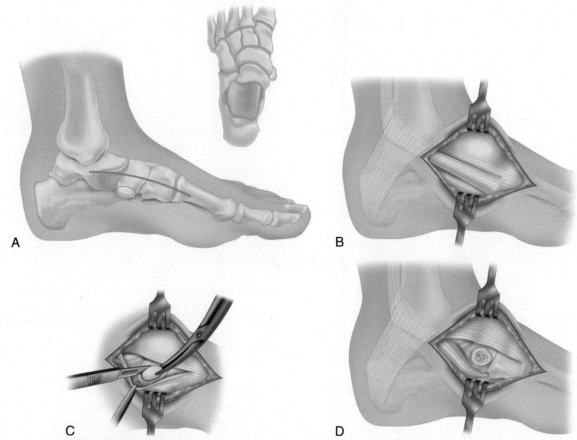

FIGURE 3.42 Kidner procedure. **A,** Incision. *Inset,* Location of accessory navicular. **B,** Exposure of posterior tibial tendon and accessory navicular. **C,** Removal of accessory navicular. **D,** Accessory navicular removed and tuberosity of navicular cut flush with adjacent cuneiform and talus. **SEE TECHNIQUE 3.11.**

bearing is allowed. At 8 weeks, full weight bearing is allowed. At 10 weeks, a firm arch support is fitted in a leather oxford shoe. It has been our experience that many patients require 6 to 12 months to be completely asymptomatic at the site of the tendon repair and advancement.

ACCESSORY NAVICULAR FUSION

TECHNIQUE 3.12

(MALICKY ET AL.)

- Approach the posterior tibial tendon in a manner similar to that described for the Kidner procedure (see Technique 3.11).
- Expose the tendon just proximal to its insertion onto the navicular, maintaining the tendon attachment to the accessory navicular bone.
- Through the dorsal aspect of the interface between the primary and accessory navicular bones, excise the intervening soft tissue to expose the bony surfaces.

- Leave the plantar distal extension of the posterior tibial tendon intact.
- Use a small saw or osteotome to remove enough of the prominent part of the primary navicular to create a flat surface at the distal plantar segment.
- Advance the accessory bone into the distal plantar aspect of the primary navicular and stabilize it with either a 2.7- or 3.5-mm lag screw. A washer can be used to better distribute the compressive forces.

POSTOPERATIVE CARE A short leg non–weight–bearing cast is worn for 6 weeks. Then progressive weight bearing is started in a removable cast boot and advanced to full weight bearing at 10 to 12 weeks.

■ PES PLANUS AND TARSAL COALITION

Although tarsal coalition has long been cited as a cause of congenital rigid pes planus, this is inaccurate. Some patients with a tarsal coalition, especially calcaneonavicular coalition, have little deformity suggestive of pes planus. Slight heel valgus and minimal loss of the longitudinal arch may be present but frequently are not among the patient's complaints. In addition, any deformity

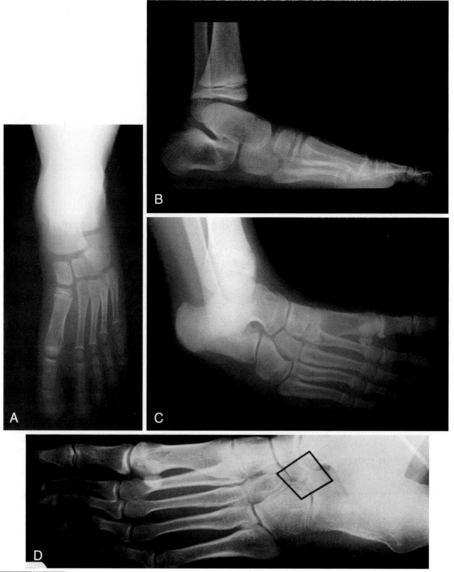

FIGURE 3.43   **A to C,** Congenital talonavicular tarsal coalition (anteroposterior, lateral, and oblique views). **D,** Calcaneonavicular incomplete tarsal coalition.

may not be rigid. This is especially true of calcaneonavicular coalition, which might allow enough subtalar motion to delude the examiner before radiographic evaluation. Most patients with tarsal coalition do have a fixed hindfoot valgus of varying severity and some loss of the normal longitudinal arch. In addition to this loss of normal longitudinal arch, many patients do not experience symptoms until their foot is close to skeletal maturity. For this reason, tarsal coalition has been included in the discussion of posterior tibial tendon insufficiency.

Tarsal coalition, rigid pes planus, and peroneal muscle spasm frequently are discussed together as essential components of peroneal spastic pes planus. However, peroneal spasm actually is an acquired or adaptive shortening of the muscle-tendon units of the peroneal muscles. Inversion stress by the examiner, producing an unsustained three-beat or four-beat clonus of the peroneal muscles, is the stretch reflex of a shortened muscle-tendon unit. That peroneal muscle tightness is the frequent *result* of tarsal coalition and not the *cause* must be emphasized.

Peroneal muscle tightness is seen in many clinical disorders other than tarsal coalition. Common among these are rheumatoid arthritis, osteochondral fracture, and infection in the subtalar joint, or neoplasm adjacent to the subtalar joint in the talus or calcaneus. The relaxed position of the subtalar joint is valgus, which places the least strain on the talocalcaneal interosseous ligament according to Lapidus. Presumably, through an ill-defined mechanism, the peroneal muscles are reflexively stimulated to evert the hindfoot, "decompressing" the subtalar joint, and with time, this position becomes fixed.

The true incidence of tarsal coalition is greater than the 1% usually quoted. Tarsal coalition appears to be inherited, probably as a unifactorial disorder of autosomal dominant inheritance with nearly full penetrance. The specific type of coalition probably represents a genetic mutation that is responsible for failure of the primitive mesenchyme to segment. Symptomatic tarsal coalitions, other than calcaneonavicular and talocalcaneal coalitions, are exceedingly rare. Talonavicular coalition (Fig. 3.43A-C) probably is much more common than calcaneocuboid, naviculocuboid, naviculocuneiform, or massive tarsal coalition, but it, too, is rare.

Specific treatment for calcaneonavicular and talocalcaneal coalitions is further discussed, but generally speaking, a trial of conservative treatment with cast or boot immobilization is indicated initially. After failing conservative treatment, surgical treatment includes bar excision (open or endoscopic) or joint arthrodesis (selective or triple). Treating physicians must also address concomitant valgus deformities through additional procedures to create a plantigrade foot.

■ CALCANEONAVICULAR COALITION

Although probably present since birth, the calcaneonavicular bar does not ossify until a person is 8 to 12 years old. Before this period, presumably because of the malleability of the cartilage surrounding the primary ossification centers of the peritalar complex, significant symptoms are rare. It is believed that, as the cartilage ossifies, hindfoot stiffness results; thus, the patient's ability to withstand the stress of vigorous childhood activity declines. The coalition might be bony (synostosis), cartilaginous (synchondrosis), or fibrous (syndesmosis). Incomplete coalitions (Fig. 3.43D), that is, cartilaginous or fibrous, usually are the more symptomatic. The 45-degree lateral oblique radiographic examination is the most useful in diagnosing calcaneonavicular coalition, whether it is complete (bony) or incomplete (cartilaginous or fibrous).

The abnormal bar runs from the anterior process of the calcaneus just lateral to the anterior facet dorsally and medially to the lateral and dorsolateral extraarticular surface of the navicular. It usually is 1.0 to 2.0 cm long × 1.0 to 1.2 cm wide. In a bar with a cartilaginous or fibrous interface, the adjacent bony margins are irregular and indistinct. The talar head might appear small and underdeveloped. Beaking of the dorsal articular margin of the talus, so common in talocalcaneal coalition, is uncommon in calcaneonavicular coalition.

The symptoms usually are vague dorsolateral foot pain centering around the sinus tarsi, difficulty walking on uneven surfaces, foot fatigue, and occasionally a painful limp. The physical examination may or may not show significant reduction of subtalar motion or flattening of the longitudinal arch, so a high index of suspicion is necessary in this patient profile. In our experience, if the condition is unilateral, careful examination of subtalar motion shows a definite difference in the two feet in most patients. In addition to varying degrees of loss of subtalar motion, tenderness usually is present in the sinus tarsi and along the course of the bar. Hindfoot valgus, some loss of the longitudinal arch, and peroneal spasm are present in most adolescent patients who are symptomatic to varying degrees.

Although a calcaneonavicular coalition may not appear until adulthood, most patients with symptomatic calcaneonavicular coalition are 8 to 12 years old, corresponding to the period in which ossification of the cartilaginous precursor occurs. Parents should be educated regarding its congenital nature, the reason for the delay in symptoms until adolescence, its hereditary pattern, and the fact that some coalitions never become symptomatic. This discussion with the patient and family members is an important part of the treatment.

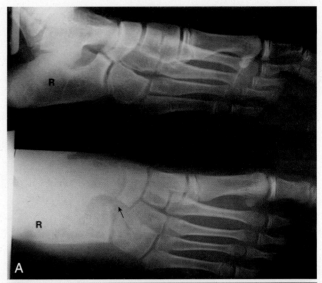
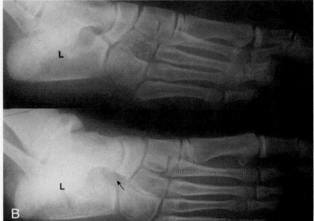

FIGURE 3.44   Resection of calcaneonavicular tarsal coalition. **A,** Before surgery. **B,** After surgery.

A trial of reduced activity or cast immobilization or both is recommended. A patient may be rendered asymptomatic for varying periods or even indefinitely after 4 to 6 weeks in a cast. Intermittent casting for short periods, with lengthy intervals of noncasting, might be all that is required. The mere presence of a tarsal coalition does not mean surgery should be recommended; if patients with tarsal coalition reach their 20s with few or no symptoms, they frequently remain asymptomatic or are only mildly symptomatic. If a trial period of casting and the use of a molded arch support do not allow an adolescent to participate in activities he or she enjoys, however, surgical treatment can be recommended with a high expectation of success in reducing or eliminating the symptoms.

For children and young adults, resection of the calcaneonavicular bar with interposition of muscle or fat at the site of resection is recommended. For adults, however, the literature is conflicting as to the efficacy of calcaneonavicular bar excision, with good results reported from 68% to 92% of patients, but with recurrence rates of 67% and osteoarthritic changes in 96% reported by some. Other authors, however, have reported restoration of subtalar motion, relief of symptoms, and improved function after resection and filling of the defect with muscle (extensor digitorum brevis) or fat (Fig. 3.44).

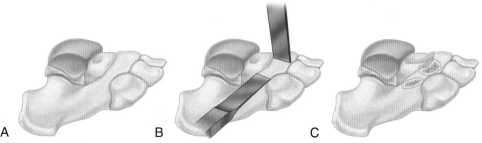

FIGURE 3.45 Resection of calcaneonavicular tarsal coalition. **A,** Before surgery. **B,** Direction of osteotome. **C,** After resection. **SEE TECHNIQUE 3.13.**

CALCANEONAVICULAR BAR RESECTION

TECHNIQUE 3.13

EXPOSURE OF BAR
- Make an Ollier incision; preserve the branches of the intermediate dorsal cutaneous branch of the superficial peroneal nerve crossing the incision, and try to preserve the sheaths of the extensor digitorum longus and peroneus tertius tendons anteriorly and the peroneal tendons posteriorly.
- Identify the muscle belly of the extensor digitorum brevis. Raise the muscle by sharp dissection from the confines of the sinus tarsi in a proximal-to-distal direction until the entire sinus tarsi and anterior process of the calcaneus are identified.

RESECTION OF BAR
- Identify the talonavicular and calcaneocuboid joints by manually rocking the forefoot-midfoot segment on the hindfoot. The bar runs from the anterior process of the calcaneus just lateral to the anterior facet anteriorly and medially to the lateral and dorsolateral margin of the navicular. If the exact location of the articular margins of the calcaneocuboid or talonavicular joints is questionable, open the capsules of these joints just enough to identify the articular surfaces.
- Use small Hohmann retractors around the waist of the bar to improve exposure. At the calcaneal origin of the bar, place a ½-inch osteotome parallel to the floor of the sinus tarsi and cut up to but not through the medial cortex of the bar. Direct the upper cut at the dorsolateral aspect of the navicular medially, plantarward, and obliquely at about 30 degrees from the vertical plane. Complete this osteotomy through the bar. By placing the osteotome in the inferior cut, fracture the bar through its medial cortex and smooth it with a rongeur. A rectangular piece of bone should be excised. In this manner, the chance of damaging the anterior facet of the subtalar joint or the inferior aspect of the head and neck of the talus is reduced (Fig. 3.45).
- Generous resection of the bar is recommended. Because the tendency is to remove less than an optimal amount of bone, we recommend a lateral oblique radiographic examination on the operating table after resection. Usually, a 1.5- to 2.5-cm segment of bar is re-

moved. Leave the lateral fourth of the articular surface of the talus uncovered by navicular to ensure adequate removal.

INTERPOSITION OF MUSCLE
- Using an absorbable suture woven through the proximal margin of the extensor digitorum brevis muscle, interpose the muscle in the depths of the defect by passing a small, straight needle medially through the defect, carrying the suture and the muscle with it into the defect.
- Bring the ends of the suture out through the skin medially, pass them through a broad felt pad, and tie them firmly.
- Deflate the tourniquet, secure hemostasis, and close the skin with absorbable sutures.
- Apply a well-padded, short leg cast in the operating room.
- The use of bone wax with Gelfoam on the raw surfaces after resection is an alternative to muscle interposition.

POSTOPERATIVE CARE The initial cast (nonwalking) remains in place 3 weeks, provided that the neurovascular status of the foot is satisfactory. At 3 weeks, the cast is removed and active plus gentle, active-assisted, inversion-eversion exercises are begun. Weight bearing to tolerance with the aid of crutches is begun; the crutches are discontinued when full weight bearing is comfortable. Although subtalar motion improves, we have not had it equal that of the uninvolved side in unilateral cases and 50% of normal is, in our opinion, a good result. The patient and parents should understand this before surgery.

ARTHRODESIS FOR CALCANEONAVICULAR COALITION

In adults, resection of a complete bony bar between the calcaneus and the navicular may not improve subtalar motion or relieve the symptoms. This is especially true if there is radiographic evidence of degenerative arthritis in the subtalar or talonavicular joints. If the findings of arthritis are mild and consist primarily of talonavicular beaking, the option of bar resection or arthrodesis is given to these patients. Salvage of the failed bar resection, regardless of age, is an arthrodesis. We prefer select arthrodeses in adult patients with degenerative changes in the peritalar joint complex.

If the hindfoot is in an acceptable position, an in situ arthrodesis is performed. If the position of the hindfoot must be changed, however, the bar is removed and the appropriate resection of the articular surfaces at the subtalar and midtarsal joints is made to reposition the hindfoot. The surgical techniques of hindfoot arthrodeses are described in other chapter.

■ TALOCALCANEAL COALITION

The talocalcaneal bridge ossifies either completely or incompletely when an individual is between 12 and 16 years old, which is later than the ossification of the calcaneonavicular bar and usually is diagnosed in older adolescents or adults. CT of a symptomatic hindfoot in children may identify the coalition earlier. The symptoms are similar to those of calcaneonavicular coalition and include foot fatigue and pain around the hindfoot on increased activity. Loss of the longitudinal arch, although present, usually is not a complaint. Peroneal spasm frequently is present, but the cardinal sign on physical examination is marked reduction or absence of subtalar motion. This is in contrast to the calcaneonavicular bar, which may allow varying degrees of subtalar motion. Tenderness in the sinus tarsi, over the talonavicular joint, along the peroneal tendons, and especially medially over the sustentaculum tali, may be present. Abnormal palpation over the enlarged middle facet ("double medial malleolus") may also be present on examination. Heel valgus and loss of the normal longitudinal arch usually occur in varying severity.

▌RADIOGRAPHIC FINDINGS

The Harris and Beath radiographic projection (i.e., posterosuperior oblique projection) passes between the sustentaculum and the neck of the talus. In a talocalcaneal coalition, the joint space is replaced by a bony bridge (Fig. 3.46) or the distinct articular margins are lost, implying a fibrous or cartilaginous bridge. This view is taken with the patient standing on the cassette, with the knees flexed enough to remove the calf shadow from the beam and the cone angled 45 degrees to the cassette and directed toward the heel. We have found in taking the coalition view that 35- to 40- to 45-degree angles to the long axis of the calcaneus are the most common angles showing the coalition (see Fig. 3.46). Jayakumar and Cowell recommended a standing lateral radiograph, from which the angles made by the posterior and medial facets with the floor are determined. The angle of inclination of the projection can be determined for the coalition view.

Other helpful radiographic signs include beaking of the head of the talus at the dorsal articular margin (Fig. 3.47), broadening or rounding of the lateral process of the talus as it impinges on the calcaneal sulcus, presence of a "true C sign," narrowing of the posterior talocalcaneal joint space, and loss of the middle subtalar joint, all seen on the lateral view of the foot (see Fig. 3.46). In addition, on the lateral oblique view, the anterior facet of the subtalar joint is asymmetric. CT scans also are helpful in characterizing the extent of coalition, especially for operative planning.

Normal variations in the osseous anatomy of the hindfoot make radiographic standardization difficult for diagnosing talocalcaneal coalition. Normally, the medial and posterior subtalar joint facets lie in planes at 35 to 45 degrees and 45 to 60 degrees to the long axis of the calcaneus, but this is highly variable (Fig. 3.48). One reason for the difficulty in diagnosing this disorder is that the bridge, which may be bony, fibrous, or cartilaginous, is not seen in ordinary radiographic projections of the foot, including the lateral oblique view, which is needed to diagnose calcaneonavicular coalitions. CT in the coronal plane at 3-mm increments is recommended. Instructions should be explicit to the radiography technician that the primary cuts of the CT should be perpendicular to the posterior and middle facets of the subtalar joint, that is, in the semicoronal plane. This

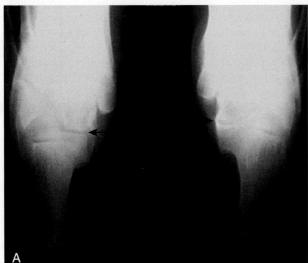
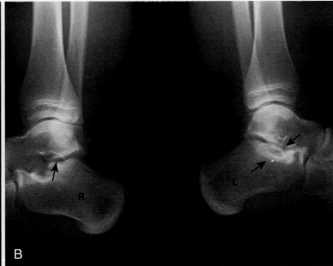

FIGURE 3.46   **A,** Harris-Beath axial calcaneal (coalition) view to identify middle facet tarsal coalition. Note normal middle facet on right and incomplete middle facet coalition on left. **B,** Lateral radiograph of hindfeet of same patient. Note normal middle and posterior facets on right but following conditions on left: loss of normal "space" at middle facet, rounding of lateral process of talus, and sclerotic semicircle in calcaneus inferior to middle facet, representing overlap of cortical margins of sustentaculum and bony bar.

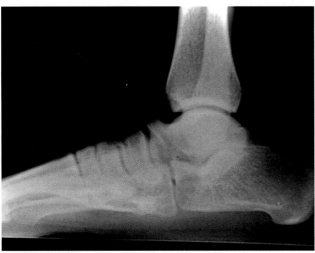

FIGURE 3.47 Note beaking of anterior aspect of neck of talus associated with middle facet tarsal coalition.

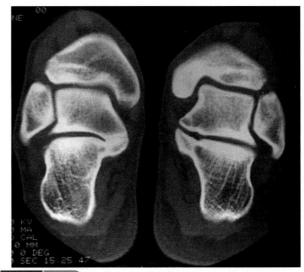

FIGURE 3.49 CT scan shows middle facet coalition.

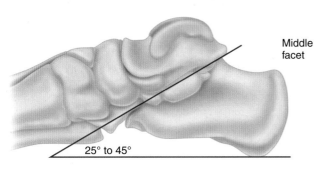

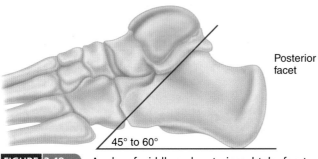

FIGURE 3.48 Angles of middle and posterior subtalar facets.

not only aids in the diagnosis of talocalcaneal coalition but also defines the exact location and margins of the coalition and shows the condition of the remaining subtalar articulations at the middle and posterior facets. Although CT sets the standard for diagnosis of talocalcaneal coalitions (Fig. 3.49), MRI may be helpful in depicting all types of coalitions, including fibrous coalitions.

▌ TREATMENT

A trial of conservative treatment is recommended, including reduced activity, 4 to 6 weeks in a short leg walking cast followed by a period of wearing molded arch supports, and possibly a corticosteroid injection within the sinus tarsi. If this form of treatment fails, operative treatment is indicated. Wilde et al. found that coalitions with more than 50% involvement of the subtalar joint were associated with more than 16 degrees of heel valgus, which resulted in poor results after resection, and he recommended subtalar fusion. More

recently, however, authors have reported comparable results with resection despite the size of the coalition. Mosca et al. reported satisfactory results and deformity correction with the use of a lateral column lengthening with or without talocalcaneal coalition resection.

In older patients, especially patients in whom degenerative changes have occurred (see Fig. 3.51), selective hindfoot arthrodesis is indicated. A triple arthrodesis has been described for this condition through either an anterolateral or an Ollier approach, supplemented by a medial approach, if needed, to expose the medial aspect of the talonavicular joint, the coalition at the sustentaculum, or both (Fig. 3.50). A subtalar fusion alone has been reported effective unless degenerative arthritic changes are present in one or both of the midtarsal joints. If subtalar arthrodesis alone is chosen, the technique is as described in other chapter. To aid with hindfoot deformity correction, resection of the coalition may be needed, allowing rotation of the calcaneus under the talus.

In a younger patient (9 to 12 years old) with symptomatic middle facet tarsal coalition, resection of the bar has gained popularity (Fig. 3.51A). This is done through a medial incision over the sustentaculum tali. This is our treatment of choice in younger patients (10 to 15 years old). For some patients who have significantly increased heel valgus or forefoot abduction in combination with a middle facet coalition, corrective osteotomies of the calcaneus can be used in addition to resection of the middle facet. Anterior lengthening osteotomy of the calcaneus is used when the deformity is primarily abduction through the midfoot. A medial displacement posterior calcaneal osteotomy is used when the deformity is primarily heel valgus without severe forefoot abduction. Alternatively, in a small cohort of patients with large, complete osseous coalitions, improved VAS scores and radiographic parameters have been reported when the coalition was not resected and osteotomies were performed around the coalition to correct foot posture. In these patients, the osseous edema at the coalition is not the pain source, but the severe valgus foot posture causes the symptoms.

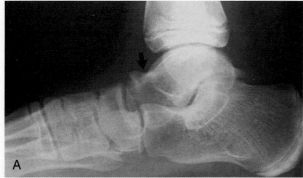
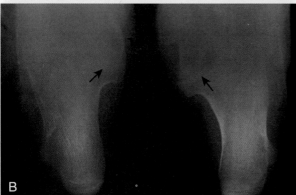
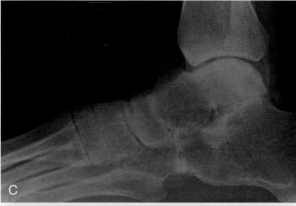
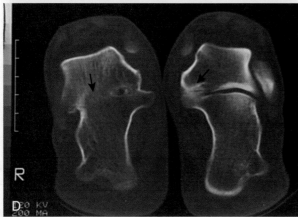

FIGURE 3.50 **A,** Standing lateral radiograph of right foot. Note middle facet tarsal coalition with talar beaking. **B,** Note middle facet coalition bilaterally. **C,** Several years after triple arthrodesis. **D,** CT scans after triple arthrodesis of right foot; left foot has not been treated.

RESECTION OF A MIDDLE FACET TARSAL COALITION

TECHNIQUE 3.14

- Begin an incision at the proximal margin of the navicular, curving it slightly dorsally, passing distal to the tip of the medial malleolus 1 to 2 cm plantar to its distal tip. At that point, curve the incision slightly plantarward, ending 3 to 4 cm proximal to the tip of the medial malleolus. The neurovascular bundle should course obliquely across the proximal end of the incision.
- When skin, subcutaneous tissue, and superficial veins (which may be large) are exposed, palpate the sustentaculum tali about 2 cm plantarward from the tip of the medial malleolus.
- The flexor digitorum longus tendon passes over the central portion of the coalition. Open the sheath and retract it dorsally or plantarly (Fig. 3.52A).
- Incise the periosteum of the coalition, defining its proximal and distal margins. Expose the entire coalition and a limited area of the posterior facet to avoid injury with the osteotome. The FHL tendon is at the plantar margin of the coalition with the coalition over it.
- With the proximal and distal margins and the dorsal and plantar margins of the facet exposed, begin the resection. Use of a ¼- to ½-inch osteotome is helpful in determining the margins of the resection; however, use a 3- to 4-mm burr for final resection until cartilage is present on the talus and calcaneal surfaces (Fig. 3.52B). The most common error is not extending the resection distally and proximally sufficiently to view cartilage on both sides of the joint. Cartilage should be seen throughout the entire coalition after resection, leaving no areas of fibrous or bony connection. Subtalar stress should reveal some motion at the subtalar joint.
- Use bone wax on the opposing surfaces of the middle facet and take a free fat graft locally if available or through a small incision in the thigh and hold in place with small sutures through the bone of the adjacent periosteum of the middle facet.
- Apply a well-padded, short leg, non–weight-bearing cast.

POSTOPERATIVE CARE The cast and sutures are removed in 10 to 12 days. The patient should begin active range of motion of the ankle, subtalar, and midtarsal joints if the wound has healed. A non–weight-bearing, removable, short leg cast is worn for another 2 to 3 weeks. Partial weight bearing is allowed at 4 weeks, and full weight bearing is allowed at 6 weeks.

DISORDERS OF THE ACHILLES TENDON

The Achilles tendon is the largest and most powerful tendon in the ankle, formed from the fibers of two muscle units: the gastrocnemius muscle, which attaches above the knee to the

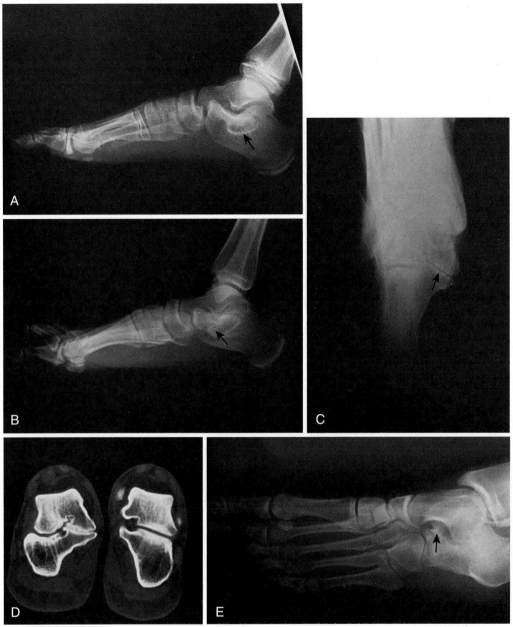

FIGURE 3.51   **A,** Lateral radiograph of immature foot with middle facet tarsal coalition. **B,** Lateral radiograph of patient in late 20s showing adaptive changes in middle facet. **C,** Harris axial calcaneal view. **D,** CT scan confirms degenerative changes in middle and posterior facets; note adaptive changes of entire shape of calcaneus. **E,** Oblique radiograph of same foot as in **B** and **D,** showing coalition extending distal to middle facet.

posterior aspect of the medial and lateral femoral condyles, and the soleus muscle, which originates from the upper part of the posterior tibia, fibula, and interosseous membrane. The gastrocnemius muscle is most effective in plantarflexion of the ankle with the knee extended, whereas the soleus muscle is most effective in plantarflexion of the ankle with the knee flexed. After coursing through the calf in the superficial posterior compartment, the fibers of the Achilles tendon rotate 90 degrees toward the insertion into the calcaneal tuberosity, with the gastrocnemius fibers lying lateral and the soleus fibers lying medial to the insertion point.

Vascularity is supplied to the tendon through the paratenon on the deep surface of the tendon, through muscular arterial branches within the gastrocsoleus complex proximally, and through small interosseous vessels at the insertion of the tendon into the calcaneus distally. There is a zone of relative avascularity 2 to 6 cm proximal to its insertion into the calcaneus. The vascular arrangement for the Achilles tendon is satisfactory for the low demand of the tendon sites in normal conditions, but increased demand may lead to inadequate vascularity, leading to subsequent degeneration and fibrosis of the involved segment of tendon.

In the classification of Achilles tendon disorders, it is helpful to divide the conditions into locality (i.e., insertional and noninsertional) and acuity. It also is helpful to distinguish "tendinitis" from "tendinosis." Tendinitis typically refers to an

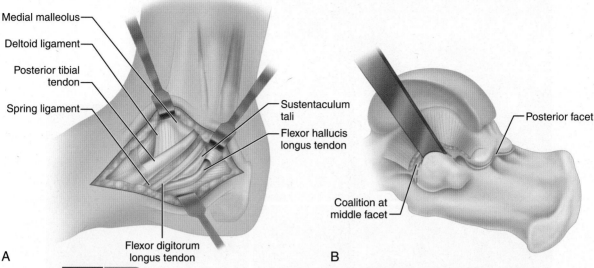

Medial malleolus

Deltoid ligament

Posterior tibial tendon

Spring ligament

Sustentaculum tali

Flexor hallucis longus tendon

Flexor digitorum longus tendon

A

Posterior facet

Coalition at middle facet

B

FIGURE 3.52   Resection of middle facet tarsal coalition. **A,** Sheath is opened and retracted dorsally or plantarly. **B,** Coalition is removed with osteotome until it is flush with posterior facet. **SEE TECHNIQUE 3.14.**

acute, reversible inflammatory process with healing potential, whereas tendinosis refers to a chronic, irreversible process characterized by fibrous degeneration without reparative, inflammatory cells. These terms are used to describe two distinct pathologic processes, but clinically these terms represent differing ends of a continual spectrum. *Tendinopathy* is a broad term used to describe both tendinitis and tendinosis.

Prolonged conservative treatment is necessary for all Achilles tendon disorders. Simple measures include a heel lift placed in the shoe, dorsiflexion night splints, oral or topical antiinflammatory medications, comprehensive stretching exercises for the calf, daily ice application, and/or a protective silicone pad to allow the patient to wear closed-back shoes. Other modalities include formal physical therapy with dry needling, Astym, heavy slow resistance exercises, and eccentric training. Ankle immobilization in a 3D walking boot or short leg walking cast may be necessary to resolve acute inflammation.

As in the treatment of plantar fasciitis, there is likely a place for extracorporeal shock wave therapy (ECSWT) in the treatment of this condition. A systematic review showed satisfactory (but limited) evidence supporting the use of low-energy ECSWT for chronic insertional and noninsertional Achilles tendinopathy.

Other reported modalities include injection treatments such as platelet-rich plasma (PRP), autologous blood, corticosteroids, prolotherapy, sclerosing agents, and protease inhibitors. The basic biologic principles for injection treatments seem sound, but our detailed understanding of the complex processes continues to evolve, and the clinical studies supporting their efficacy remain inconclusive.

INSERTIONAL ACHILLES TENDINOPATHY

Insertional tendinopathy may be characterized by one or a combination of conditions, including retrocalcaneal bursitis, pretendinous bursitis, or insertional Achilles tendinopathy with or without calcification. To most effectively treat the patient's symptoms, it is important for the examiner to distinguish between these similar but differing pain sources.

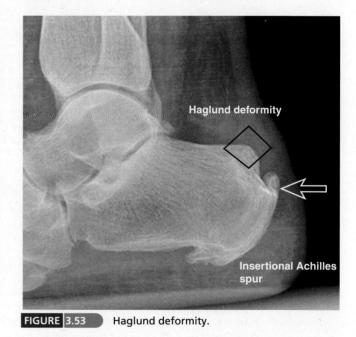

Haglund deformity

Insertional Achilles spur

FIGURE 3.53   Haglund deformity.

The term *Haglund deformity* is often used incorrectly to represent any swelling or enlargement around the insertion of the Achilles, but a true Haglund deformity refers to a large exostosis off the posterosuperior aspect of the calcaneal tuberosity located anterior to the Achilles tendon (Fig. 3.53). Protecting the tendon from this tuberosity, the retrocalcaneal bursa lies between the tuberosity and the Achilles tendon just anterior and proximal to the Achilles' insertional footprint. It is theorized that increased or repetitive abrasion of the tendon against the tuberosity creates inflammation of retrocalcaneal bursa (retrocalcaneal bursitis). With prolonged inflammation and worsening symptoms, degenerative changes occur and osteophytes form within the tendon.

In addition to a Haglund deformity and its associated retrocalcaneal bursitis, a superficial bursitis (pretendinous) may cause symptoms. This superficial bursa separates the Achilles

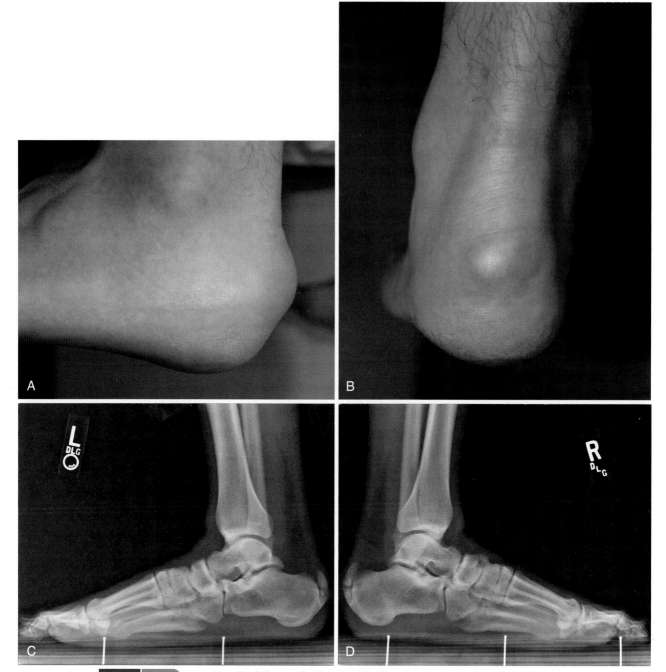

FIGURE 3.54 Insertional Achilles tendinitis. **A** and **B,** Clinical appearance. **C** and **D,** Radiographs show intratendinous calcification.

tendon from the overlying skin (Fig. 3.54). With insertional thickening from tendinosis and calcification, this pretendinous bursa becomes inflamed by chronic irritation from a shoe heel counter. Modification of shoe wear or a silicone sleeve may relieve the pretendinous symptoms.

■ DIAGNOSIS

The patient rarely gives a history of acute injury in this condition; rather it is a slow, insidious process of gradual enlargement and pain at the insertion of the Achilles tendon. Progressive difficulty with wearing closed-back shoes and pain after a period of rest, such as when first arising in the morning, are noted. Pain only when wearing shoes may indicate a pretendinous bursitis; pain

when first arising in the morning is more consistent with retrocalcaneal bursitis or Achilles tendinitis. Direct palpation over the retrocalcaneal bursa just anterior to the Achilles tendon, centralized over the Achilles insertion, or more superficially over the pretendinous bursa can further aid in making an accurate diagnosis. In prolonged or severe cases, all aspects of insertional tendinopathy (retrocalcaneal bursitis, Achilles tendinopathy, and pretendinous bursitis) can exist concomitantly. Examination often reveals a significant contracture of the gastrocsoleus complex, especially with the knee in extension. Radiographic evaluation should include a standing lateral view of the heel to evaluate for the presence of calcific spurs and the presence of a large posterosuperior process of the calcaneal tuberosity; however, the size of the Haglund deformity in symptomatic patients has not been statistically different from control groups.

■ TREATMENT

Depending on the nature of the symptoms (e.g., retrocalcaneal bursitis associated with Haglund deformity versus pretendinous bursitis associated with chronic tendinosis), several different procedures have been described for the treatment of insertional Achilles tendinopathy. Surgical procedures are indicated only after failure of conservative treatment.

In early disease, treatment for retrocalcaneal bursitis by removing the Haglund deformity does not necessarily accompany tendon debridement. Recalcitrant retrocalcaneal bursitis without tendinosis can be treated with open or endoscopic calcaneal exostectomy. A few case series also have described a dorsal closing wedge calcaneal osteotomy technique that decompresses the tuberosity impingement.

In the later stages of disease, insertional Achilles tendinosis often requires more traditional techniques with tendon debridement, calcaneal exostectomy, with or without augmentation with tendon transfers. Good results have been reported with these procedures, but these open techniques require large incisions with significant wound complications and prolonged recovery. Despite the prolonged recovery, many patients are able to return to sports after these procedures. In a small series of runners treated with open procedures, Rousseau et al. found that 67% were able to return to the same level of sport at an average of 8 months after an exostectomy, and 78% were able to return to the same level of sport at an average of 10 months after reconstruction procedures. In an effort to lessen the recovery and improve the underlying pathology, success has been reported with *isolated* gastrocnemius lengthening in insertional and noninsertional tendinopathy, but when compared with controls, patients do exhibit continued plantarflexion weakness 18 months after this procedure. Although technically more difficult, similar success also has been reported through endoscopic techniques.

If debridement of the tendon for insertional Achilles tendon disease and tendinitis is necessary, the question arises about how much tendon can be removed before risk of rupture. Evaluation of anatomic parameters of the insertion of the Achilles tendon found that the average height of the insertion measured 19.8 mm, the average width at the proximal aspect of the insertion measured 23.8 mm, and distally it measured 32.1 mm. With release of the tendon from superior to inferior, as much as 50% of the tendon could be resected safely. Hunt et al. prospectively compared patients treated for chronic insertional Achilles tendinopathy augmented with FHL transfer with those who did not have FHL augmentation. Both groups had improved function and pain scores without any differences in complications, but the FHL group did demonstrate greater plantar flexion strength. Hence, a FHL transfer may not be necessary for primary cases.

The FHL can be harvested through a single posterior incision behind the medial malleolus or through a second incision at the knot of Henry. Because of interconnections between the flexor hallucis longus and flexor digitorum longus tendons in the midfoot, an anastomosis between these tendons is not necessary when harvesting through a single incision. These interconnections allow the flexor digitorum longus muscle to move the distal flexor hallucis longus stump, flexing the hallux interphalangeal joint. The use of the flexor digitorum tendon to augment the Achilles repair has also been described with positive results.

CALCANEAL OSTEOTOMY FOR HAGLUND DEFORMITY

TECHNIQUE 3.15

- Place the patient prone and after administration of a general or local anesthetic make a longitudinal lateral incision 1 cm lateral to the Achilles tendon, extending distally from 3 to 4 cm proximal to the superior tuberosity of the calcaneus to 2 to 3 cm distal to the superior tuberosity of the calcaneus.
- Plantarflex the ankle joint and, by sharp and blunt dissection, identify the Achilles tendon.
- Place a right-angle retractor between the Achilles tendon and posterior and superior borders of the calcaneal tuberosity. With the foot plantarflexed this usually affords enough exposure to remove the superior border of the calcaneal tuberosity without raising any of the Achilles tendon off the calcaneus. However, the Achilles tendon has such an extensive insertion into the posterior and plantar aspect of the calcaneal tuberosity that raising a 1- to 2-cm long portion of the tendon may be necessary to resect the bone adequately.
- Remove the superior aspect of the tuberosity with a microsagittal saw or an osteotome. Placing several drill holes along the proposed osteotomy site makes this resection easier.
- Lavage the wound and close in layers. Apply a well-padded, short leg, non–weight-bearing cast with the ankle in approximately 20 degrees of plantarflexion.

POSTOPERATIVE CARE To aid with wound healing, the patient remains non–weight bearing until the sutures are removed at around 3 weeks. Once the incision has healed, a removable weight-bearing walking boot is applied, and active plantarflexion and dorsiflexion exercises are begun. Depending on the patient's level of discomfort, one heel lift may be added to the walking boot to lessen the forces across the Achilles. This lift is discontinued after 2 weeks. The walking boot is discontinued as pain allows and strength returns around 6 to 8 weeks from surgery.

DEBRIDEMENT OF THE TENDON FOR INSERTIONAL ACHILLES TENDON DISEASE

TECHNIQUE 3.16

(MCGARVEY ET AL. CENTRAL SPLITTING APPROACH)
- Place the patient prone after adequate administration of a general anesthetic.
- Starting approximately 2 cm above the insertion, make a midline longitudinal incision that extends roughly 6 cm distally.
- Avoid excessive skin handling and carry the dissection down full thickness to the tendon.
- Through the midline, incise the tendon and reflect the central attachment medially and laterally to expose the central aspect of the tendon and its osseous insertion.

- Identify and resect calcific or degenerative portions of the tendon.
- Resect the retrocalcaneal bursa.
- Use an osteotome or microsagittal saw to remove the posterosuperior calcaneal tuberosity (Haglund deformity) (Fig. 3.55).
- The tendon split is closed with an absorbable suture.
- If a significant amount of tendon was removed from its insertion, reattach the Achilles with suture anchor(s).
- If a significant amount of tendon was debrided (>50%), consider augmenting the repair with a tendon transfer.
- After thorough irrigation, close the skin with nonabsorbable, interrupted suture and apply a plantarflexed splint.

See also Video 3.2.

POSTOPERATIVE CARE To aid with wound healing, the patient does not bear weight until the sutures are removed at around 2 to 3 weeks after surgery. Once the incision has healed, a removable weight-bearing walking boot with two heel wedges is applied and active plantarflexion and dorsiflexion exercises are begun, but no passive dorsiflexion or aggressive strengthening is allowed. After 4 to 5 weeks from surgery, one wedge is removed. After another 1 to 2 weeks, the second wedge is removed. At 6 to 8 weeks after surgery, patients begin strengthening and weaning out of the boot with the guidance of a physical therapist.

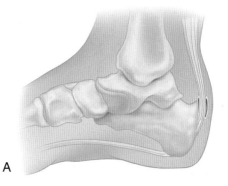

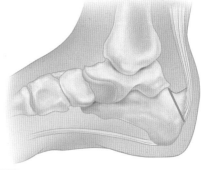

FIGURE 3.55 Central tendon splitting approach for treatment of Achilles tendinopathy. **SEE TECHNIQUE 3.16.**

NONINSERTIONAL ACHILLES TENDINOPATHY

Noninsertional tendinosis typically occurs in the watershed area of the Achilles tendon, 2 to 6 cm proximal to its insertion into the calcaneus. Noninsertional disorders occur as three main types: peritendinitis without tendinosis, which involves inflammation primarily of the paratenon and peritendinous structures; peritendinitis with tendinosis, which involves inflammation of the paratenon and degenerative changes within the Achilles tendon; and tendinosis, which involves thickening and degenerative changes within the Achilles tendon without inflammation of the paratenon.

Acute peritendinitis causes pain and swelling, but chronic tendinosis can be a relatively asymptomatic condition characterized by a bulbous nodularity that moves with passive flexion and extension of the ankle (Fig. 3.56). As seen on radiographs, calcification within the tendon may ensue from chronic, degenerative tendinosis. MRI is helpful in evaluating the extent of the degenerative changes especially in preoperative planning and counseling.

Similar to insertional Achilles tendon disorders, treatment may be prolonged and difficult. Surgical management is indicated for patients in whom conservative treatment of at least 6 months has failed. Through open, percutaneous, and endoscopic techniques surgical treatments include ventral paratenon stripping, open tendon debridement, and tendon reconstruction procedures with tendon transfers. In extensive disease, reconstruction procedures have excellent results and remain the gold standard but are accompanied by

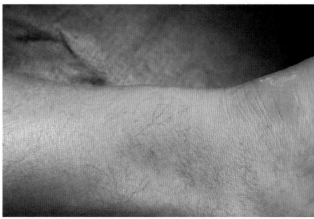

FIGURE 3.56 Bulbous nodularity in patient with chronic noninsertional Achilles tendinitis.

significant recovery times and potential complications. With less morbidity and good results, a gastrocnemius recession is becoming more popular as an alternative surgical treatment. Other authors have reported good results and shortened recovery with endoscopic debridement of ventral paratenon adhesions.

As discussed with insertional Achilles tendon reconstruction, surgically treated patients with extensive disease (>50% of the tendon volume) may be candidates for tendon transfer augmentation. Most literature supports the use of flexor hallucis longus tendon transfers, but similar outcomes have been reported with flexor digitorum longus transfers. The flexor hallucis longus can be harvested through a single- or double-incision technique (Fig. 3.57). Martin et al. reported

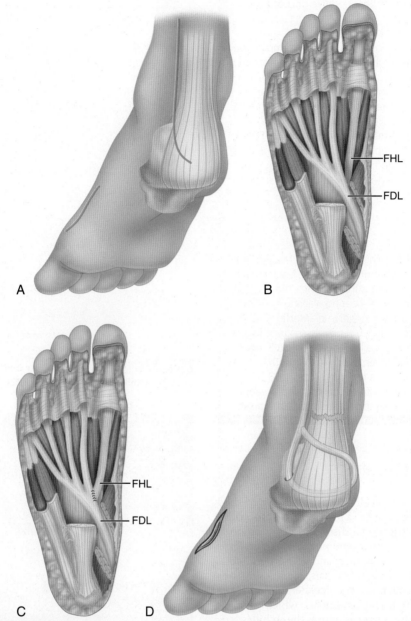

FIGURE 3.57 **A,** Incisions for exposure and harvest of flexor hallucis longus tendon. **B,** Plantar view of flexor digitorum longus (*FDL*) and adjacent flexor hallucis longus (*FHL*) tendon. **C,** Anastomosis of distal stump of FHL tendon to FDL tendon. **D,** FHL is pulled through transverse drill hole in calcaneus. **SEE TECHNIQUE 3.17.**

decreased pain in 42 of 44 patients treated with complete excision of the diseased Achilles tendon and transfer of the FHL tendon. Richardson et al. demonstrated decreased hallux pressure and FHL weakness after a single incision FHL transfer, but minimal patient morbidity was noted. Furthermore, no differences were noted in the 1st and 2nd metatarsal head pressures when compared with the unaffected foot.

Schon et al. prospectively reported the results of surgical treatment in 46 patients with insertional or midsubstance tendinosis. After failed conservative treatment, patients were treated with Achilles debridement and FHL transfer. At 24 months after surgery, significant improvement was recorded in visual analogue scale (VAS) scores, Short Form Health Survey (SF-36) physical scores, Ankle Osteoarthritis Scale, and performance of a single-leg heel rise.

FLEXOR HALLUCIS LONGUS TRANSFER FOR CHRONIC NONINSERTIONAL ACHILLES TENDINOSIS

TECHNIQUE 3.17

- Place the patient prone on the operating table after administering a satisfactory general anesthetic.

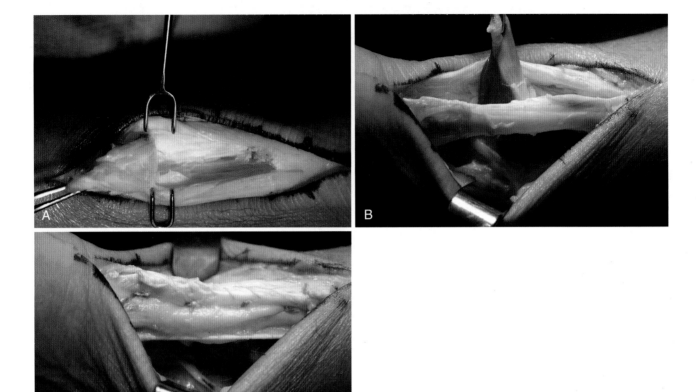

FIGURE 3.58 Flexor hallucis longus transfer for chronic noninsertional Achilles tendinosis. **A,** Exposure of involved portion of tendon. **B,** Harvest of flexor hallucis longus tendon. **C,** Flexor hallucis longus muscle belly sutured into defect. **SEE TECHNIQUE 3.17.**

- Make an incision just medial to the Achilles tendon for a total length of approximately 10 cm centered over the diseased section of tendon (Fig. 3.57A).
- Carefully incise the paratenon and remove any inflammatory peritendinitis with a rongeur.
- Retract the medial border of the tendon posteriorly with a double skin hook retractor for access to the deep involved portion of the tendon (Fig. 3.58A).
- Debride the area of degeneration sharply until normal tendon is present. If less than 50% of the tendon is involved, close the wound with interrupted 2-0 braided, nonabsorbable suture. Do not excessively strip the vascular supply of the mesotenon on the deep surface of the Achilles tendon. If substantially more than 50% of the tendon is involved, flexor hallucis longus transfer may be indicated.
- Make a longitudinal incision just deep to the Achilles tendon. Numerous small veins are present in the area and must be cauterized.
- Develop the interval between the flexor hallucis longus and peroneal tendons. Take care to avoid the neurovascular structures by staying at or lateral to the flexor hallucis longus tendon.
- After identifying the flexor hallucis longus tendon, make a longitudinal incision over the medial aspect of the dorsal arch of the abductor hallucis muscle. Deepen the incision with plantar retraction of the abductor hallucis muscle.
- Identify the master knot of Henry proximally. Avoid the medial plantar nerve and artery, which generally lie just deep and lateral to the flexor hallucis longus tendon.
- Dissect distally to allow sufficient harvest of the tendon, depending on just how much will be needed to augment the repair. If the entire insertion of the Achilles tendon is removed, a longer tendon graft will be needed.
- With the toes in flexion, suture the flexor digitorum longus tendon and flexor hallucis longus tendon together with interrupted 2-0 Vicryl suture (Fig. 3.57C).
- Harvest the flexor hallucis longus tendon (Fig. 3.58B). Release all connections between the flexor hallucis longus and the flexor digitorum longus and deliver the flexor hallucis longus into the posterior calf incision.
- For noninsertional Achilles tendinosis debridement, sew the flexor hallucis longus muscle belly and tendon into the defect created by the debridement (Fig. 3.58C).
- Use successively larger drill bits to drill a tunnel from medial to lateral in the tuberosity of the calcaneus. Generally a ⅜-inch tunnel is satisfactory to allow passage of the tendon with ease.
- For insertional Achilles tendinosis, after complete debridement of the Achilles tendon insertion, weave (Pulvertaft) the flexor hallucis longus tendon through the Achilles tendon and then pass it through the bone tunnel and suture it onto itself with interrupted no. 2 Ethibond or nonabsorbable sutures (Fig. 3.57D).

- If complete debridement of the Achilles tendon has been done, tension the graft with the ankle in moderate equinus provided that the ankle can be brought to neutral after final suturing of the graft. This helps to provide sufficient push-off power postoperatively.
- Alternatively, an interference-type absorbable screw can be used in the bone tunnel to secure the flexor hallucis longus tendon to the calcaneus.
- Close the paratenon with interrupted 2-0 absorbable sutures and close the skin in a routine fashion.

POSTOPERATIVE CARE Without tendon transfer, postoperative care is as described for Technique 3.15. With FHL tendon transfer, postoperative care is as described for Technique 3.16, in which the reconstruction is protected by a boot with heel wedges that are slowly removed so that the patient begins shoe wear around 8 weeks and gradual return to activities 3 to 4 months from surgery.

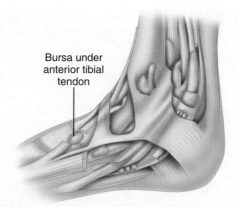

FIGURE 3.59 Bursa beneath insertion of anterior tibial tendon.

DISORDERS OF THE ANTERIOR TIBIAL TENDON

Tenosynovitis and rupture are the most common disorders of the anterior tibial tendon. However, compared with the peroneal tendons and especially the posterior tibial tendon, clinical problems with this tendon are rare. In general, the anterior tibial tendon loses continuity in two situations. In the first situation, a patient older than 45 years of age has a predisposing disease that contributes to attritional rupture; this spontaneous rupture has been associated with inflammatory arthritis, steroid injections, and diabetes. In the second situation, a young adult forcefully dorsiflexes the acutely plantarflexed foot against resistance, such as in soccer or American football. Distance runners most often experience tenosynovitis rather than rupture.

The tendon typically ruptures at one of two locations: its insertion into the adjacent surface of the medial cuneiform (Fig. 3.59) or beneath the superomedial limb of the inferior extensor retinaculum (Fig. 3.60, #6). This second location is relatively avascular and is associated with attritional ruptures. Synovitis around the ankle joint may further constrict the tendon in the retinacular envelope, further contributing to ischemic changes and attritional tendon ruptures.

DIAGNOSIS

In complete ruptures, the presenting complaint is weakness of dorsiflexion of the foot and, to a lesser degree, pain over the anterior aspect of the ankle. On physical examination, the extrinsic toe extensors are used to dorsiflex the foot, which can mislead the examiner. Depending on the chronicity of the rupture, there may or may not be a palpable defect in the tendon. The tendon may have healed in a lengthened position by scar in continuity. In chronic ruptures, contracture of the long toe extensors may create toe clawing.

Beischer et al. described the clinical features of distal anterior tibial tendinosis in 29 patients: nocturnal burning pain localized to the medial midfoot, point tenderness over the insertion of the anterior tibial tendon, and often subtle swelling over the distal tendon. They developed an examination technique to aid in diagnosis of distal tendinosis of the

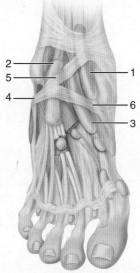

FIGURE 3.60 *1*, Sheath of anterior tibial tendon; *2*, sheath of extensor digitorum longus; *3*, sheath of extensor hallucis longus; *4*, inferior extensor retinaculum; *5*, superomedial arm of inferior extensor retinaculum; *6*, inferomedial arm of inferior extensor retinaculum.

anterior tibial tendon. The ankle is plantarflexed, the hindfoot everted, and the midfoot abducted and pronated in an attempt to passively stretch the anterior tibial tendon. Reproduction or aggravation of the patient's pain at the insertion of the anterior tibial tendon constitutes a positive test. According to Beischer et al., the test has a sensitivity of 90% and a specificity of 95%. The positive predictive value was found to be 95% and the negative predictive value 90% for distal anterior tibial tendinosis that was confirmed with MRI. In tenosynovitis, pain over the anterior ankle and foot is the primary complaint. Crepitance is common in florid tenosynovitis. Night pain also may be present from passive plantarflexion, placing the inflamed tendon on stretch.

TREATMENT
■ TENOSYNOVITIS

Tenosynovitis is treated by oral antiinflammatory medications and immobilization in a removable or nonremovable walking cast. The benefits of the prefabricated, removable cast are obvious, but the removable cast should be worn continuously for

3 weeks except while bathing and another 3 weeks while ambulating. When the disease is resistant (rarely), a corticosteroid or protein-rich plasma (PRP) injection judiciously placed within the tendon sheath but *not* within the tendon is the basic conservative management. Ultrasound guidance assists with injection accuracy. Synovectomy of this tendon is seldom required, except when associated with one of the inflammatory arthritides. If tenosynovectomy is required, the sheath of the anterior tibial tendon is situated so that one or both limbs of the inferior extensor retinaculum can be preserved (Fig. 3.60).

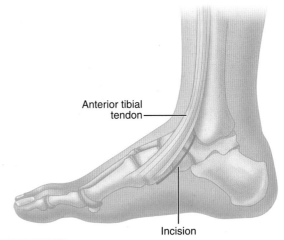

FIGURE **3.61** Note that incision does not cross ankle joint and courses medial to anterior tibial tendon. **SEE TECHNIQUE 3.18.**

SYNOVECTOMY OF THE ANTERIOR TIBIAL TENDON

TECHNIQUE 3.18

- Beginning just distal to the ankle joint, carry the incision medial and posterior to the anterior tibial tendon 5 to 6 cm distally. Stay 2 to 3 mm medial to the tendon almost to its insertion (Fig. 3.61).
- Isolate the communicating branches of the saphenous vein as they course plantarward and preserve as many of them as possible. The terminal branch or branches of the saphenous nerve may lie just deep to the saphenous vein.
- Raise the anterior flap no more than is necessary to expose the tendon. Open the sheath; debride it and the synovium. By dorsiflexing the ankle and pulling distally on the tendon, most of the synovium (even that proximal to the ankle) can be removed.
- Incise the superomedial band of the inferior anterior retinaculum if necessary; resuturing it is unnecessary and technically difficult.
- Obtain hemostasis. Close the skin only and apply a bulky compression dressing and a short leg walking cast.

POSTOPERATIVE CARE Crutches are used the first 5 to 7 days, and weight bearing to tolerance is permitted. The cast is changed at 12 to 16 days, when the sutures are removed. Another cast is applied and is worn for 4 to 6 weeks, after which time a compressive ankle corset is worn for an additional 4 to 6 weeks.

■ INSERTIONAL TENDINOSIS

Grundy et al. reported good results after debridement and repair of the distal anterior tibial tendon with extensor hallucis longus augmentation in patients with more than 50% tendon involvement in whom nonoperative treatment had failed.

DEBRIDEMENT AND REPAIR OF THE DISTAL ANTERIOR TIBIAL TENDON

TECHNIQUE 3.19

(GRUNDY ET AL.)
- After administration of a combination of general anesthetic and either a local anesthetic, popliteal block, or ankle block, place the patient supine on the operating table with a sandbag under the ipsilateral hip. Apply and inflate a thigh tourniquet.
- Make a curvilinear incision over the anterior tibial tendon, taking care to protect the cutaneous nerve.
- Open the tendon sheath and examine the tendon for evidence of tendinosis and a split tear (Fig. 3.62A).
- Excise any degenerated tendon, exostosis of the medial cuneiform at the tendon insertion, and prominent osteophytes of the adjacent midfoot joints (first tarsometatarsal, naviculocuneiform, talonavicular).
- If more than 50% of normal tendon remains after debridement, repair the longitudinal split with no. 0 Ethibond sutures. Use a Bio-Corkscrew FT suture anchor with no. 2 FiberWire (Arthrex, Naples, FL) at the tendon insertion into the medial cuneiform.
- If less than 50% of normal tendon remains after debridement, augment the tendon with an extensor hallucis longus tendon transfer.
- Make an incision longitudinally over the dorsolateral aspect of the first metatarsophalangeal joint and identify the extensor hallucis brevis and longus. Scrape their surfaces with a no. 15 scalpel blade to facilitate tendon adhesion.
- Suture the extensor hallucis longus to the extensor hallucis brevis (Fig. 3.62B) with no. 0 polydioxanone (PDS) and no. 0 polyglactin 910 (Vicryl) with the hallux interphalangeal joint held in 20 degrees of dorsiflexion.
- Identify the extensor hallucis longus tendon in the proximal incision and transect it immediately proximal to the site of tenodesis to the extensor hallucis brevis tendon.
- Pull the extensor hallucis longus tendon into the proximal incision and tag its cut end with a Krackow suture.
- Close the distal incision.
- Drill a 4.5-mm hole in the medial cuneiform from dorsal to plantar.
- Pass the extensor hallucis longus tendon through the split in the remaining anterior tibial tendon and then through the drill hole from plantar to dorsal (Fig. 3.62C,D)

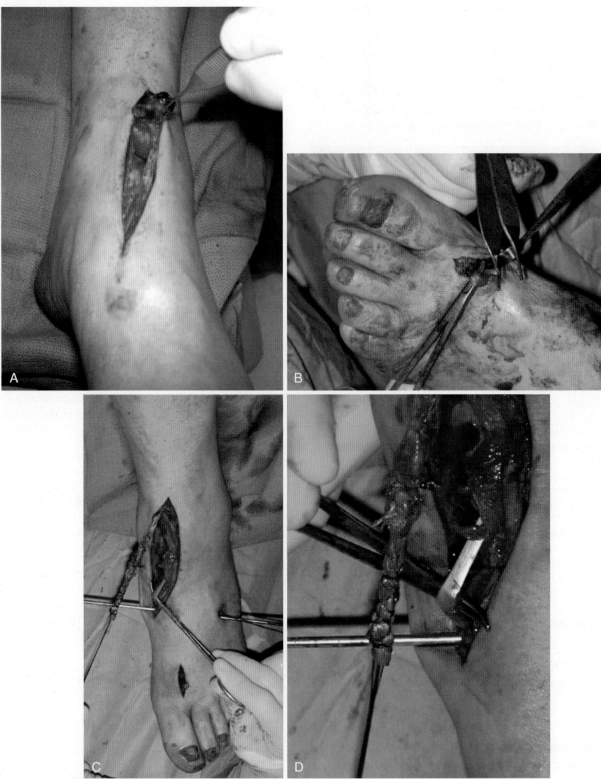

FIGURE 3.62 Repair of chronic anterior tibial tendon rupture. **A,** Ruptured anterior tibial tendon. **B,** Extensor hallucis longus tendon identified distally and anastomosed to extensor hallucis brevis before transection. **C,** Extensor hallucis longus passed through drill hole in cuneiform. **D,** Close-up of the transfers. (From Coughlin MJ, Schon LC: Disorders of tendons. In Coughlin MJ, Mann RA, Saltzman CL, editors: *Surgery of the foot and ankle*, 8th ed, Philadelphia, 2007, Elsevier.) **SEE TECHNIQUE 3.19.**

- Secure the extensor hallucis longus tendon with a 5.5-mm Bio-Interference screw under firm but not maximal tension with the ankle held in a plantigrade position.
- Repair the remaining anterior tibial tendon with no. 0 Vicryl sutures, close the wound in layers with interrupted sutures, and apply a well-padded plaster splint with the ankle plantigrade.

POSTOPERATIVE CARE The leg is kept elevated, and the dressing is left undisturbed for 2 weeks, at which time the sutures are removed and a full lightweight weight-bearing below-knee cast is applied. This cast is worn for an additional 4 weeks. At 6 weeks, a controlled ankle motion walker with a custom full-length medial longitudinal arch support orthosis is fitted and physical therapy is begun. After 4 weeks, the walker is discontinued and the patient can wear normal shoes with the orthosis and gradually return to normal activities.

■ COMPLETE RUPTURE

Operative treatment of a rupture of the anterior tibial tendon is determined entirely by the patient's symptoms and degree of functional impairment. In low-demand patients, this impairment can be tolerated well as opposed to that caused by posterior tibial tendon rupture. A short leg brace with a 90-degree downstop for 3 to 6 months may allow enough "healing" of the tendon that the patient will not desire operative treatment. However, in more active patients, surgical management of acute and chronic ruptures demonstrated better outcomes than conservative management. In a systematic review, techniques involving direct repair, turn-down tibialis anterior, semitendinosus autograft, extensor digitorum longus autograft, or plantaris autograft showed better outcomes than extensor hallucis longus autograft reconstruction techniques. Huh et al. demonstrated successful treatment with allograft reconstruction in chronic ruptures. Michels et al. reported good results in 12 patients with a minimally invasive reconstruction with semitendinosus autograft. The technique involves minimal disturbance of the extensor retinaculum, which minimizes recovery time, adhesions, and wound problems.

REPAIR OF COMPLETE RUPTURE OF THE ANTERIOR TIBIAL TENDON

TECHNIQUE 3.20

- Use the same incision as for synovectomy (see Technique 3.18).
- If the tendon is ruptured beneath the inferomedial limb of the inferior extensor retinaculum, incise this band and advance the tendon as far distally as possible.
- Drill a hole in the medial cuneiform from dorsal to plantar and raise the inferior flap and abductor hallucis muscle plantarward enough to see the drill bit emerge. The

hole usually must be enlarged incrementally to ¼ inch or ⁵⁄₁₆ inch.
- With a Bunnell weave of 0 nonabsorbable suture on free straight needles, pass the tendon through this hole. This step is made easier by passing one end of the suture at a time using the straight needle. Pull the tendon into the hole and, while dorsiflexing the ankle 20 to 30 degrees, suture the edge of the tendon to the adjacent periosteum and deep fascia.
- If the tendon is ruptured beneath the superomedial limb of the inferior extensor retinaculum, incise this limb. The tendon may be more difficult to advance at this level. However, by slowly passing a hemostat or small tendon passer proximally through the sheath, it usually can be advanced. If not, rather than crossing the ankle joint with the incision, make a small (2- to 3-cm) incision anteromedially above the ankle and identify the tendon at the anteromedial border of the tibia.
- Pass a long, curved clamp along the tendon from proximal to distal. Grasp the end of this clamp with another clamp *end on* and reverse the direction. Discard the initial clamp, grasp the tendon, and bring it into the distal wound.
- If this method of passing the tendon is difficult, redirect the clamp proximal to distal. Grasp a rubber urinary catheter, bringing it proximally. Suture the tendon to the catheter and pull the tendon distally into the inferior wound.
- If the tendon cannot reach the medial cuneiform, use the navicular as the bony insertion. The same technique is used as for the medial cuneiform insertion, but the dissection plantarward is more tedious as a result of the intervening posterior tibial tendon. Stay plantar to this tendon, dissecting the abductor hallucis plantarward and being aware of the long toe flexor tendons laterally as they cross one another. The tendon is more difficult to suture at this location once passed through the navicular.
- Using a small, free, curved cutting needle is helpful (a no. 7 Murphy needle is suggested). Pass the tendon through the middle of the navicular and dorsiflex the ankle as it is sutured under tension to the inferior surface of the bone.
- Bring the abductor hallucis fascia and muscle dorsally to their normal positions and attach them with absorbable sutures.

TENDON RECONSTRUCTION WITH AUTOGENOUS TENDON GRAFT (SAMMARCO ET AL.)

- If the tendon ends cannot be approximated or the tendon cannot be apposed onto its insertion site, use an interpositional graft to bridge the gap and reinforce the repair. Autogenous tendon graft sources include the plantaris (preferred), the extensor digitorum, the peroneus tertius, and Achilles tendons; a semitendinosus allograft also can be used.
- If the plantaris is absent and the extensor digitorum or peroneus tertius tendon is used as graft, harvest 8 to 10 cm of tendon and suture the remaining free segment of the distal part of the tendon to the intact extensor digitorum communis tendons.
- Because these grafts are much smaller in diameter than the anterior tibial tendon, fold the grafts over two or three times to achieve a satisfactory diameter (Fig. 3.63).
- Repair the extensor retinaculum to prevent bowstringing and adhesion of the reconstructed tendon to the subcutaneous tissue.

See also Video 3.3.

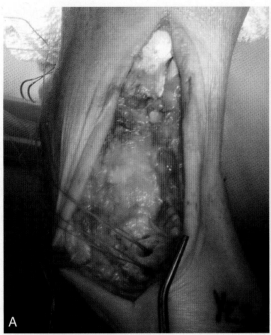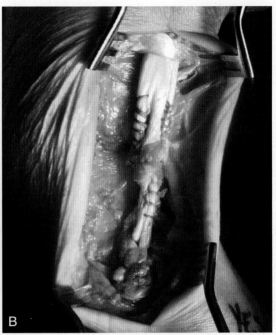

FIGURE 3.63 Tendon reconstruction with autogenous tendon graft. **A,** Remaining portion of anterior tibial tendon after excision of degenerated portion and interposed scar tissue. Suture anchors have been placed. **B,** Tripled interpositional plantaris tendon graft used to reconstruct defect in anterior tibial tendon. (From Sammarco VJ, Sammarco GJ, Henning C, Chaim S: Surgical repair of acute and chronic tibialis anterior tendon ruptures, *J Bone Joint Surg* 91A:325, 2009.) **SEE TECHNIQUE 3.20.**

POSTOPERATIVE CARE A short leg cast with the ankle in 0 degrees of dorsiflexion is worn for 4 to 6 weeks; weight bearing in the cast is allowed after 3 weeks. The duration of cast immobilization is determined in part by the perceived quality of the repair. Patients with an autograft-augmented reconstruction wear the cast for 6 weeks after surgery. Once the cast is discontinued, the patient is allowed to bear full weight in a boot with a hinged ankle joint that allows full dorsiflexion but prevents planar flexion. Plantarflexion is gradually increased, and the boot is eventually discontinued 10 to 12 weeks after surgery.

MINIMALLY INVASIVE TENDON RECONSTRUCTION WITH SEMITENDINOSUS AUTOGRAFT

TECHNIQUE 3.21

(MICHELS ET AL.)
- If 5 degrees of dorsiflexion cannot be achieved, perform a gastrocnemius recession.
- Harvest the semitendinosus tendon with a tendon stripper (as in an anterior cruciate ligament reconstruction).
- Make a small longitudinal incision above the superior extensor retinaculum, leaving the extensor retinaculum intact.

- With severe adhesions to the retinaculum, limit the opening of the extensor retinaculum to a window that avoids bowstringing and minimizes reoccurrence of adhesions.
- Pull the proximal tendon end out the proximal incision and debride the degenerative portion.
- Suture the semitendinosus autograft into the proximal end using a Pulvertaft weave.
- Make a second incision, localized with fluoroscopy over the medial cuneiform.
- Identify the distal tendon end and elevate the periosteum from the medial side of the medial cuneiform.
- Drill a tunnel for an interference screw from medial to lateral under fluoroscopic guidance.
- Use a clamp with a looped suture end to pull the anastomosed tendon distally (Fig. 3.64A).
- If necessary to create enough space for the graft, use dissecting scissors to release the scar tissue beneath the extensor retinaculum.
- Hold the ankle in maximal dorsiflexion and the foot in maximal supination to determine the final length of tendon graft.
- Pass the graft and secure it in the bony tunnel with an interference screw (Fig. 3.64B).

POSTOPERATIVE CARE For the first 2 weeks, non–weight bearing is enforced with cast immobilization in neutral position. During the following 4 weeks, weight bearing is allowed in an ankle-foot orthosis, and gentle dorsiflexion and plantarflexion exercises are started. At 6 weeks postoperatively, weight bearing without an orthosis is allowed and exercises against resistance are continued with physical therapy for 3 to 4 months postoperatively.

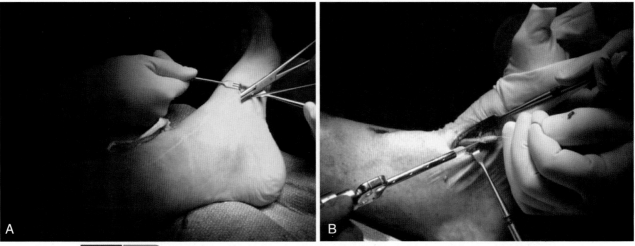

FIGURE 3.64 Minimally invasive tendon reconstruction with semitendinosus autograft. **A,** Anastomosed tendon is pulled distally. **B,** Tendon is secured in bony tunnel with an interference screw. **SEE TECHNIQUE 3.21.**

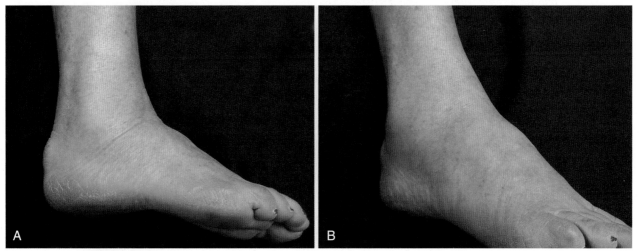

FIGURE 3.65 **A** and **B,** Clinical appearance of peroneal tenosynovitis; note swelling just posterior to lateral malleolus.

DISORDERS OF THE PERONEAL TENDONS

Disorders of the peroneal tendons fall primarily into three types. The first is peroneal tendinitis or peroneal tendon tears *without* subluxation of the peroneal tendons. This condition is seen primarily in middle-aged athletes during repetitive activities or in patients with chronic underlying hindfoot malalignment. A second type of peroneal pathology is hallmarked by associated *instability* of the peroneal tendons at the level of the superior peroneal retinaculum. This condition frequently is seen in athletes after acute ankle injury, causing rupture of the superior peroneal retinaculum and instability of the tendons, but it also may be present in more chronic settings. Frequently, it is associated with chronic lateral ankle instability. The third type is stenosing tenosynovitis of the peroneus longus tendon, which may be associated with a painful os peroneum, an enlarged peroneal tubercle, or a pathologic process at the cuboid joint, including complete encasement of the peroneus longus tendon in a bony tunnel at the level of the cuboid. Associated physical findings often include a cavovarus foot and limitation of eversion.

DIAGNOSIS

The diagnosis of peroneal pathology is made primarily on clinical evaluation of the patient. Evaluation with the patient standing is essential to determine biomechanical abnormalities of the hindfoot, including a varus or, less commonly, valgus hindfoot. Symptoms include swelling (Fig. 3.65), tenderness, popping, and crepitance just posterior to the lateral malleolus as the two tendons course beneath the superior peroneal retinaculum. Fluid often is palpable within the tendon sheath. Manual testing of eversion strength may reveal weakness, but more commonly eversion strength is painful but maintained. Selective testing of the peroneus longus tendon is done with the ankle in active eversion while the examiner pushes up on the plantarflexed first metatarsal head.

Diagnosis of peroneal tendon pathology may be aided by plain radiographs (bone avulsion) (Figs. 3.66 and 3.67), bone scans, CT (Fig. 3.68), tenography, MRI (Fig. 3.69), or ultrasound, but clinical awareness coupled with a detailed history and physical examination should suggest the diagnosis. With peroneal tendon instability, radiographs may show bony avulsion of the superior peroneal retinaculum (SPR) attachment

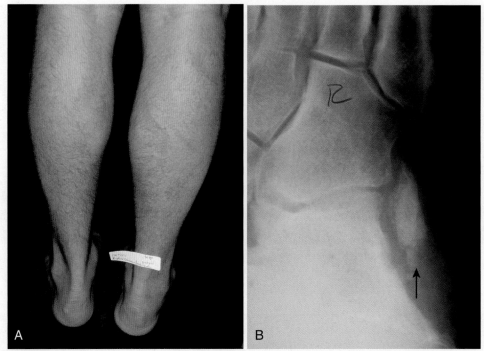

FIGURE 3.66 **A,** Sixty-one-year-old man with rupture of peroneus longus tendon and varus of right foot. Peroneus brevis tendon had longitudinal split tear but was intact. **B,** Note hypertrophic os peroneum and its proximal migration after rupture. He also had lateral ankle instability compared with opposite side. **SEE VIDEO 3.4.**

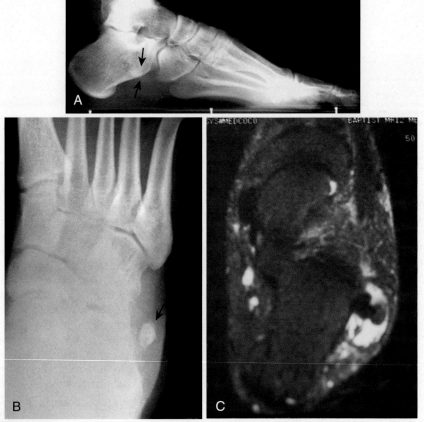

FIGURE 3.67 **A** and **B,** Radiographs of patient with tear of peroneus longus and retraction of sesamoid bone (os peroneum). **C,** T2-weighted MRI of type I tear of both peroneus longus and peroneus brevis tendons. Peroneus brevis disease was best seen at inferior aspect of lateral malleolus, and peroneus longus disease was best seen at lateral border of foot near cuboid groove.

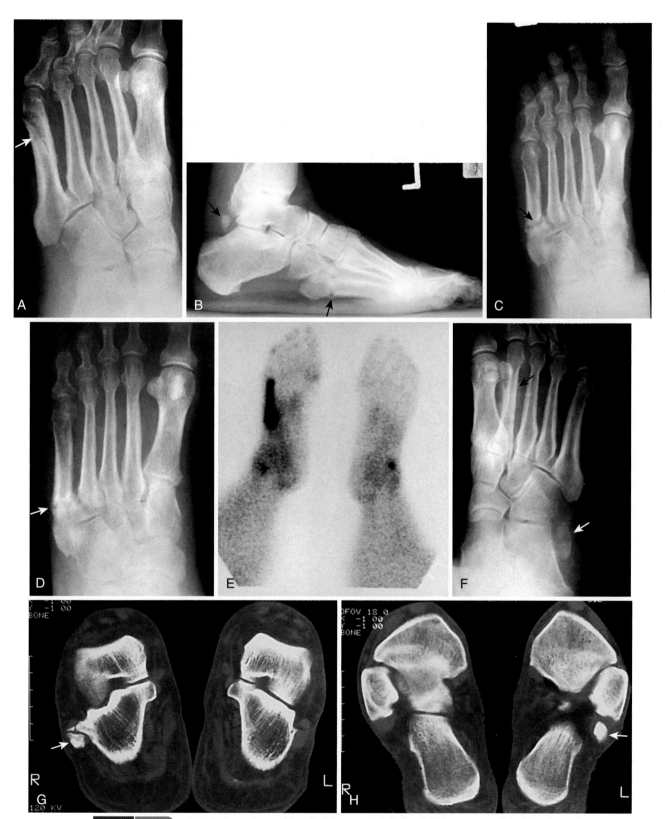

FIGURE 3.68   **A,** Elderly patient with spiral fracture of shaft of fifth metatarsal. **B,** Standing lateral view 15 months later. *Posterior arrow* indicates avulsed os peroneum from rupture of peroneus longus. *Plantar arrow* indicates second fracture at base of fifth metatarsal; oblique fracture has healed. Note cavus and varus posture of heel. **C,** Eighteen months after initial fracture and extended period of casting, fracture is uniting. Note new stress fracture at base of fifth metatarsal. **D,** Twenty-one months after initial fracture, union progressed sufficiently that patient is pain free; note osteopenia of fifth metatarsal. **E,** Bone scan shows uptake isolated to fifth metatarsal. **F,** *Proximal arrow* indicates bony avulsion by peroneus longus on *opposite* foot; *distal arrow* indicates stress fracture. **G,** CT scan; note in right foot bony fragment laterally at level of sustentaculum tali. **H,** CT scan shows bony fragment farther posteriorly with peroneus longus more proximal on left.

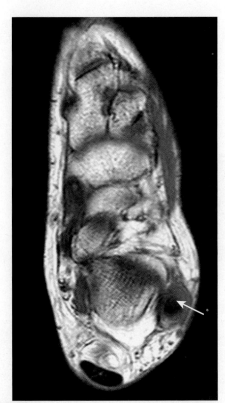

FIGURE 3.69   MRI appearance of peroneal tendon rupture *(arrow)* with tenosynovitis.

from the lateral malleolus, known as the *fleck sign*. CT depicts the bony characteristics of the peroneal tubercle, cuboid groove, and os peroneum. Dynamic ultrasound aids with identification of subluxation and tears. Preoperative MRI may be helpful in determining the amount of expected debridement and location of any pathologic process; however, MRI has moderate sensitivity (60% to 83%) in detecting tears and should be used as an adjunct to clinical examination and history in diagnosis. Furthermore, MRI findings most correlate with peroneal tendon symptomology. Approximately 35% of asymptomatic patients demonstrate peroneal tendon pathology on MRI. Peroneal tendon symptoms from encroachment after calcaneal fractures are discussed in other chapter.

TREATMENT
■ PERONEAL TENDINITIS
Peroneal tendinitis occurring as an isolated entity without direct observable evidence of peroneal subluxation is uncommon. Krause and Brodsky found that many patients with a diagnosis of primary peroneal tendinitis did not have clinical instability, but subluxation of the tendons was found intraoperatively. Every effort should be made to look for and correct subluxation of the peroneal tendons as described in the next section.

Conservative treatment of isolated peroneal tendinitis can be effective. Cast or boot immobilization, oral antiinflammatory medications, and subsequent physical therapy can relieve tendinitis symptoms. However, for long-term benefit, biomechanical corrections need to be made to the foot, generally with an orthosis or use of an ankle brace for 4 to 6 months after resolution of the acute inflammation.

For patients who do not respond to conservative treatment, tenosynovectomy with repair and stabilization as

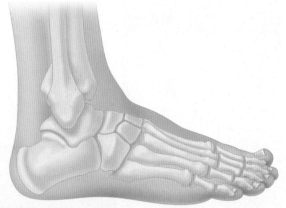

FIGURE 3.70   Incision for tenosynovectomy for tear of peroneal tendons. **SEE TECHNIQUE 3.22.**

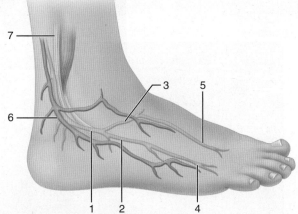

FIGURE 3.71   Lateral aspect of foot and ankle. *1,* Sural nerve dividing into lateral branch (*2*), forming dorsolateral cutaneous nerve (*4*) and medial branch (*3*) uniting with intermediate dorsal cutaneous nerve (*5*) of superficial peroneal nerve; *6,* shorter saphenous vein; *7,* peroneal tendons. **SEE TECHNIQUE 3.22.**

needed is indicated. Surgical findings vary, constituting a progression from clear fluid and relatively normal-appearing tendons and tendon sheaths to small linear tears in one or both tendons (usually the brevis) to thickened, fibrotic tendon sheaths and grayish-appearing but intact tendons.

SYNOVECTOMY OF THE PERONEAL TENDONS

TECHNIQUE 3.22

- With a bolster beneath the ipsilateral hip and the foot held in equinovalgus, begin an incision 10 to 12 cm proximal to the tip of, and 1 cm posterior to, the subcutaneous border of the fibula. Continue the incision distally and slightly obliquely to accommodate the bulbous posterior aspect of the lateral malleolus. Curve the incision gently 1 cm distal to the tip of the lateral malleolus toward the base of the fifth metatarsal for another 3 to 4 cm (Fig. 3.70). The sural nerve and small saphenous vein course just posterior to the tendons and are subcutaneous at this level (Fig. 3.71).

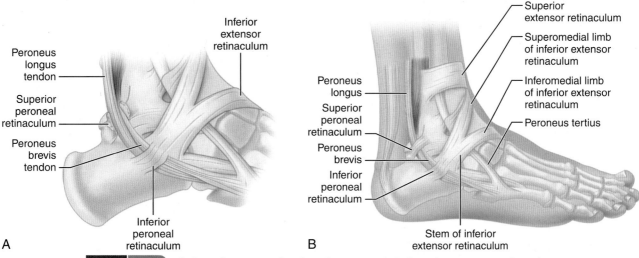

FIGURE 3.72 **A,** Superior peroneal retinaculum opened. **B,** Superior extensor retinaculum. **SEE TECHNIQUE 3.22.**

- Open the sheath of the peroneal tendons proximally and trace the tendons to the superior peroneal retinaculum (Fig. 3.72).
- If the tendons appear normal both proximal and distal to this structure, incise only half of the retinaculum (about 1 cm or less).
- If this pulley is thickened or the sheath is thickened, suggesting that excursion is impaired, incise the entire retinaculum and inspect the inferior peroneal retinaculum. In tenosynovitis, it is unusual to have to release both. Be careful at the septum that goes from the fibula to the superior peroneal retinaculum and separates the peroneus longus and brevis because an accessory peroneal tendon may be present in a separate compartment. Release this septum and inspect the peroneus brevis while looking for any accessory slips of either tendon.
- After a complete tenosynovectomy, sharply debride portions of the tendon sheath using a small rongeur. Inspect the tendons for the presence of attritional, longitudinal fissuring (Fig. 3.73A), which is most commonly located on the deep surface of the peroneus brevis tendon. If the tear involves less than 50% of the tendon, remove the smaller section of the tendon completely. Tubularize the remaining viable portion with a running 3-0 absorbable, braided suture.
- If more than 50% of the peroneus brevis tendon is disrupted and fissured, the remaining section generally is too small to be tubularized and the entire diseased segment of the peroneus brevis is resected.
- Tenodese (side-to-side) the peroneus longus and brevis tendons both proximally and distally (Fig. 3.73B,C). The tenodesis should be well proximal to the level of the superior peroneal retinaculum, 3 to 4 cm proximal to the ankle joint, generally at the musculotendinous junction of the peroneus brevis.
- Complete the repair using 2-0 nonabsorbable, braided sutures. Distally, leave the tendon sheaths for both the brevis and longus open and suture the brevis and longus tendons together with 2-0 nonabsorbable sutures. Other than the superior peroneal retinaculum, which is repaired

with 2-0 absorbable sutures, leave the remainder of the tendon sheath open and close the skin and subcutaneous tissues.

POSTOPERATIVE CARE A posterior plaster splint is applied over a bulky dressing in the operating room. The patient is seen 2 weeks postoperatively at which time the sutures are removed. If the wound is healed, early active motion without resistance is started to prevent adhesions of the tendons within the sheath. Only partial weight bearing is allowed for an additional 2 to 4 weeks, depending on the severity of the tendinopathy and the amount of repair required. More aggressive strengthening is allowed, with a planned return to full activities at 3 months, depending on the return of motion and calf strength.

■ SUBLUXATION OF THE PERONEAL TENDONS

Peroneal tendon instability is discussed separately for emphasis; however, it should be recognized that peroneal tendinitis, tears, and instability often occur together, and a combination of techniques is required for complete resolution.

If instability is recognized early, non–weight-bearing casting with the foot in neutral to slight inversion may be helpful in allowing the superior peroneal retinaculum to adhere to the posterolateral aspect of the fibula. Most often, however, patients with chronic laxity of the superior peroneal retinaculum develop a pouch between the normal attachment of the superior peroneal retinaculum and the fibula that allows subluxation of the peroneal tendons, especially the peroneus brevis. This may be demonstrated clinically by resisted eversion of the ankle with the examiner's fingers placed on the peroneal tendon sheath at the level of the superior peroneal retinaculum. Patients often complain of a pop associated with pain in the region. Once the condition is fully developed and is chronic, it has been our experience that conservative treatment to prevent subluxation of the tendons with the associated tendinitis rarely is successful. Many techniques have been described for the treatment of chronic subluxation of the peroneal tendons.

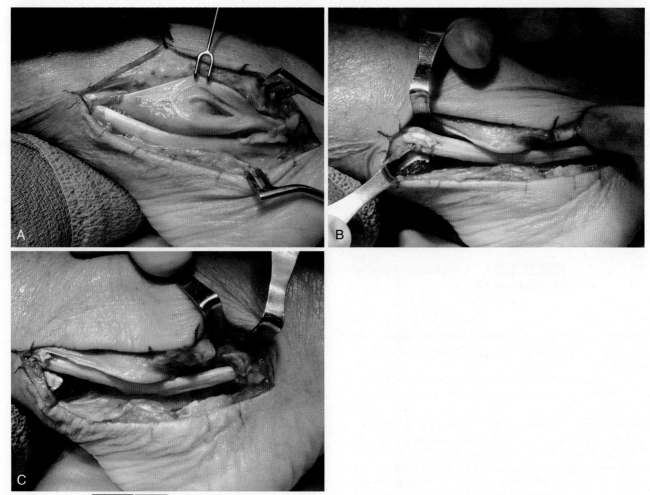

FIGURE 3.73 Debridement of peroneus brevis tendon and tenodesis to peroneus longus tendon. **A,** Longitudinal fissuring of tendon. **B** and **C,** Proximal and distal tenodesis. **SEE TECHNIQUE 3.22.**

As the main stabilizer for the peroneal tendons, repair of the superior peroneal retinaculum (SPR) to the posterior lateral fibula remains the surgical focus. Adding further stability, deepening procedures of the posterior fibular sulcus also prevent recurrent dislocation. Although common wisdom suggests that a shallow or convex posterior sulcus of the fibula is associated with peroneal tendon instability, Adachi et al. demonstrated no significant difference in the morphologic shape of the posterior lateral malleolus in patients with and without dislocation of the peroneal tendons. A fibrocartilage rim located on the posterolateral aspect of the lateral malleolus adds depth to the retromalleolar groove, placing less emphasis on the bony morphology. Porter et al. reported no recurrent subluxation or dislocation and a return to sports by 3 months after fibular groove deepening and retinacular reconstruction in 13 athletes, and Maffulli et al. described anatomic reattachment of the retinaculum with soft-tissue anchors in 14 patients, all of whom returned to their normal activities with no further episodes of tendon subluxation. Cho et al. compared retinacular repair alone (16 patients) to retinacular repair with a groove-deepening procedure (15 patients) and found no difference between the groups, but a power analysis was not completed in the statistical analysis. With continued evolution of minimally invasive surgery and tendinoscopy, several authors

have described tendonscopic repair of the superior peroneal retinaculum.

In mostly level V evidence, low-lying peroneal brevis muscle belly also has been described as contributing to tendon instability by decreasing the retromalleolar groove volume. Anecdotally, excising low-lying muscle belly decreases the risk of subluxation. Because MRI has poor sensitivity in detecting this anomaly, peroneal brevis low-lying muscle belly is most commonly identified at the time of surgery.

FIBULAR GROOVE DEEPENING AND REPAIR OF THE SUPERIOR RETINACULUM

TECHNIQUE 3.23

(RAIKIN)
- Approach the peroneal tendons through a curvilinear incision over the path of the peroneal tendon, immediately posterior to the fibula (Fig. 3.74A).

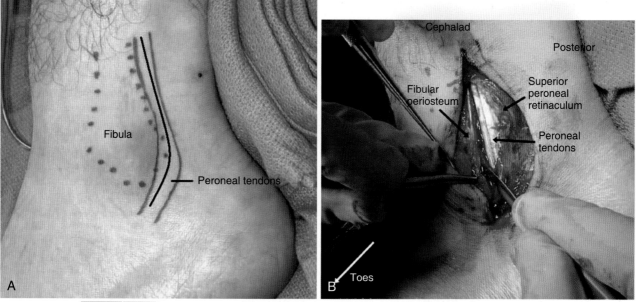

FIGURE 3.74 Repair of subluxation of peroneal tendons. **A,** Incision *(solid black line)* between peroneal tendons *(solid blue lines).* **B,** Incision into retinaculum, leaving 1-mm rim of retinacular tissue attached to fibula. (From Raikin SM: Intrasheath subluxation of the peroneal tendons: surgical technique, *J Bone Joint Surg* 91A[Suppl 2 pt 1]:146, 2009.) **SEE TECHNIQUE 3.23 AND VIDEO 3.1.**

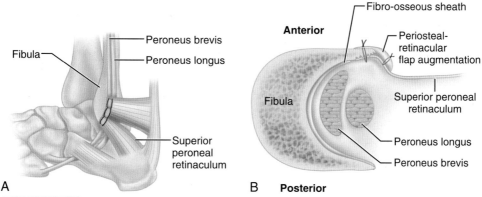

FIGURE 3.75 Repaired peroneal retinaculum attached under deep anterior surface of groove with pants-over-vest suture repair. (From Raikin SM: Intrasheath subluxation of the peroneal tendons: surgical technique, *J Bone Joint Surg* 91A[Suppl 2 pt 1]:146, 2009.) **SEE TECHNIQUE 3.23 AND VIDEO 3.1.**

- Inspect for a peroneus quartus tendon or low-lying muscle belly of the peroneus brevis, and, if found, remove the accessory peroneal tendon or a portion of the distal muscle of the peroneus brevis.
- After completion of any repair of the peroneus brevis and tenosynovectomy as indicated, inspect the posterolateral sulcus and the peroneal tendons on the posterior aspect of the fibula. In most instances, this groove is shallow or even convex.
- To deepen the grove, use a small osteotome to elevate the cartilaginous surface of the sulcus from its most lateral margin, leaving it attached at its most medial margin (Fig. 3.74B).
- Elevate the cartilaginous flap out of the bed for a total of 1.5 to 2.0 cm in length.
- With a curet or a gouge, remove the underlying cancellous bone to a depth of 4 to 5 mm. Depress the osteocartilaginous flap back into the groove.

- Treat the remaining cancellous surfaces generously with bone wax.
- Recess the peroneus longus and brevis tendons back into the groove. Roughen the posterolateral ridge of the fibula with a small rasp and suture the posterior flap of the superior peroneal retinaculum to the fibular ridge, completing the reconstruction (Fig. 3.75).
- Use 2-0 nonabsorbable suture for repair of the superior peroneal retinaculum. The remainder of the peroneal tendon sheath is left open.
- If insufficient tissue is available for reconstruction of the superior peroneal retinaculum, additional options include detachment of the calcaneofibular ligament from its fibular attachment and rerouting the peroneal tendons beneath it and lateral to the subtalar capsule. The calcaneofibular ligament also can be taken off its calcaneal attachment. A posterior bone block procedure

can be done with an osteotomy of the lateral fibula, rotation of the bone block, and fixation with small fragment compression screws. In the absence of any other reconstruction options, a slip of the Achilles tendon can be harvested and brought anteriorly in place of the superior peroneal retinaculum and sutured to the posterolateral fibula. Finally, in the case of the chronic split of the peroneus brevis tendon, the anterior half of the split can be rerouted through the fibula (as in a Chrisman-Snook operation) with the proximal limb passing over the peroneal tendons after its course through the bone tunnel in the fibula and attached to the lateral aspect of the calcaneus.

POSTOPERATIVE CARE Postoperative care is the same as that after primary repair of the peroneal tendons (see Technique 3.24).

■ INTRASHEATH PERONEAL TENDON SUBLUXATION

This condition, originally described by Bassett in 1985, involves subluxation of the peroneal tendons within the peroneal tendon sheath without subluxation over the posterolateral fibular groove. Subluxation of the tendons occurs as the foot is brought into extension and eversion. Popping or snapping of the peroneal tendons is noted on physical examination, but the tendons do not sublux around the posterolateral fibular ridge. Dynamic sonography aids with diagnosis. We have had some success in treating this condition with the previously described methods. When conservative treatment fails, surgical management consists of using the SPR to add intrasheath stability. A segment of the SPR (approximately half) is left with its posterior attachment and is brought up between the two tendons and sutured to the posterolateral aspect of the fibula, in effect creating separate tendon sheaths for the longus and brevis tendons at the proximal level of the SPR (Fig. 3.76). Raikin described a technique for correction of this disorder and reported good-to-excellent results in 13 of 14 patients with intrasheath subluxation of the peroneal tendons (see Technique 3.23).

■ TEARS AND RUPTURES OF THE PERONEAL TENDONS

The tendons may have a single, longitudinal tear, multiple or large longitudinal tears, or complete ruptures. To aid with surgical decision-making, tears of the peroneus brevis are classified into two types: grade I, tears that involve 50% or less of the peroneus brevis cross section, and grade II, tears that involve more than 50% of the tendon. Grade I tears generally are debrided and repaired with tubularization. In grade II tears insufficient viable tendon remains for repair; the diseased segment is excised, and the remaining proximal and distal limbs are tenodesed to the peroneus longus or connected by allograft reconstruction.

Steel and DeOrio evaluated 26 patients at an almost 3-year average follow-up after operative treatment of peroneal tendon tears. Over half had complaints of scar tenderness, lateral ankle swelling, numbness over the lateral ankle, pain at rest, or shoe wear limitations. Only 5 of 26 patients were able to return to participation in sports with no limitations; an additional 7 patients returned to participation in some sport or recreational activity. At an average follow-up of 6.5 years, 17 of 18 patients treated by Demetracopoulos et al. with debridement and primary repair of peroneal tears returned to full sports activity without limitations and no reoperations. More recently, Steginsky et al. retrospectively described 71 patients who had primary repair of the peroneus brevis tendon; 59 (83%) returned to regular exercise but only 62% returned to their previous level of activity. Mook et al. described allograft reconstruction of 14 nonrepairable tears, avoiding tenodesis. At an average follow-up of 17 months, no complications were reported and all patients had returned to their previous levels of activity. In a cadaver model, allograft reconstruction restored distal peroneal brevis tendon tension significantly better than tenodesis.

Rarely, both tendons may have significant tears or complete ruptures, making tenodesis impractical. Redfern and Myerson described an algorithm to aid in choosing surgical treatment for severe, concomitant peroneal tendon tears (type III) (Fig. 3.77). These tears are further classified into type IIIa, in which no proximal muscle excursion is present, and type IIIb, in which proximal muscle excursion exists. They recommended tendon transfer for IIIa, allograft reconstruction or tendon transfer for IIIb, and staged procedures with silicone rods for scarred tendon beds. Jockel and Brodsky described eight patients with severe concomitant tears that were treated with single-stage flexor hallucis longus transfer with good results. Comparable results have been demonstrated with the transfer of flexor digitorum longus or flexor hallucis longus for concomitant tears. Both groups had a high satisfaction rate with improved outcome scores but still demonstrated strength and balance deficits compared to the contralateral extremity. Wapner et al. reported satisfactory results in seven patients who had a staged procedure using Hunter rods for chronic ruptures with scarred peroneal sheaths.

REPAIR OF RUPTURE OF THE PERONEAL TENDONS

TECHNIQUE 3.24

- If physical examination localizes the site of rupture to the lateral aspect of the hindfoot distal to the superior peroneal retinaculum, the entire incision described for tenosynovectomy may not be necessary. Usually, however, it is required for suture of the proximal end of the ruptured tendon to the remaining intact tendon.
- If both tendons are ruptured, which is uncommon in traumatic injuries, attempt to repair both with 2-0 or 0 nonabsorbable suture, again not repairing the superior peroneal retinaculum.
- If the peroneus longus tendon has an attritional rupture beneath the cuboid, resect the distal end 1 to 2 cm plantarward along with its sesamoid, if present (Figs. 3.78 and 3.79).
- Suture the proximal end of the peroneus longus to the peroneus brevis under moderate tension while the foot is held in mild equinovalgus.

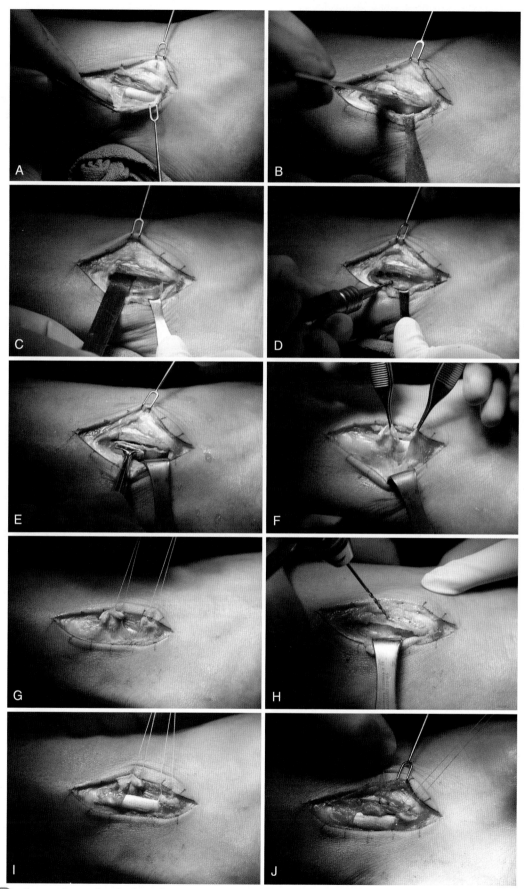

FIGURE 3.76 Groove deepening for intrasheath peroneal tendon subluxation. **A,** Detachment of superior peroneal retinaculum. **B,** Osteotomy of posterior fibula. **C,** Elevation of posterior fibular bone for groove deepening. **D,** Removal of cancellous bone with burr. **E,** Bone tamp used to impact bone flap into deepened groove. **F and G,** Separation of superior peroneal retinaculum into two segments to place superior limb between subluxating peroneal tendons. **H,** Holes drilled into lateral fibula for attachment of retinaculum. **I,** Superior limb of retinaculum passed deep to peroneus longus, inferior limb passed over peroneus longus. **J,** Completed repair.

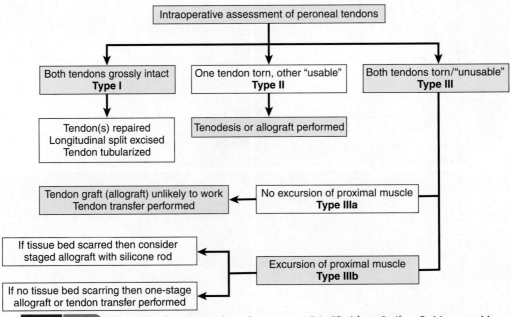

Intraoperative assessment of peroneal tendons

| Both tendons grossly intact **Type I** | One tendon torn, other "usable" **Type II** | Both tendons torn/"unusable" **Type III** |

Tendon(s) repaired
Longitudinal split excised
Tendon tubularized

Tenodesis or allograft performed

Tendon graft (allograft) unlikely to work
Tendon transfer performed ← No excursion of proximal muscle **Type IIIa**

If tissue bed scarred then consider staged allograft with silicone rod

Excursion of proximal muscle **Type IIIb**

If no tissue bed scarring then one-stage allograft or tendon transfer performed

FIGURE 3.77 Algorithm for peroneal tendon surgery. (Modified from Redfern D, Meyerson M: The management of concomitant tears of the peroneus longus and brevis tendons, *Foot Ankle Int* 25:695, 2004.)

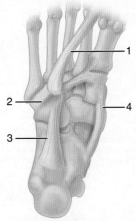

FIGURE 3.78 Plantar surface of foot. *1,* Reflected peroneus longus with intratendinous sesamoid; *2,* cuboid groove for peroneus longus; *3,* long calcaneocuboid ligament; *4,* posterior tibial tendon. **SEE TECHNIQUE 3.24.**

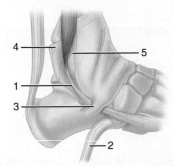

FIGURE 3.79 Plantar surface of foot. *1,* Peroneus brevis tendon; *2,* reflected peroneus longus tendon with sesamoid; *3,* inferior peroneal retinaculum with dividing septum; *4,* deep surface of superior peroneal retinaculum; *5,* sulcus of fibula for peroneal tendons. **SEE TECHNIQUE 3.24.**

POSTOPERATIVE CARE The postoperative care is the same as after tenosynovectomy, but a double-upright brace with limited ankle motion and an outside T-strap is worn for 3 to 6 months if a tendon was repaired end to end at an attritional rupture site.

PERONEAL TENDON REPAIR-RECONSTRUCTION

TECHNIQUE 3.25

(SOBEL AND BOHNE)
- Position the patient supine on the operating table with a sandbag under the ipsilateral greater trochanter.
- Make a curved 7 cm incision through the skin and subcutaneous tissue along the posterior third of the fibula off its central prominence.
- Expose the superior peroneal retinaculum and elevate full-thickness flaps. Subluxation of the anterior portion of the peroneus brevis tendon sometimes can be demonstrated with the superior peroneal retinaculum exposed. Determine the competence of the superior peroneal retinaculum.
- Sharply incise the peroneal sheath near its anterior attachment to the fibula (Fig. 3.80A).
- When surgically treating peroneal tendon injuries, do not violate the synovial and vascular attachments to the peroneal tendons. Proximal traction on the peroneus longus tendon can cause subluxation of the anterior portion of a split peroneus brevis tendon.

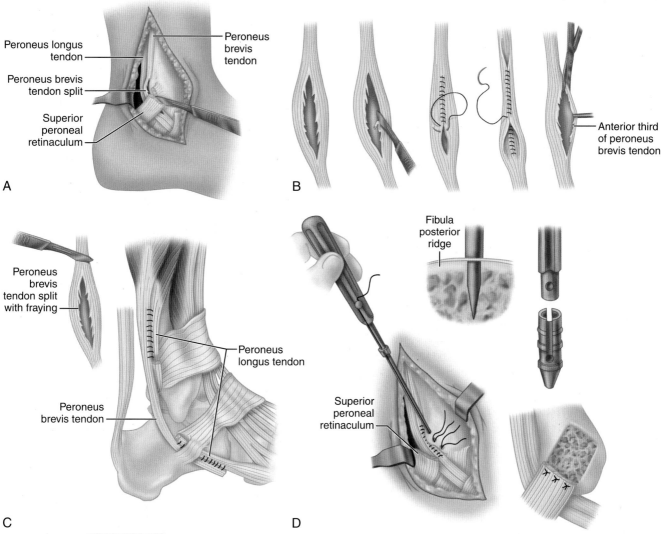

FIGURE 3.80 Peroneal tendon repair-reconstruction. **A,** Incision in superior peroneal retinaculum along posterior ridge of fibula to expose peroneal tendons. **B,** Peroneus brevis split is debrided along margins of split, sutured along split, then tubularized. Alternatively, if split is very anterior within tendon, it simply can be debrided. **C,** Severely degenerated peroneus brevis tendon split can be resected and remaining tendon tenodesed proximally and distally to peroneus longus tendon. **D,** Suture anchors can be used for superior peroneal retinaculum repair. **SEE TECHNIQUE 3.25 AND VIDEO 3.4.**

- Inspect the peroneus brevis tendon; if attrition or a split is evident, debride the attenuated or degenerated tissue and repair and tubulate the tendon (Fig. 3.80B).
- If the peroneus brevis muscle belly is low lying and encroaching on the peroneal tunnel, remove it to create more space for the peroneal tendons within the fibular groove. If an anomalous peroneus quartus tendon encroaches on the fibular groove, remove it also. Failure to identify and remove anomalous tissue allows an overpacking phenomenon that places excessive stress on the superior peroneal retinaculum.
- Other surgical treatment options that can be undertaken at this time are (1) excision of the diseased peroneus brevis segment and suture of the proximal and distal stumps to the peroneus longus tendon (an option that should be reserved for patients in whom the peroneus tendon is severely degenerated); (2) resection of a thickened area of the peroneus brevis tendon, leaving the tendon in continuity

(Fig. 3.80C); (3) use of the anterior half of the split peroneus brevis tendon for a modification of the Chrisman-Snook or other tendon-weaving reconstructive procedure; and (4) transfer of the flexor hallucis longus tendon to repair combined tears of the peroneus brevis and peroneus longus tendons. Creation of a proper gliding tunnel for such a free tendon transfer is accomplished by inserting a Hunter rod in the area of the peroneal tendons in a first procedure and by doing a tendon transfer in a second procedure.
- Remove the sharp posterior ridge of the fibula with a rongeur and file the area smooth to create a fresh bony bed for the repair of the superior peroneal retinaculum. Careful anatomic reconstruction of this structure may be necessary to ensure stability of the tendons within the groove. Advance the superior peroneal retinaculum into the fresh bony bed on the posterior aspect of the fibula

and firmly secure it to the fibula with an Acuflex anchor or suture it to the periosteum.

- Create a posteriorly based trapdoor by using the periosteum anteriorly and the repaired superior peroneal retinaculum. Turn the trapdoor back and suture it on top of the superior peroneal retinaculum to reinforce it.
- Distal extension of the incision with anterior retraction of full-thickness flaps allows primary repair of the attenuated anterior talofibular and calcaneofibular ligaments.
- After the repair, test for peroneal tendon subluxation by placing eversion stress and tension on the peroneus longus tendon. Test the tightness of the lateral ankle ligament repair with gentle anterior drawer testing and compare with the preoperative laxity under anesthesia. Failure to recognize concurrent lateral ankle instability can lead to recurrent laxity and subsequent peroneal tendon injury.
- Perform routine closure and apply a compressive soft-tissue dressing and a posterior splint or cast.

POSTOPERATIVE CARE   The patient does not bear weight for 2 weeks. At that time, a short leg walking cast is applied and is worn for 4 weeks. After the cast is removed, an air splint is applied and is worn for another 4 weeks, at which time peroneal strengthening exercises are begun.

■ DISTAL PERONEAL LONGUS TENDINITIS ASSOCIATED WITH OS PERONEUM: THE PAINFUL OS PERONEUM SYNDROME

Patients occasionally may have localized inflammation and tendinitis at the peroneus longus tendon as it curves around the tunnel through the posterolateral aspect of the cuboid (Fig. 3.81A,B). The os peroneum in this area may be painful and may appear sclerotic on plain radiographs (Fig. 3.81C to E). Prolonged immobilization in a cast is recommended, as well as oral antiinflammatory medication. A very proximal position of the os peroneum or migration from its normal position, lateral and plantar to the cuboid tunnel, may indicate rupture of the peroneus longus tendon distal to the cuboid tunnel. MRI may show rupture of the peroneus longus tendon (Fig. 3.81F). In either event, chronic reproducible tenderness in the plantarlateral aspect of the lateral midfoot in the region of the peroneal groove despite conservative treatment may be an indication for debridement of the peroneus longus tendon, removal of the os peroneum, and, if necessary, tenodesis of the peroneus longus to the peroneus brevis.

DEBRIDEMENT OF THE PERONEUS LONGUS TENDON, REMOVAL OF OS PERONEUM, AND TENODESIS OF PERONEUS LONGUS TENDON TO PERONEUS BREVIS TENDON

TECHNIQUE 3.26

- Place the patient in a lateral decubitus position on a sandbag. Prepare and drape the limb in the usual fashion. Use a thigh tourniquet for better exposure.

- Make an incision over the lateral aspect of the foot longitudinally for approximately 4 cm. Take care to protect the branches of the sural nerve that cross the peroneal tendon sheath in the region.
- Reflect the abductor digiti quinti muscle and fascia plantarly, exposing the peroneus longus tendon from the inferior peroneal retinaculum and peroneal tubercle of the calcaneus to the peroneal tunnel in the lateral plantar aspect of the cuboid.
- Excise the os peroneum.
- If the remainder of the tendon appears normal other than tenosynovitis, perform a tenosynovectomy.
- Repair small tears in the peroneus longus tendon, and if the cuboid tunnel is constricted, enlarge it with a small osteotome and rasp, using bone wax to cover the exposed cancellous surfaces.
- Alternatively, if the tendon appears to be degenerated or there is insufficient tendon left for repair after excision of the os peroneum, perform a side-to-side tenodesis with the peroneus brevis, leaving the tendon sheath open.
- Thoroughly irrigate the wound, obtain meticulous hemostasis, close the subcutaneous tissue in a routine fashion, and apply a bulky, short leg non–weight-bearing cast.

POSTOPERATIVE CARE   The non–weight-bearing cast is worn for 4 weeks, and then protected weight bearing in a walking boot is allowed. Gentle range-of-motion exercises of the ankle and subtalar joints are done. Formal physical therapy is started at 8 weeks after surgery.

INJURIES OF THE FLEXOR TENDONS
FLEXOR HALLUCIS LONGUS TENDINITIS AND IMPINGEMENT

Injuries to the flexor tendons are not common, especially in comparison with injuries and disorders of the posterior tibial and peroneal tendons. Flexor hallucis longus tendinitis has been thought to occur primarily in dancers and athletes whose sports require repetitive forefoot push-off, but some authors have suggested that flexor hallucis longus tendinitis is not rare among nonathletes and should be considered in the differential diagnosis of posteromedial ankle pain. Michelson and Dunn described the varied clinical presentations in 81 patients with flexor hallucis longus tendon pathologic processes. The most common presenting symptom was pain with activity, most often posterior ankle pain (50% of patients). Heel pain and midfoot pain were reported in 28% and 27%, respectively. Tenderness of the tendon usually was elicited at its musculotendinous junction behind the medial malleolus (approximately 60%) or where it crossed the flexor digitorum longus tendon at the knot of Henry (approximately 40%). Restriction of flexor hallucis longus excursion was demonstrated in 37% of patients by limited first metatarsophalangeal joint dorsiflexion with the ankle dorsiflexed (flexor hallucis longus stretch test). Of plain radiographs available for 50 patients, 70% were completely normal, 14% demonstrated an os trigonum, and 8% showed mild degenerative changes

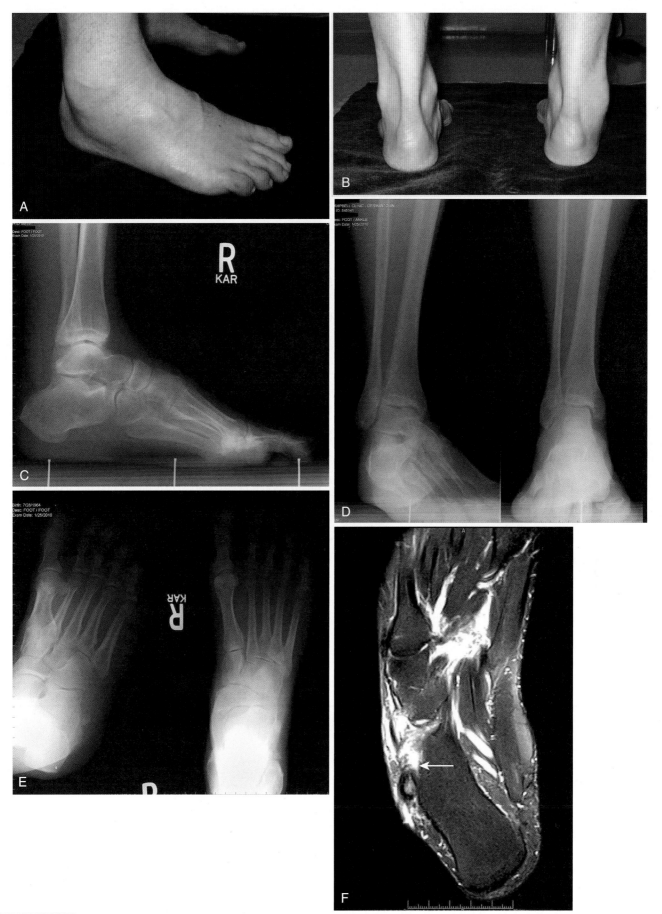

FIGURE 3.81 Painful os peroneus syndrome. **A** and **B**, Note subtle cavovarus foot and swelling inferior to lateral malleolus on right. Left foot was treated 3 years earlier for same problem. **C** to **E**, Sclerotic appearance of os peroneum on radiographs. **F**, MRI shows closing wedge calcaneal osteotomy and dorsiflexion osteotomy of first metatarsal.

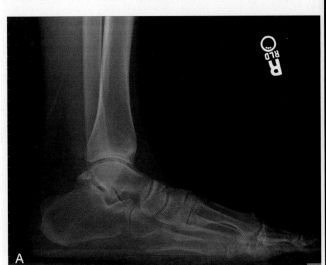

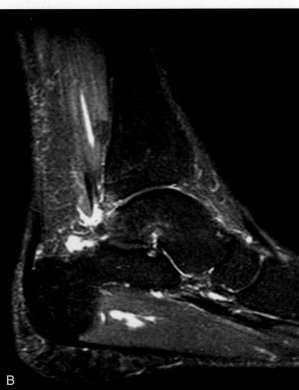

in the first metatarsophalangeal joint; 82% of magnetic resonance images showed synovitis associated with the flexor hallucis longus tendon.

■ DIAGNOSIS

On physical examination, careful differentiation should be made between posterior compression syndrome, which involves an elongated Stieda (trigonal) process or an enlarged os trigonum in the posterior aspect of the ankle, flexor hallucis longus tendinitis, and compression tendinopathy with stenosis of the flexor hallucis longus tendon sheath in the posterior aspect of the ankle. Reproduction of pain in the posterior aspect with forced plantarflexion is more suggestive of a posterior ankle compression syndrome. Flexor hallucis longus tendinitis is characterized by pain posterior to the medial malleolus and often is misdiagnosed as posterior tibial tendinitis. The tendon may be palpated posterior to the ankle. The diagnosis is confirmed if pain is reproduced with passive extension of the great toe with compression of the posteromedial tendon sheath of the flexor hallucis longus in the posterior aspect of the ankle. MRI may be helpful in the diagnosis of this disease, often showing fluid around the flexor hallucis longus tendon and occasionally intratendinous degenerative changes (Fig. 3.82). Plain lateral standing radiographs of the ankle are helpful in differentiating a painful os trigonum from flexor hallucis longus tendinitis.

■ TREATMENT

Conservative management consists of rest, modification of dance technique or sporting activity, oral antiinflammatory medication, and stretching exercises. Most authors have reported conservative treatment to be largely unsuccessful, but Michelson and Dunn reported successful nonoperative treatment in 64% of patients with a stretching program and short-term

immobilization; all patients treated operatively with decompression and synovectomy had successful outcomes. Operative treatment has been reported to achieve good or excellent results in 82% to 100% of patients. Open and endoscopic techniques for os trigonum excision and flexor hallucis longus release have produced excellent results. In a recent systematic review of ballet dancers, similar results were found with endoscopic and open approaches for flexor hallucis longus tendinopathy and posterior ankle impingement syndrome treatment.

RELEASE OF THE FIBROOSSEOUS TUNNEL

TECHNIQUE 3.27

(HAMILTON ET AL.)

A medial approach was recommended when both tendinitis and posterior impingement are present; the lateral approach is used for treatment of isolated posterior impingement without tendinitis.

MEDIAL APPROACH

- For the medial approach, make a 4-cm curvilinear incision posterior to the malleolus at the level of the superior border of the calcaneus, following the course of the underlying neurovascular bundle.
- Retract the neurovascular bundle posteriorly with a blunt retractor and identify the underlying tunnel by motion of the great toe.

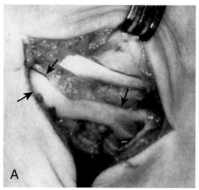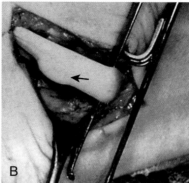

FIGURE 3.83 **A,** Flexor hallucis longus constricted at entrance of fibroosseous tunnel. Tendon is completely free with ankle and great toe in neutral. Flexor digitorum longus anterior to flexor hallucis longus. **B,** Large nodule within fibroosseous tunnel. Despite size of nodule, there is free excursion of tendon after release of tunnel. **SEE TECHNIQUE 3.27.**

■ Release the tunnel, proximal to distal, to the level of the sustentaculum tali and debride or repair as needed (Fig. 3.83A). Nodules on or within the flexor hallucis tendon usually are not excised because after the fibroosseous tunnel has been released the excursion of the tendon is no longer restricted (Fig. 3.83B).

■ Evaluate functional hallux rigidus intraoperatively to ensure complete release and free excursion of the tendon.

■ Retract the released tendon posteriorly with the neurovascular bundle and remove the os trigonum on the lateral side of the entrance of the fibroosseous tunnel.

■ Examine the ankle in full plantarflexion and remove remaining bone or soft-tissue impingement. The ankle should be in a neutral position of flexion and extension during closure so that the skin is aligned properly.

LATERAL APPROACH

■ Because of increased external rotation of the lower extremities of dancers, the patient should be placed in a lateral decubitus position on the operating table for the lateral approach to this procedure.

■ Make a curvilinear incision at the posterior aspect of the ankle mortise in line with the posterior border of the peroneal tendons. Take care to avoid the sural nerve.

■ Perform a capsulotomy with the ankle in slight dorsiflexion and identify the lateral tubercle or os trigonum lateral to the tunnel.

■ Assess adequate osseous decompression by plantarflexing the foot and palpating for any bone-on-bone impingement. Occasionally, loose bodies, calcaneal protuberances, or portions of the posterior part of the tibia need to be debrided.

POSTOPERATIVE CARE A compression dressing should be applied and weight bearing allowed as tolerated with crutches. The dressing is removed in 1 week. An active range of motion is initiated as tolerance to pain permits. At 2 weeks, the patient begins physical therapy consisting of progressive active and passive range-of-motion and strengthening exercises. Swimming is encouraged after the wound has healed. The patient is progressed to higher lev-

els of activity under supervision of a physical therapist. An average of 6 months should be expected for full recovery.

FLEXOR HALLUCIS LONGUS TEAR

If the flexor hallucis longus is torn proximal to the metatarsophalangeal joint so that the repair site will not move through the pulley system, repair may be justified; however, the exposure in the plantar surface of the forefoot proximal to the metatarsophalangeal joint is difficult. Floyd et al. suggested repair of the flexor hallucis longus in the foot. We do not repair this tendon within the pulley system of the hallux; with an intact flexor hallucis brevis in the forefoot-midfoot area, repair of the flexor hallucis longus probably is not needed for function. However, if repair is chosen, the following exposure is recommended.

REPAIR OF FLEXOR HALLUCIS TEAR

TECHNIQUE 3.28

■ Begin a plantar longitudinal incision on the sole of the foot between the first and second metatarsals just lateral and distal to the fibular sesamoid. Continue this incision proximally 4 to 5 cm (Fig. 3.84).

■ Bluntly remove the fibrous connections between the slips of plantar fascia to the first and second toes.

■ Using small, blunt-tipped dissecting scissors, expose the common digital nerve and accompanying vessels to the first web space (Fig. 3.85). Retract these laterally and toward the distal part of the wound to expose the lateral head of the flexor hallucis brevis tendon (Fig. 3.86).

■ Develop this plane between the two muscle bellies throughout the length of the wound and acutely flex the great toe. The distal tendon stump should appear in the wound. (This should guide the surgeon toward the proximal course of the retracted tendon, particularly if dark hematoma or scar directs the way.)

■ Use a tendon passer or hemostat to probe proximally along the suspected path with the ankle in equinus. The tendon should not retract past the navicular because of

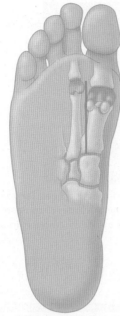

FIGURE **3.84**   Incision on plantar surface of foot for repair of flexor hallucis longus. **SEE TECHNIQUE 3.28.**

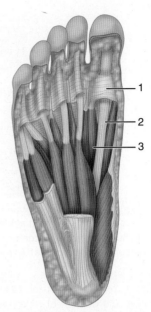

FIGURE **3.86**   *1,* Pulley of flexor hallucis longus at first metatarsophalangeal joint; *2,* flexor hallucis longus; *3,* lateral head of flexor hallucis brevis. **SEE TECHNIQUE 3.28.**

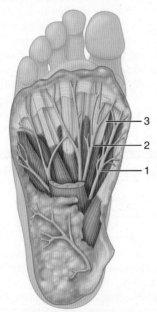

FIGURE **3.85**   *1,* Medial proper branch of medial plantar nerve to tibial side of hallux; *2,* common digital branch of medial plantar nerve to first web; *3,* flexor hallucis longus tendon. **SEE TECHNIQUE 3.28.**

not "accordion" the tendon any more than is necessary to have adequate tension to approximate the tendon ends.

- Close the skin with 2-0 or 3-0 nylon. Simple sutures are desirable, but vertical mattress sutures are acceptable if the approximation is offset. Apply a bulky soft-tissue wrap and a short leg cast with mild equinus at the ankle and neutral position of the hallux. The cast should extend distal to the toes.

POSTOPERATIVE CARE The patient is kept non–weight bearing for 3 weeks with the ankle in mild equinus; then the foot is brought to neutral position at the ankle and another short leg cast is applied, extending past the toes. Weight bearing to tolerance in the cast is allowed. Sutures are removed at the time of cast change. The short leg walking cast is removed at 6 weeks, and active toe flexion is begun both at the interphalangeal and metatarsophalangeal joints while one or the other joint is blocked manually. With repair of the tendon 2 cm or more proximal to the metatarsophalangeal joint, the interphalangeal joint should recover independent flexion.

FLEXOR DIGITORUM LONGUS TENDON INJURY

Repair of an isolated injury of the flexor digitorum longus in the toes or in the midfoot is not indicated. If a deep plantar laceration near the midfoot-hindfoot junction occurs proximal to the junction of the quadratus plantae and flexor digitorum longus and the flexor hallucis longus also is lacerated (usually with concomitant medial or lateral plantar nerve injury), then repair may be indicated along with the other structures.

the tethering by the cross connection with the flexor digitorum longus at this level.

- Once the tendon is located and brought into the wound and with the ankle plantarflexed, pass a straight needle through the skin and flexor hallucis longus tendon and into the skin on the other side.
- Flex the toe and repair the tendon end to end with a double right-angle stitch using 2-0 nonabsorbable materials wedged to a tapered, atraumatic needle. Do

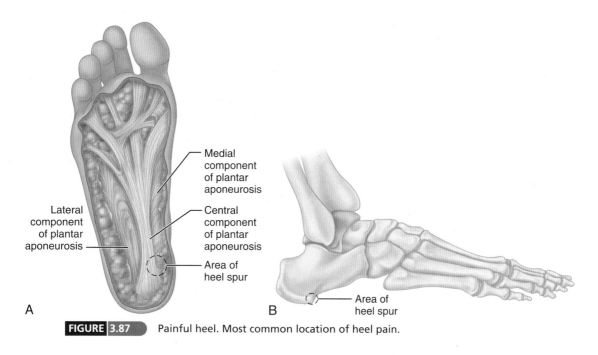

FIGURE 3.87 Painful heel. Most common location of heel pain.

PAINFUL HEEL

In 1922, Stiell stated, "painful heel appears to be a condition which is seldom efficiently treated, for the simple reason that the causation is not exactly diagnosed." Forty-three years later Lapidus and Guidotti stated, "the name of *painful heel* is used deliberately in preference to any other more precise etiologic diagnosis, since the cause of this definite clinical entity still remains unknown." Now, nearly 100 years later, we still do not know the precise, inclusive cause of pain beneath the antero-medial prominence of the calcaneal tuberosity (Fig. 3.87). A variety of other causes of heel pain are better understood, such as heel cord tendinitis, retrocalcaneal bursitis, and poste-rior tibial tendinitis, but plantar heel pain remains enigmatic. Despite being poorly understood, plantar heel pain is very common, creating frustration for both physician and patient. Tong and Furia reported that more than 2 million patients are treated for plantar fasciitis every year in the United States and estimated the cost of treatment in 2007 as ranging from $192 to $376 million.

ETIOLOGY

The differential diagnosis of plantar heel pain should include heel pad atrophy, plantar fasciitis (plantar fasciopathy), entrapment of the first branch of lateral plantar nerve, cal-caneal stress fracture, plantar calcaneal bursitis, and tarsal tunnel syndrome. Other more uncommon etiologies include rheumatoid arthritis, ankylosing spondylitis, and Reiter syn-drome. In addition, especially in patients with diabetes, deep soft-tissue abscess should be considered. In men younger than 40 years of age with bilateral painful heels, ankylosing spondylitis and Reiter syndrome should be ruled out. Women with bilateral symptoms should be evaluated for rheumatoid arthritis.

Degenerative changes with increasing age are the most constant findings in the elastic adipose tissue of the heel pad. Aging also brings about a gradual reduction in collagen and water content, as well as elastic fibrous tissue. This degenera-tive process in the calcaneal heel pad can account in part for soreness under the heel, which is more consistent with heel pad atrophy.

Another possible cause of symptoms involves the wind-lass mechanism of the plantar fascia as the toes are dorsi-flexed. The plantar fascia originates from the anteromedial plantar aspect of the calcaneal tuberosity and inserts through several slips into the plantar plates of the metatarsophalangeal joints, the flexor tendon sheaths, and the bases of the proxi-mal phalanges of the digits. It is under constant traction as it is pulled distally around the drum of the windlass (metatarsal heads). This tightening of the cable, so to speak, elevates the longitudinal arch and in so doing places traction on the origin of the plantar fascia (Fig. 3.88).

Another finding that supports this theory is that the most dense, unyielding section of the plantar aponeurosis origi-nates from the location on the tuberosity of the calcaneus where the most common point of local tenderness is found during physical examination. It is not farfetched to com-pare this to "tennis elbow." In fact, this entity has been called "tennis heel," in which repetitive traction and aging produce microscopic tears, myxoid degeneration with disorientation of collagen fibers, and angiofibroblastic hyperplasia in the origin of the plantar fascia.

Other than the plantar fascia origin, a neurogenic cause of painful heel syndrome involving entrapment of the first branch of the lateral plantar nerve to the abductor digiti minimi was proposed by Schon and Baxter. After review-ing this in the laboratory and clinically, they concluded that a few patients (1% to 2%) have a neurogenic pathologic condition associated with painful heel syndrome. They dif-ferentiated neurogenic causes from others by localizing ten-derness along the lateral plantar nerve inferior to the flexor retinaculum as the nerve approaches the calcaneal tuberos-ity. Patients with plantar fasciitis describe tenderness only at the medial tubercle, but patients with a neurogenic compo-nent have tenderness all along this nerve. Schon and Baxter emphasized release of the deep fascial edge of the abductor hallucis muscle.

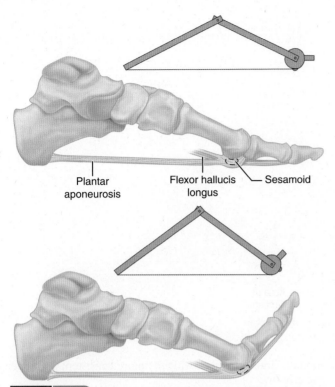

FIGURE 3.88 Painful heel. Windlass mechanism, placing tension on origin of plantar fascia (see text).

Significant research has been done in the past few years regarding the consequences of surgical treatment for plantar fasciitis. The role of the plantar fascia as a supporting structure of the longitudinal arch of the foot also has been extensively studied, and it has been found to be the most important static support for the arch. Significant changes have been shown to occur in the longitudinal arch after sectioning of the plantar fascia. These laboratory studies help us to understand the clinical picture of arch pain in patients who have had either rupture or surgical release of the plantar fascia.

It is important to note the association between chronic heel pain and heel cord tightness. Gastrocnemius contractures have been associated with plantar fasciitis, but on the other hand it must be stressed that an overly aggressive lengthening may result in a particularly difficult type of heel overload and pain. Chilvers et al. described heel overload associated with heel cord insufficiency in nine patients after heel cord lengthening. They identified diabetes and an insensate heel as risk factors.

CLINICAL AND RADIOGRAPHIC FINDINGS

Most often, patients with heel pain are between 40 and 70 years of age and have unilateral symptoms in a normally arched foot. Obesity is a predisposing factor, and the symptoms are even more difficult to control when a patient is overweight. It is uncertain if pes planus or pes cavus predisposes to this condition. Decreased ankle dorsiflexion and decreased knee extension are associated with plantar heel pain.

The major complaint is pain beneath the heel that is worse on rising in the morning or after sitting for a while. After a few steps the pain diminishes, and the patient is reasonably comfortable during the day. Toward the end of the day, the discomfort becomes more of an aching that is relieved by absence of weight bearing.

The most common physical finding is localized tenderness at the inferomedial aspect of the calcaneal tuberosity. If the symptomatic heel is compared with the asymptomatic one, mild swelling and erythema often are apparent. The duration of symptoms varies from a few weeks to several months or even years. Radiographs reveal a calcaneal spur in about 50% of patients, but the exact significance of this finding is uncertain. The size and shape of plantar heel spurs do not correlate with patients' symptoms. Because MRI can reliably delineate both the soft-tissue and bony anatomy of the foot, it can be helpful in the evaluation of recalcitrant or atypical heel pain. Although it rarely changes the management, MRI may demonstrate other pathologic processes such as plantar fascia tearing, calcaneal edema, or space-occupying lesions.

TREATMENT

Rarely does a patient with a painful heel require surgery to relieve the symptoms. Orthoses, night splints, specific plantar fascia stretching regimen, oral nonsteroidal antiinflammatory agents, local injections, extracorporeal shockwave therapy, and low-level laser therapy all have been reported to be successful. More commonly, corticosteroid injections have been used successfully, but other injections such as PRP, micronized dehydrated human amnion/chorion membrane (dHACM), botulinum toxin, and whole blood also have relieved symptoms. Rupture of the plantar fascia has been reported after corticosteroid injection so patients should be warned of this complication. Furthermore, corticosteroids may provide only brief, temporary relief. A prospective, randomized controlled trial comparing intralesional autologous blood injection with corticosteroid injection found that the blood injection was effective in reducing pain and tenderness but that corticosteroid was superior in onset of relief. At 6-month follow-up, both groups maintained improved VAS scores. In another prospective trial, Monto randomized 43 patients to corticosteroid or PRP injections. At 3 months, both showed improved AOFAS scores; however, the corticosteroid group steadily declined to baseline levels while the PRP group improvement persisted at 2 years. Others have reported similar results in which both corticosteroid and PRP injections statistically improve VAS scores, but the improvement after a corticosteroid injection appears to be temporary. Reports in the literature indicate that more than 90% of patients with plantar fasciitis can be successfully treated nonoperatively. At our institution, the most common foot complaint in adults is a painful heel, yet surgery for this disorder is extremely rare. In a survey of AOFAS members, 74% of respondents prefer surgery or extracorporeal shockwave therapy (ECSWT) for patients with symptoms present for more than 10 months. High-energy ECSWT has been reported to be effective for plantar fasciitis, but level 1 evidence also demonstrates no difference between plantar fascia–specific stretching and shockwave therapy as *initial* treatment. For chronic plantar fasciitis, a meta-analyses of randomized controlled trials and quasi-randomized trials supported the use of ECSWT. Other reported treatments include botulinum toxin A, radiofrequency electromagnetic field therapy, percutaneous electrolysis, and low-level laser therapy, but no large randomized trials have confirmed their effectiveness. Jastifer et al. reported the use of low-level laser therapy in 30 patients with recalcitrant plantar fasciitis. At 6-month and 12-month follow-up, VAS and foot function index scores were improved significantly.

In some patients, symptoms persist over an extended time despite all forms of conservative management. If the patient is made fully aware of the possibility that no improvement may occur after surgery, then surgery can be recommended. Recommended procedures include neurolysis of a single nerve, gastrocnemius lengthening, partial plantar fasciectomy (open and endoscopic), and exostectomy of the calcaneus. If the procedure chosen does not involve removing the calcaneal spur, if present, the patient must be informed of this before surgery to avoid confusion, disappointment, and possibly a poor result from a psychologic perspective alone. Isolated gastrocnemius recession has been shown to improve symptoms of plantar fasciitis with less morbidity than traditional open, partial plantar fascia release.

Ward and Clippinger described a proximal medial longitudinal arch incision for plantar fascia release and reported that this limited, noninvasive procedure allowed release of the central cord of the plantar fascia while leaving the lateral 35% to 50% intact, reducing the recovery time required after an open procedure. Because no dissection was done through the underlying flexor digitorum brevis muscle, no neurolysis or tendinous release over the course of the nerve to the abductor digiti minimi was necessary. The incisional scar caused no complaints.

The use of endoscopy for plantar fascia release also is based on limited release of the central cord of the fascia. Although earlier reports in the orthopaedic literature emphasized complications of this procedure, more recent studies have reported that endoscopic plantar fasciotomy is an effective procedure with reproducible results, a low complication rate, and little risk of iatrogenic nerve injury. Anatomic dissections have shown that, if properly performed, endoscopic plantar fascia release appears to be a reasonably safe procedure. Saxena reported excellent or good results with single-portal endoscopic release in 16 athletic patients, all of whom returned to sports (primarily running) within 3 months of surgery. Half of patients with a body mass index of more than 27 had poor results. We have no experience with endoscopic technique and prefer open plantar fascia and nerve release.

Most patients with heel pain syndrome who ultimately require surgery have some evidence of entrapment of the first branch of the lateral plantar nerve. For these few patients, the procedure described below, which includes decompression of the first branch of the lateral plantar nerve, removal of the insertion of a portion of the plantar fascia, and removal of the heel spur, seems to be more of a complete procedure than a simple incision of the plantar fascia with the endoscopic method. Because release of the plantar fascia from the tuberosity of the calcaneus, removal of any calcaneal spur, neurolysis of the nerve to the abductor digiti minimi, release of the flexor digitorum brevis, and excision of the anterior tuberosity of the calcaneus can all be done through one incision, only one procedure is described. Several authors have reported good results after neurolysis of the nerve to the abductor digiti minimi combined with partial plantar fascia release.

PLANTAR FASCIA AND NERVE RELEASE

TECHNIQUE 3.29

(SCHON; BAXTER)

- A tourniquet is not required for this procedure but can be used if desired. Place the patient supine so that the affected foot can be rotated externally. A 2.5× loupe magnification routinely is used for the surgery. If no tourniquet is used, the patient may be put in a slight Trendelenburg position to reduce venous backflow. Prophylactic intravenous antibiotics can be used at the discretion of the surgeon.
- Make an oblique 3- to 4-cm incision along the medial aspect of the heel overlying the course of the first branch of the lateral plantar nerve and the proximal edge of the belly of the abductor hallucis muscle (Fig. 3.89A). The starting point of the incision can be located by bisecting a longitudinal axial line that runs 1 cm from the posterior edge of the medial malleolus. Direct the incision obliquely in a distal and plantar direction, ending at the junction of the plantar and medial skin.
- Carry sharp dissection through the subcutaneous fat, paying careful attention to the superficial branch of the calcaneal nerves. Occasionally, before the superficial fascia of the abductor is encountered, subcutaneous fascia is seen and often is confused with the abductor hallucis fascia.
- Identify the superficial fascia of the abductor hallucis and insert a self-retaining retractor into the wound.
- Identify the plantar fascia by passing a Freer elevator from the medial distal edge of the abductor in a plantar and lateral direction. Insert a small lamina spreader with teeth at this junction of the abductor fascia and plantar fascia and place a Senn retractor distally between the two arms of the lamina spreader for better exposure of the plantar fascia.
- Once exposure is complete, sharply release the superficial fascia of the abductor (Fig. 3.89B).
- Identify the deep fascia of the abductor, using a Freer elevator. This fascia is concave and must be identified clearly before the release is performed.
- Using a Senn retractor, pull the abductor muscle superiorly and release the deep fascia of the abductor with a scalpel (Fig. 3.89C). Beneath this fascia there is fat, an artery, a vein, and the first branch of the lateral plantar nerve. Place the Senn retractor superiorly and pull the abductor muscle distally to permit complete release of the deep fascia of the abductor from this direction and thus release the lateral plantar nerve (Fig. 3.89D). In about 20% of patients the nerve can be seen without dissection. It is not recommended to routinely dissect out the nerve because this may cause unnecessary bleeding and trauma to the structures. Careful release of fascia is warranted when a sharp edge of the medial caudal border of the quadratus plantae is palpated (Fig. 3.89E).
- Attention now should be turned to the inferior aspect of the wound, where the plantar fascia can be seen medially. Resect a 2- to 3- × 4-mm rectangle of medial plantar fascia (Fig. 3.89F). An entire plantar fasciotomy may be performed in some nonathletic patients who have pain throughout the entire insertion of the plantar fascia medially and laterally. If the entire plantar fascia is to be released, insert a lamina spreader in the resected area and cut the remaining portion of the plantar fascia.
- If a large spur is present preoperatively and is thought to contribute to symptoms, resect the spur by gently reflecting the flexor digitorum brevis off the exostosis. Place a Freer elevator superior and inferior to the spur and transect it with a ¼-inch osteotome. Take care not to damage the first branch of the lateral plantar nerve that lies just superior to the spur. After the spur is cut, remove it with a rongeur and smooth the bone edges. Several authors recommend packing thrombin or bone wax at the cut edge of the bone.

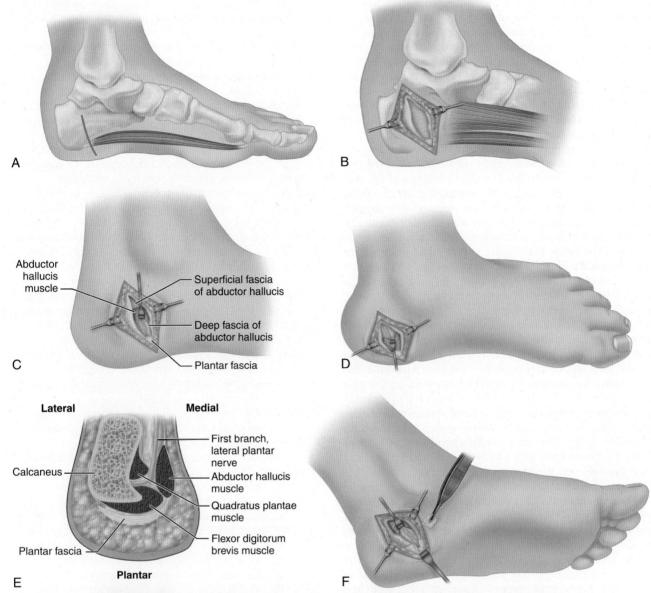

FIGURE 3.89   Plantar fascia and nerve release. **A,** Incision is made over first branch of lateral plantar nerve. **B,** Superficial fascia of abductor hallucis muscle is released. **C,** Abductor hallucis muscle is reflected proximally. **D,** Abductor hallucis muscle is retracted distally. **E,** Cross-sectional anatomy of heel along course of first branch of lateral plantar nerve. **F,** Resection of small medial portion of plantar fascia. (From Schon LC: Plantar fascia and Baxter's nerve release. In Myerson M, editor: *Current therapy in foot and ankle surgery*, St. Louis, 1993, Mosby.) **SEE TECHNIQUE 3.29.**

- Check the release by placing a small, curved hemostat deep to the deep fascia of the abductor and gently spreading it, palpating for any tight bands.
- Irrigate the wound copiously and achieve hemostasis. Close the skin with 4-0 nylon mattress sutures. Apply a compression dressing consisting of 4- × 4-inch sponge gauzes, 4-inch Kerlix bandage, 4-inch Kling bandage, and then a 4-inch elastic bandage.

POSTOPERATIVE CARE   The patient is kept non–weight bearing for 2 weeks after surgery. The sutures are then removed, and gradual weight bearing to tolerance is begun. Resumption of heel cord stretching and increased activity are encouraged.

TWO-PORTAL ENDOSCOPIC PLANTAR FASCIA RELEASE

TECHNIQUE 3.30

(BARRETT ET AL.)

- After administration of an intravenous sedative and local anesthesia, prepare and drape the patient in the usual manner. Exsanguinate the foot and inflate a pneumatic ankle tourniquet.
- Make a reference point for incision immediately anterior and inferior to the inferior aspect of the medial calcaneal

tubercle, as viewed on a non–weight-bearing lateral projection.

- Make a 5-mm vertical stab incision and bluntly dissect to the level of the plantar fascia (Fig. 3.90A). Because direct observation through this small incision is impossible, palpation is necessary.
- The Endotrac (Instratek, Houston, TX) consists of a fascial elevator, hook probe, slotted obturator-cannula system, and two blade handles for disposable hook and triangle blades.
- Palpate the medial investment of the plantar fascia with the fascial elevator.
- Create a channel immediately inferior to the plantar fascia with the fascial elevator (Fig. 3.90B). Introduce the obturator-cannula system into this channel and advance it across the inferior surface of the plantar fascia to the lateral aspect of the foot.
- Palpate the obturator and make a 5-mm vertical incision over its tip, allowing the obturator-cannula to be passed through the skin.
- Remove the obturator from the slotted cannula, leaving the cannula in place.
- Introduce the endoscope medially and the fascial probe laterally.
- Using the endoscope, view the entire inferior surface of the plantar fascia on the monitor. Double marks on the interior wall of the cannula indicate the approximate location of the medial plantar fascia investment. Proceeding laterally, a single mark indicates the approximate location of the medial intermuscular septum. The first two marks are 9 mm and 11 mm from the medial dermis, respectively, whereas the third mark is 13.5 mm from the midpoint of the first two marks. These marks correspond to average dermal and medial band widths obtained from cadaver dissections and should be used only as guides.
- While viewing the medial investment of the plantar fascia through the endoscope, use the probe to palpate its fibers. Introduce the retrograde knife to this anatomic reference point and sever the medial band of the plantar fascia (Fig. 3.90C).
- Insert the endoscope laterally and the fascial probe medially to allow a 180-degree perspective. If any remaining plantar fascial fibers are palpated, introduce the triangle blade medially to release them. It is important to see the complete thickness of the plantar fascia on the video monitor to ensure a proper release (Fig. 3.90D).
- After fasciotomy, irrigate the area with sterile saline and remove the slotted cannula.
- Approximate the two incisions with two 5-0 Prolene sutures and infiltrate the area with 0.5% bupivacaine and 1 mL of dexamethasone to decrease postoperative discomfort. Apply a sterile compressive gauze dressing and deflate the tourniquet.

POSTOPERATIVE CARE Patients are allowed full weight bearing immediately after surgery but should avoid excessive ambulation. The dressings are removed on the third day after surgery, and sterile cloth adhesive bandages are applied. The patient may return to regular shoes fitted with an orthotic appliance as soon as tolerated.

SINGLE-PORTAL ENDOSCOPIC PLANTAR FASCIA RELEASE

TECHNIQUE 3.31

(SAXENA)
- Make an incision on the medial aspect of the foot, 1 cm distal to the medial tubercle of the calcaneus just above the junction of the plantar skin. Dorsiflex the hallux to identify the medial portion of the plantar fascia, and make the incision within the slightly oblique skin lines that run dorsal-proximal to plantar-distal.
- Use a hemostat to bluntly dissect down to the plantar fascia.
- Use a fascial elevator to separate the subcutaneous layer from the plantar fascia on the inferior heel and introduce an obturator cannula from medial to lateral in the pathway created by the fascial elevator.
- Remove the obturator and place a 30-degree 4.0-mm endoscope within the cannula to view the plantar fascia superiorly.
- Remove the endoscope and apply the cannulated depth gauge with a stop device. Reintroduce the endoscope with the depth gauge from medial to lateral.
- Identify the medial half of the central plantar fascia band by rotating the cannula 180 degrees and viewing this location externally by transillumination on the inferior heel.
- Note the measurement corresponding to the appropriate level of transection, usually 7 to 8 on the depth gauge.
- Withdraw the endoscope, remove the depth gauge, and attach a disposable cannulated knife with the stop device at the appropriate number to allow transection of the medial half of the central plantar fascia. Reinsert the endoscope and use the knife to transect the fascia. Dorsiflexing the toes can aid in the transection.
- After transection, examine the cut ends of the plantar fascia, as well as the first plantar muscle layer. When appropriate fasciotomy is confirmed, remove all instrumentation and irrigate the surgical site.
- Use small scissors to transect any palpable taut fibers of the medial band under direct vision.
- Close the incision with one or two horizontal mattress sutures.

POSTOPERATIVE CARE A short below-knee cast boot is worn for 4 weeks, with the sutures removed at about 2 weeks. Patients are kept non–weight bearing on crutches for the first 2 weeks and are advised to use a foot orthosis during initiation of weight bearing. Physical therapy, consisting of stretching, massage, ultrasound, and gradual strengthening is begun at 4 weeks. Running is resumed when the patient can tolerate 30 to 40 minutes of continuous walking and has no daily symptoms.

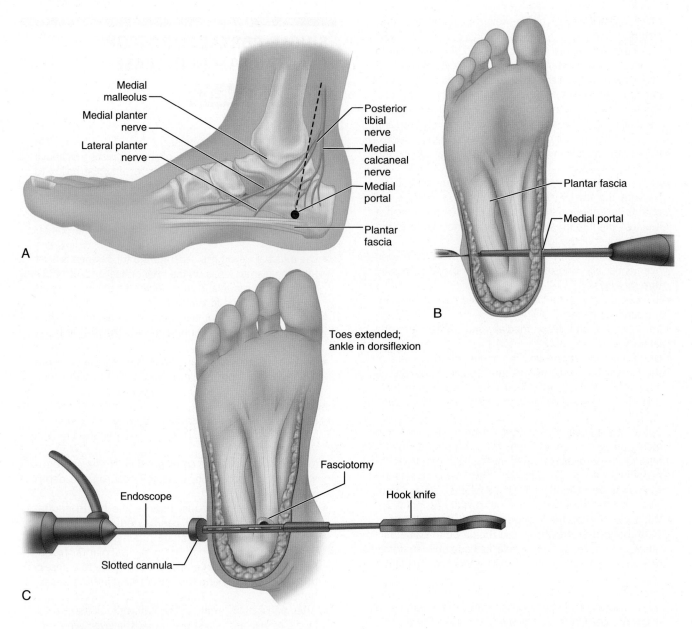

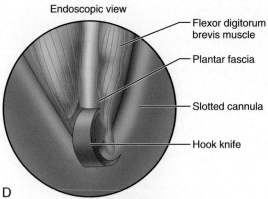

FIGURE 3.90 Endoscopic plantar fascia release with two-portal technique (see text). **A,** Medial portal is determined by extending line distally along posterior aspect of medial malleolus, where it intersects with medial origin of plantar fascia at calcaneal tuberosity. **B,** Lateral portal is made by placing blunt trocar superficial and perpendicular to plantar fascia. **C,** With ankle dorsiflexed and toes extended, medial aspect of plantar fascia is released with hook knife. **D,** When appropriate amount of plantar fascia is released, underlying flexor digitorum brevis muscle can be seen. (From Ferkel RD, Hommen JP: Arthroscopy of the ankle and foot. In Coughlin MJ, Mann RA, Saltzman CL, editors: *Surgery of the foot and ankle,* 8th ed, Philadelphia, 2007, Elsevier.) **SEE TECHNIQUE 3.30.**

REFERENCES

DISORDERS OF TENDONS

Posterior and Anterior Tibial Tendons

Acevedo J, Vora A: Anatomical reconstruction of the spring ligament complex: "internal brace" augmentation, *Foot Ankle Spec* 6:441, 2013.

Bernasconi A, Sadile F, Welck M, et al.: Role of tendoscopy in treating stage II posterior tibial tendon dysfunction, *Foot Ankle Int* 39:433, 2018.

Cao HH, Tang KI, Lu WZ, et al.: Medial displacement calcaneal osteotomy with posterior tibial tendon reconstruction for the flexible flatfoot with symptomatic accessory navicular, *J Foot Ankle Surg* 53:539, 2014.

Cha SM, Shin HD, Kim KC, Lee JK: Simple excision vs the Kidner procedure for type 2 accessory navicular associated with flatfoot in pediatric population, *Foot Ankle Int* 34:167, 2013.

DeOrio JK, Shapiro SA, McNeil RB, Stansel J: Validity of the posterior tibial edema sign in posterior tibial tendon dysfunction, *Foot Ankle Int* 32:189, 2011.

Ellington JK, McCormick J, Marion C, et al.: Surgical outcome following tibialis anterior tendon repair, *Foot Ankle Int* 31:412, 2010.

Gianakos AL, Ross KA, Hannon CP, et al.: Functional outcomes of tibialis posterior tendoscopy with comparison to magnetic resonance imaging, *Foot Ankle Int* 36:812, 2015.

Grundy JR, O'Sullivan RM, Beischer AD: Operative management of distal tibialis anterior tendinopathy, *Foot Ankle Int* 31:212, 2010.

Haleem AM, Pavlov H, Bogner E, et al.: Comparison of deformity with respect to the talus in patients with posterior tibial tendon dysfunction and controls using multiplanar weight-bearing imaging or conventional radiography, *J Bone Joint Surg Am* 96:1, 2014.

Harkin E, Pinzur M, Schiff A: Treatment of acute and chronic tibialis anterior tendon rupture and tendinopathy, *Foot Ankle Clin N Am* 22:819, 2017.

Huh J, Boyette DM, Parekh SG, Nunley JA: Allograft reconstruction of chronic tibialis anterior tendon ruptures, *Foot Ankle Int* 36(10):1180, 2015.

Ikoma K, Ohashi S, Maki M, et al.: Diagnostic characteristics of standard radiographs and magnetic resonance imaging of ruptures of the tibialis posterior tendon, *J Foot Ankle Surg* 55:542, 2016.

Khazen G, Khazen C: Tendoscopy in stage I posterior tibial tendon dysfunction, *Foot Ankle Clin* 17:399, 2012.

Liang ZC, Lui TH: Endoscopically assisted reconstruction of posterior tibial tendon for stage 2 posterior tibial tendon dysfunction, *Arthrosc Tech* 8:e237, 2019.

Michels F, van der Bauwhede J, Oosterlinck D, et al.: Minimally invasive repair of the tibialis anterior tendon using a semitendinosus autografts, *Foot Ankle Int* 35:264, 2014.

Miyamoto W, Takao M, Yamada K, et al.: Reconstructive surgery using interference screw fixation for painful accessory navicular in adult athletes, *Arch Orthop Trauma Surg* 132:1423, 2012.

Monteagudo M, Maceira E: Posterior tibial tendoscopy, *Foot Ankle Clin N Am* 20:1, 2015.

O'Connor K, Baumhauer J, Houck JR: Patient factors in the selection of operative versus nonoperative treatment for posterior tibial tendon dysfunction, *Foot Ankle Int* 31:197, 2010.

Parsons S, Naim S, Richards PJ, McBride D: Correction and prevention of deformity in type II tibialis posterior dysfunction, *Clin Orthop Relat Res* 468:1025, 2010.

Ryssman DB, Jeng CL: Reconstruction of the spring ligament with a posterior tibial tendon autograft: technique tip, *Foot Ankle Int* 38:452, 2016.

Schepull T, Kvist J, Norman H, et al.: Autologous platelets have no effect on the healing of human Achilles tendon ruptures: a randomized single-blind study, *Am J Sports Med* 39:38, 2011.

Tickner A, Throng S, Martin M, et al.: Management of isolated anterior tibial tendon rupture: a systematic review and meta-analysis, *J Foot Ankle Surg* 58:213, 2019.

Wake J, Marin K: Posterior tibial tendon endoscopic debridement for stage I and II posterior tibial tendon dysfunction, *Arthros Tech* 6:e2019, 2017.

ADOLESCENT AND ADULT PES PLANUS

Aiyer A, Dall GF, Shub J, et al.: Radiographic correction following reconstruction of adult acquired flat foot deformity using the Cotton medial cuneiform osteotomy, *Foot Ankle Int* 37:508, 2016.

Apostle KL, Coleman NW, Sangeorzan BJ: Subtalar joint axis in patients with symptomatic peritalar subluxation compared to normal controls, *Foot Ankle Int* 35:1153, 2014.

Aynardi MC, Saloky K, Foush EP, et al.: Biomechanical evaluation of spring ligament augmentation with the fibertape device in a cadaveric flatfoot model, *Foot Ankle Int* 40:596, 2019.

Baxter JR, Demetracopoulos CA, Prado MP, et al.: Lateral column lengthening corrects hindfoot valgus in a cadaveric flatfoot model, *Foot Ankle Int* 36:705, 2015.

Brodell JD, MacDonald A, Perkins JA, et al.: Deltoid-spring ligament reconstruction in adult acquired flatfoot deformity with medial peritalar instability, *Foot Ankle Int* 40:753, 2019.

Chan JY, Greenfield ST, Soukup DS, et al.: Contribution of lateral column lengthening to correction of forefoot abduction in stage IIb adult acquired flatfoot deformity reconstruction, *Foot Ankle Int* 36:1400, 2015.

Cody EA, Williamson ER, Burket JC, et al.: Correlation of talar anatomy and subtalar joint alignment on weightbearing computed tomography with radiographic flatfoot parameters, *Foot Ankle Int* 37:874, 2016.

Conti MS, Garfinkel JH, Kunas GC, et al.: Postoperative medial cuneiform position correlation with patient-reported outcomes following Cotton osteotomy for reconstruction of the stage II adult-acquired flatfoot deformity, *Foot Ankle Int* 40:491, 2019.

Cöster MC, Rosengren BE, Bremander A, Karlsson MK: Surgery for adult acquired flatfoot due to posterior tibial tendon dysfunction reduces pain, improves function and health related quality of life, *Foot Ankle Surg* 21:286, 2015.

Demetracopoulos CA, Nair P, Malzberg A, et al.: Outcomes of a stepcut lengthening calcaneal osteotomy for adult-acquired flatfoot deformity, *Foot Ankle Int* 36:749, 2015.

Ebaugh MP, Larson DR, Reb CW, et al.: Outcomes of the extended Z-cut osteotomy for correction of adult acquired flatfoot deformity, *Foot Ankle Int* 40:914, 2019.

Ellis SJ, Deyer T, Williams BR, et al.: Assessment of lateral hindfoot pain in acquired flatfoot deformity using weightbearing multiplanar imaging, *Foot Ankle Int* 31:361, 2010.

Ellis SJ, Williams BR, Wagshul AD, et al.: Deltoid ligament reconstruction with peroneus longus autograft in flatfoot deformity, *Foot Ankle Int* 31:781, 2010.

Ellis SJ, Yu JC, Johnson AH, et al.: Plantar pressures in patients with and without lateral foot pain after lateral column lengthening, *J Bone Joint Surg* 92A:81, 2010.

Ettinger S, Mattinger T, Stukenborg-Colsman C, et al.: Outcomes of Evans versus Hintermann calcaneal lengthening osteotomy for flexible flatfoot, *Foot Ankle Int* 40:661, 2019.

Ettinger S, Sibai K, Stukenborg-Colsman C, et al.: Comparison of anatomic structures at risk with 2 lateral lengthening calcaneal osteotomies, *Foot Ankle Int* 39:1481, 2018.

Garras DN, Hansen PL, Miller AG, Raikin SM: Outcome of modified Kidner procedure with subtalar arthroereisis for painful accessory navicular associated with planovalgus deformity, *Foot Ankle Int* 33:934, 2012.

Giannini S, Cadossi M, Mazzotti A, et al.: Bioabsorbable calcaneo-stop implant for the treatment of flexible flatfoot: a retrospective cohort study at a minimum follow-up of 4 years, *J Foot Ankle Surg* 56:776, 2017.

Grier KM, Walling AK: The use of tricortical autograft versus allograft in lateral column lengthening for adult acquired flatfoot deformity: an analysis of union rates and complications, *Foot Ankle Int* 31:760, 2010.

Gross CE, Huh J, Gray J, et al.: Radiographic outcomes following lateral column lengthening with a porous titanium wedge, *Foot Ankle Int* 36:953, 2015.

Haddad SL, Myerson MS, Younger A, et al.: Symposium: adult acquired flatfoot deformity, *Foot Ankle Int* 32:95, 2011.

Iossi M, Johnson JE, McCormick JJ, Klein SE: Short-term radiographic analysis of operative correction of adult acquired flatfoot deformity, *Foot Ankle Int* 34:781, 2013.

Jegal H, Park YU, Kim JS, et al.: Accessory navicular syndrome in athletes vs general population, *Foot Ankle Int* 37:862, 2016.

Jeng CL, Bluman EM, Myerson MS: Minimally invasive deltoid ligament reconstruction for stage IV flatfoot deformity, *Foot Ankle Int* 32:21, 2011.

Jeng CL, Rutherford T, Hull MG, et al.: Assessment of bony subfibular impingement in flatfoot patients using weight-bearing CT scans, *Foot Ankle Int* 40:152, 2019.

Kendal AR, Khalid A, Ball T, et al.: Complications of minimally invasive calcaneal osteotomy versus open osteotomy, *Foot Ankle Int* 36:685, 2015.

Kheir E, Borse V, Sharpe J, et al.: Medial displacement calcaneal osteotomy using minimally invasive technique, *Foot Ankle Int* 36:248, 2015.

Kido M, Ikoma K, Hara Y, et al.: Effect of therapeutic insoles on the medial longitudinal arch in patients with flatfoot: a three-dimensional loading computed tomography study, *Clin Biomech (Bristol, Avon)* 29:1095, 2014.

Kunas GC, Do HT, Aiyer A, et al.: Contribution of medial cuneiform osteotomy to correction of longitudinal arch collapse in stage IIb adult-acquired flatfoot deformity, *Foot Ankle Int* 39:885, 2018.

Louwerens JW, Valderrabano V, Winson I: Minimal invasive surgery (MIS) in foot and ankle surgery, *Foot Ankle Surg* 17:51, 2011.

Memeo A, Verdoni F, Rossi L, et al.: Flexible juvenile flat foot surgical correction: a comparison between two techniques after ten years' experience, *J Foot Ankle Surg* 58:203, 2019.

Mengiardi B, Pinto C, Zanetti M: Spring ligament complex and posterior tibial tendon: MR anatomy and findings in acquired adult flatfoot deformity, *Semin Musculoskelet Radiol* 20:104, 2016.

Nery C, Lemos AVKC, Raduan F, et al.: Combined spring and deltoid ligament repair in adult-acquired flatfoot, *Foot Ankle Int* 39:903, 2018.

Netto CC, Grace KC, Soukup D: Correlation of clinical evaluation and radiographic hindfoot alignment in stage II adult acquired flatfoot deformity, *Foot Ankle Int* 39, 2018, 771-771.

Niki H, Hirano T, Okada H, Beppu M: Outcome of medial displacement calcaneal osteotomy for correction of acquired flatfoot, *Foot Ankle Int* 33:940, 2012.

Ormsby N, Jackson G, Evans P, et al.: Imaging of the tibionavicular ligament, and its potential role in adult acquired flatfoot deformity, *Foot Ankle Int* 39:629, 2018.

Park H, Hwang JH, Seo JO, Kim HW: The relationship between accessory navicular and flat foot: a radiologic study, *J Pediatr Orthop* 35:739, 2015.

Probasco W, Haleem AM, Yu J, et al.: Assessment of coronal plane subtalar joint alignment in peritalar subluxation via weight-bearing multiplanar imaging, *Foot Ankle Int* 36, 2015.

Pourghasem M, Kamali N, Farsi M, et al.: Prevalence of flatfoot among school students and its relationship with BMI, *Acta Orthop Traumatol Turcica* 50:554, 2016.

Saunders SM, Ellis SJ, Demetracopoulos CA, et al.: Comparative outcomes between stepcut lengthening calcaneal osteotomy vs traditional Evans osteotomy for stage IIB adult-acquired flatfoot deformity, *Foot Ankle Int* 39:18, 2018.

Scott R, Berlet G: Calcaneal Z osteotomy for extra-articular correction of hindfoot valgus, *J Foot Ankle Surg* 52:406, 2013.

Sensiba PR, Coffey MJ, Williams NE, et al.: Inter- and intraobserver reliability in the radiographic evaluation of adult flatfoot deformity, *Foot Ankle Int* 31:141, 2010.

Sherman TI, Guyton GP: Minimal Incision/minimally invasive medializing displacement calcaneal osteotomy, *Foot Ankle Int* 39:119, 2017.

Soukup DS, MacMahon A, Burket JC, et al.: Effect of obesity on clinical and radiographic outcomes following reconstruction of stage II adult acquired flatfoot deformity, *Foot Ankle Int* 37:245, 2016.

Steginsky B, Vora A: What to do with the spring ligament, *Foot Ankle Clin N Am* 22:515, 2017.

Steiner CS, Gilgen A, Zwicky L, et al.: Combined subtalar and naviculocuneiform fusion for treating adult acquired flatfoot deformity without medial arch collapse at the level of the naviculocuneiform joint, *Foot Ankle Int* 40(1):42, 2019.

Vander Griend R: Lateral column lengthening using a "Z" osteotomy of the calcaneus, *Tech Foot Ankle Surg* 7:257, 2008.

Vosseller JT, Ellis SJ, O'Malley MJ, et al.: Autograft and allograft unite similarly in lateral column lengthening for adult acquired flatfoot deformity, *HSS J* 9:6, 2013.

Williams BR, Ellis SJ, Deyer TW, et al.: Reconstruction of the spring ligament using a peroneus longus autograft tendon transfer, *Foot Ankle Int* 31:567, 2010.

Williamson ER, Chan JY, Burket JC, et al.: New radiographic parameter assessing hindfoot alignment in stage II adult-acquired flatfoot deformity, *Foot Ankle Int* 36:417, 2015.

Zanolli DH, Glisson RR, Nunley 2nd JA, Easley ME: Biomechanical assessment of flexible flatfoot correction: comparison of techniques in a cadaver model, *J Bone Joint Surg* 96A:e45, 2014.

Zanolli DH, Glisson RR, Utturkas GM, et al.: Calcaneal "Z" osteotomy effect on hindfoot varus after triple arthrodesis in a cadaver model, *Foot Ankle Int* 35:1350, 2014.

RIGID FLATFOOT AND TARSAL COALITION

Aibinder WR, Young EY, Milbrandt TA: Intraoperative three-dimensional navigation for talocalcaneal coalition resection, *J Foot Ankle Surg* 56:1091, 2017.

Aldahshan W, Hamed A, Elsherief F, et al.: Endoscopic resection of different types of talocalcaneal coalition, *Foot Ankle Int* 39:1082, 2018.

Cass AD, Camasta CA: A review of tarsal coalition and pes planovalgus: clinical examination, diagnostic imaging, and surgical planning, *J Foot Ankle Surg* 49:274, 2010.

Chou LB, Halligan BW: Treatment of severe, painful pes planovalgus deformity with hindfoot arthrodesis and wedge-shaped tricortical allograft, *Foot Ankle Int* 28:569, 2007.

Gantsoudes GD, Roocroft JH, Mubarak SJ: Treatment of talocalcaneal coalitions, *J Pediatr Orthop* 32:301, 2012.

Hubert J, Hawellek T, Beil FT, et al.: Resection of medial talocalcaneal coalition with Interposition of a pediculated flap of tibialis posterior tendon sheath, *Foot Ankle Int* 39:935, 2018.

Javier Masquijo J, Vazquez I, Allende V, et al.: Surgical reconstruction for talocalcaneal coalitions with severe hindfoot valgus deformity, *J Pediatr Orthop* 37:293, 2017.

Khoshbin A, Law PW, Caspi L, Wright JG: Long-term functional outcomes of resected tarsal coalitions, *Foot Ankle Int* 34:1370, 2013.

Klammer G, Espinosa N, Iselin LD: Coalitions of the tarsal bones, *Foot Ankle Clin* 23:435, 2018.

Lisella JM, Bellapianta JM, Manoli 2nd A: Tarsal coalition resection with pes planovalgus hindfoot reconstruction, *J Surg Orthop Adv* 20:102, 2011.

Mahan ST, Prete VI, Spencer SA, et al.: Subtalar coalitions: does the morphology of the subtalar joint involvement influence outcomes after coalition excision? *J Foot Ankle Surg* 56:797, 2017.

Mahan ST, Spencer SA, Vezeridis PS, Kasser JR: Patient-reported outcomes of tarsal coalitions treated with surgical excision, *J Pediatr Orthop* 35:583, 2015.

Moraleda L, Gantsoudes GD, Mubarak SJ: C sign: talocalcaneal coalition or flatfoot deformity? *J Pediatr Orthop* 34:814, 2014.

Mosca VS, Bevan WP: Talocalcaneal tarsal coalitions and the calcaneal lengthening osteotomy: the role of deformity correction, *J Bone Joint Surg* 94A:1584, 2012.

Quinn EA, Peterson KS, Hyer CF: Calcaneonavicular coalition resection with pes planovalgus reconstruction, *J Foot Ankle Surg* 55:578, 2016.

Rocchi V, Huang MT, Bomar JD, et al.: The "double medial malleolus": a new physical finding in talocalcaneal coalition, *J Pediatr Orthop* 38:239, 2018.

SUBTALAR ARTHROEREISIS

Chong DY, Macwilliams BA, Hennessey TA, et al.: Prospective comparison of subtalar arthroereisis with lateral column lengthening for painful flatfeet, *J Pediatr Orthop B* 24:345, 2015.

Martinelli N, Bianchi A, Martinkevich P, et al.: Return to sport activities after subtalar arthroereisis for correction of pediatric flexible flatfoot, *J Pediatr Orthop B* 27:82, 2018.

Metcalfe SA, Bowling L, Reeves ND: Subtalar joint arthroereisis in the management of pediatric flexible flatfoot: a critical review of the literature, *Foot Ankle Int* 32:1127, 2011.

Ortiz CA, Wagner E, Wagner P: Arthroereisis: what have we learned? *Foot Ankle Clin* 23:415, 2018.

Scharer BM, Black BE, Sockrider N: Treatment of painful pediatric flatfoot with Maxwell-Brancheau subtalar arthroereisis implant: a retrospective radiographic review, *Foot Ankle Spec* 3:67, 2010.

van Ooij B, Vos CJ, Saouti R: Arthroereisis of the subtalar joint: an uncommon complication and literature review, *J Foot Ankle Surg* 51:114, 2012.

ACHILLES TENDON

Akoh CC, Phisitkul P: Minimally invasive and endoscopic approach for the treatment of noninsertional Achilles tendinopathy, *Foot Ankle Clin* 24:495, 2019.

Alfredson H, Spang C, Forsgren S: Unilateral surgical treatment for patients with midportion Achilles tendinopathy may result in bilateral recovery, *Br J Sports Med* 48:1421, 2014.

Baltes TP, Zwiers R, Wiegerinck JI, van Dijk CN: Surgical treatment for midportion Achilles tendinopathy: a systematic review, *Knee Surg Sports Traumatol Arthrosc* 25:1817, 2017.

Barg A, Ludwig T: Surgical strategies for the treatment of insertional Achilles tendinopathy, *Foot Ankle Clin* 24:533, 2019.

Bedi HS, Jowett C, Ristanis S, et al.: Plantaris excision and ventral paratendinous scraping for Achilles tendinopathy in an athletic population, *Foot Ankle Int* 37:386, 2016.

Beyer R, Kongsgaard M, Kjaer BH, et al.: Heavy slow resistance versus eccentric training as treatment for Achilles tendinopathy, *Am J Sports Med* 43:1704, 2015.

Bulstra GH, van Rheenen TA, Scholtes VA: Can we measure the heel bump? Radiographic evaluation of Haglund's deformity, *J Foot Ankle Surg* 54:338, 2015.

Bussin ER, Cairns B, Bovard J, et al.: Randomized controlled trial evaluating the short term analgesic effect of topical diclofenac on chronic Achilles tendon pain: a pilot study, *BMJ Open* 7:e05126, 2017.

Chimenti RL, Cychosz CC, Hall MM, et al.: Current concepts review update: insertional Achilles tendinopathy, *Foot Ankle Int* 38:1160, 2017.

de Cesar Netto C, Chinanuvathana A, Fonseca LFD, et al.: Outcomes of flexor digitorum longus (FDL) tendon transfer in the treatment of Achilles tendon disorders, *Foot Ankle Surg* 25:303, 2019.

de Jong S, de Vos RJ, Weir A, et al.: One-year follow-up of platelet-rich plasma treatment in chronic Achilles tendinopathy: a double-blind randomized placebo-controlled trial, *Am J Sports Med* 39:1623, 2011.

de Jong S, van den Berg C, de Vos RJ, et al.: Incidence of midportion Achilles tendinopathy in the general population, *Br J Sports Med* 45:1026, 2011.

de Vos RJ, Weir A, Tol JL, et al.: No effects of PRP on ultrasonographic tendon structure and neovascularisation in chronic midportion Achilles tendinopathy, *Br J Sports Med* 45:387, 2011.

de Vos RJ, Weir A, van Schie HT, et al.: Platelet-rich plasma injection for chronic Achilles tendinopathy: a randomized controlled trial, *J Am Med Assoc* 303:144, 2010.

Ettinger S, Razzaq R, Waizy H, et al.: Operative treatment of the insertional Achilles tendinopathy through a transtendinous approach, *Foot Ankle Int* 37:288, 2016.

Georgiannos D, Lampridis V, Vasiliadis A, et al.: Treatment of insertional Achilles pathology with dorsal wedge calcaneal osteotomy in athletes, *Foot Ankle Int* 38:381, 2017.

Gross CE, Hsu AR, Chahal J, Holmes Jr GB: Injectable treatments for noninsertional Achilles tendinosis: a systematic review, *Foot Ankle Int* 34:619, 2013.

Gurdezi S, Kohls-Gatzoulis J, Solan MC: Results of proximal medial gastrocnemius release for Achilles tendinopathy, *Foot Ankle Int* 34:1364, 2013.

Hedgewald KW, Doyle MD, Todd NW, Rush SM: Minimally invasive approach to Achilles tendon pathology, *J Foot Ankle Surg* 55:166, 2016.

Hunt KJ, Cohen BE, Davis H, et al.: Surgical treatment of insertional Achilles tendinopathy with or without flexor halluces longus tendon transfer: a prospective, randomized study, *Foot Ankle Int* 36:998, 2015.

Indino C, D'Ambrosi R, Usuelli FG: Biologics in the treatment of Achilles tendon pathologies, *Foot Ankle Clin* 24:471, 2019.

Irwin TA: Current concepts review: insertional Achilles tendinopathy, *Foot Ankle Int* 31:933, 2010.

Kang S, Thordarson DB, Charlton TP: Insertional Achilles tendinitis and Haglund's deformity, *Foot Ankle Int* 33:487, 2012.

Kearney R, Costa ML: Insertional Achilles tendinopathy management: a systematic review, *Foot Ankle Int* 31:689, 2010.

Kiewiet NJ, Holthusen SM, Bohay DR, Anderson JG: Gastrocnemius recession for chronic noninsertional Achilles tendinopathy, *Foot Ankle Int* 34:481, 2013.

Krogh T, Ellingsen T, Christensen R: Ultrasound guided injection therapy of Achilles tendinopathy with PRP or saline, *Am J Sports Med* 44:1990, 2016.

Leduc S, Walling AK: Posterior midline approach for treatment of Achilles calcific insertional tendonopathy, *Tech Foot Ankle* 9:271, 2010.

Lohrer H, Davis S, Nauck T: Surgical treatment for Achilles tendinopathy—a systematic review, *BMC Musculoskelet Disord* 17:207, 2016.

Lui TH: Treatment of chronic noninsertional Achilles tendinopathy with endoscopic Achilles tendon debridement and flexor hallucis longus transfer, *Foot Ankle Spec* 5:195, 2012.

Lui TH, Lo CY, Siu YC: Minimally invasive and endoscopic treatment of Haglund syndrome, *Foot Ankle Clin* 24:515, 2019.

Maffulli N, Del Buono A, Testa V, et al.: Safety and outcome of surgical debridement of insertional Achilles tendinopathy using a transverse (Cincinnati) incision, *J Bone Joint Surg* 93B:1503, 2011.

McCormack JR, Underwood FB, Slaven EJ, Cappaert TA: Eccentric exercise versus eccentric exercise and soft tissue treatment (Astym) in the management of insertional Achilles tendinopathy: a randomized controlled trial, *Sports Health* 8:230, 2016.

McGarvey WC, Palumbo RC, Baxter DE, et al.: Insertional Achilles tendinosis: surgical treatment through a central tendon splitting approach, *Foot Ankle Int* 23:19, 2002.

Molund M, Lapinskas SR, Nilsen FA, et al.: Clinical and functional outcomes of gastrocnemius recession for chronic Achilles tendinopathy, *Foot Ankle Int* 37:1091, 2016.

Monto RR: Platelet rich plasma treatment for chronic Achilles tendinosis, *Foot Ankle Int* 33:379, 2012.

Nawoczenski DA, Barske H, Tome J, et al.: Isolated gastrocnemius recession for Achilles tendinopathy: strength and functional outcomes, *J Bone Joint Surg* 97A:99, 2015.

Nawoczenski DA, DiLiberto FE, Cantor MS, et al.: Ankle power and endurance outcomes following isolated gastrocnemius recession for Achilles tendinopathy, *Foot Ankle Int* 37:766, 2016.

Nunley JA, Ruskin G, Horst F: Long-term clinical outcomes following the central incision technique for insertional Achilles tendinopathy, *Foot Ankle Int* 32:850, 2011.

Rousseau R, Gerometta A, Fogerty S, et al.: Results of surgical treatment of calcaneus insertional tendinopathy in middle and long distance runners, *Knee Surg Sports Traumataol Arthrosc* 23:2494, 2015.

Saxena A, Hong BK, Hofer D: Peritenolysis and debridement for main body (mid-portion) Achilles tendinopathy in athletic patients: results of 107 procedures, *J Foot Ankle Surg* 56:922, 2017.

Schon LC, Shores JL, Faro FD, et al.: Flexor hallucis longus tendon transfer in treatment of Achilles tendinosis, *J Bone Joint Surg* 95A:54, 2013.

Shakked RJ, Raikin SM: Insertional tendinopathy of the Achilles: debridement, primary repair, and when to augment, *Foot Ankle Clin* 22:761, 2017.

Silbernagel KG, Brorsson A, Lundberg M: The majority of patients with Achilles tendinopathy recover fully when treated with exercise along: a 5-year follow-up, *Am J Sports Med* 39:607, 2011.

Singh A, Calafi A, Diefenbach C, et al.: Noninsertional tendinopathy of the Achilles, *Foot Ankle Clin* 22:745, 2017.

Sullivan J, Burns J, Adams R, et al.: Musculoskeletal and activity-related factors associated with plantar heel pain, *Foot Ankle Int* 36:37, 2015.

Taylor J, Dunkerley S, Silver D, et al.: Extracorporeal shockwave therapy (ESWT) for refractory Achilles tendinopathy: a prospective audit with 2-year follow up, *Foot* 26:23, 2016.

Tickner A, Throng S, Martin M, et al.: Management of isolated anterior tibial tendon rupture: a systematic review and meta-analysis, *J Foot Ankle Surg* 58:213, 2019.

Verrall G, Schofield S, Brustad T: Chronic Achilles tendinopathy treated with eccentric stretching program, *Foot Ankle Int* 32:843, 2011.

Vega J, Baduell A, Malagelada F, et al.: Endoscopic Achilles tendon augmentation with suture anchors after calcaneal exostectomy in Haglund syndrome, *Foot Ankle Int* 39:551, 2018.

Wagner P, Wagner E, Ortiz C, et al.: Achilles tendoscopy for non- insertional Achilles tendinopathy: a case series study, *Foot Ankle Surg*, 2019 May 18, [Epub ahead of print].

Yan R, Gu Y, Ran J, et al.: Intratendon delivery of leukocyte-poor PRP improves healing compared with leukocyte-rich PRP in a rabbit Achilles tendinopathy model, *Am J Sports Med* 45:1909, 2017.

Yeo A, Kendal N, Jayaraman S: Ultrasound-guided dry needling with percutaneous paratenon decompression for chronic Achilles tendinopathy, *Knee Surg Sports Traumatol Arthros* 24:2118, 2016.

PERONEAL TENDONS

Cho J, Kim JY, Song DG, Lee WC: Comparison of outcome after retinaculum repair with and without fibular groove deepening for recurrent dislocation of the peroneal tendons, *Foot Ankle Int* 35:683, 2014.

Demetracopoulos CA, Vineyard JC, Kiesau CD, Nunley 2nd JA: Long-term results of debridement and primary repair of peroneal tendon tears, *Foot Ankle Int* 35:252, 2014.

Jockel JR, Brodsky JW: Single-stage flexor tendon transfer for the treatment of severe concomitant peroneus longus and brevis tendon tears, *Foot Ankle Int* 34:666, 2013.

Lui TH, Tse LF: Peroneal tendoscopy, *Foot Ankle Clin N Am* 20:15, 2015.

Mirmiran R, Squire C, Wassell D: Prevalence and role of a low-lying peroneus brevis muscle belly in patients with peroneal tendon pathologic features: a potential source of tendon subluxation, *J Foot Ankle Surg* 54:872, 2015.

Miyamoto W, Takao M, Miki S, Giza E: Tendoscopic repair of the superior peroneal retinaculum via 2 portals for peroneal tendon instability, *Foot Ankle Int* 36(10):1243, 2015.

Mook WR, Parekh SG, Nunley JA: Allograft reconstruction of peroneal tendons: operative technique and clinical outcomes, *Foot Ankle Int* 34:1212, 2013.

O'Neil JT, Pedowitz DI, Kerbel YE, et al.: Peroneal tendon abnormalities on routine magnetic resonance imaging of the foot and ankle, *Foot Ankle Int* 37:743, 2016.

Pellegrini MJ, Glisson RR, Matsumoto T, et al.: Effectiveness of allograft reconstruction vs tenodesis for irreparable peroneus brevis tears: a cadaveric model, *Foot Ankle Int* 37:803, 2016.

Raikin SM, Schick FA, Karanjia HN: Use of a Hunter rod for staged reconstruction of peroneal tendons, *J Foot Ankle Surg* 55:198, 2016.

Rapley JH, Crates J, Barber A: Mid-substance peroneal tendon defects augmented with an acellular dermal matrix allograft, *Foot Ankle Int* 31:136, 2010.

Rietveld A, Boni BM, Hagemans FMT, et al.: Results of treatment of posterior ankle impingement syndrome and flexor hallucis longus tendinopathy in dancers: a systematic review, *J Dance Med Sci* 22:19, 2018.

Seybold JD, Campbell JT, Jeng CL, et al.: Outcome of lateral transfer of FHL or FDL for concomitant peroneal tendon tears, *Foot Ankle Int* 37:576, 2016.

Steginsky B, Riley A, Lucas DE, et al.: Patient-reported outcomes and return to activity after peroneus brevis repair, *Foot Ankle Int* 37:178, 2016.

Stockton KG, Brodsky JW: Peroneus longus tears associated with pathology of the os peroneum, *Foot Ankle Int* 35:346, 2014.

Valerio VL, Seijas R, Alvarez P, et al.: Endoscopic repair of posterior ankle impingement syndrome due to os trigonum in soccer players, *Foot Ankle Int* 36(1):70, 2015.

Vosseller JT, Dennis ER, Bronner S: Ankle injuries in dancers, *J Am Acad Orthop Surg* 27:582, 2019.

Zhenbo Z, Jin W, Haifeng G, et al.: Sliding fibular graft repair for the treatment of recurrent peroneal subluxation, *Foot Ankle Int* 35:496, 2014.

Ziai P, Sabeti-Aschraf M, Fehske K, et al.: Treatment of peroneal tendon dislocation and coexisting medial and lateral ligamentous laxity in the ankle joint, *Knee Surg Sports Traumatol Arthrosc* 19:1004, 2011.

FLEXOR TENDONS

Corte-Real NM, Moreira RM, Guerra-Pinto F: Arthroscopic treatment of tenosynovitis of the flexor hallucis longus tendon, *Foot Ankle Int* 33:1108, 2012.

Lui TH: Arthroscopic synovectomy for zone 2 flexor hallucis longus tenosynovitis, *Arthrosc Tech* 4:ee403, 2015.

Miyamoto W, Takao M, Matsushita T: Hindfoot endoscopy for posterior ankle impingement syndrome and flexor hallucis hallucis longus tendon disorders, *Foot Ankle Clin* 20:139, 2015.

Ogut T, Ayhan E: Hindfoot endoscopy for accessory flexor digitorum longus and flexor hallucis longus tenosynovitis, *Foot Ankle Surg* 17:e7, 2011.

Rungprai C, Tennant JN, Phisitkul P: Disorders of the flexor hallucis longus and os trigonum, *Clin Sports Med* 34:741, 2015.

PAINFUL HEEL (PLANTAR FASCIITIS)

Abbassian A, Kohis-Gatzoulis J, Solan MC: Proximal gastrocnemius release in the treatment of recalcitrant plantar fasciitis, *Foot Ankle Int* 33:14, 2012.

Ahmad J, Ahmad SH, Jones K: Treatment of plantar fasciitis with botulinum toxin, *Foot Ankle Int* 38(1):1, 2017.

Ahmad J, Karim A, Daniel JN: Relationship and classification of plantar heel spurs in patients with plantar fasciitis, *Foot Ankle Int* 37(9):994, 2016.

Al-Abbad H, Simon JV: The effectiveness of extracorporeal shock wave therapy on chronic Achilles tendinopathy: a systematic review, *Foot Ankle Int* 34:33, 2013.

Aqil A, Siddiqui MR, Solan M, et al.: Extracorporeal shock wave therapy is effective in treating chronic plantar fasciitis: a meta-analysis of RCTs, *Clin Orthop Relat Res* 471:3645, 2013.

Bader L, Park K, Gu Y, O'Malley MJ: Functional outcome of endoscopic plantar fasciotomy, *Foot Ankle Int* 33:37, 2012.

Barrett SL: Endoscopic plantar fasciotomy: surgical technique, *Tech Foot Ankle Surg* 10:56, 2011.

Bolivar YA, Munuera PV, Padillo JP: Relationship between tightness of the posterior muscles of the lower limb and plantar fasciitis, *Foot Ankle Int* 34:42, 2013.

Brook J, Dauphinee DM, Korpinen J, Raw IM: Pulsed radiofrequency electromagnetic field therapy: a potential novel treatment of plantar fasciitis, *J Foot Ankle Surg* 51:312, 2012.

Cazzell S, Stewart J, Agnew PS, et al.: Randomized controlled trial of micronized dehydrated human amnion/chorion membrane (dHACM) injection compared to placebo for the treatment of plantar fasciitis, *Foot Ankle Int* 39(1):1151, 2018.

Celik D, Kus G, Sirma SÖ: Joint mobilization and stretching exercise vs steroid injection in the treatment of plantar fasciitis: a randomized controlled study, *Foot Ankle Int* 37:150, 2016.

Chimutengwende-Gordon M, O'Donnell P, Singh D: Magnetic resonance imaging in plantar heel pain, *Foot Ankle Int* 31:865, 2010.

Cottom JM, Maker JM: Endoscopic debridement for treatment of chronic plantar fasciitis: an innovative surgical technique, *J Foot Ankle Surg* 55(3):655, 2016.

David JA, Sankarapandian V, Christopher PR, Chatterjee A, Macaden AS: Injected corticosteroids for treating plantar heel pain in adults, *Cochrane Database Syst Rev* 6:CD009348, 2017.

De Prado M, Cuervas-Mons M, De Prado V, Golanó P, Vaquero J: Does the minimally invasive complete plantar fasciotomy result in deformity of the Plantar arch? A prospective study, *Foot Ankle Surg*, 2019 Apr 27. pii: S1268-7731.

DiGiovanni BF, Moore AM, Ziotnicki JP, Pinney SJ: Preferred management of recalcitrant plantar fasciitis among orthopaedic foot and ankle surgeons, *Foot Ankle Int* 33:507, 2012.

El Shazly O, El Beltagy A: Endoscopic plantar fascia release, calcaneal drilling and calcaneal spur removal for management of painful heel syndrome, *Foot (Edinb)* 20:121, 2010.

Fernández-Roriguez T, Fernández-Rolle Á, Truyols-Domínguez S, Benítez-Martínez JC, Casaña-Granell J: Prospective randomized trial of electrolysis for chronic plantar heel pain, *Foot Ankle Int* 39(9):1039, 2018.

Ficke B, Elattar O, Naranje SM, Araoye I, Shah AB: Gastrocnemius recession for recalcitrant plantar fasciitis in overweight and obese patients, *Foot Ankle Surg* 34(6):471, 2018.

Gibbons R, Mackie KE, Beveridge T, Hince D, Ammon P: Evaluation of long-term outcomes following plantar fasciotomy, *Foot Ankle Int* 39:1312, 2018.

Iborra-Marcos Á, Ramos-Álarez JJ, Rodriguez-Fabián G, et al.: Intratissue percutaneous electrolysis vs corticosteroid infiltration for the treatment of plantar fasciosis, *Foot Ankle Int* 39(6):704, 2018.

Ibrahim MI, Donatelli RA, Schmitz C, et al.: Chronic plantar fasciitis treated with two sessions of radial extracorporeal shock wave therapy, *Foot Ankle Int* 31:391, 2010.

Jastifer JR, Catena F, Doty JF, et al.: Low-level laser therapy for the treatment of chronic plantar fasciitis: a prospective study, *Foot Ankle Int* 35:566, 2014.

Jain SK, Suprashant K, Kumar S, Yadav A, Kearns SR: Comparison of plantar fasciitis injected with platelet-rich plasma vs corticosteroids, *Foot Ankle Int* 39(7):780, 2018.

Jiménez-Pérez AE, Gonzalez-Arabio D, Diaz AS, Maderuelo JA, Ramos-Pascua LR: Clinical and imaging effects of corticosteroids and platelet-rich plasma for the treatment of chronic plantar fasciitis: a comparative non randomized prospective study, *Foot Ankle Surg* 25(3):354, 2019.

Johannsen F, Konradsen L, Herzog R, Rindom Krogsgaard M: Plantar fasciitis treated with endoscopic partial plantar fasciotomy-One-year clinical and ultrasonographic follow-up, *Foot (Edinb)* 39:50, 2019.

MacInnes A, Roberts SC, Kimpton J, Pillai A: Long-term outcome of open plantar fascia release, *Foot Ankle Int* 37:17, 2016.

Malahias MA, Cantiller EB, Kadu VV, Müller S: The clinical outcome of endoscopic plantar fascia release: a current concept review, *Foot Ankle Surg.* pii: S1268-7731, 2018.

Mahindra P, Yamin M, Selhi HS, et al.: Chronic plantar fasciitis: effect of platelet-rich plasma, corticosteroid, and placebo, *Orthopedics* 39:e285, 2016.

Maskill JD, Bohay DR, Anderson JG: Gastrocnemius recession to treat isolated foot pain, *Foot Ankle Int* 31:19, 2010.

Metzner G, Dohnalek C, Aigner E: High-energy extracorporeal shock-wave therapy (ESWT) for the treatment of chronic plantar fasciitis, *Foot Ankle Int* 31:790, 2010.

Mishra BN, Poudel RR, Banskota B, Shrestha BK, Banskota AK: Effectiveness of extra-corporeal shock wave therapy (ESWT) vs methylprednisolone injections in plantar fasciitis, *J Clin Orthop Trauma* 10(2):401, 2019.

Miyamoto W, Takao M, Uchio Y: Calcaneal osteotomy for the treatment of plantar fasciitis, *Arch Orthop Trauma Surg* 130:151, 2010.

Molund M, Husebye EE, Hellesnes J, Nilsen F, Hvaal K: Proximal medial gastrocnemius recession and stretching versus stretching as treatment of chronic plantar heel pain, *Foot Ankle Int* 39(12):1423, 2018.

Monto RR: Platelet-rich plasma efficacy versus corticosteroid injection treatment for chronic severe plantar fasciitis, *Foot Ankle Int* 35:313, 2014.

Nakale NT, Strydom A, Saragas NP, Ferrao PNF: Association between plantar fasciitis and isolated gastrocnemius tightness, *Foot Ankle Int* 39(3):271, 2018.

Peterlein CD, Funk JF, Hölscher A, et al.: Is botulinum toxin A effective for the treatment of plantar fasciitis? *Clin J Pain* 28:527, 2012.

Purcell RL, Schroeder IG, Keeling LE, et al.: Clinical outcomes after extracorporeal shock wave therapy for chronic plantar fasciitis in a predominantly active duty population, *J Foot Ankle Surg* 57(4):654, 2018.

Shetty SH, Dhond A, Arora M, Deore S: Platelet-rich plasma has better long-term results than corticosteroids or placebo for chronic plantar fasciitis: randomized control trial, *J Foot Ankle Surg* 58(1):42, 2019.

Taş S, Bek N, Onur R, Korkusuz F: Effects of body mass index on mechanical properties of the plantar fascia and heel pad in asymptomatic participants, *Foot Ankle Int* 38(7):779, 2017.

Tong KB, Furia J: Economic burden of plantar fasciitis treatment in the United States, *Am J Orthop* 39:227, 2010.

Tsikopoulos K, Vasiliadis HS, Mavridis D: Injection therapies for plantar fasciopathy ("plantar fasciitis"): a systematic review and network meta-analysis of 22 randomised controlled trials, *Br J Sports Med* 50:1367, 2016.

Yin MC, Ye J, Yao M, et al.: Is extracorporeal shock wave therapy clinical efficacy for relief of chronic, recalcitrant plastar fasciitis? A systematic review and meta-analysis of randomized placebo or active-treatment controlled trials, *Arch Phys Med Rehabil* 95:1585, 2014.

The complete list of references is available online at ExpertConsult.inkling.com.

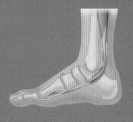
METATARSOPHALANGEAL JOINT INSTABILITY
ETIOLOGY

Deformity of the lesser toes, particularly of the second toe, sometimes is related to instability of the metatarsophalangeal joint. This disorder, which ranges in severity from synovitis of the metatarsophalangeal joint to dislocation and chronic deformity (hammer toe, claw toe, or crossover toe), has become a well-recognized problem. Lesser toe deformities are frequent in women older than the age of 50 years who wear constrictive high-heeled shoes and in athletes with chronic overuse and hyperextension of the toes. Coughlin's extensive review of crossover toe deformity (which commonly involves some element of metatarsophalangeal synovitis) found the following associative factors: women older than age 50 years, hallux valgus, and degenerative changes in the first metatarsophalangeal joint. The most consistent physical finding was the presence of a positive drawer sign or Lachman test (Fig. 4.1). Although the commonly held belief is that instability and synovitis are associated with an excessively long second metatarsal, this has been called into question. The traditional technique of measurement of second metatarsal length described by Morton involves a line drawn across the articular surfaces of metatarsals 1 and 3 (Fig. 4.2A). The Hardy and Clapham method (Fig. 4.2B) gives a different analysis of second metatarsal length. Weber et al., in a cadaver study evaluating the length of the second metatarsal, found a significant correlation between increased forefoot pressure and medial deviation of the second toe. Bhutta et al. found that a correlation between second metatarsal length as a causative factor and a metatarsophalangeal pathologic process depends

largely on the method of measurement. This question is not a trivial one because the treatment decision often involves whether to shorten the metatarsal. Hallux valgus often is associated with metatarsophalangeal joint instability, but the most likely causes of instability are attritional changes in the lateral collateral ligament, capsule, and plantar plate. These changes more likely are caused by chronic synovitis and not by pressure from the deformity of the hallux. Other causes of instability include chronic synovitis from systemic arthritis, neuromuscular disease causing muscular imbalance, and acute traumatic disruptions of the plantar plate and collateral ligaments.

ANATOMY AND BIOMECHANICS

The most common site of synovitis, instability, and development of fixed toe deformity is the second metatarsophalangeal joint. Normal toe position depends on dynamic and static restraints. The most powerful extension force on the joint is delivered by the extensor digitorum longus tendon, which extends the metatarsophalangeal joint through a fibroaponeurotic sling that attaches plantarly to the plantar plate and capsule and suspends the phalanx (Fig. 4.3). The extensor digitorum longus tendon is able to extend the interphalangeal joints of the toe only when the metatarsophalangeal joint is in a neutral or flexed position. If a toe is held in an extended position, such as in a high-heeled shoe, the extensor digitorum longus becomes a deforming force on the metatarsophalangeal joint.

Flexion of the metatarsophalangeal joint primarily is a function of the intrinsic muscles. The second toe is unique in that there are two dorsal interossei and no plantar interossei. Normally, the axis of the pull of these muscles

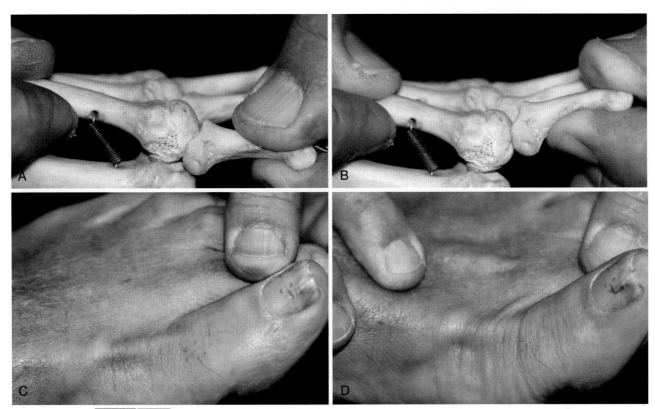

FIGURE 4.1 Lachman test of metatarsophalangeal joint stability. **A,** Starting position. **B,** Positive Lachman test of metatarsophalangeal joint. **C,** Starting position for examination. **D,** Positive test with visible and palpable subluxation of joint. (**A** and **B** from Thompson FM, Hamilton WG: Problems of the second metatarsophalangeal joint, Orthopedics 10:83, 1987.)

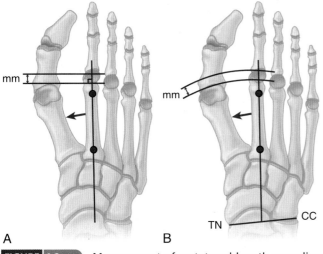

FIGURE 4.2 Measurement of metatarsal length according to the methods of Morton **(A)** and Hardy and Clapham **(B)**. CC, Calcaneocuboid joint; TN, talonavicular joint.

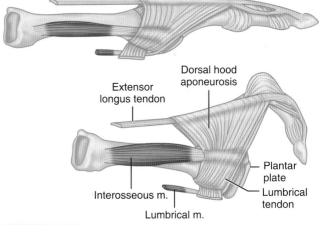

FIGURE 4.3 Anatomy of extrinsic and intrinsic musculature of metatarsophalangeal joint.

is plantar to the center of rotation of the metatarsophalangeal joint. As the metatarsophalangeal joint becomes chronically extended, however, the line of action moves dorsal to the center of rotation of the metatarsophalangeal joint, and these tendons become a deforming force for dorsal subluxation.

The lumbrical muscle is located on the medial side of the joint and axis and acts as an unopposed adductor of the toe. Although the lumbrical muscle normally passes plantar to the transverse intermetatarsal ligament and acts as a plantar flexor of the metatarsophalangeal joint, with chronic extension deformity it becomes ineffective as a plantar flexor.

Static restraints for joint stability include the collateral ligaments and the plantar plate, coupled with dynamic pull from the intrinsic muscles. The plantar plate, which originates partially as a thin synovial attachment in continuity with the periosteum of the metatarsal metaphysis, provides most of the stabilizing force. A firm fibrocartilaginous attachment inserts onto the base of the proximal phalanx adjacent to the articular cartilage. A cadaver study determined that the plantar plate is approximately 2 cm long, 1 cm wide, and 2 to 5 mm thick. The medial and lateral borders of the plate are thicker than the central portion, except for a broad thickened portion directly plantar to the metatarsal head.

The plantar plate has a number of important attachments, including the collateral ligaments, the plantar fascia, the fibrous sheath of the flexor tendons, the interossei tendons, and the deep transverse metatarsal ligament. Several cadaver studies have evaluated the effects on joint stability of sectioning various structures around the lesser metatarsophalangeal joints. Reported contributions to dorsal translation stability for the plantar plate have ranged from 19% to 34% and for the collateral ligaments, 37% to 46%. Wang et al. found that bilateral sectioning of the deep transverse metatarsal ligament produced significant instability of the lesser metatarsophalangeal joints. Each of the collateral ligaments that insert onto the plantar plate has two distinct portions: the proper collateral ligament, which inserts at the base of the proximal

phalanx, and the accessory collateral ligament, which inserts onto the plantar plate (Fig. 4.4). Barg et al. found that insufficiency of the accessory collateral ligament leads to the most severe instability.

Chronic irritation of the joint and subsequent synovitis and joint effusion cause attritional degeneration, lengthening, and eventual rupture of these structures, especially the lateral collateral ligament and plantar plate, and subsequent instability. On the basis of their research and the research of other authors, Doty and Coughlin concluded that the plantar plate is the primary stabilizing structure that is the first to fail. The collateral ligaments also may fail in time, contributing to the transverse and sagittal plane malalignment of the toe.

DIAGNOSIS

Patients with synovitis and instability of the metatarsophalangeal joint usually have an insidious, slowly progressive course of metatarsalgia, especially when wearing high-heeled shoes. Occasionally, neuritic symptoms may be present in the second web space, with radiation into the second and third toes. It must be emphasized that pain in this area is far more likely to be from the metatarsophalangeal joint than from an associated interdigital neuroma. Some patients, especially athletes, may remember an acute hyperextension injury to the foot that began the cycle of pain. Initially, pain occurs with weight bearing, but as the problem progresses, some patients have pain with rest. In the later stages of deformity, patients may have an antalgic gait pattern and compensate by shifting weight to the lateral column of the foot.

On examination, a hammer toe or crossover toe may or may not be present. Usually, some swelling of the joint manifests by the loss of contour of the long extensor tendon compared with the adjacent toes. Often a palpable effusion is present in the joint (Fig. 4.5). Tenderness may be present in the dorsofibular side of the joint or the plantar plate directly beneath and just proximal to the metatarsal head. The Lachman (drawer) test is helpful in assessing dorsal-plantar instability (see Fig. 4.1). Limited motion of the joint usually is apparent, especially in flexion, compared with the contralateral toe. Clinical staging of instability defines the severity of the subluxation and is rated on a scale of 0 to 4 (Table 4.1). Interestingly, Klein et al. found that a positive

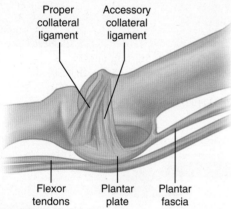

Proper collateral ligament   Accessory collateral ligament

Flexor tendons   Plantar plate   Plantar fascia

FIGURE 4.4 Location of plantar plate, flexor tendons, and collateral ligaments in relation to metatarsophalangeal joint. (Redrawn from Doty JF, Coughlin MJ: Metatarsophalangeal joint instability of the lesser toes and plantar plate deficiency, J Am Acad Orthop Surg 22:235, 2014.)

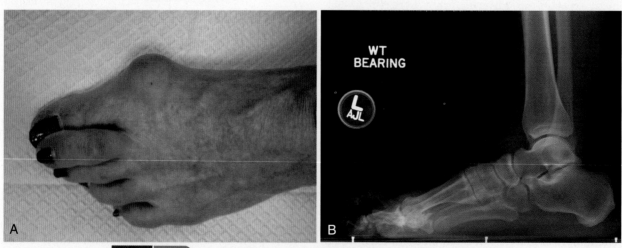

WT BEARING

FIGURE 4.5 **A** and **B,** Effusion in joint of patient with hammer toe deformity.

TABLE 4.1

Clinical Staging System for Metatarsophalangeal Joint Instability

STAGE	ALIGNMENT	PHYSICAL EXAMINATION
0	No malalignment, prodromal phase with pain	Joint pain, swelling, diminished toe purchase, negative drawer test
1	Mild malalignment, widening of the web space, medial deviation	Joint pain, swelling, diminished toe purchase, mildly positive drawer test (<50% subluxation)
2	Moderate malalignment; medial, lateral, or dorsal deformity; hyperextension	Joint pain, diminished swelling, no toe purchase, moderately positive drawer test (>50% subluxation)
3	Severe malalignment, dorsal deformity, toes may overlap, possible hammer toe	Joint and toe pain, little swelling, no toe purchase, dislocatable on drawer test
4	Severe malalignment, dislocation, fixed hammer toe	No toe purchase, dislocated toe

From Coughlin MJ, Baumfeld DS, Nery C: Second MTP joint instability: grading of the deformity and description of surgical repair of capsular insufficiency, Phys Sportsmed 39:132, 2011.

drawer test and deviation of the *third* metatarsophalangeal joint suggested a high-grade tear of the *second* metatarsophalangeal joint plantar plate (Fig. 4.6).

The paper pull-out test can be used to evaluate toe strength and dynamic digital purchase on the ground. A narrow strip of paper is placed between the affected toe and the ground. The patient grasps the paper by plantarflexing the toe, resisting the examiner's attempts to pull the paper from beneath the toe. The test is positive when the patient is unable to resist this pull.

As deformity progresses, a plantar callus may develop. Although the diagnoses of metatarsophalangeal joint instability and plantar plate rupture are made primarily by clinical examination, MRI using a small receiver coil, as described by Yao et al., can be used for evaluation (Fig. 4.7). Yamada et al. assessed direct and indirect MRI features related to plantar plate tears. They noted that when classic signs of a plantar plate tear could not be detected on MRI, indirect signs such as a pseudoneuroma sign, changes at the interosseous tendon-collateral ligament complex, and distance between the plantar plate and proximal phalanx were strongly associated with a tear. Ultrasound imaging has been found to have comparable sensitivity to MRI in the identification of lesser metatarsophalangeal joint plantar plate tears (Fig. 4.8). Gregg et al. prospectively evaluated 160 patients with symptoms of plantar plate tears using ultrasonography and MRI; the sensitivity of MRI with surgical correlation was 87%, and ultrasound demonstrated a sensitivity of 96%. Feuerstein et al. found that, although both static and dynamic ultrasound techniques were highly sensitive, the sensitivity and accuracy of ultrasound examination were better with dynamic techniques.

TREATMENT

In the early stages of synovitis when minimal deformity is present, a single intraarticular cortisone injection, oral antiinflammatory agents, metatarsal supports, taping of the toe in a neutral position, and use of stiff-soled shoes may eliminate pain and prevent deformity. The addition of a spring steel plate to the orthosis or directly to the sole of the shoe may help to eliminate extension forces on the toe. Peck et al., in a study of 154 patients with lesser metatarsophalangeal joint instability, found that 64% were managed nonoperatively with these methods and 36%

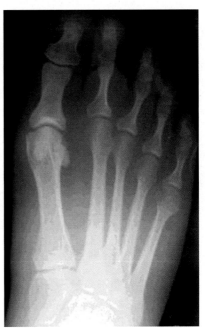

FIGURE 4.6 High-grade tear of second metatarsophalangeal joint plantar plate in patient with deviation of third metatarsophalangeal joint.

were managed operatively with a combination of a flexor-to-extensor transfer, a Weil osteotomy, and a Stainsby procedure (which involved removal of the base of the proximal phalanx). They reported no significant difference in improvement between patients treated operatively and those treated nonoperatively. When significant deformity or instability is present, however, conservative treatment may be insufficient.

For chronic synovitis of the joint that is unresponsive to conservative treatment when no significant instability is present, extensor longus lengthening, dorsal capsulotomy, and synovectomy are indicated. Very occasionally, a second web space neuroma is present and should be resected if preoperative symptoms suggest neuritic pain.

If the joint subluxates more than 50%, a stabilizing procedure should be added to the synovectomy. Attritional rupture of the plantar plate has been reported to occur primarily at the attachment on the plantar aspect

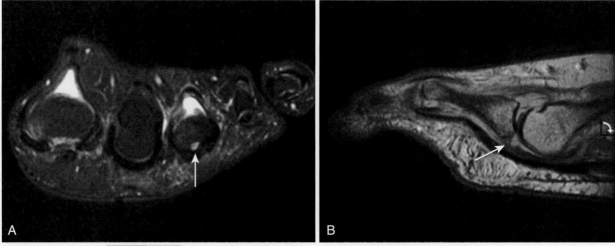

FIGURE 4.7   **A** and **B,** Small receiver coil used for MRI evaluation of instability.

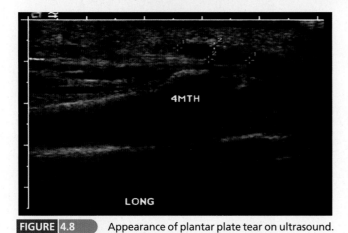

FIGURE 4.8   Appearance of plantar plate tear on ultrasound.

of the proximal phalanx. Direct repair of the plantar plate to the base of the proximal phalanx using a plantar approach to the metatarsophalangeal joint has been reported, but no long-term outcome studies are available. Plantar plate repair through a dorsal approach is now our preferred treatment method for this condition, as it has been found to anatomically restore ligamentous support in the lesser metatarsophalangeal joints. Although tedious, it can be accomplished with correction of the primary problem: disruption of all or a portion of the plantar plate. Flint et al. in a prospective case series of 138 plantar plate tears reported 80% good to excellent satisfaction scores after dorsal plantar plate repair. Devices are now available that significantly improve the technique, making it faster and easier to perform. Two suture configurations generally are used in the dorsal approach, the horizontal mattress stitch or a luggage-tag stitch (Fig. 4.9). In a biomechanical cadaver study, Finney et al. found the horizontal mattress stitch to be a superior configuration to the luggage-tag stitch, trending toward a higher load-to-failure force.

Although we believe that in most patients a Weil osteotomy is important, Saltzman has described a technique that does not call for the routine use of the osteotomy.

The Weil shortening osteotomy corrects what is often the underlying problem, excessive metatarsal length, but also significantly improves visualization of the plantar plate. It is important not to overshorten the second metatarsal, because this will limit the ability to obtain tension on the repair. Removing a small slice of bone from the osteotomy and then restoring most of the length usually is sufficient to decompress the joint. Flexor-to-extensor transfer is still a very useful technique, especially in severe dislocations where there is little remaining plantar plate for repair. Garg et al. described a modification of the Weil osteotomy, a "segmental" osteotomy (Fig. 4.10), that effectively shortens the metatarsal and reduces the plantar load under the metatarsal head. Although technically easier than the Weil osteotomy, the segmental osteotomy had frequent complications, including transfer metatarsalgia, floating toe, infection, and wound healing problems.

Flexor-to-extensor transfer or rerouting of the extensor digitorum brevis tendon underneath the second intermetatarsal ligament has been reported to be effective in the treatment of crossover second toe deformity, as has transfer of the flexor digitorum longus. Myerson and Jung reported combining flexor digitorum longus tendon transfer with proximal interphalangeal resection arthroplasty, proximal interphalangeal fusion, and/or Weil osteotomy of the metatarsal. Although many patients were pleased with the pain relief obtained, frequent complications, such as residual extension contractures at the metatarsophalangeal joint, medial deviation of the joint, and stiffness of the toe, resulted in 14% of patients being dissatisfied with the procedure. It cannot be emphasized enough that with lesser toe surgery, preoperative counseling regarding patient expectations is mandatory.

Percutaneous distal metatarsal osteotomies without soft-tissue procedures have been described for treatment of mild to moderate metatarsophalangeal joint instability with comparable results to open procedures. Authors cite as advantages reduced operating times and lower rates of complications (2.9% metatarsalgia) compared with traditional open techniques. However, delayed and nonunions have been reported, as well as the potential for injury to the metatarsal epiphyseal blood supply.

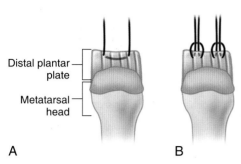

FIGURE 4.9 **A,** Horizontal mattress stitch. **B,** Luggage-tag stitch. (From Finney FT, Lee S, Scott J, et al: Biomechanical evaluation of suture configurations in lesser toe plantar plate repairs, Foot Ankle Int 39(7):836, 2018.)

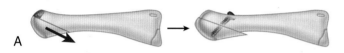

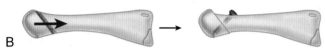

FIGURE 4.10 **A and B,** Segmental osteotomy for correction of metatarsophalangeal instability (see text).

PRIMARY PLANTAR PLATE REPAIR THROUGH A DORSAL APPROACH

Although direct repair of a plantar plate detachment can be technically challenging, it can provide stability to the joint. Cooper and Coughlin described an approach for adequate exposure of the plantar plate, and Gregg et al. reported the results of plantar plate repair combined with Weil osteotomy.

TECHNIQUE 4.1

- Make a dorsal incision over the related interspace and a longitudinal capsulotomy at the affected metatarsophalangeal joint.
- Divide the extensor digitorum brevis and make a Z-tenotomy of the extensor digitorum longus.
- After full collateral release of the metatarsophalangeal joint, use a microsagittal saw to remove a small wedge of bone.
- Provisionally fix the toe in a maximally shortened position with a 1.2-mm Kirschner wire.
- Pull on the toe to expose the plantar plate.
- If the plantar plate is partially or completely detached from the base of the proximal phalanx, freshen the plantar rim of the proximal phalanx.
- With a 1.6-mm Kirschner wire, drill two holes from the dorsal cortex to the plantar rim of the proximal phalanx, medially and laterally (Fig. 4.11A).
- Pass a {1/10} Ethibond suture across the plantar plate proximal to the disruption and back through the holes in the proximal phalanx (Fig. 4.11B).

- Fix the Weil osteotomy in optimal position with a 1.3-mm titanium "twist-off" screw (DePuy/Johnson & Johnson, Leeds, UK).
- Tie the two suture ends over the dorsal phalangeal cortex to advance the plantar plate onto the base of the proximal phalanx.
- Pass a 1.6-mm Kirschner wire through the toe and across the metatarsophalangeal joint, holding the toe in a neutral position.

POSTOPERATIVE CARE The foot is kept elevated. The wound is inspected at 7 to 10 days. Weight bearing is allowed in a multipurpose medical/surgical shoe for the first 6 weeks after surgery. The Kirschner wire is removed at 4 weeks.

PRIMARY PLANTAR PLATE REPAIR THROUGH A DORSAL APPROACH

TECHNIQUE 4.2

(COUGHLIN)
- Place the patient supine on the operating table; place and inflate a tourniquet.
- Make a dorsal longitudinal incision just inferior to the tendons of the extensor digitorum longus and brevis to expose the affected second metatarsophalangeal joint.
- Partially release the collateral ligament off of the proximal phalanx of the metatarsophalangeal joint to improve exposure.
- Use a sagittal saw to make a Weil osteotomy (Fig. 4.12A). Make the cut parallel to the plantar aspect of the foot, starting at a point 2 to 3 mm below the top of the metatarsal articular surface.
- Push the capital fragment proximally about 10 mm and fix it with a temporary vertical Kirschner wire to hold it in a retracted position.
- Place a second vertical Kirschner wire in the base of the proximal phalanx. Place a special miniature joint distractor (Arthrex, Inc., Naples, FL) over the vertical wires and spread them to expose the plantar plate (Fig. 4.12B).
- Evaluate and grade the plantar plate.
- Repair longitudinal tears (grade 3) with a side-to-side interrupted nonabsorbable suture.
- Repair transverse tears (grades 1 and 2) by placing nonabsorbable suture in the distal plantar plate. Roughen the distal plantar edge of the proximal phalanx with a burr or curet to prepare a surface for reimplantation of the plantar plate.
- Transfix the distal plantar plate just proximal to the transverse tear using a small curved needle or special curved Micro SutureLasso (Arthrex, Inc., Naples, FL) or suture punch (Mini Scorpion, Arthrex) to pass the suture within the restricted metatarsophalangeal joint surgical area of exposure.
- Use a 1.6-mm drill to create two parallel holes medially and laterally on the proximal phalanx, directed from the dorsal cortex of the proximal phalanx to its plantar rim.

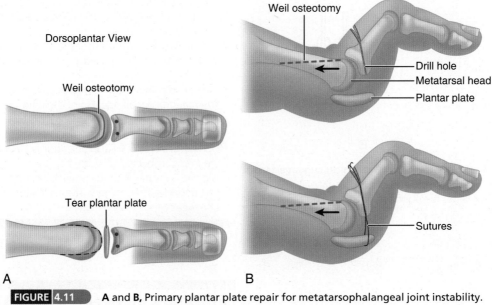

Dorsoplantar View

Weil osteotomy

Tear plantar plate

Weil osteotomy

Drill hole
Metatarsal head
Plantar plate

Sutures

FIGURE 4.11   **A** and **B,** Primary plantar plate repair for metatarsophalangeal joint instability.
SEE TECHNIQUE 4.2.

This allows passage of a suture, plantar to dorsal, to fix the plantar plate to its insertion point at the plantar base of the phalanx (Fig. 4.12C).

- Reduce the Weil osteotomy, shortening the toe only 1 to 2 mm. Fix the toe in optimal position with one or two small compression screws.
- Hold the toe reduced on the metatarsal articular surface, in 15 degrees of plantarflexion and with tension on the sutures, which have been pulled through the holes in the proximal phalanx. Tie the sutures over the dorsal phalangeal cortex, advancing the plantar plate onto the base of the proximal phalanx.
- Perform a lateral soft-tissue reefing with 2-0 nonabsorbable sutures to repair the lateral collateral ligament release.
- Close the wound in usual fashion and apply a gauze-and-tape compression dressing with the toe held in 10 to 15 degrees of plantarflexion.

POSTOPERATIVE CARE The dressing is changed at 1 and 2 weeks after surgery and then discontinued. The foot is placed in a compression wrap with a dynamic toe exercise strap. Ambulation is allowed in a postoperative shoe with weight bearing only on the heel. Comfortable shoes are permitted at 6 weeks after surgery. Passive and active range-of-motion exercises are begun at 2 weeks to recondition the short and long flexors and extensors of the lesser toes.

PERCUTANEOUS DISTAL LESSER TOE OSTEOTOMY FOR GRADE 0-I METATARSOPHALANGEAL JOINT INSTABILITY

This minimally invasive distal osteotomy of the lateral metatarsal bones without a soft-tissue procedure has been used for treatment of biomechanical metatarsalgia and metatarsophalangeal joint instability when the involved joint is still reducible and there is no structural toe deformity. The advantages of this technique include being simple, not requiring a fixation device or immobilization, and it can be done with an ankle block. Although there is the potential for nonunion, osteonecrosis of the metatarsal head, and infection, none of these occurred in a study by Magnan et al. This technique is not recommended in stiff, Coughlin grade III metatarsophalangeal joint dislocations.

TECHNIQUE 4.3

(MAGNAN ET AL)
- After ankle block anesthesia is administered, make a short skin incision on the dorsum of the distal metatarsal metaphysis close to the metatarsal head (Fig. 4.13A, B).
- With a scissor inserted through the small incision, detach the periosteum at the site of the osteotomy.
- Using a 2.3-mm micromotorized bone cutter, perform the osteotomy in a single plane 45 degrees from dorsal to plantar and distal to proximal on the metatarsal axis, moving down the lateral cortex of the metatarsal neck proximal to the metatarsal head (Fig. 4.13C–F).
- Manually mobilize the toe and metatarsal head to check that the osteotomy is complete and to release all periosteal attachments that may hinder shortening and raising the distal metatarsal fragment.

POSTOPERATIVE CARE An adhesive bandage is used to keep the toes aligned with flexion of the metatarsophalangeal joint and is changed every week for 6 weeks. Immediate full weight bearing is allowed 1 day postoperatively in a postoperative shoe with a flat, rigid sole. Normal shoes are allowed after 4 weeks, and exercise of the joint is encouraged.

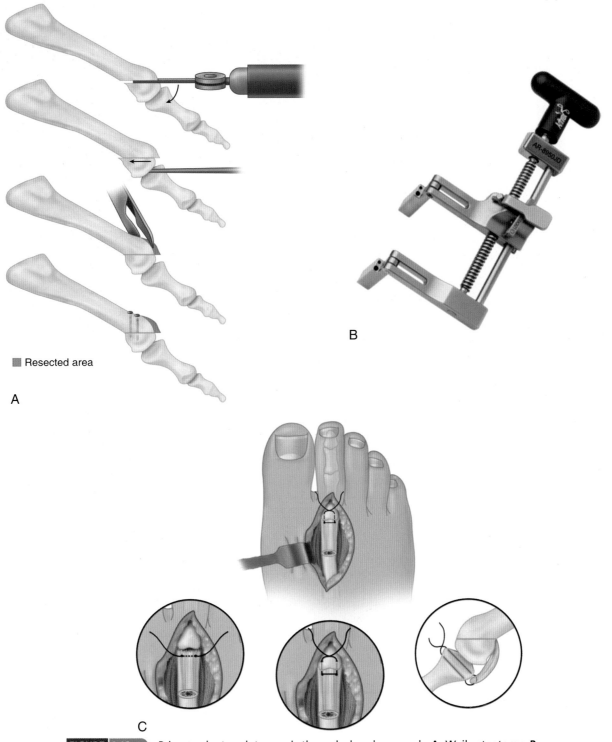

■ Resected area

A

B

C

FIGURE 4.12 Primary plantar plate repair through dorsal approach. **A,** Weil osteotomy. **B,** Miniature joint distractor (Arthrex, Inc., Naples, FL). **C,** Fixation of plantar plate to its insertion point at plantar base of phalanx. **SEE TECHNIQUE 4.2.**

AXIAL PLANE DEFORMITY OF THE METATARSOPHALANGEAL JOINT

One of the more challenging deformities of the forefoot is the medially or laterally deviated toe. Medial deviation is most often seen in crossover toe deformities, with or without associated hallux valgus, and sometimes involves multiple toes, not just the second. The valgus second toe deformity also may be associated with hallux valgus and also may involve multiple toes. In both cases, attention to the lesser toe deformity is critical because failure to correct this may lead to recurrence of the hallux deformity.

In the mildest cases of either varus or valgus deformity, simple release of the contracted collateral ligament may be all that is

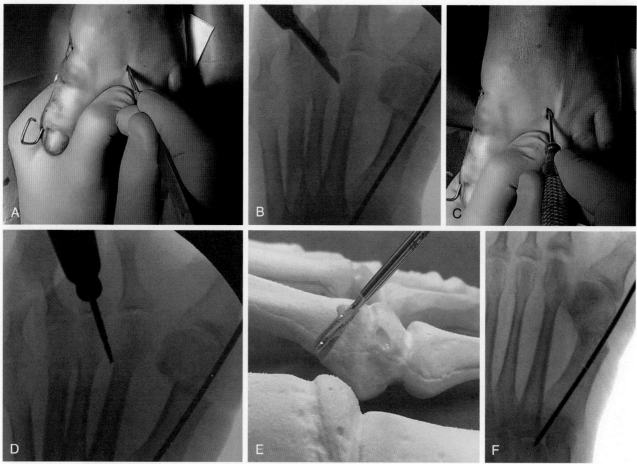

FIGURE 4.13 Percutaneous distal osteotomy of the lesser metatarsals. **A** and **B**, Incision. **C-E**, Osteotomy performed with micromotorized bone-cutter. **F**, Completion of osteotomy confirmed fluoroscopically. (From Magnan B, Bonetti I, Negri S, et al: Percutaneous distal osteotomy of lesser metatarsals (DMMO) for treatment of metatarsalgia with metatarsophalangeal instability, Foot Ankle Surg 24:400, 2018.) **SEE TECHNIQUE 4.3.**

necessary. Imbrication of the opposite side may provide an additional measure of correction. For varus deformity, satisfactory results have been reported with the use of the extensor digitorum brevis tendon rerouted underneath the transverse metatarsal ligament. It is important to note that a competent intermetatarsal ligament is a prerequisite for this procedure. Ellis et al. described an extensor digitorum brevis reconstructive technique combined with a medial collateral ligament and partial plantar plate release for correction of multiplanar deformity of the second metatarsophalangeal joint. Also, while a shortening osteotomy of the metatarsal may be necessary to correct the deformity and instability of the metatarsophalangeal joint, this osteotomy will prevent the use of the extensor digitorum brevis transfer.

Klinge et al. described a modification of the Weil osteotomy to address this issue, and we have found it to be particularly successful and powerful in procedures involving varus or valgus angulation of the toe not corrected with simple ligament balancing. It is our preferred procedure of the following three, but we still find it useful to be familiar with a number of techniques to deal with this challenging problem. As a technical tip, when managing complex forefoot deformity, it can be useful to use a proximal thigh tourniquet and general anesthesia so that the ankle tourniquet does not produce tension on the long extensor and flexor tendons to the toe while attempting to balance alignment of the toe.

Finally, the complexity of this problem gives rise to the question of whether a simple arthrodesis might suffice in patients with more severe or recurrent deformities. Although we have no experience with this procedure, Joseph et al. reported a statistically significant reduction in pain, improvement in alignment, and full return to unrestricted weight-bearing activities in 31 patients with metatarsophalangeal joint fusions. Complications were, however, relatively frequent: 13% with nonunions, 6% with implant breakage, and 3% with soft-tissue infection.

MODIFIED WEIL OSTEOTOMY

TECHNIQUE 4.4   *Figure 4.14*

(KLINGE ET AL.)
- First, restore first ray alignment with either a modified McBride procedure (see Technique 2.1) or a transarticular soft-tissue release, followed by a chevron or scarf osteotomy (see Techniques 2.3 and 2.11). If needed to correct residual hallux valgus interphalangeus, an Akin procedure (see Technique 2.15) can be done.

- To ameliorate extensor overrecruitment and extrinsic-intrinsic imbalance (tightness), transect the long extensor to the second ray proximally and cut the short extensor distally, just proximal to its insertion.
- Perform a complete medial or lateral capsular and collateral ligament release to the level of, but not including, the plantar plate for varus or valgus deformities, respectively.
- If residual metatarsophalangeal joint contracture remains, perform a modified Weil three-step shortening osteotomy (see Technique 4.12) to further decompress the joint, allow congruent reduction, and restore dorsal-plantar competence.
- If adjacent lesser rays remain malaligned or of an inappropriate length, similar procedures should be done on them.
- For persistent coronal plane metatarsophalangeal joint drift and malalignment, obtain more anatomic realignment by displacing the metatarsal head in the coronal plane before fixation.
- Use a dental pick, anteater rongeur, or Freer elevator to adjust and maintain proper metatarsal head position while coronal plane alignment is checked clinically and radiographically. Make coronal plane adjustments as necessary.
- For fixation, place a single 2-mm solid cortical screw in lag fashion across the osteotomy site after satisfactory reduction. Slightly offset the screw trajectory from the pure sagittal plane in the direction of translation to maximize central purchase within the metatarsal head. Take care to ensure that the metatarsal head shift resulted in a purely translational rather than an angular (coronal plane) realignment, making adjustments as necessary before fixation until the final metatarsophalangeal joint alignment is deemed anatomically congruent.
- Evaluate the foot clinically and with fluoroscopy to ensure satisfactory alignment of the metatarsals and congruent reduction of the metatarsophalangeal joints.
- When bony realignment is completed, transfer the short extensor to the long extensor for effective intrinsicplasty and close all incisions.

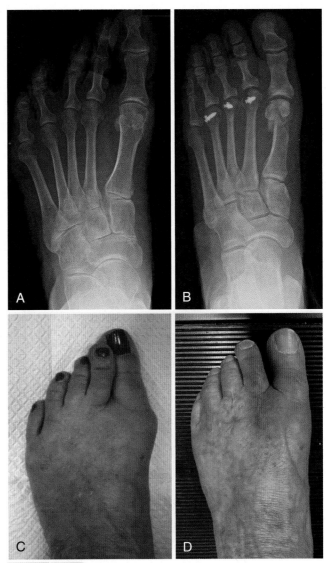

FIGURE 4.14 Weil osteotomy. **A,** Preoperative views showing varus deformity of second through fourth metatarsophalangeal joints. **B,** Correction with medializing Weil osteotomies and medial collateral ligament releases. **C** and **D,** Preoperative and postoperative clinical photographs after Weil osteotomy. **SEE TECHNIQUE 4.4.**

CORRECTION OF MULTIPLANAR DEFORMITY OF THE SECOND TOE WITH METATARSOPHALANGEAL RELEASE AND EXTENSOR BREVIS RECONSTRUCTION

TECHNIQUE 4.5

(ELLIS ET AL.)
- Make an incision over the dorsal aspect of the metatarsophalangeal joint and identify the extensor digitorum brevis and longus tendons.
- Lengthen the extensor digitorum longus with a Z-plasty technique and release the extensor digitorum brevis 0.5 cm proximal to the metatarsophalangeal joint.

- Release the dorsal capsule and the medial collateral ligament.
- If not reduced, release the plantar plate on the contracted side (Fig. 4.15A) until the metatarsophalangeal joint is reduced on the anteroposterior fluoroscopic view taken with the ankle in neutral and the foot and toes plantigrade to simulate gentle weight bearing.
- Because the authors noted that such a release tended to overcorrect the deformity once the reconstruction was added, they have subsequently performed the release sequentially until the multiplanar subluxation was nearly but not fully corrected on fluoroscopy.
- If full correction is obtained with release of one third the width of the plantar plate or less, a tendon reconstruction is not added.
- If tendon reconstruction is necessary, leave the extensor digitorum brevis tendon attached distally; this eliminates the need for it to heal to bone at the proximal phalanx.

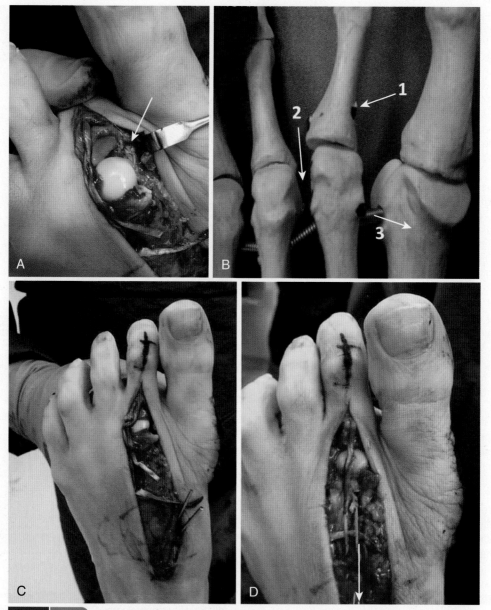

FIGURE 4.15 Metatarsophalangeal release and extensor brevis reconstruction. **A,** Second metatarsophalangeal joint after plantar plate release *(arrow)*, but before extensor digitorum brevis reconstruction. **B,** Path of extensor digitorum brevis tendon: through proximal phalanx *(1)*, under soft tissue dorsal to transverse ligament on lateral side of joint *(2)*, and through neck of second metatarsal *(3)*. **C,** Extensor digitorum brevis tendon has been passed through proximal phalanx and metatarsal. Position of toe before (**C**) and after (**D**) tensioning shows correction of second toe varus. **D,** *Arrow* below nonabsorbable suture shows vector of tensioning used before reconstruction is secured to screw post in metatarsal shaft. (From Ellis SJ, Young EM, Endo Y, et al: Correction of multiplanar deformity of the second toe with metatarsophalangeal release and extensor brevis reconstruction, Foot Ankle Int 34:792, 2013.) **SEE TECHNIQUE 4.5.**

- Pass the extensor digitorum brevis tendon through a drill hole in the proximal phalanx from dorsal-medial to plantar-lateral and under the soft tissue dorsal to the transverse metatarsal.
- Pass the tendon back up through a second drill hole from plantar-lateral to dorsal-medial through the metatarsal neck, replicating the plantar course of the involved lateral collateral ligament (Fig. 4.15B).

- Tension the tendon appropriately with the toe in a corrected position (Fig. 4.15C) and secure it over a small screw post (2 or 2.4 mm) placed in the metatarsal shaft (Fig. 4.15D).
- If the toe remains slightly extended at the metatarsophalangeal joint, add a plantar dermodesis.

FLEXOR-TO-EXTENSOR TRANSFER

TECHNIQUE 4.6

- On each toe to be corrected, make a transverse plantar incision at the proximal flexion crease of the toe (Fig. 4.16A), taking care to preserve the digital arteries and nerves.
- Retract the skin and subcutaneous tissue with small hooked retractors and expose the underlying flexor tendons and their fibrous sheaths.
- Open the proximal 3 to 4 mm of pulley to expose the flexor digitorum longus immediately under it. This is best done by opening the pulley to one side and dissecting over the underlying tendons, removing a small segment of pulley. This dissection is made easier by the use of magnification loupes and a small round-end knife. Topographically, this dissection is located at about the middle third of the proximal phalanx. The central tendon should be the flexor digitorum longus; gentle, passive flexion and extension of the distal interphalangeal joint while the proximal interphalangeal joint is held straight confirms this.

- While lifting the flexor digitorum longus tendon, the vinculum longum, if present, appears under tension and should be severed after electrocautery.
- Make a second transverse plantar incision at the distal interphalangeal joint and perform a tenotomy of the flexor digitorum longus, taking care not to violate the plantar plate of this joint (Fig. 4.16A,B).
- Returning to the proximal incision, hook (but do not clamp) the flexor digitorum longus with a small hemostat and deliver the distal segment into the wound. If the vincula between the two incisions are tenacious, this step might require force.
- When the flexor digitorum longus is delivered from the proximal incision, inspect the wound again to ensure that the two lateral slips of the flexor digitorum brevis are intact (Fig. 4.16C).
- Careful inspection of the flexor digitorum longus shows a shallow, linear furrow running longitudinally along its plantar surface. Using small forceps, hold one side of the delivered tendon at its free end, while an assistant holds the other, and split the tendon longitudinally along this natural cleavage plane for 1.5 to 2.5 cm (Fig. 4.16D).

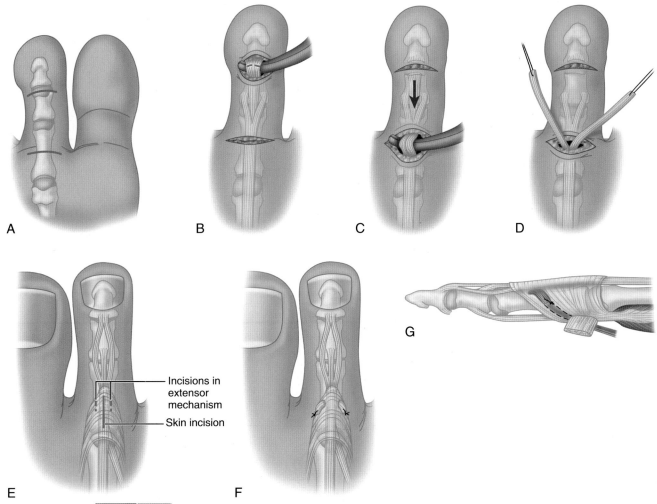

A   B   C   D

E

Incisions in extensor mechanism

Skin incision

F

G

FIGURE **4.16**   **A-G,** Flexor-to-extensor tendon transfer to dorsum of second toe. **SEE TECHNIQUE 4.6.**

- Pull the tendon distally with the ankle plantarflexed to see clearly both sides of the tendon during this step and to prevent inadvertent sectioning of half of the tendon. Other helpful points are to hold the two segments apart only enough to fit a small pair of straight scissors in the axilla of dissection and to use the tips of the scissors.
- Moisten the tendon with saline and make a second skin incision longitudinally in the midline on the dorsum of the proximal phalanx, 1.5 to 2 cm in length (Fig. 4.16E). The dorsal digital veins usually are to each side of this incision, but if they are in line with the incision, cauterize them.
- By sharp dissection, identify the trailing edge of each lateral band of the extensor mechanism while the skin is retracted, including the superficial veins and nerves to either side, using two-pronged skin hooks.
- Make 3- to 4-mm longitudinal incisions into the extensor mechanism halfway between the midline dorsally and the trailing edge of the lateral band plantarward on each side. These incisions should be at the level of the middiaphysis of the proximal phalanx (see Fig. 4.16E).
- Pass a small hemostat through one incision in the extensor mechanism to emerge into the plantar incision, staying close to bone. This technique avoids the digital neurovascular bundle.
- Grasp one slip of the split flexor digitorum longus at its tip with a hemostat and bring it into the dorsal wound through the extensor mechanism.
- Repeat the same procedure on the other side of the phalanx, always ensuring that the slips remain plantar to the deep transverse intermetatarsal ligament.
- With an assistant holding the ankle joint at 90 degrees (neutral dorsiflexion and plantarflexion), tighten the tendon slips sufficiently to hold the metatarsophalangeal joint at neutral to 5 degrees of plantarflexion (Fig. 4.16F,G).
- An alternative technique is to overlap the tendon slips dorsally. Occasionally, the flexor digitorum longus needs to be split further linearly. If so, the tendon slips must be returned to the plantar incision to avoid severing one half.

- With the tendon slips held at the desired tension, use 3-0 or 4-0 nonabsorbable sutures to fasten each slip of the flexor digitorum longus under tension to the extensor mechanism, while the assistant continues to hold the ankle in neutral position.
- Loop the tip of each slip back on itself and secure it to the trailing edge of each side of the lateral band and to itself. Section any excess tendon.
- Alternatively, suture the two tendon slips to one another over the dorsum of the phalanx. This leaves a small knot beneath the skin (Fig. 4.17).
- With the ankle extended to neutral, the metatarsophalangeal joint should rest in the neutral or slightly flexed position and the proximal interphalangeal joint should rest in the neutral position or in a position with less than 10 degrees of flexion.
- If the same procedure is being done for the central three digits, correct the second toe first because it usually is the most severely affected. The flexor digitorum longus of the third and fourth digits will have been pulled distally through the common tendon in the midsole as the second toe flexor digitorum longus is sutured under tension. This makes tension adjustment easier in the third and fourth toes.
- In a modification of the technique, after distal release of the flexor digitorum longus, it can be put through a hole in the proximal phalanx and sutured to the extensor at the appropriate tension.
- Before closing the skin, remove any tourniquet and obtain hemostasis by cautery or compression. Close the wounds with 4-0 monofilament nylon or suture of the surgeon's choice.

POSTOPERATIVE CARE A short leg, well-padded cast extending past the toes is applied in the operating room. The foot is elevated for 48 to 72 hours, and bathroom privileges are allowed. Crutches are optional, and weight bearing to tolerance is allowed. The patient usually is off crutches within 1 week. The cast is removed and replaced at 2 weeks, and at 4 weeks, a deep, wide toe box, soft-vamp shoe is allowed. Active toe exercises are encouraged at 6 weeks.

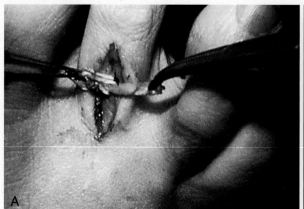
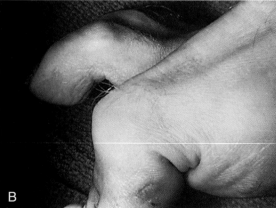

FIGURE 4.17   Flexible hammer toe. **A,** During transfer of flexor to extensor tendon. **B,** After surgery. Note small knot beneath skin. **SEE TECHNIQUE 4.6.**

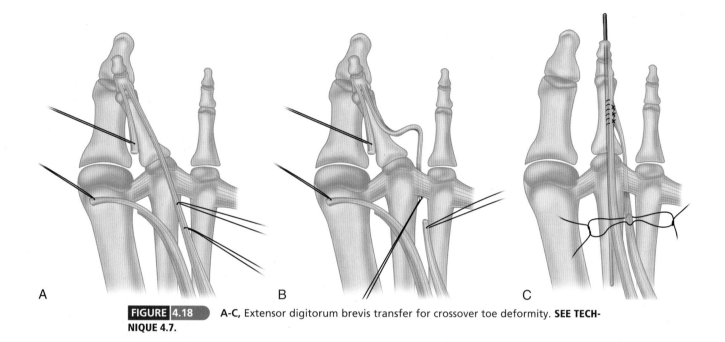

FIGURE 4.18 A-C, Extensor digitorum brevis transfer for crossover toe deformity. **SEE TECHNIQUE 4.7.**

EXTENSOR DIGITORUM BREVIS TRANSFER FOR CROSSOVER TOE DEFORMITY

TECHNIQUE 4.7

(HADDAD)

- Begin a dorsal approach just distal to the proximal interphalangeal joint, with a gentle curve at the level of the metatarsophalangeal joint along the lateral border of the metatarsal shafts and extending 5 cm proximal to the metatarsophalangeal joint.
- Dissect the dorsal digital nerves free and protect them during dissection to preserve postoperative sensation.
- Identify the extensor digitorum brevis to the musculotendinous junction proximally and place two stay sutures (3.0 Ethibond) on either side of the proposed sectioning of the tendon. Note that this is a proximal sectioning, near the musculotendinous junction (Fig. 4.18A).
- Section the tendon.
- Identify the extensor digitorum brevis tendon distally to its insertion and free it from the capsular aponeurosis (extensor hood) proximally to the transverse metatarsal ligament.
- Completely section the medial collateral ligament and the dorsal capsule of the metatarsophalangeal joint; make sure that the medial sectioning does not violate the plantar plate.
- Use a McGlamry elevator or gouge to strip the volar plate at its origin. This will allow the plate to scar to the metatarsal proximal to its current insertion, assisting with stability.
- Examine the lateral collateral ligament for rupture. If it is attenuated, excise redundant tissue. Place, but do not tie, permanent sutures in a figure-of-eight configuration to repair the lateral collateral ligament.
- If a hammer toe deformity is present, perform minimal resection of the distal and proximal condyle to stimulate proximal interphalangeal fusion.
- Suture the distal extensor digitorum brevis tendon to the plantar lateral base of the proximal phalanx with a permanent suture to eliminate a rotary force on the toe after transfer.
- Identify the transverse metatarsal ligament between the second and third metatarsal heads. It is critical not to mistake the more dorsal fascia for the transverse metatarsal ligament because it does not have the integrity of this structure. Use a lamina spreader to place tension on this ligament.
- Place a 90-degree right-angle clamp from proximal to distal deep to the transverse metatarsal ligament.
- Pass the extensor digitorum brevis tendon from distal to proximal deep to the transverse metatarsal ligament by grasping the previously placed stay suture (Fig. 4.18B).
- Tie the sutures repairing the lateral collateral ligament.
- Place a 0.062-inch Kirschner wire across the metatarsophalangeal joint to hold the joint reduced. This takes the tension off the lateral collateral ligament repair by placing the toe in some valgus and plantarflexion.
- Tie the tendon transfer end to end, completing the anastomosis (Fig. 4.18C).
- Release the tourniquet and evaluate vascularity of the digit before closing the incision with a layered closure using 4-0 Monocryl and 4-0 nylon.

POSTOPERATIVE CARE The pin is removed at 6 weeks after surgery, and the toe is taped into slight valgus for an additional 6 weeks.

CLOSING WEDGE OSTEOTOMY OF THE PROXIMAL PHALANX FOR CORRECTION OF AXIAL DEFORMITY

For residual deformity in the axial plane, an osteotomy at the proximal metaphysis of the proximal phalanx can provide realignment of either valgus or varus malalignment of the toe. The technique described by Kilmartin and O'Kane is described. We prefer to use a 2- or 3-mm burr to make the osteotomy, leaving the opposite cortex intact, "greenstick" the osteotomy closed, and fix the basilar osteotomy with the Kirschner wire inserted to provide stability for the proximal interphalangeal resection done for hammer toe correction.

TECHNIQUE 4.8

(KILMARTIN AND O'KANE)

- Make a 3-cm "lazy-S" incision extending from the midpoint of the second toe proximal phalanx medially into the metatarsophalangeal joint.
- Deepen the incision to bone, passing medial and plantar to the extensor tendon.
- Divide the joint capsule to expose the base of the phalanx only; do not extend the capsular incision onto the metatarsophalangeal joint.
- Use a power saw to make a cut where the flare of the base of the phalanx meets the shaft. Make the first osteotomy cut parallel with the base of the phalanx, passing through the dorsal, plantar, and medial cortices but leaving the lateral cortex intact.
- Make the second distal cut parallel with the distal end of the toe so that the distal cut converges with the proximal cut, leaving the lateral cortex intact (Fig. 4.19). This creates a triangular wedge, generally 3 to 4 mm wide at the base.
- Feather the lateral cortex and close the osteotomy with finger pressure.
- Close the deep structures with 3-0 Vicryl interrupted sutures and the skin with 4-0 Monocryl subcuticular sutures.

POSTOPERATIVE CARE The second toe is "buddy taped" to the first toe with up to six 12-mm-wide strips of adhesive surgical tape, which are placed dorsally and plantarly on the hallux and second toe. The tape is kept in place for 2 weeks. A stiff-soled postoperative shoe is worn for 2 weeks, and then patients are allowed to return to wearing running shoes and to slowly return to normal activities.

HAMMER TOE AND CLAW TOE

The term *hammer toe* is used most often to describe an abnormal flexion posture of the proximal interphalangeal joint of one of the lesser four toes (Fig. 4.20). The flexion deformity may be fixed (i.e., not passively correctable to the neutral position) or flexible (i.e., passively correctable). If the flexion contracture at this middle joint of the digit is severe and

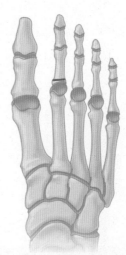

FIGURE 4.19   Closing wedge osteotomy of proximal phalanx for correction of axial deformity. **SEE TECHNIQUE 4.8.**

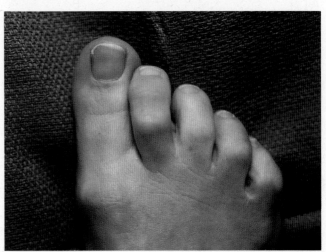

FIGURE 4.20   Fixed flexion contracture of proximal interphalangeal joint with flexible metatarsophalangeal and distal interphalangeal joints.

of long duration, the metatarsophalangeal joint usually is deformed in the opposite direction (i.e., extension). The distal joint usually stays supple, but it also may develop a flexion or an extension deformity. The terms *claw toe* and *hammer toe* are differentiated from one another by the following: claw toes frequently are caused by neuromuscular diseases, and often a similar deformity is present in all toes, whereas in hammer toe deformity only one or two toes are involved; claw toes always have extension deformity at the metatarsophalangeal joint, but in hammer toe deformity, extension of the metatarsophalangeal joint may or may not be present; and claw toes often have a flexion deformity at the distal interphalangeal joint, but this usually does not occur in hammer toes (Fig. 4.21).

ETIOLOGY

Claw toes can be caused by neuromuscular diseases. The intrinsic muscles of the foot, specifically the interossei, pass plantar to the axis of rotation of the metatarsophalangeal joint, causing flexion of this joint. Loss of intrinsic function of the foot leads to an imbalance, allowing the extensor digitorum

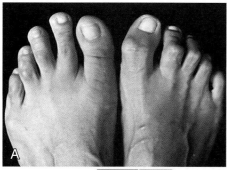
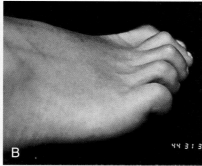
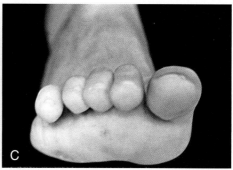

FIGURE 4.21 **A,** Claw toes, right foot, secondary to medial and lateral plantar nerve laceration. **B,** Metatarsophalangeal joints of second and third toes could not be flexed to neutral position, and none could be flexed past neutral. **C,** Extension posture of claw toes increases plantar pressure on metatarsal heads.

longus to extend the metatarsophalangeal joint and the flexor digitorum longus to flex the interphalangeal joints. Although the long extensors of the toes may extend the interphalangeal joints with the metatarsophalangeal joint in neutral, when an extension posture of the metatarsophalangeal joint develops, the long extensor loses its excursion and no longer can extend the interphalangeal joints. The powerful flexors of the toe, specifically the long flexor, which attaches to the base of the distal phalanx, accentuate the deformity, causing flexion of the interphalangeal joints.

Although the causes of claw toe deformity can be easily understood, most hammer toes have no underlying intrinsic imbalance. The use of electrodes to evaluate the phasic activity of the intrinsic muscles of the foot found no activity of the intrinsic muscles during the first 35% of the gait cycle. With quiet standing, intrinsic muscle activity was absent. Hammering of the toes usually is accentuated by standing, and the lack of activity of the intrinsics during quiet standing implies that loss of intrinsic function is not the cause of the deformity.

Factors commonly thought to contribute to hammer toe deformity include the long-term use of poorly fitting shoes. Crowding of the toes within an excessively tight toe box causes some deformation of the metatarsophalangeal and interphalangeal joints that over time can lead to flexible and eventually fixed deformities at these joints. Anatomic factors that can cause lesser toe deformities include a "two-bone toe" and a long second ray, which may result in buckling of the toe, and hallux valgus, causing pressure against the second toe. Other factors include connective tissue disorders and trauma.

CLINICAL FINDINGS

Three areas may be painful in hammer toe deformity. The most common area is the dorsum of the proximal interphalangeal joint, where a hard corn caused by pressure from the toe box or vamp of the shoe develops. When a flexion posture or end-bearing posture of the distal interphalangeal joint is present, a painful callus develops just plantar to the nail end. This is called an *end corn*. Finally, a painful callus may develop beneath the metatarsal head if the proximal phalanx subluxates dorsally. In a patient with decreased sensibility, such as occurs in diabetes mellitus or myelomeningocele, ulceration and deep infection can develop at one or more of these areas of pressure, complicating the treatment plan and endangering the toe or foot. Sometimes the dorsofibular side of the second metatarsophalangeal joint is tender (Fig. 4.22).

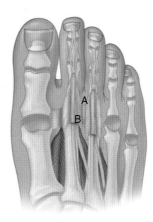

FIGURE 4.22 Site of tenderness with interdigital neuroma of second web space *(A).* Site of tenderness in idiopathic synovitis of second metatarsophalangeal joint: dorsofibular capsule and fibular collateral ligament *(B).*

TREATMENT

Conservative treatment of hammer toe usually is disappointing. Various pads and strappings are commercially available to reduce the deformity and relieve pressure over painful points. If the deformity is not of long duration and an extension deformity at the metatarsophalangeal joint is not present, daily manipulations and taping the toe so that the metatarsophalangeal joint is not extended occasionally can correct the flexion deformity at the proximal interphalangeal joint. This is because the extensor digitorum longus can forcefully extend the middle phalanx only if the metatarsophalangeal joint is in neutral or some degree of flexion. Recurrence is likely, however, when the passive stretching and taping cease, and most patients with symptomatic hammer toe eventually require surgery. The following procedures are not all of the operations available for treating hammer toes; rather, they are the most commonly recommended procedures that have follow-up data to support the recommendations (Table 4.2).

■ SOFT-TISSUE PROCEDURES (GIRDLESTONE; TAYLOR; PARRISH; MANN AND COUGHLIN)

The use of soft-tissue procedures alone without bone shortening or arthrodesis may or may not result in permanent correction. In a skeletally immature foot with symptomatic flexible hammer toe or in a young adult foot with dynamic flexible

TABLE 4.2

Procedures for Hammer Toe Deformities

DEFORMITY	CHARACTERISTICS	TREATMENT
Flexible hammer toe	No fixed contracture at MTP or PIP joint	Usually nonoperative; rarely, flexor-to-extensor transfer using FDL
Fixed hammer toe with fixed extension of MTP	Fixed flexion contracture at PIP; MTP subluxation in extension	Resection of condyles of proximal phalanx, dermodesis; lengthening of EDL, tenotomy of EDB; MTP capsulotomy, collateral ligament sectioning
Fixed hammer toe with MTP subluxation	Fixed flexion contracture at PIP; MTP subluxation in extension	Plantar plate repair after Weil osteotomy
Crossover toe	Fixed flexion contracture at PIP; MTP subluxation in varus or valgus	Resection of condyles of proximal phalanx, dermodesis; collateral ligament/capsular repair; EDB transfer
Mallet toe	Fixed flexion contracture at DIP	Resection of condyles of middle phalanx, dermodesis; FDL tenotomy

DIP, Distal interphalangeal joint; *EDB*, extensor digitorum brevis; *EDL*, extensor digitorum longus; *FDL*, flexor digitorum longus; *MTP*, metatarsophalangeal joint; *PIP*, proximal interphalangeal joint.

deformities of one or more toes (prominent hammering only with weight bearing) that interfere with shoe wear, flexor-to-extensor transfer is indicated, based on the assumption that the flexor digitorum longus contributes to deformity. The role of the flexor digitorum longus in causing flexion contracture at the proximal interphalangeal joint has been questioned, but several authors have advocated the procedure for flexible hammer toes.

A soft-tissue procedure is most reliable in patients with planovalgus or normal arches as opposed to cavus feet. In addition, patients should be younger than 30 years old, have no deformity at the metatarsophalangeal joint (can flex the joints beyond neutral position), and have no fixed flexion deformity at the proximal interphalangeal joints. In other words, a symptomatic, idiopathic, mild, flexible hammer toe deformity in a young patient is most likely to benefit from flexor-to-extensor transfer. To decrease the frequency of "floating toe" after flexor digitorum longus transfer, Boyer and DeOrio modified the technique by placing the plantar incision for harvest of the flexor digitorum longus longitudinally at the metatarsophalangeal joint crease rather than transversely, using larger (0.54-mm) Kirschner wires for fixation, using absorbable sutures for tenodesis, and passing the transferred tendon deep to the dorsal hood rather than superficial to it. They reported no floating toe deformities in their 38 patients (79 toes) and an 89% patient satisfaction rate.

■ BONE AND JOINT PROCEDURES

The most commonly used procedures for the correction of hammer toe are resection of the proximal interphalangeal joint, resection of the base of the proximal phalanx, resection of the distal third or fourth of the proximal phalanx, complete proximal phalangectomy, and arthrodesis of the proximal interphalangeal joint. Schrier et al. compared outcomes after proximal interphalangeal joint resection with those after arthrodesis and found no difference between the two procedures; both had good results in regard to pain and activity scores.

The following recommendations are not unique, and they are not intended to be absolute or universal in the surgical treatment of hammer toe. Only a symptomatic toe should undergo surgery. An unattractive deformity is not a strong enough indication for surgical correction. Hammer toe encompasses a spectrum of deformities, and the indicated procedure varies, depending on the stage of the deformity when first seen and the diagnosis, as follows:

■ MILD DEFORMITY

No fixed contracture at the metatarsophalangeal or proximal interphalangeal joint is evident. The deformity increases on weight bearing. In a young adult with a mild deformity, a flexor-to-extensor transfer using the flexor digitorum longus is recommended, as previously described.

■ MODERATE DEFORMITY

There is a fixed flexion contracture at the proximal interphalangeal joint and no extension contracture at the metatarsophalangeal joint. In moderate deformity, resection of the head and neck of the proximal phalanx and dermodesis are recommended. A percutaneous extensor digitorum longus tenotomy is performed in the presence of extensor tightness with the ankle held in the neutral position. A Kirschner wire may be needed to maintain reduction. We have found that resection of only the head of the proximal phalanx without arthrodesis has been more successful. Arthrodesis with permanent implantable devices is used primarily for revision surgery. Patients are counseled before surgery that some "molding" of the toe to fit comfortably between the adjacent toes can be expected. In our experience, most patients prefer to have some limited mobility of the proximal interphalangeal joint as opposed to a completely fused proximal interphalangeal joint.

In recent years, there has been a focus on alternative fixation techniques for hammer toe correction, with the goal of reducing the development of recurrent deformity of the toe. In their extensive review of 1115 procedures, Kramer et al. concluded that Kirschner wire fixation resulted in good maintenance of correction with a relatively low complication rate; they suggested that Kirschner wires remain an effective, low-cost method of fixation for hammer toe correction. Obrador et al. reported the use of two intramedullary implants for fixation to avoid complications reported with Kirschner wire fixation. Both implants provided good alignment, improved function, and pain relief; however, the devices were more expensive than Kirschner wires, and the authors noted the need for more cost-benefit studies. A recent literature review by Guelfi et al. found that complications and reoperations after use of various intramedullary fixation devices were similar to those (0 to 8.6%) after Kirschner wire fixation. However, they too acknowledged the higher price of these implants.

Good results have been reported in 90% of patients with the use of an absorbable intramedullary pin for proximal interphalangeal joint arthrodesis. Cited advantages of this technique include avoidance of pins penetrating the skin, less restriction on activity, and a decrease in complications such as floating toe. The authors cautioned, however, that the 2-mm absorbable pins may not provide adequate fixation in larger, longer toes.

▍SEVERE DEFORMITY

There is a fixed flexion contracture at the proximal interphalangeal joint, with a fixed extension contracture at the metatarsophalangeal joint. (Subluxation or dislocation of the proximal phalanx on the metatarsal head may be present in addition to the fixed extension contracture at the metatarsophalangeal joint and fixed flexion contracture at the proximal interphalangeal joint.) In severe deformity without subluxation or dislocation of the metatarsophalangeal joint, it is necessary to resect the head and neck of the proximal phalanx through a dorsal elliptical skin window (and dermodesis), lengthen the extensor digitorum longus, tenotomize the extensor digitorum brevis, and perform a dorsal capsulotomy at the metatarsophalangeal joint. If the extension posture of the metatarsophalangeal joint is not corrected after extensor tenotomy and dorsal capsulotomy, both collateral ligaments should be sectioned, the joint should be brought to neutral position, and the extensor digitorum longus should be repaired in its lengthened position. The metatarsophalangeal joint must be reduced not only in the anteroposterior plane but also in the mediolateral plane, and the reduction of the proximal interphalangeal and metatarsophalangeal joints must be maintained with a longitudinal Kirschner wire. (A carefully applied soft dressing that holds the toe in the corrected position may preclude the use of a Kirschner wire; this dressing must be changed frequently as swelling subsides.) In severe deformity with subluxation or dislocation of the metatarsophalangeal joint, a metatarsophalangeal joint arthroplasty or distal metatarsal osteotomy (Weil) may be needed to decompress the metatarsophalangeal joint (see Technique 4.12).

CORRECTION OF MODERATE HAMMER TOE OR CLAW TOE DEFORMITY

TECHNIQUE 4.9

- Make an elliptical incision over the proximal interphalangeal joint that measures 5 to 6 mm wide and has a 2- or 3-mm lateral extension on either side (Fig. 4.23A,B).
- Remove the skin only initially and cauterize the vessels (Fig. 4.23C).
- Remove a slightly smaller segment of extensor tendon and dorsal capsule of the proximal interphalangeal joint, leaving a 2-mm remnant of extensor tendon attached to the base of the middle phalanx. The proximal end of the extensor tendon usually retracts beneath the proximal skin flap, but it can be easily pulled distally at the appropriate time.

- Flex the proximal interphalangeal joint about 20 degrees while putting traction on the distal and middle phalanges.
- Using a small-blade knife, section the collateral ligaments from outside in on both sides of the joint by placing the blade between the skin and the ligament and turning the cutting edge toward the joint. The proximal interphalangeal joint can be flexed to 90 degrees (Fig. 4.23D), and the head and neck of the proximal phalanx is clearly exposed (Fig. 4.23E).
- With a rongeur or small-blade power saw, remove the head and neck of the proximal phalanx and smooth any sharp points of bone with a rasp or rongeur (Fig. 4.23F).
- Extend the toe to neutral position at the proximal interphalangeal joint and feel for tightness with abutment of the articular surface of the middle phalanx on the distal end of the proximal phalangeal remnant. If it feels tight, remove 2 or 3 mm more of bone.
- Use a 3-0 or 4-0 nonabsorbable suture to enter the proximal skin edge and pass through the proximal end of the extensor tendon.
- Enter the distal remnant of the extensor tendon on its joint surface and exit through the skin. By canting the stitch, a few degrees of lateral deformity also would be corrected.
- Suture the corners of the wound with a simple stitch (Fig. 4.23G). An initial mattress stitch can be used if deemed appropriate.
- A supportive forefoot dressing to the tips of the toes is crucial (Fig. 4.24).
- This technique usually holds the proximal interphalangeal joint in acceptable alignment with only a few degrees of flexion.
- If needed, perform a percutaneous extensor digitorum longus tenotomy over the neck of the metatarsal, avoiding the dorsal veins (see Fig. 4.23F).
- When the ankle is held in neutral position, if the metatarsophalangeal joint rests in extension, the tenotomy is performed. The toe is flexed at least 60 to 70 degrees at the metatarsophalangeal joint to allow the metatarsophalangeal joint to flex to neutral position with the ankle joint at neutral in a moderate hammer toe deformity.
- Occasionally, an extensor digitorum brevis tenotomy also is required. At the neck of the metatarsal, the extensor digitorum brevis tendon is immediately lateral and slightly plantarward to the extensor digitorum longus.
- Use a soft dressing (2-inch gauze is helpful) and ½-inch tape to hold the toe in the desired position, wrapping it to an adjacent toe.

POSTOPERATIVE CARE Weight bearing to tolerance is allowed after 48 to 72 hours of elevation of the foot. A wooden-soled shoe is worn for 4 weeks. The sutures are removed at 12 to 16 days, and a carefully applied dressing maintains the toe in the corrected position for another 2 weeks. At 4 weeks, the dressing and taping usually can be discontinued, but they should be continued another 2 to 4 weeks if the deformity has any tendency to recur. The proximal interphalangeal joint usually retains a few degrees of active motion and is gently flexed, which seems to be more pleasing than a fused, straight toe at the proximal interphalangeal joint.

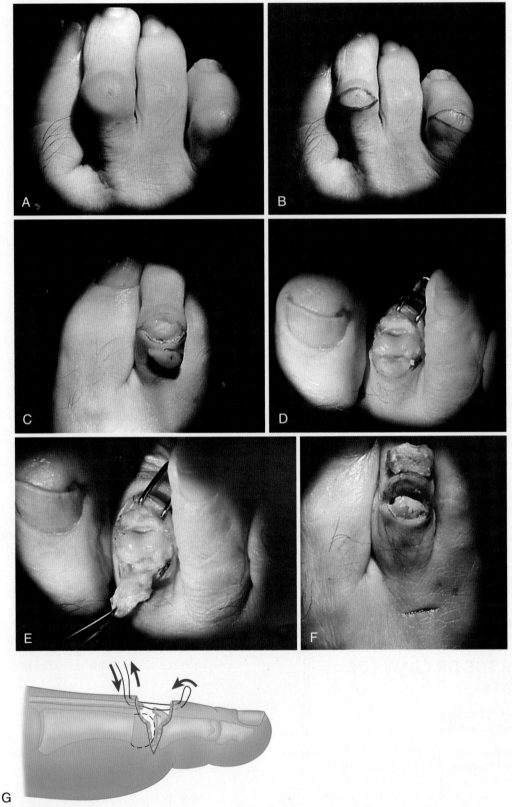

FIGURE 4.23 **A,** Moderate hammer toe deformity with fixed contracture at proximal inter-phalangeal joint but only extensor tightness at metatarsophalangeal joint with no fixed extension contracture. **B,** Dorsal elliptical incision over proximal interphalangeal joint. **C,** Superficial dissection leaving dorsal veins visible to make cauterization easier. **D,** Dorsal capsule, both collateral ligaments, and extensor tendon are sectioned transversely, and toe is acutely flexed. **E,** Extensor tendon is dissected proximally to junction of middle and distal thirds of proximal phalanx. **F,** Distal 25% to 30% of proximal phalanx is excised and rests on middle phalanx. Small dorsal incision for extensor tenotomy. **G,** Closure of wound. **SEE TECHNIQUE 4.9.**

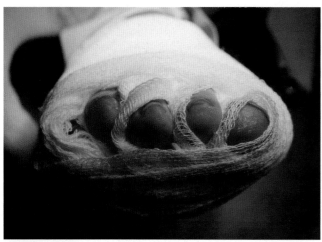

FIGURE 4.24 Postoperative dressing must be conforming and binding enough to hold toe in exact position; if not, Kirschner wire should be used. **SEE TECHNIQUE 4.9.**

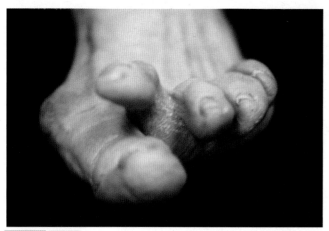

FIGURE 4.25 Severe crossover hammer toe deformity. **SEE TECHNIQUE 4.10.**

CORRECTION OF SEVERE DEFORMITY

Because a severe deformity by definition has a fixed extension contracture at the metatarsophalangeal joint and a fixed flexion contracture at the proximal phalangeal joint, both joints require correction (Fig. 4.25).

TECHNIQUE 4.10

- Begin at the metatarsophalangeal joint with a straight or angled incision centered over the fibular aspect of the metatarsophalangeal joint (Fig. 4.26A).
- Cauterize or retract the branches of the dorsal venous arch returning from the toe to expose the extensor tendons.
- The extensor digitorum brevis is slightly fibular and deep to the extensor digitorum longus. The extensor digitorum brevis joins the extensor digitorum longus and extensor expansion at the neck of the metatarsal (Fig. 4.26B). Before this confluence, dissect the extensor digitorum brevis from the extensor digitorum longus and remove a 2- to 3-mm segment of extensor digitorum brevis.

- Perform a Z-plasty lengthening of the extensor digitorum longus. The use of a small blade (No. 67 Beaver or similar cutting edge) is helpful.
- From the proximal part of the skin incision until the extensor digitorum longus joins with the extensor expansion, make a longitudinal incision into the extensor digitorum longus, exiting at a right angle at the junction of the extensor digitorum longus and the extensor expansion. Sever the tendon proximally at a right angle in the opposite direction.
- Lift the tendon away from other soft-tissue attachments. This maneuver lengthens the extensor digitorum longus by 8 to 12 mm (Fig. 4.26C).
- Usually, if the extension contracture is less than 20 to 30 degrees and there is no dorsal subluxation of the proximal phalanx on the metatarsal head, firmly flex the toe 30 to 40 degrees. If the toe rests in neutral position at the metatarsophalangeal joint with the ankle at 90 degrees, this is all that is required at this joint except suturing the extensor digitorum longus in its lengthened position with 3-0 or 4-0 absorbable suture after the proximal interphalangeal joint has been corrected.
- If after the just-described procedure the toe still rests in 10 to 20 degrees of extension, perform a dorsal capsulotomy transversely while the toe is flexed 40 to 50 degrees (Fig. 4.26C, inset). This much flexion of the toe pulls the extensor expansion distally, giving better exposure of the dorsal capsule. The capsule may vary from a thin, filmy, pliable, synovial-like covering to a dense, thick, fibrous encapsulation of the joint, depending on the chronicity of the deformity, the number of recurrent synovial inflammatory episodes, and the congruency of the joint.
- When the capsule is divided, flex the toe acutely again and return the ankle to 90 degrees, observing the resting posture of the toe. If the posture is acceptable (neutral to 10 degrees of metatarsophalangeal joint extension with the ankle at 90 degrees), all that is needed is to suture the extensor digitorum longus in its lengthened position.
- If the toe still has an unacceptable extension posture, acutely flex the toe and use a small blade to incise the collateral ligaments on both sides of the metatarsal head down to, but not through, the plantar plate of the metatarsophalangeal joint. This should allow the toe to assume a neutral to slightly flexed position at the metatarsophalangeal joint even if the toe was subluxed dorsally (Fig. 4.26D).
- Suture the extensor digitorum longus after correcting the proximal interphalangeal joint contracture.

■ CORRECTION OF SEVERE DEFORMITY WITH DISLOCATION OF THE METATARSOPHALANGEAL JOINT

Severe deformity with dislocation of the metatarsophalangeal joint is difficult to correct. All of the aforementioned recommendations are applicable—extensor digitorum longus lengthening, extensor digitorum brevis tenotomy, dorsal capsulotomy, and bilateral collateral ligament release—but, in addition, decompression of the metatarsophalangeal joint usually is required. This can be done on the phalangeal or metatarsal side of the joint; however, because of the difficulty

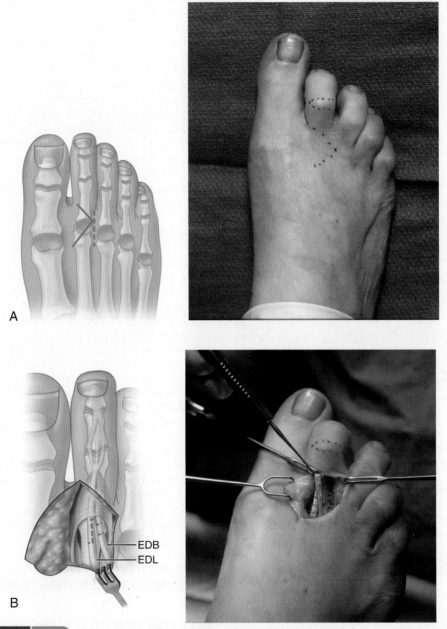

A

B

EDB
EDL

FIGURE 4.26   **A-D,** Technique for correction of severe hammer toe deformity. EDB, extensor digitorum brevis; EDL, extensor digitorum longus. **SEE TECHNIQUE 4.10.**

Continued

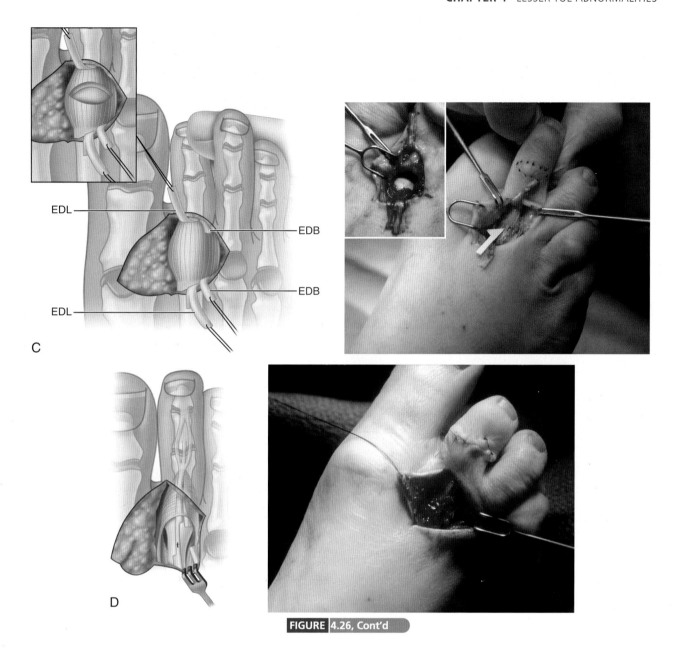

EDL

EDB

EDB

EDL

C

D

FIGURE 4.26, Cont'd

in maintaining the position of the toe, even with pinning of the reduced joint for several weeks, and the probability of a metatarsal head plantar callus developing laterally, resecting the base of the proximal phalanx is not preferred. Decompression on the metatarsal side of the joint can be achieved with a metatarsophalangeal joint arthroplasty or shortening (Weil) osteotomy of the distal metatarsal.

METATARSOPHALANGEAL JOINT ARTHROPLASTY

TECHNIQUE 4.11

- For metatarsophalangeal joint arthroplasty, resect (contour) the metatarsal head 3 to 4 mm, including its plantar projection (Fig. 4.27). This resection does not return the joint to normal, but it usually restores 10 to 20 degrees of motion in an acceptable plane, and the toe remains reduced on the metatarsal head.
- Contouring the metatarsal head enough to allow reduction of the toe and passively moving the toe 30 to 40 degrees without grating or forceful impingement of the adjacent surfaces should provide an acceptable result in a difficult deformity. The position must be held 3 to 4 weeks with a medullary pin (Fig. 4.28).
- Pin the metatarsophalangeal joint in 10 degrees of extension with the ankle held at 90 degrees. Ensure that the joint is reduced in the mediolateral plane, again while holding the ankle at 90 degrees.
- A *word of caution* concerning palpable grating of the "arthroplasty": if after contouring the metatarsal head the metatarsophalangeal joint still feels tight, with the proximal phalanx grating on the contoured metatarsal head, more bone should be removed until the grating stops.

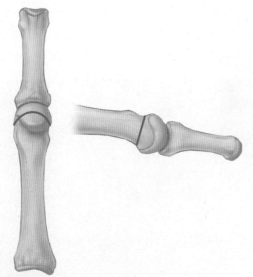

FIGURE 4.27 Resection (contouring) of metatarsal head for correction of severe hammer toe deformity with dislocation of metatarsophalangeal joint. **SEE TECHNIQUE 4.11.**

- The technique of pinning varies, but one suggestion is to insert the pin antegrade through the middle and distal phalanges, exiting in the midline 2 to 3 mm plantar to the nail (Fig. 4.29A). Reverse the pin to drive it retrograde through the remaining portion of the shaft of the proximal phalanx (the head and neck of the phalanx have been resected through a separate dorsal elliptical incision over the proximal interphalangeal joint) (Fig. 4.29B).
- Exit the articular surface of the proximal phalanx near its center, and, while standing at the head of the table holding the toe reduced at the metatarsophalangeal joint (as the patient would see the toe), have an assistant drill the pin into the metatarsal.
- Finding the medullary canal of the proximal phalanx occasionally is difficult. Take a free 0.062-inch or 0.045-inch Kirschner wire or a small straight hemostat and open the canal of the proximal phalanx. This allows the Kirschner wire to find its way without exiting the cortex before reaching the proximal articular surface.
- In moderate or severe deformity, the metatarsophalangeal joint is not pinned until the proximal interphalangeal joint contracture is corrected. This technique is the same as described in Technique 4.10.
- Remove the tourniquet and obtain hemostasis.
- Resuture the extensor digitorum longus in a lengthened position end to end. Bring the ankle joint to 90 degrees and put just enough tension on the proximal end of the extensor digitorum longus to bring it out to its resting length. Where the severed ends of the extensor digitorum longus overlap, excise the overlapping proximal portion and continue the repair with 3-0 or 4-0 absorbable suture.
- Close the skin with 4-0 or 5-0 nonabsorbable suture and place a forefoot dressing, taking care not to constrict the vascularity of the toe.
- In a chronically dislocated toe, reducing contractures at the metatarsophalangeal and proximal interphalangeal joints may place tension on the neurovascular bundles. Particularly vulnerable is the reoperated toe, with its attendant scarring

and compromised dorsal venous return. If the toe looks vascularly impaired, remove the Kirschner wire and allow the toe to "settle" in a shortened position. This places additional demands on the dressing, which must be meticulously applied to hold the toe in an acceptable position.
- A patient who requires extensive dissection on adjacent joints of the same toe must be advised preoperatively that loss of the toe from vascular compromise could occur.

POSTOPERATIVE CARE Postoperative care is the same as for a moderate deformity except that the Kirschner wire almost always is used in a severe deformity, unless compromised vascularity prevents it. The Kirschner wire is removed at 3 to 4 weeks, and the toe is maintained in the corrected position at the metatarsophalangeal and proximal interphalangeal joints with a gauze wrap and ½-inch tape. A wooden-soled shoe usually is worn for 4 weeks, and a deep, wide, soft shoe is worn for another 4 to 6 weeks. Weight bearing to tolerance is allowed after the foot is kept elevated for 48 to 72 hours. The use of crutches is optional.

■ CORRECTION OF A DISLOCATED SECOND METATARSOPHALANGEAL JOINT WITH SHORTENING METATARSAL OSTEOTOMY

As an alternative to contouring or resection arthroplasty of the second metatarsal head for a dislocated second metatarsophalangeal joint, a shortening osteotomy of the metatarsal head and neck region is reasonable, and satisfactory results have been described. An advantage of this technique is that it preserves the articular surface while decompressing the joint, making this a more popular procedure. This procedure is especially useful if the length of the second metatarsal is excessive in relation to the first and third metatarsals. Reports in the literature suggest a small incidence of transfer metatarsalgia or recurrent instability. Stiffness of the metatarsophalangeal joint may occur postoperatively but is usually not a cause of patient dissatisfaction. Complications including floating toe, recurrence of metatarsalgia, and transfer metatarsalgia have been reported in 7% to 15% of patients. Strategies to reduce the frequency of these complications include removal of a slice of bone to prevent excessive plantar translation, repair of the plantar plate when indicated or possible (see Technique 4.1), transfer of the long flexor tendon dorsally, and, occasionally, transarticular pinning across the metatarsophalangeal joint for temporary stabilization.

SHORTENING METATARSAL (WEIL) OSTEOTOMY

TECHNIQUE 4.12

(WEIL)
- Make a 3-cm longitudinal incision over the second metatarsophalangeal joint.

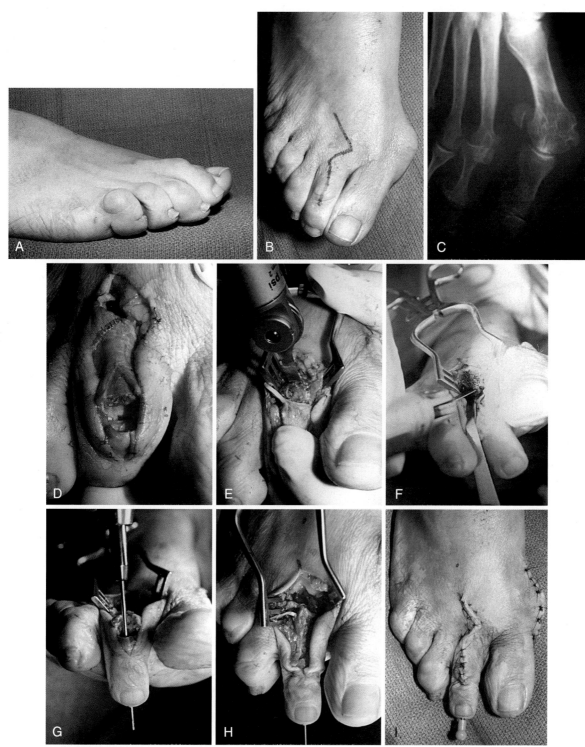

FIGURE 4.28 Reconstruction for severe hammer toe deformity with dislocation of metatarsophalangeal joint. **A** and **B,** Clinical appearance and planned operative incision. **C,** Radiographic evaluation of dislocation. **D,** After resection of proximal phalanx, dorsal capsulotomy at metatarsophalangeal joint, and extensor tendon lengthening. **E,** Resection of distal portion of metatarsal head. **F,** Plantar condylectomy of metatarsal head. **G,** Antegrade pinning through proximal interphalangeal joint with 0.045-inch Kirschner wire. **H,** Retrograde pinning through proximal phalanx across metatarsophalangeal joint. **I,** Postoperative appearance. **SEE TECHNIQUE 4.11.**

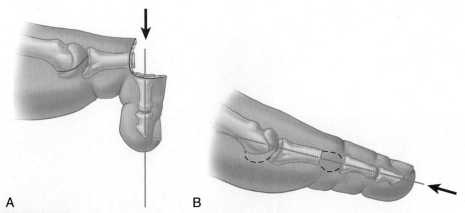

FIGURE 4.29 Pinning of metatarsophalangeal joint after contouring. **A,** Pin inserted antegrade through middle and distal phalanges. **B,** Pin reversed and driven retrograde through remaining portion of shaft of phalanx. **SEE TECHNIQUE 4.11.**

- After identification of the metatarsal head and neck, incise the joint capsule.
- Dissect the collateral ligaments of the metatarsophalangeal joint from the base of the proximal phalanx.
- Partly reduce the dislocation of the metatarsophalangeal joint and plantarflex the toe for optimal exposure of the metatarsal head.
- Use a small sagittal saw to create the osteotomy. The plane of the osteotomy should be parallel to the ground from the dorsal portion of the metatarsal head proximally (Fig. 4.30). Before this first cut is complete, create a second cut parallel to the first, removing a slice of bone 2 to 3 mm thick, depending on the amount of shortening desired.
- Shift the plantar fragment proximally to achieve the requisite amount of shortening measured preoperatively on dorsoplantar radiographs. The shortening should range from 3 to 8 mm and is determined by the length of the involved and adjacent metatarsals and by the severity of the dislocation. Attempt to make the lengths of the metatarsals equal.
- Secure the osteotomy with a single screw from the minifragment AO/ASIF set. Measure the length of the screw precisely and evaluate with intraoperative radiographs. Take care to countersink the screw head.
- Remove the resulting dorsal protuberance over the metatarsal head remnant.
- Consider advancing the Kirschner wire holding the proximal interphalangeal joint correction across the metatarsophalangeal joint and performing the osteotomy under fluoroscopic guidance. The wire must be 0.062 inch or greater to transfix the metatarsophalangeal joint or risk of pin breakage is great.

POSTOPERATIVE CARE If fixation is secure, a lightly compressive forefoot dressing is applied and the patient is allowed to bear weight as tolerated in a postoperative stiff-soled shoe. The bandages are replaced 2 weeks after surgery and are worn for 4 weeks. If radiographs show satisfactory healing, a supportive, stiff-soled running shoe may be worn 4 to 6 weeks after surgery.

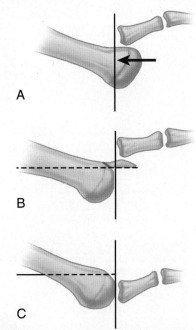

FIGURE 4.30 Weil osteotomy. **A,** Before surgery. **B,** After proximal displacement of metatarsal head. **C,** After resection of distal tip of dorsal fragment. **SEE TECHNIQUE 4.12.**

■ AMPUTATION FOR SEVERE DEFORMITY

Removal of the second toe has been recommended for severe hammer toe deformity in low-demand elderly patients. Gallentine and DeOrio reported amputation at the metatarsophalangeal joint of 17 toes in 12 patients, 10 of whom were satisfied with their outcomes and two of whom were satisfied with reservations. Associated hallux valgus was not corrected surgically, and at an average follow-up of 33 months, progression of deformity did not appear to be a problem.

MALLET TOE
ETIOLOGY

Mallet toe refers to a flexion posture of the distal interphalangeal joint (Fig. 4.31); it can occur as an isolated deformity or in conjunction with hammer toe deformity at the proximal interphalangeal joint (Fig. 4.32). The cause of mallet toe

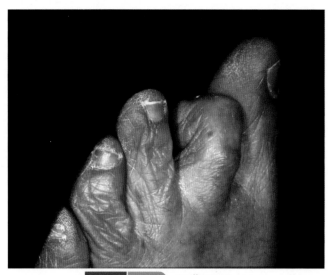

FIGURE 4.31 Mallet toe.

is uncertain; however, it occurs most often in the second toe, which is frequently the longest toe. This projection of the second toe distal to the other toes can cause pressure at the tip of the toe and buckling at the distal interphalangeal joint in a shoe with a narrow or short toe box. With time, this flexion posture can attenuate the terminal extensor tendon until it no longer can extend the distal joint. The flexor digitorum longus, in the absence of a strong antagonist, holds the distal interphalangeal joint in flexion until the deformity becomes fixed. Mallet toe is common in diabetic patients with peripheral neuropathy; the exact reason is uncertain. In feet with normal sensibility, the most frequent complication of a mallet toe is a painful end corn just beneath the nail (Fig. 4.33). The end corn results from chronic pressure at the tip of the toe, which is habitually flexed into the sole of the shoe. In diabetic patients, the corn can ulcerate and progress to a deep infection before the patient is aware of the problem. As in congenital hammer toe, congenital mallet toe usually requires no treatment.

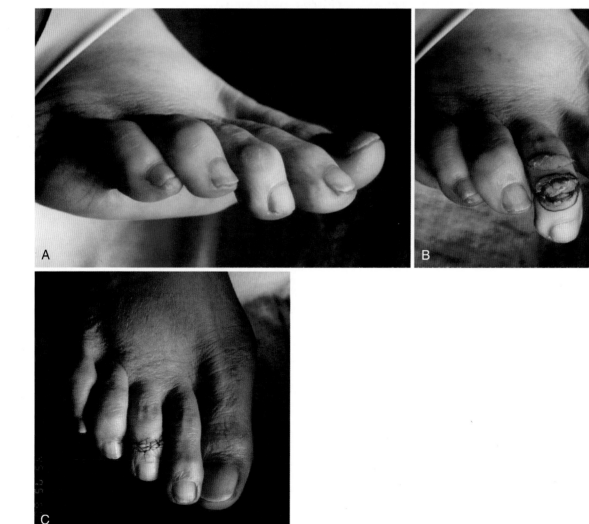

FIGURE 4.32 Mallet deformity of third and fourth digits; hammer toe deformity of second digit. **A,** Mallet deformity of third toe with dorsal callus. **B,** Dorsal elliptical skin excision. **C,** Mallet toe correction by dermodesis and hemiphalangectomy.

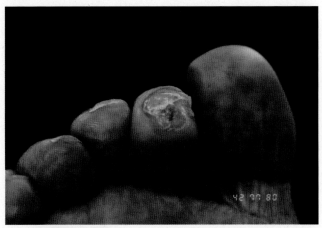

FIGURE 4.33   Mallet toe with painful end corn.

TREATMENT

The use of pads and splints for conservative treatment of mallet toe is difficult and generally unrewarding. Extra-depth shoes can be helpful, along with the use of a toe crest to relieve pressure at the tip of the toes by elevating them. If symptoms warrant surgical treatment, the alternatives are (1) flexor tenotomy at the distal interphalangeal flexion crease, (2) subtotal or total resection of the middle phalanx with dorsal dermodesis (a tenotomy of the flexor digitorum longus can be added if the bony resection and dermodesis do not hold the toe in the corrected position), or (3) amputation of the distal half of the distal phalanx to include the nail and the matrix.

Transfer of the deforming flexor digitorum longus to the extensor mechanism to correct a flexion deformity this far distal is technically difficult with little to recommend it over simpler and more dependable procedures. In elderly patients, a flexor tenotomy at the distal interphalangeal flexion crease may be all that is needed to relieve the symptoms. The flexor tenotomy usually is combined with manual correction of any fixed flexion contracture at this joint. The wound is closed with one or two sutures, and a wooden-soled shoe is recommended until the sutures are removed at 2 weeks. The patient is encouraged to wear adequately long shoes with wide toe boxes after the sutures are removed. We also have used this procedure in diabetic patients because of its simplicity. The tenotomy is performed percutaneously in the office in the midline of the distal interphalangeal crease. A compression forefoot dressing is applied, and the foot is elevated for 5 minutes by placing it on the opposite knee, which has been flexed with the patient supine. One or two sutures are used for hemostasis if needed.

If the mallet deformity is of long duration and fixed in severe flexion, resection of a portion or all of the middle phalanx, tenotomy of the flexor digitorum longus, and dorsal dermodesis are necessary to maintain correction. A terminal Syme procedure, analogous to that described for the hallux, also can be used for a severe fixed flexion contracture at the distal interphalangeal joint (Technique 4.14; Fig. 4.34). A flexor tenotomy should not be necessary, because the symptomatic end-bearing pulp of the toe is brought dorsally to close the wound. In most instances, we prefer the resection dermodesis procedure for a severe mallet toe with an end corn because it preserves the nail. Coughlin reported a slightly higher satisfaction rate with successful arthrodesis of

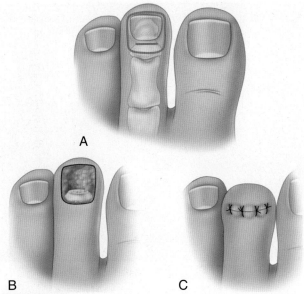

A

B   C

FIGURE 4.34   Terminal Syme procedure. **A,** Incision. **B,** After removal of nail matrix and distal half of distal phalanx, ensuring no nail matrix remains. **C,** Closure, bringing pulp dorsally. **SEE TECHNIQUE 4.14.**

the distal interphalangeal joint after resection of the head of the middle phalanx.

RESECTION DERMODESIS

TECHNIQUE 4.13

- Make a 5- to 6-mm transverse incision in the flexion crease of the distal interphalangeal joint, avoiding the neurovascular bundles at the ends of the incision.
- Use a small, single-pronged hook to bring the flexor digitorum longus into the wound and sharply divide it.
- Center a dorsal, transverse, elliptical incision over the distal interphalangeal joint and resect the skin in the ellipse (Fig. 4.35A). Short (2- to 3-mm) extensions of the elliptical incision on each side facilitate exposure of the collateral ligaments, which are divided along with the terminal extensor tendon and dorsal capsule (Fig. 4.35B).
- Acutely flex the distal phalanx and remove the head and neck of the middle phalanx (Fig. 4.35C and D).
- If a tourniquet has been used, secure hemostasis before wound closure. (By spreading longitudinally with scissors or a small hemostat, the flexor digitorum longus can be exposed through the dorsal incision after bony resection; however, if the tenotomy is performed first, as described, the amount of bone that needs to be resected to correct the deformity is better gauged.)
- Alternatively, after resection of the head and neck of the distal phalanx, remove the base of the distal phalanx with a small saw or rongeur (Fig. 4.35E).
- Use a 0.045-inch Kirschner wire to secure the position of the arthrodesis (Fig. 4.35F); remove it in 3 to 4 weeks.
- Close the dorsal incision with a horizontal mattress stitch in the center and simple sutures on each side.

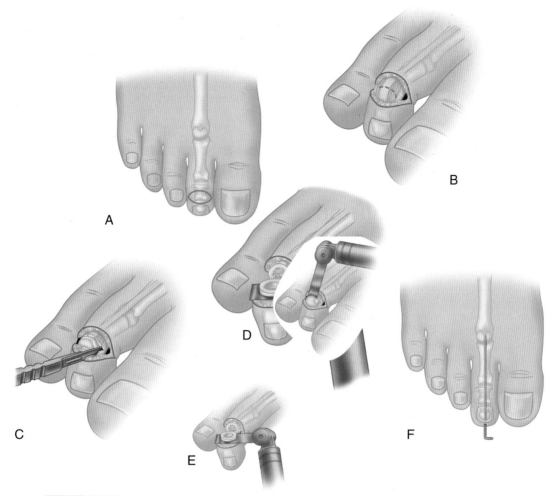

FIGURE 4.35 Resection dermodesis. **A,** Elliptical skin incision. **B,** Extensor tendon and dorsal capsule are excised. **C,** Collateral ligaments are severed, exposing condyles of middle phalanx. **D,** Condyles of middle phalanx are excised in supracondylar region with rongeur. **E,** Articular surface of distal phalanx is excised. **F,** Placement of Kirschner wire. **SEE TECHNIQUE 4.13.**

- Close the plantar wound with simple interrupted sutures and apply a dressing that maintains the toe in the desired position by splinting it to an adjacent toe.

POSTOPERATIVE CARE The sutures are removed at 2 weeks, and the affected toe is kept splinted with a soft dressing to an adjacent toe for another week.

TERMINAL SYME PROCEDURE

TECHNIQUE 4.14

- Make an incision that encircles the nail of the affected toe to include 2 to 3 mm of nail fold on each side and distally and 3 to 4 mm proximally to ensure complete removal of the nail matrix (see Fig. 4.34A).

- Carry the incision to bone proximally. Skirt the side and tip of the tuft of the phalanx until the pulp tissue is freed from the distal half of the distal phalanx. Do not disturb the flexor digitorum longus tendon.
- Using a small bone biter or rongeur, remove the exposed bone (usually the distal half).
- Carefully inspect the proximal margin of the wound to ensure no matrix tissue remains (see Fig. 4.34B).
- Bring the pulp flap dorsally and suture it to the proximal skin margin with interrupted 4-0 nonabsorbable sutures (see Fig. 4.34C).

POSTOPERATIVE CARE The postoperative care is essentially the same as for resection dermodesis, but the dressing can be removed at 2 weeks when the sutures are removed. No splinting is necessary because the distal interphalangeal joint is stable.

COMBINED HAMMER TOE AND MALLET TOE DEFORMITY WITH ASSOCIATED DOUBLE CORNS

Combined hammer toe and mallet toe deformity with associated double corns differs from the traditional claw toe deformity in that there is minimal to no extension deformity at the metatarsophalangeal joint. Large prominent corns usually are over the proximal and distal interphalangeal joints. The approximately 10% recurrence rate after combined distal interphalangeal and proximal interphalangeal resection arthroplasties has been attributed to inadequate bone resection.

COMPLICATIONS AND REVISION SURGERY OF HAMMER TOE DEFORMITIES

Certainly, the most immediate complication of lesser toe surgery is postoperative ischemia of the toe. Fortunately, this is rare in patients with adequate vascularity preoperatively. It seems to be more common in revision procedures and in patients who are active smokers. The patients should be counseled before surgery about this potential problem. We do not use epinephrine in forefoot blocks if a tourniquet is to be used. If a toe exhibits ischemia in the immediate postoperative period, the dressing can be loosened and the Kirschner wire removed if needed. Often the toe will have some venous engorgement and not true ischemia, which can be managed with observation only. Boyce and Dhukaram described three patients in whom glyceryl trinitrate patches successfully reversed ischemic episodes after correction of toe deformities.

Unfortunately, not all hammer toe operations produce a nicely aligned, painless toe that is comfortable in a variety of shoes. Decision making for a patient with a less than perfect outcome begins with a thorough analysis of the problem. Were there unrealistic expectations to begin with? What are the specific complaints of the patient? Has there been sufficient time for the particular problem to resolve? Where is the deformity and is there satisfactory structural support for a revision procedure?

Many of the previously discussed procedures may be appropriate for a revision situation, but care must be taken to correct the specific problem(s). Probably the most common problem is the development of varus or valgus deformity at the proximal interphalangeal joint after a hammer toe procedure. This often is the result of an overly aggressive resection of the head of the proximal phalanx. Bone overgrowth after the resection can produce deformity as well. The patient should understand before any hammer toe procedure that some mild residual deformity often occurs as the toe "molds" into a position between the adjacent toes. Postoperative swelling and edema in the toe can be protracted, and the final size and shape of the toe often are not completely defined for about a year after the procedure.

For recurrent deformity, an internal stent often can be helpful in producing lasting deformity correction. We have been pleased with the results of using an absorbable intramedullary device for this purpose. It is important to correct any metatarsophalangeal joint instability before revision of the toe deformity. Konkel et al. recently reported improved results with the use of stiffer poly-L-lactate absorbable pins over those obtained with more flexible polydioxanone absorbable pins.

Boffeli et al. proposed a two-pin Kirschner wire fixation technique as an option, noting improved stability against rotational and bending forces and decreased potential for pin-related complications. Only two complications (loose or broken implant) were encountered in 91 digits (2.20%) in their study. At our institution, we use this technique for joint arthrodesis of the fifth toe.

PROXIMAL INTERPHALANGEAL JOINT ARTHRODESIS WITH AN ABSORBABLE INTRAMEDULLARY PIN

TECHNIQUE 4.15

(KONKEL ET AL.)

- After mild to moderate sedation is obtained with an ankle block and an Esmarch ankle tourniquet is applied, make a 2-cm dorsal longitudinal incision over the proximal interphalangeal joint and carry dissection down to the bone.
- Release the extensor hood, capsule, synovium, and collateral ligaments; do not cut the volar plate or expose or release the flexor tendon.
- Use a mini–oscillating saw to cut the cartilage and subchondral bone from the distal proximal phalanx at a right angle to the longitudinal axis of the proximal phalanx and remove it from the field.
- Use the mini–oscillating saw to cut the cartilage and subchondral bone at right angles to the longitudinal axis of the middle phalanx and remove this piece from the field.
- If the proximal interphalangeal joint is easily corrected with the bone ends apposed without tension, no further resection is necessary. If it is not easily corrected, remove more of the distal proximal phalanx as needed to correct the deformity without force. Avoid excessive resection to minimize the risk of an unstable construct.
- Use a 2-mm drill retrograde to drill through the middle phalanx and into the distal phalanx, taking care to avoid drilling through the tuft of the distal phalanx. Be sure to hold the distal phalanx straight and aligned to the longitudinal axis of the middle phalanx during retrograde drilling.
- Use a 2-mm smooth spike to slightly overream the areas of drilling proximally and distally to allow rod insertion.
- Carefully measure the lengths of the drillings with a depth gauge and cut a 2-mm absorbable pin to the proper length; bevel the cut ends to avoid sharp edges.
- Insert the pin into the middle phalanx.
- While holding the dorsal phalanx straight in relation to the middle phalanx, slide the distal pin through the intramedullary canal of the middle phalanx and into the distal phalanx until the distal interphalangeal joint is straight and the pin is secure in the distal phalanx.
- Use a moderate-size needle holder or hemostat to bend and curl the pin until its distal tip enters the hole drilled in the proximal phalanx. The raw bone ends of the middle phalanx and proximal phalanx should be opposed as the pin is placed into the proximal phalanx.

- Release the toe and check for position. Bring the foot and ankle into standing position; if the toe is hyperextended at the metatarsophalangeal joint, use a No. 11 scalpel blade to make a percutaneous extensor tenotomy proximal to the metatarsophalangeal joint. If the toe is flexed, release the Esmarch tourniquet before closure to relax flexion. Flexor tendon release is not necessary.
- Close the wound in layers with 3-0 Dexon used for the extensor hood and subcutaneous tissue and 4-0 nylon running suture for the skin. Apply a soft dressing with a 4-inch elastic wrap to hold the toe in the corrected position.

POSTOPERATIVE CARE An open-toe postoperative shoe is used constantly for the first 2 weeks. The patient is advised to elevate the foot above the heart as much as possible for the first 48 hours and to keep the dressings clean, dry, and intact during the first 2 weeks. After the first 2 weeks, a light dressing is worn until all eschars are gone and the wound is completely healed. There are no restrictions on weight bearing. At 10 to 14 days the sutures are removed and adhesive strips are applied; 10 days after suture removal, showers are allowed with air drying. No soaking or tub baths are allowed for the first 6 weeks. Comfort shoes with extra depth are recommended for the next 4 to 6 weeks, with any shoes allowed at 10 to 14 weeks.

CORNS (HELOMATA AND CLAVI)
ETIOLOGY AND CLINICAL FINDINGS

Corns are hyperkeratotic lesions occurring over bony prominences and involving the stratum corneum, or horny layer, of the skin. Clinically, corns usually are classified as hard or soft. Both types are caused by pressure from unyielding structures. In hard corns, the phalangeal condyle beneath the skin and an unyielding shoe toe box over the skin generate pressure and friction. With time, a painful lesion develops, usually over the dorsolateral aspect of the proximal interphalangeal joint of the fifth toe. The lesion is firm, dry, and tender. Surrounding erythema and heat are present if the corn is acutely irritated, and a bursa may develop (Fig. 4.36). A wart should not be mistaken for a hard corn (Fig. 4.37).

In contrast, a soft corn usually is interdigital. An *interdigital* corn probably is a more descriptive term than a *soft* corn. There are two types of interdigital corns, the most common of which is in the distal portion of the web and involves the base of the distal phalanx of the shorter toe and abuts the head of the proximal phalanx of the longer toe. Occasionally, a dystrophic nail can produce the pressure necessary for an interdigital corn to develop. A slightly less common, but more troublesome, soft corn occurs in the base of the web space, most commonly in the fourth web space (Fig. 4.38A). These corns are associated with an abnormally short fifth metatarsal and occasionally are associated with hallux valgus, which causes adduction pressure on the fifth toe from the shoe (Fig. 4.38B,C). They result from pressure imposed by the lateral side of the base of the fourth proximal phalanx or the medial condyle of the head of the fifth proximal phalanx, or both. Moisture softens the hyperkeratotic area, and occasionally

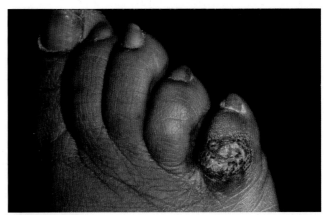

FIGURE 4.36 Acutely inflamed hard corn over dorsolateral surface of fifth toe with swelling, heat, and erythema.

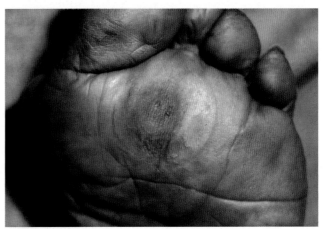

FIGURE 4.37 Lesion appeared to be plantar keratosis until pared down to reveal wart.

a sinus develops between the central part of the corn and the web space. When this happens, suppuration usually follows (Fig. 4.39). In a diabetic or any immunocompromised patient, this relatively minor lesion can produce catastrophic problems.

The plantar corn is another example of a hard corn (heloma durum and clavus durus). Patients occasionally present with a circumscribed plug of keratin that recently has been plucked from the center of these isolated, hyperkeratotic lesions. They are located beneath a metatarsal head, usually of the lesser toes, just plantar to the prominent fibular side of the condyle of the metatarsal head, which projects more plantar than the tibial side. If the lesion occurs beneath the first metatarsal head, it usually is under the tibial sesamoid. Mann and DuVries referred to a plantar corn that failed to respond to conservative treatment as an intractable plantar keratosis, or a localized invaginated callus, and distinguished between localized and diffuse lesions (Fig. 4.40). Plantar hyperkeratotic lesions are common in older people, causing pain, mobility impairment, and functional limitation. One study found plantar hyperkeratotic lesions in 60% of 301 patients older than the age of 70 years, most often in women and those with hallux valgus or other toe deformities. Correction of the hallux valgus deformity alone, without lesser metatarsal osteotomy, has been reported to improve painful plantar callosities under the lesser metatarsals.

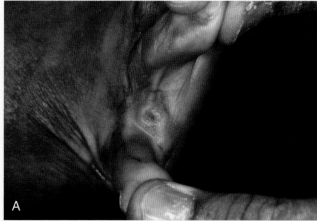

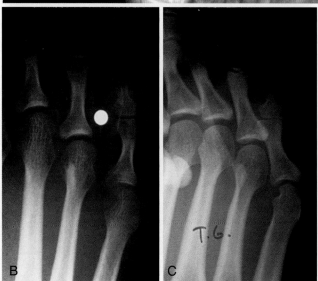

FIGURE 4.38 **A,** Fourth web space interdigital corn. **B,** Corresponding radiograph with marker overlying corn. Note two-boned fifth toe and abnormally short fifth metatarsal. **C,** Oblique view showing apposition of base of fourth proximal phalanx and head of fifth proximal phalanx.

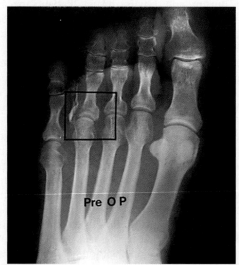

FIGURE 4.39 Infected soft corn. Note opaque material for sinogram and lytic changes at base of proximal phalanx *(box)*.

Finally, a rare lesion is the neurovascular corn, which is very painful and usually is located beneath the first or fifth metatarsal head. It frequently is confused with a plantar wart. Gentle paring of the lesion reveals poorly demarcated edges with blood vessels that lie parallel to the plantar surface of the foot, however, as opposed to the vertical orientation of vessels in a plantar wart.

TREATMENT

Keratotic lesions should be managed nonoperatively until the patient has tried a variety of self-help aids widely available in foot care sections of retail stores. (We keep a small variety of these aids in the office for instruction and initial treatment.) We have had some success using a sleeve with a friction-absorbing pad consisting of medical-grade paraffin (Silipos). If this fails to relieve symptoms or is time-consuming for the patient on a daily basis, surgical treatment is warranted. Lee et al. reported that over 90% of patients with lesser metatarsal callosities had improvement of their pain after correction of the hallux valgus deformity. Although symptoms associated with lesser metatarsal callosities may improve, deformity of the lesser toe at the metatarsophalangeal joint must be corrected at the time of hallux valgus correction to obtain complete long-term relief.

■ HARD CORN

Because the most common location of a hard corn is over the dorsolateral side of the proximal interphalangeal joint of the little toe, the procedure for this location is described; however, it can be used in other lesser toes.

HARD CORN TREATMENT

TECHNIQUE 4.16

- Use local anesthesia and a local tourniquet if needed, to make a dorsolateral incision skirting the medial border of the corn, beginning 5 to 6 mm proximal to the nail and extending proximally 1.5 cm.
- Remove the bony prominence on the dorsolateral aspect of the condyle of the proximal phalanx by sharp dissection with a small-blade knife, and, with a rongeur or small sagittal saw, resect any bony prominence from the adjacent side of the middle phalangeal base.
- Palpation of this area after removing the prominence is more revealing than inspection to determine the completeness of removal. Ensure that no bony prominence remains, even if this means resecting the entire head and neck of the proximal phalanx.
- Resection of the head and neck of the proximal phalanx more reliably prevents recurrence, and it is the most commonly used procedure at this clinic. Instability at the resected proximal interphalangeal joint occurs, however. This annoyance has been lessened by appropriate dressings worn for 3 to 4 weeks and then tape splinting for an additional 3 to 4 weeks. If only the bony prominence is removed, it is wise to inform the patient of possible recurrence and later need for resection arthroplasty.

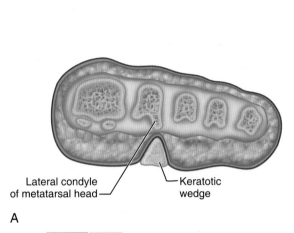

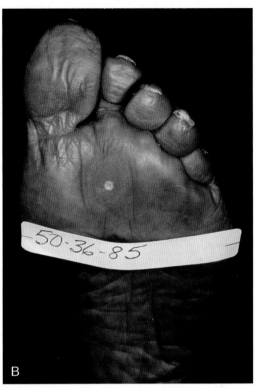

Lateral condyle
of metatarsal head —

— Keratotic
wedge

A

B

FIGURE 4.40 Plantar keratosis. **A,** Intractable plantar keratosis; note prominent lateral condyle of second metatarsal head. **B,** Intractable plantar keratosis beneath second metatarsal head.

POSTOPERATIVE CARE A wooden-soled shoe or any shoe with the toe box removed laterally is worn for 3 to 4 weeks, at which time a shoe with a wide toe box usually is comfortable.

A note of caution: Enlargement of the toe frequently persists for weeks or even months after the procedure. Swelling is visible because of the lack of a soft-tissue envelope of the toes; acute or chronic edema has no place to hide. This swelling resolves for the most part, but informing the patient preoperatively of enlargement of the toe for an extended period prevents misunderstanding.

■ SOFT CORN (INTERDIGITAL CORN)

Soft corns usually are located in the fourth interdigital space and are caused by underlying pressure from the medial flare of the base of the distal phalanx of the fifth toe abutting the proximal interphalangeal joint of the fourth toe. This problem can be resolved surgically by removing the underlying bony problem. Usually only one side of the opposing prominence requires removal; however, in severe cases, resection of both sides may be necessary. A "web corn," or a soft corn located deep in the fourth web space, is caused when the lateral condyle of the base of the proximal phalanx of the fourth toe and the medial side of the head of the proximal phalanx of the fifth toe pinch the adjacent skin surfaces together. Appreciating bony prominences by palpation and inspection often is difficult. Separating the toes draws the corn into the center of the web space, when actually, in a shod, weight-bearing position, the corn is superficial to the lateral base of the proximal phalanx of the fourth toe. A callosity develops, and this callosity can ulcerate and become infected by the normal flora occupying the moist interdigital web space. The usual treatment is to wash the web spaces twice a day with household soap; dry the web completely; and apply an antifungal, antibacterial powder and lamb's wool or a self-adherent rubber web spacer (doughnut), which can be found in any foot care section in a retail store.

If the corn remains painful, becomes infected again, or ulcerates despite preventing bony impingement, or if the patient tires of the time and care necessary to control the corn, operative treatment is justified.

A web space corn can be most troublesome, and recurrence is likely if adequate bone is not removed. Resecting the lateral flare of the base of the proximal phalanx of the fourth toe flush with the diaphysis or removing the head and neck of the proximal phalanx of the fifth toe may be curative. Occasionally, however, both may need resecting. If the hyperkeratotic area of ulceration is located more on the fifth toe side of the web, the head and neck of the proximal phalanx of the fifth toe should be resected through either a dorsal, transverse, elliptical incision over the proximal interphalangeal joint or a dorsolateral, gently curved incision. If the center of the hyperkeratotic area or ulceration is more on the fourth phalangeal side of the web, however, the lateral flare of the base of the fourth phalanx should be resected flush with the diaphysis. Either way, the web space should be palpated after the resection to determine whether there will be any residual bony impingement. If the resection seems inadequate, the opposite bony offender must be resected. The toes are kept dressed for 3 weeks, holding them in the proper position, followed by 3 weeks of taping the toes together loosely with lamb's wool between them.

Ulcers should not be closed because they heal quickly when the bony pressure is removed. The surgical portion

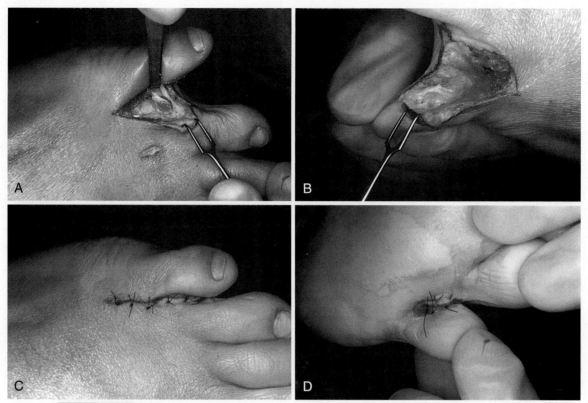

FIGURE 4.41 **A,** Exposure of web space and resection of lateral base of fourth phalanx. **B,** Exposure and resection of medial aspect of proximal fifth toe. Dorsal **(C)** and plantar **(D)** appearance of closure. **SEE TECHNIQUE 4.17.**

of the wound can be closed. Surgery should never be done through a moist, weeping ulcer. The web space can be treated with drying agents, antibacterial solutions, and a spacer such as lamb's wool until the web space is dry.

For a recurrent or intractable interdigital corn, a partial, simple syndactylization can be effective. Placing the digital limbs of the incision on the adjacent plantar sides of the toes retains some of the cosmetic cleft the patient sees from the dorsal aspect of the toe.

PARTIAL SYNDACTYLIZATION FOR INTRACTABLE INTERDIGITAL CORN

TECHNIQUE 4.17

- Make a dorsal longitudinal incision extending to the plantar portion of the interdigital space.
- Extend the two limbs into the adjacent sides of the plantar third of the opposing toes.
- Resect the lateral flare of the base of the proximal phalanx of the fourth toe (Fig. 4.41A) and the medial portion of the head of the proximal phalanx of the fifth toe (Fig. 4.41B).
- Close the wound beginning proximally and extending distally, suturing the dorsal limbs together (Fig. 4.41C).
- Excise a small amount of skin at the apex of the dorsal skin flaps, including the web corn if necessary.

- Close the plantar limbs, partially syndactylizing the toe (Fig. 4.41D).

POSTOPERATIVE CARE A soft compressive dressing is applied, and a broad-spectrum antibiotic is given for 2 days. Sutures are removed at 2 weeks. With lamb's wool in the interdigital space overlying the incision, the toes are buddy taped for an additional 2 weeks.

PLANTAR CORN (INTRACTABLE PLANTAR KERATOSIS)

A plantar corn usually can be made asymptomatic by conservative care. Patient education and physician assiduity are essential for the method to succeed. If a lengthy course of conservative care fails, the following procedures have given the best results. Regardless of the procedure chosen, recurrence or transfer of the lesion occurs in 10% to 15% of patients, emphasizing the need for using all conservative measures before surgery. Careful physical and radiographic evaluation of the callus and the metatarsal head are essential in choosing the correct procedure. For a small, intractable plantar keratosis, arthroplasty usually is preferred. A diffuse callosity in which the involved metatarsal head is more prominent or plantarflexed relative to the adjacent heads may require dorsiflexion osteotomy. For a diffuse callosity in which the radiograph shows an abnormally long metatarsal, a shortening osteotomy may be indicated.

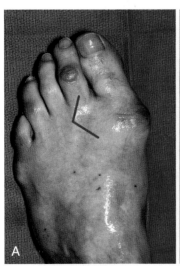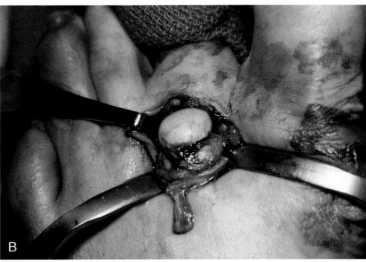

FIGURE 4.42   Arthroplasty of metatarsophalangeal joint. **A,** Incision over second metatarsophalangeal joint with apex at joint level. **B,** Acute flexion of second toe after sectioning of collateral ligaments. **SEE TECHNIQUE 4.18.**

ARTHROPLASTY OF THE METATARSOPHALANGEAL JOINT

Arthroplasty is indicated for a small, isolated, intractable plantar keratosis beneath the lateral condyle of one of the second to fifth metatarsals, resulting in a reported 85% to 90% satisfaction rate. Complications of the procedure include dorsal contracture of the metatarsophalangeal joint, with hammering of the affected toe, fracture of the metatarsal head, osteonecrosis of the metatarsal head, and medial or lateral drift of the toe and limitation of motion of the metatarsophalangeal joint.

TECHNIQUE 4.18

(MANN AND DUVRIES)
- Make a hockey-stick incision, starting in the web space, and carry it down over the metatarsal head and distal third of the metatarsal shaft (Fig. 4.42A).
- Identify the transverse metatarsal ligament on both sides of the involved metatarsal head and cut the ligament.
- Retract the extensor tendon to one side and enter the metatarsophalangeal joint through a longitudinal incision.
- Sever the collateral ligaments and firmly plantarflex the involved toe while pushing dorsally on the distal metatarsal shaft (Fig. 4.42B).
- Remove 2 to 3 mm of the distal portion of the metatarsal head with a thin, small osteotome or power saw with a 4-mm blade.
- By placing traction on the toe while it is flexed and pushing dorsally under the distal metatarsal, the plantar lip of the condyle is visible. Remove the plantar lip so that approximately 50% of the metatarsal head is excised.
- Smooth the metatarsal head with a rongeur or rasp and reduce the joint.

POSTOPERATIVE CARE   A wooden-soled shoe is worn for 4 weeks, and active range-of-motion exercises are begun. Usually about 25% of joint motion is lost after this procedure, but this rarely is of clinical significance. Transfer lesions beneath an adjacent metatarsal head occur in fewer than 5% of patients.

We have modified this procedure in several ways. An extension posture to the metatarsophalangeal joint frequently is present and must be relieved by dorsal capsulotomy (also by a collateral ligament incision, if necessary). The toe is held in the proper position on the metatarsal head by the dressing or a small Kirschner wire. It is not necessary to remove the articular surface of the metatarsal head if the metatarsal is lifted dorsally with a curved Hohmann retractor and the toe acutely flexed more than 90 degrees. This allows exposure of the plantar projection of the metatarsal head so that only the projecting plantar portion of the condyle is osteotomized flush with the metatarsal shaft. A small key elevator placed behind the plantar condyles of the metatarsal heads may prevent migration of the fragment after osteotomy.

This procedure can be done through a plantar approach with a longitudinal incision set a few millimeters medial to the weight-bearing portion of the metatarsal head and 4 to 5 cm long. When deep to the skin and subcutaneous tissue, the neurovascular bundle is retracted medially, and the sheath of the flexor tendons is incised longitudinally. The flexor tendons are retracted laterally, and the plantar plate is incised longitudinally. This gives excellent exposure of the projecting condyle and allows removal without disrupting the dorsal capsule, collateral ligaments, deep transverse intermetatarsal ligaments, or articular surface of the metatarsal head.

The plantar plate is closed with 3-0 absorbable sutures after the curved needle is bent more acutely to facilitate passage in a tight space. The flexor tendons are allowed to resume their normal course, and the pulley is not repaired. The skin is closed with nonabsorbable 2-0 or 3-0 monofilament nylon. The sutures are removed after 14 to 21 days. Weight bearing to tolerance in a postoperative stiff-soled shoe is allowed immediately.

We have found the plantar incision useful in many instances of foot surgery; it affords excellent exposure that would have been unobtainable through a dorsal incision and results in no more incisional complications than the dorsal approach.

■ EXCESSIVE METATARSAL LENGTH AND DIFFUSE PLANTAR KERATOSIS AND METATARSALGIA

Many procedures have been developed for diffuse plantar keratoses associated with metatarsalgia and a long metatarsal. Because of satisfactory results in the literature, several options for treatment are presented. Our experience with metatarsal osteotomy for plantar keratoses has been unsatisfactory because of complications, and all conservative measures should be exhausted. Resection of the plantar aspect of the metatarsal head, although less likely to yield a bad result, may cause symptoms to shift to the adjacent metatarsal head. In some patients, especially women who must wear fashionable shoes, intractable pain under a long second metatarsal requires surgical intervention. We recommend the Weil osteotomy for these patients (see Technique 4.12) because it has fewer complications and better results than other shortening osteotomies. There is less chance of transfer symptoms to adjacent metatarsal heads than with shortening osteotomies of the metatarsal shaft. In addition, the Weil osteotomy incorporates the metaphyseal bone, so there is less chance of delayed union or nonunion. With a dorsiflexion osteotomy through the metaphyseal bone at the base of the metatarsal, controlling the amount of dorsiflexion and the relative position of the metatarsal head can be difficult, and this procedure is not as effective in shortening the metatarsal as others.

Although we prefer the Weil osteotomy to treat excessive length of the metatarsal associated with metatarsalgia and diffuse plantar callosity with or without instability of the metatarsophalangeal joint, the following two procedures are included based on reported satisfactory results.

DORSAL CLOSING WEDGE OSTEOTOMY OF THE METATARSALS FOR INTRACTABLE PLANTAR KERATOSIS

TECHNIQUE 4.19

- Use an Esmarch wrap exsanguination to ankle level after administering an ankle block regional anesthetic for hemostasis and analgesia.
- If the keratosis is beneath the second metatarsal (most commonly), begin the incision 1 cm proximal to the articulation of the second metatarsal with the intermediate cuneiform and continue it distally over the second metatarsal for 3 cm. This articulation is palpable by lifting up and down on the second metatarsal head while palpating the base of the metatarsal. This articulation is recessed proximally about 0.5 cm to the third metatarsal base and about 1 cm to the first metatarsal base.
- Incise just the skin because a branch of the superficial peroneal nerve, extensor hallucis brevis, deep peroneal

nerve, and accompanying dorsalis pedis artery all may be encountered through this incision. The same incision placed more laterally in the third or fourth metatarsal is not anatomically encumbered.
- Identify the joint.
- Using motion or a straight needle, measure 6 to 7 mm distal to the joint and score the bone at this point.
- Remove a dorsal wedge 2 mm wide and penetrate the plantar cortex just enough to allow the wedge to be closed by pushing dorsally on the second metatarsal head.
- The osteology of the base of the second metatarsal is such that it is shaped on its plantar surface similar to the keel of a boat. The apex of this keel is slightly lateral to the midline of the dorsal base. Aim the osteotome or power saw (4-mm blade) slightly (10 to 20 degrees) lateral when making the dorsal-to-plantar cut. The height of the base of the second metatarsal is about 1.5 cm.
- Hold the osteotomy with crossed Kirschner wires or a 2.7-mm screw. If the screw is used, it is helpful to drill the near cortex before the osteotomy and place the screw dorsomedial to plantar-lateral to ensure bony purchase.
- Remove the tourniquet wrap, obtain hemostasis, and apply a short leg cast to extend beyond the toes over a soft compression dressing.

POSTOPERATIVE CARE Weight bearing is not allowed on the cast for 3 weeks, and only partial weight bearing is allowed for another 3 weeks. If union is apparent at 6 weeks, a stiff-soled shoe is permitted. If not, a short leg walking cast is worn another 4 weeks. Union may require 3 to 5 months.

For a well-localized, intractable keratosis beneath the tibial sesamoid, Mann and DuVries recommended resecting the sesamoid or skiving off its plantar half. An alternative treatment is a dorsal closing wedge (2 to 3 mm) proximal osteotomy of the first metatarsal with pin fixation. In either instance, a short leg cast is recommended for 6 weeks, with partial weight bearing allowed in the last 3 weeks.

BUNIONETTE (TAILOR'S BUNION)

The bony prominence on the lateral side of the fifth metatarsal head often is called a *tailor's bunion*, referring to the position in which tailors would sit on the floor with their legs crossed, forcing the lateral border of the foot against the floor (Fig. 4.43). It often is seen in splay foot combined with hallux valgus, or the head of the fifth metatarsal may be congenitally or traumatically enlarged. Also, the shaft may be angulated laterally, making the fifth metatarsal head more prominent (Fig. 4.44). Standard weight-bearing views of the foot, including dorsoplantar, lateral, and oblique, should be obtained for measurement of the 4-5 intermetatarsal angle (4-5 IMA). This angle is formed by two lines that bisect the fourth and fifth metatarsals (Fig. 4.45). The normal 4-5 IMA is less than 6.5 to 8 degrees; the average 4-5 IMA is 6.5 degrees in normal feet and 9.6 degrees in feet with a symptomatic bunionette. Bunionettes also are classified based on these weight-bearing radiographs (Fig. 4.46): type I, enlargement of the fifth metatarsal head or a

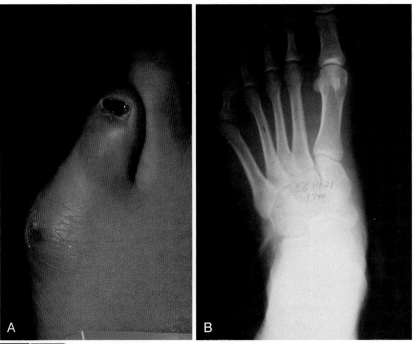

FIGURE 4.43 **A** and **B**, Bunionette with metatarsus quintus valgus and fifth toe varus.

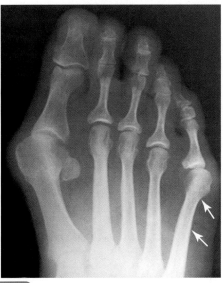

FIGURE 4.44 Bunionette–hallux valgus–splay foot complex. Note lateral angulation of shaft of fifth metatarsal at distal third *(arrows)*.

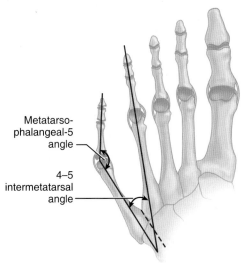

FIGURE 4.45 Measurement of metatarsophalangeal-fifth and fourth-fifth intermetatarsal angles for evaluation of bunionette deformity. (Redrawn from Cohen BE, Nicholson CW: Bunionette, J Am Acad Orthop Surg 15:300, 2007.)

lateral exostosis; type II, abnormal lateral bend to the distal fifth metatarsal with a normal 4-5 IMA; and type III, an increased 4-5 IMA (>8 degrees) that results in a widened forefoot. Type III is the most common deformity. Other angles that may be useful are the lateral deviation angle (Fig. 4.47), which is formed by a line from the center of the metatarsal head and neck to the metatarsal base and a line along the medial cortex of the fifth metatarsal (normal, 2.6 degrees; with bunionette, 8 degrees), and the fifth metatarsophalangeal angle (see Fig. 4.45), which usually is more than 14 degrees in symptomatic patients. Shimobayashi et al. analyzed the radiographic morphologic characteristics of the entire foot in patients with symptomatic bunionette deformity and found that the third, fourth, and fifth metatarsal heads were more displaced laterally in patients with deformity than those without deformity. In addition, all intermetatarsal angles were larger in patients with deformity compared with normal feet. They suggest assessing the entire foot for width and splaying of all metatarsals, not just the fifth, which may represent only one cause of the deformity.

Constricting shoes are the main source of discomfort. With continuous pressure over this bony prominence, a bursa develops and enlarges because of chronic irritation

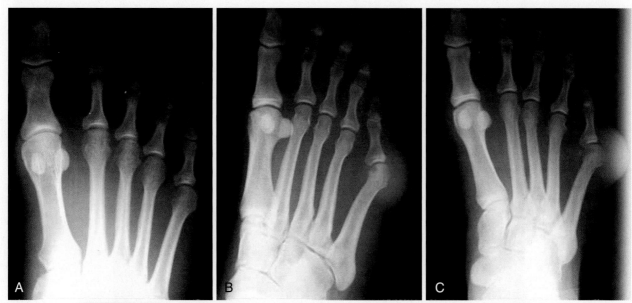

FIGURE 4.46 Classification of bunionette deformity. **A,** Type I, lateral prominence of metatarsal head. **B,** Type II, lateral bowing of fifth metatarsal. **C,** Type III, widening of fourth-fifth intermetatarsal angle. (From Cohen BE, Nicholson CW: Bunionette, J Am Acad Orthop Surg 15:300, 2007.)

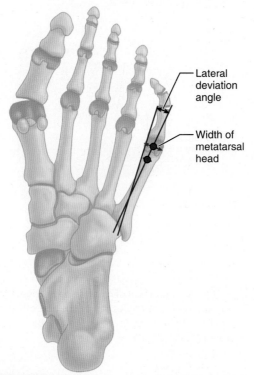

Lateral
deviation
angle

Width of
metatarsal
head

FIGURE 4.47 Measurement of lateral deviation angle in evaluation of bunionette deformity. (Redrawn from Cohen BE, Nicholson CW: Bunionette, J Am Acad Orthop Surg 15:300, 2007.)

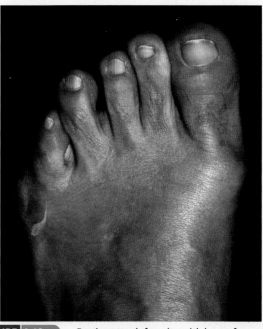

FIGURE 4.48 Bunionette deformity with bursa formation.

(Fig. 4.48). Ulceration may ensue. An intractable keratosis may develop over a prominent bunionette because of shoe pressure. In diabetes, advanced Charcot-Marie-Tooth disease, or certain types of spinal dysraphism with poor sensibility, this complication can result in loss of the entire fifth ray or even the foot.

In addition to a symptomatic bursa over the lateral aspect of the prominent fifth metatarsal head, a diffuse callus or localized intractable keratosis can develop beneath the plantar aspect of the fifth metatarsal head (Fig. 4.49).

TREATMENT

Treatment with metatarsal pads or bars, wide toe box shoes, semirigid shoe inserts with a relief (or "well") beneath the plantar aspect of the condyle, or ⅛- to ¼-inch foam rubber between the prominence and the shoe may relieve the symptoms. If surgical treatment becomes necessary, the choices are (1) resection of the lateral third of the fifth metatarsal head, (2) osteotomy of the fifth metatarsal (Fig. 4.50), and (3) resection of the fifth metatarsal head.

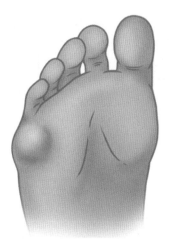

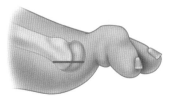

FIGURE 4.51 Plantar aspect of fifth metatarsal head should be removed in addition to lateral flare.

FIGURE 4.49 Callus beneath fifth metatarsal head. If extension deformity is present at fifth metatarsophalangeal joint, painful callus may develop beneath fifth metatarsal head.

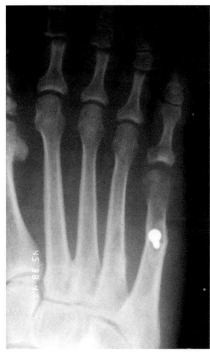

FIGURE 4.50 Diaphyseal osteotomy for metatarsus quintus varus.

■ RESECTION

PARTIAL RESECTION OF THE LATERAL CONDYLE OF THE FIFTH METATARSAL HEAD

Partial resection of the lateral condyle of the fifth metatarsal head probably is the most commonly used procedure. It relieves the pressure symptoms and allows a slightly greater variety of shoe wear. The cosmetic correction is not always pleasing, however. Causes of failure may include inadequate resection, metatarsophalangeal joint subluxation, and forefoot splaying. The patient must be warned

before surgery that only the painful bony prominence will be removed and that the width of the forefoot will not be altered appreciably. In addition, if there is a painful callosity beneath the metatarsal head, the plantar aspect of the condyle also should be removed (Fig. 4.51). The presence of a plantar keratosis suggests that an osteotomy of the metatarsal may be necessary for satisfactory correction of the deformity.

TECHNIQUE 4.20

- Make a dorsolateral or straight lateral (preferred) incision extending from the junction of the middle and distal thirds of the fifth metatarsal shaft to the midshaft of the proximal phalanx.
- Incise only the skin.
- If the dorsolateral incision is used, identify and protect the dorsolateral cutaneous branch of the sural nerve (Fig. 4.52A,B).
- The straight lateral incision should pass between this nerve dorsally and the proper digital branch of the lateral plantar nerve to the fifth toe plantarward.
- The tendon of insertion of the abductor digiti minimi passes just plantar to the midline of the lateral aspect of the fifth metatarsal head. If the periosteal and capsular incision is in a straight line 2 or 3 mm dorsal to the midline, this tendon is preserved. This is important because the fifth toe can subluxate or dislocate medially if the tendon of insertion is lost (Fig. 4.53).
- By sharp dissection, elevate the capsule dorsally and plantarward until the fifth metatarsal head can be made visible by delivering it laterally as the phalanx is pushed medially. More metatarsal head can be removed than is intended if the medial edge of the articular cartilage is not exposed. Approximately 35% to 40% of the metatarsal head usually is removed to excise the bony prominence. A thin osteotome or a small blade on a power saw is mandatory.
- Score the proximal margin of the proposed osteotomy and direct the cut in a dorsal distal-to-plantar proximal direction (Fig. 4.52C,D).
- Reduce the phalanx over the remaining part of the fifth metatarsal head and palpate the lateral flare of the base of the phalanx. If this produces a projecting bony prominence that may cause symptoms, excise the prominence with a rongeur or bone-biter in the same manner as a web corn is treated medially.
- This procedure removes the origin and possibly the insertion of the lateral collateral ligament of this joint. Consequently, an imbricating capsular closure and preservation of the abductor digiti minimi insertion are imperative (Fig. 4.52E).

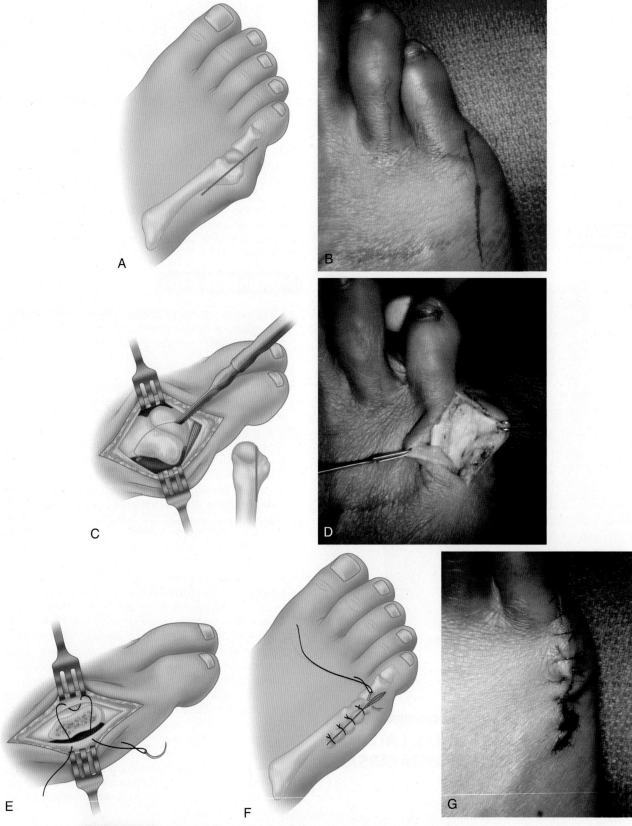

FIGURE 4.52   Bunionette removal. **A** and **B,** Skin incision. **C** and **D,** Excision of lateral prominence of fifth metatarsal head to include 40% of articular surface. **E,** Capsular closure, carefully preserving abductor digiti minimi insertion. **F** and **G,** Skin closure. **SEE TECHNIQUE 4.20.**

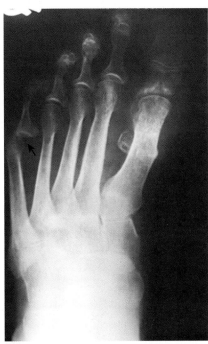

FIGURE 4.53 Medial dislocation of fifth toe after bunionette excision. **SEE TECHNIQUE 4.20**.

- Before closing the capsule, round off the bone edges with a rasp, and if a plantar callus coexists beneath the metatarsal head, smooth the plantar projection of the condyle flush with the shaft.
- Close the skin with interrupted, nonabsorbable sutures (Fig. 4.52F,G).
- The dressing should hold the fifth toe in slight abduction to release the tension on the capsular repair.

POSTOPERATIVE CARE Bathroom privileges and weight bearing to tolerance are allowed the first postoperative day in a firm-soled shoe with open toe box. The fifth toe is kept in a dressing that holds it in the proper position for 2 weeks. The sutures are removed at 2 weeks, and a spacer is placed in the fourth web space to prevent strain on the lateral capsular repair. The spacer is used for an additional 4 weeks, and fashionable shoes are allowed at 6 weeks.

RESECTION OF THE FIFTH METATARSAL HEAD FOR BUNIONETTE DEFORMITY

We do not recommend this procedure for initial operative treatment of bunionette deformity, and generally reserve it for an insensitive foot with callus formation and ulceration beneath the fifth metatarsal head in conjunction with a bunionette.

TECHNIQUE 4.21

- Make a midlateral incision over the distal third of the metatarsal to expose the metatarsal head and remove it obliquely 5 mm proximal to the capsular insertion at the head-neck junction (Fig. 4.54).

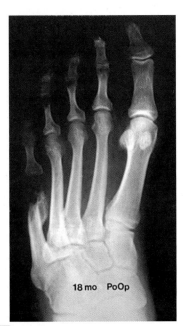

FIGURE 4.54 Resection of fifth metatarsal head. Metatarsal head is removed by oblique osteotomy well proximal to head-neck junction. **SEE TECHNIQUE 4.21**.

- Close the capsule with absorbable sutures and the skin with nonabsorbable sutures.

POSTOPERATIVE CARE Weight bearing to tolerance in a wooden-soled shoe is allowed immediately, but elevation of the extremity is encouraged for 48 to 72 hours. The patient usually is able to wear a lace-up shoe with a metatarsal pad at 4 weeks.

■ OSTEOTOMY OF THE METATARSAL

If the metatarsal at the distal shaft or neck is significantly deviated laterally, an osteotomy may be indicated. Only 2 to 3 mm to include the lateral eminence and 1 to 2 mm of articular cartilage of the metatarsal head should be removed, however. Otherwise, bony contact at the osteotomy site would be poor because of reduced surface area. The osteotomy can be made distally or proximally. Cooper and Coughlin described a subcapital oblique osteotomy, similar to the Weil osteotomy, for bunionette correction. They recommended this procedure for type I deformity in which there is a prominent lateral eminence of the fifth metatarsal head without significant increase in the fourth-to-fifth intermetatarsal angle or lateral bowing of the metatarsal shaft.

The chevron osteotomy is useful in metatarsus quintus valgus or in a splay foot with symptomatic bunionette and lateral splaying of the entire fifth ray. It is technically demanding because of small bony contact and because the cuts must be precise and calculated. It is a useful procedure, however, that can be used not only to narrow the forefoot slightly and relieve lateral pressure but also to reduce pressure plantarward if a concomitant symptomatic fifth metatarsal head callus is present. In this case, the head fragment is rotated dorsally 2 to 3 mm and shifted medially. More recently, an alternative distal transverse osteotomy with longitudinal pin fixation has been described by several authors. We do not have adequate experience with this procedure to recommend it over the chevron osteotomy, but it is included here because of its simplicity and

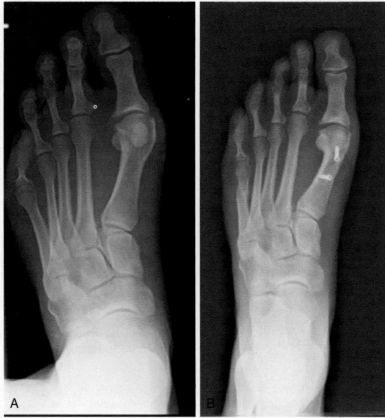

FIGURE 4.55 **A,** Preoperative radiograph of bunionette deformity. **B,** Postoperative radiograph at 3 months. (From Teoh KH, Hariharan K: Minimally invasive distal metatarsal metaphyseal osteotomy of the fifth metatarsal for bunionette correction. *Foot Ankle Int.* 39:450, 2018.)

the good outcomes (80% to 86% excellent or good) reported at long-term follow-up (3 to 8 years). The most frequent complication appears to be skin irritation or infection around the pin.

Minimally invasive and percutaneous techniques also have been described for distal osteotomy of the metatarsal for the correction of bunionette deformity. These techniques have been suggested to reduce complications because of the limited surgical exposure. Magnan et al. reported a 93% patient satisfaction rate with no nonunions, recurrences, osteonecrosis, or deep infection after 30 consecutive percutaneous fifth metatarsal distal osteotomies for bunionette correction. Laffenêtre et al. reported a 97.5% satisfaction rate in their patients after a percutaneous technique without pin fixation (Fig. 4.55).

SUBCAPITAL OBLIQUE OSTEOTOMY FOR BUNIONETTE DEFORMITY

The subcapital linear osteotomies are stabilized with a single Kirschner wire, and no soft-tissue procedures are done. Deformity correction was comparable with that reported with traditional open distal osteotomies.

TECHNIQUE 4.22

(COOPER AND COUGHLIN)
- After administration of an appropriate dose of perioperative antibiotics, perform a regional popliteal anesthetic block and use an Esmarch bandage to exsanguinate the

foot. Tie the Esmarch bandage about the ankle to serve as a tourniquet.
- Make a longitudinal skin incision centered over the lateral eminence of the metatarsal head, starting proximal to the lateral eminence and extending distally to the midportion of the proximal phalanx. Take care to protect the distal branches of the sural nerve.
- Incise the capsule of the fifth metatarsophalangeal joint in a L-shape along the dorsal and proximal margin, forming a flap; detach this flap from the periosteum dorsally and the abductor digiti quinti muscle proximally and reflect it distally and plantarward to expose the joint and lateral eminence.
- With a sagittal saw, resect the lateral eminence in a line parallel with the lateral border of the fifth metatarsal diaphysis.
- Make an oblique osteotomy from lateral to medial, starting 2 to 3 mm plantar to the dorsal margin of the metatarsal head articular cartilage, with the orientation parallel to the plantar surface of the foot (Fig. 4.56).
- Shift the capital fragment medially 2 to 4 mm, taking care not to overshift the metatarsal head and create an unstable construct.
- Secure the osteotomy with two dorsal-plantar 2-mm miniframgent screws oriented from dorsal-lateral to plantar-medial to capture the fragment.
- Shave the overhanging lateral bone with the saw and repair the lateral joint capsule with absorbable sutures through a drill hole in the metatarsal neck.

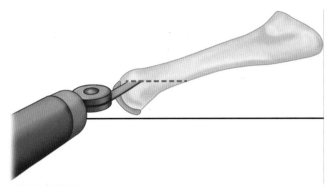

FIGURE 4.56   Subcapital oblique osteotomy for bunionette deformity. Saw cut is made from the lateral aspect, oriented from dorsal and distal to plantar and proximal. The blade is parallel to the plantar foot. (Redrawn from Cooper MT, Coughlin MJ: Subcapital oblique osteotomy for correction of bunionette deformity: medium-term results, Foot Ankle Int 34:1376, 2013.) **SEE TECHNIQUE 4.22.**

POSTOPERATIVE CARE The patient is allowed immediate heel weight bearing in a postoperative hard-soled shoe, unless other concomitant procedures prohibit this. The postoperative shoe is worn for 6 weeks, at which point the patient is transitioned to regular shoe wear with gradual resumption of normal activities.

TRANSVERSE MEDIAL SLIDE OSTEOTOMY FOR BUNIONETTE DEFORMITY

TECHNIQUE 4.23

- After induction of general anesthesia and application of a tourniquet, make a lateral approach to the fifth metatarsal neck. Local or block anesthesia also can be used in carefully selected patients.
- Make the osteotomy cuts with a standard pneumatic saw with a 9.5 × 25 × 0.4-mm blade. Incline the osteotomy in the lateral to medial direction so that it is perpendicular to the fourth ray if the length of fifth metatarsal bone is to be maintained. Incline the osteotomy in a distal-proximal direction up to 25 degrees if shortening of the metatarsal or decompression of the metatarsophalangeal joint is necessary (as in patients with mild arthritis). If lengthening of the fifth metatarsal is necessary (rare), incline the osteotomy in a proximal-distal direction up to 15 degrees.
- Insert a 1.6-mm Kirschner wire retrograde through the lateral soft tissues of the toe and pass it through the medullary canal into the base of the fifth metatarsal to act as a buttress to prevent loss of position of the distal fragment.
- Cut the wire, leaving it protruding distally.

POSTOPERATIVE CARE A hard-soled postoperative shoe is worn for 6 weeks, at which time the wire is removed in the outpatient surgery department.

OBLIQUE DIAPHYSEAL OSTEOTOMY OF THE FIFTH METATARSAL FOR SEVERE SPLAY FOOT OR METATARSUS QUINTUS VALGUS

A long, oblique, diaphyseal osteotomy of the fifth metatarsal for severe splay foot or metatarsus quintus valgus can correct a great degree of deformity. Although delayed union and even nonunion are more common than with osteotomies in the metaphyseal head segment, good or excellent results, with no delayed unions or nonunions, have been reported with longitudinal diaphyseal osteotomy, lateral condylectomy, and distal metatarsal joint soft-tissue realignment. If diaphyseal osteotomy is chosen, internal fixation with 2.7-mm screws using lag technique for compression, cast immobilization for 6 to 8 weeks (4 of which are non–weight bearing), and reduced activity level for 3 to 4 months are recommended. Vienne et al. reported good or excellent results in 97% of 33 feet treated with diaphyseal realignment osteotomy and compression screw fixation.

TECHNIQUE 4.24

(COUGHLIN)
- Make a longitudinal incision centered on the dorsolateral aspect of the fifth metatarsal extending from the base of the fifth metatarsal to the middle of the proximal phalanx. Protect the dorsolateral cutaneous nerve during dissection.
- Reflect the abductor digiti quinti muscle plantarward to expose the fifth metatarsal diaphysis. Leave the soft-tissue attachments to the medial aspect intact.
- Expose the metatarsophalangeal joint capsule and make an L-shaped incision along the dorsal and proximal aspects to expose the lateral eminence.
- After the capsule is detached, use a sagittal saw to resect the lateral condyle of the metatarsal head.
- Distract the metatarsophalangeal joint by applying distal traction to the fifth toe and release the medial capsule of the metatarsophalangeal joint so that it can be realigned after the osteotomy is made.
- Use a sagittal saw to make an osteotomy in the fifth metatarsal diaphysis. For pure lateral keratosis, direct the cut from lateral to medial, with the obliquity oriented from a dorsal-proximal to a plantar-distal direction (Fig. 4.57A). If plantar and lateral keratoses are present, angle the saw blade slightly upward to elevate the fifth metatarsal head (Fig. 4.57B). For a pure plantar keratosis, when more elevation of the distal fragment is desired, increase the obliquity of the osteotomy.
- Before completing the osteotomy, drill fixation holes in the proximal and distal fragments. Because the diaphysis is so narrow, placement of the holes after osteotomy can be difficult.
- Complete the osteotomy and rotate the distal fragment medially so that it is parallel with the fourth metatarsal (Fig. 4.57C), using the fixation hole as the axis for rotation. It is important that the osteotomy is rotated rather than translated to ensure maximal bony contact; rotation also maintains metatarsal length.

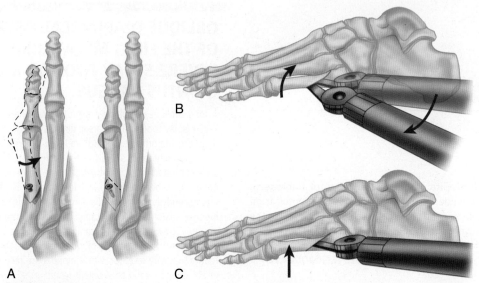

FIGURE 4.57 Diaphyseal osteotomy. **A,** Saw cut directed from lateral to medial with obliquity oriented from dorsal-proximal to plantar-distal. **B,** In presence of plantar callosity, saw blade is directed cephalad so that fifth metatarsal is elevated when osteotomy site is rotated. **C,** Osteotomy is rotated in diaphyseal region until distal fragment is parallel with fourth metatarsal. **SEE TECHNIQUE 4.24.**

- Fix the osteotomy with a small fragment screw, screw and Kirschner wire, or multiple Kirschner wires. Alternatively, use one or two dorsoplantar 2.4- or 2.7-mm titanium compression screws.
- Realign the fifth toe by reefing the lateral capsule to the fifth metatarsal metaphyseal periosteum and the abductor digiti quinti. If tissue is insufficient to attach the metatarsophalangeal capsule, place interrupted sutures through holes drilled in the metaphysis. This capsular plication allows significant correction of axial malalignment or malrotation.
- Close the incision in the usual manner and apply a gauze and tape dressing.

POSTOPERATIVE CARE The dressing is changed weekly for 6 weeks. Ambulation is allowed in a wooden-soled shoe. Casting is recommended for unreliable patients or patients who are unsteady when walking.

CHEVRON OSTEOTOMY OF THE FIFTH METATARSAL FOR BUNIONETTE DEFORMITY

TECHNIQUE 4.25

- Begin the incision laterally in the midline 1 cm distal to the fifth metatarsophalangeal joint and extend it proximally in line with the metatarsal shaft for 3 to 4 cm (Fig. 4.58A). Enter the metatarsophalangeal joint through a midlateral or L-shaped capsulotomy, exposing the entire fifth metatarsal head (Fig. 4.58B).

- Sublux the toe medially to improve exposure.
- Expose the distal 2 cm of metatarsal shaft dorsally, laterally, and enough plantarward to see clearly the plantar limb of the proposed osteotomy. Leave the soft tissue intact medially. Use sharp dissection for exposure so that periosteal elevation does not become necessary.
- Remove the lateral 1 to 2 mm of lateral eminence (Fig. 4.58C).
- Make a centering hole with a 0.045-inch Kirschner wire 5 mm proximal to the articular surface of the metatarsal head and equal distances from the dorsal and plantar cortices. This hole serves as the apex of the osteotomy.
- Using a 4-mm blade on a power saw, start the dorsal limb of the osteotomy angled 30 to 40 degrees from the midlateral longitudinal axis of the fifth metatarsal. Proceed cautiously with little pushing of the saw. The area for the double-limb osteotomy is constrained, so precision is necessary.
- The plantar limb of the osteotomy is cut, again about 30 degrees to the midline. Exposure of the distal shaft dorsally, laterally, and plantarward affords more control and precision over the cuts (Fig. 4.58D). As in the first metatarsal chevron osteotomy, the cuts should be at right angles to the shaft.
- Translate the fifth metatarsal head medially 2 to 4 mm depending on the size of the metatarsal. If there is a plantar callosity, tilt the metatarsal head dorsally 2 to 3 mm (Fig. 4.58E).
- Because this osteotomy is not as stable as in the first metatarsal and can tilt unexpectedly medially, plantarward, or dorsally, appose the osteotomy surfaces as much as possible with the head in line with the shaft of the metatarsal and use one or two 0.045-inch Kirschner wires for stability. These wires are started proximally just dorsal and plantar to the midline of the shaft and are driven obliquely into the metatarsal head (Fig. 4.58F).

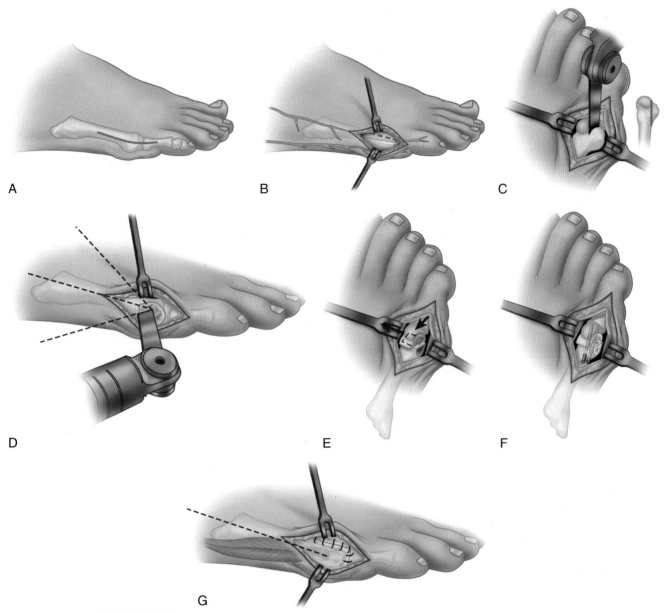

FIGURE 4.58 Chevron osteotomy of fifth metatarsophalangeal joint. **A,** Suggested incision. **B,** Inverted-L–shaped capsular incision transecting abductor digiti minimi. **C,** Amount of lateral eminence removed, not quite flush with shaft. **D,** Dorsal limb of osteotomy begins at centering hole; care is taken to prevent blade from "walking" into capital fragment distally. **E,** Translation of capital fragment medially 2 to 4 mm; it is tilted dorsally if callus is beneath fifth metatarsal head. **F,** Two small Kirschner wires improve stability. Overhanging lateral wedge of proximal fragment is removed, taking care not to enter entrance portal of Kirschner wires. **G,** Abductor digiti minimi is repositioned laterally to prevent medial subluxation of toe. **SEE TECHNIQUE 4.25.**

- Use a small rongeur to smooth the lateral overhang of the metatarsal shaft, taking care not to remove the cortex adjacent to the Kirschner wires.
- The capsular closure is important to prevent medial subluxation of the fifth toe. Using 3-0 absorbable suture while holding the toe congruously on the metatarsal head, repair the lateral capsule, bringing the tendon of the abductor digiti minimi dorsally into the midline. After completing the capsular repair, the toe should remain in proper position without any extraneous support (Fig. 4.58G).

- Apply a dressing to hold the toe in the proper position and relieve tension on the capsular repair.

POSTOPERATIVE CARE Activity is reduced for 72 hours, and the foot is elevated. A postoperative shoe is worn, and weight bearing to tolerance is allowed for 4 weeks. The dressing is changed at 1 week, being carefully reapplied to maintain proper position of the toe and relieve tension on the capsular repair. At 2 weeks, the sutures are removed and a web spacer of gauze or foam rubber and narrow tape is used to maintain the proper position of the toe. A wide

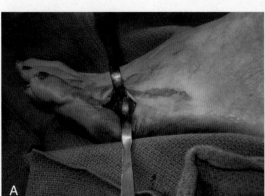
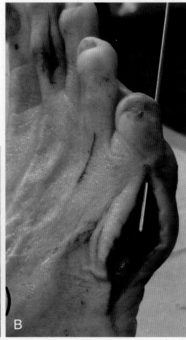
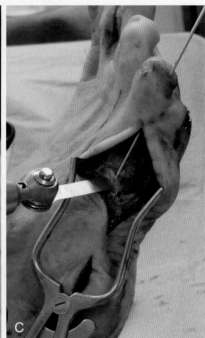

FIGURE 4.59 Kramer osteotomy for bunionette deformity. **A,** Skin incision at head-neck junction of fifth metatarsal with subperiosteal flaps elevated and retracted. **B,** Kirschner wire advanced antegrade through incision subcutaneously, exiting at toe. **C,** Kirschner wire advanced retrograde into fifth metatarsal shaft to hold segment and saw used to smooth subcutaneous contour. (From Lee DC, de Cesar Netto C, Staggers JR, et al: Clinical and radiographic outcomes of the Kramer osteotomy in the treatment of bunionette deformity, Foot Ankle Surg 24:530, 2018.) **SEE TECHNIQUE 4.26.**

toe box, firm-soled shoe can be worn at 4 weeks. The pins are removed in the office using a local anesthetic after the osteotomy has healed, usually 6 to 8 weeks after surgery. A short leg walking cast extending distal to the toes occasionally is worn for 1 month if the patient must be more active than a postoperative shoe would allow.

MINIMALLY INVASIVE KRAMER OSTEOTOMY FOR BUNIONETTE DEFORMITY

Lee et al. conducted a retrospective study of 38 patients who were treated with a Kramer osteotomy for bunionette deformity. The mean 4-5 intermetatarsal angle improved from 8.3 degrees preoperatively to 4.4 degrees postoperatively ($P < 0.01$) and the mean metatarsophalangeal joint angle improved from 13.6 degrees preoperatively to 0.4 degrees at final follow-up ($P < 0.01$). They reported five delayed unions and one nonunion.

TECHNIQUE 4.26

(KRAMER, LEE)
- After a regional ankle block is administered, make a small, 1- to 2-cm, skin incision at the head-neck junction of the fifth metatarsal.
- Using blunt dissection, carry the incision down to the periosteum.
- Raise subperiosteal flaps dorsally and plantarly and retract (Fig. 4.59A).
- Using a microsagittal saw, make an oblique osteotomy in the fifth metatarsal (15 to 20 degrees), creating slight shortening of the fifth metatarsal and medial displacement of the distal segment.
- Advance a 0.062-inch Kirschner wire antegrade through the incision subcutaneously along the lateral edge of the fifth metatarsal and phalanges, exiting the skin at the end of the toe (Fig. 4.59B).
- Grasp the Kirschner wire distally and advance it proximally to the level of the osteotomy. Desired correction is obtained by medial translation.
- Advance the Kirschner wire retrograde into the medullary canal of the fifth metatarsal shaft until cortical purchase is achieved within the fifth metatarsal base.
- Remove the small dorsal triangular shelf on the proximal fragment of the fifth metatarsal using a saw, creating a smooth contour (Fig. 4.59C).

POSTOPERATIVE CARE Heel weight bearing is allowed in a postoperative shoe. Kirschner wires are removed at 10 to 14 days as well as the sutures. Patients are allowed increasing weight bearing as tolerated with limited activity.

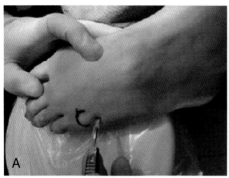
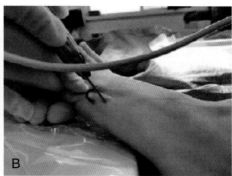
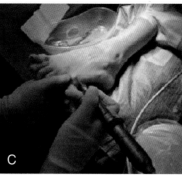

FIGURE 4.60 Minimally invasive distal metatarsal metaphyseal osteotomy. **A,** Stab incision. **B,** Burr position at beginning of osteotomy. **C,** Burr position at end of osteotomy. (From Teoh K, Hariharan K: Minimally invasive distal metatarsal osteotomy (DMMO) of the fifth metatarsal for bunionette correction, Foot Ankle Int 39(4):450, 2018.) **SEE TECHNIQUE 4.27.**

MINIMALLY INVASIVE DISTAL METATARSAL METAPHYSEAL OSTEOTOMY FOR FIFTH TOE BUNIONETTE CORRECTION

Teoh et al. evaluated their outcomes after distal metatarsal metaphyseal osteotomy using a minimally invasive technique in 19 patients, noting the technique to be safe and effective with few complications. They did note swelling of the forefoot and pain that persisted an average of 3 months after surgery compared to osteotomy with fixation and the possibility of a prominent callus over the osteotomy site.

TECHNIQUE 4.27

(TEOH ET AL.)

- Place the patient supine, with the heel hanging off the end of the operating table.
- Make a 3-mm stab incision over the dorsum of the foot at the neck of the fifth metatarsal, lateral or medial to the extensor tendon, depending on the handedness of the surgeon (Fig. 4.60A).
- Using a hemostat, dissect down to the metatarsal neck.
- Perform an extraarticular distal metatarsal osteotomy of the fifth metatarsal using a low-speed, high-torque burr. Determine the cut with the help of fluoroscopy beforehand and by feeling the plantar flare of the plantar condyle, ensuring that the burr is proximal to it. Hold the burr initially at a 45-degree angle in relation to the metatarsal shaft in the sagittal plane. Create a lateral furrow to ensure fixation of the start of the osteotomy. Make the cut from proximal plantar to distal dorsal (Fig. 4.60B), ending with the burr facing 90 degrees to the shaft in the coronal plane (Fig. 4.60C). Run sterile saline continuously over the burr to prevent thermal necrosis.
- Check that the osteotomy is complete on fluoroscopic stress views by pulling on the toe to distract the cut.
- Close the stab incision with Steri-Strips.

POSTOPERATIVE CARE The patient may bear weight in a flat shoe immediately postoperatively for 3 to 6 weeks unless other procedures were performed. The fifth toe is kept in a neutral or slightly abducted position with tape initially and a toe splint after the first week.

FREIBERG INFRACTION

In 1914, A.H. Freiberg reported six infractions (incomplete fracture of a bone without displacement of the fragments) of the second metatarsal head. Three of these had a single significant traumatic event to the toe before the symptoms developed. For this reason, Freiberg considered this disorder to be secondary to acute trauma. In 1917, Campbell reported the same condition in the third metatarsal head. Since then, several large series have been published, but the exact cause remains uncertain.

Because it is most commonly recognized in the second decade of life and radiographically resembles other examples of the osteochondroses, it presumably falls into this category: osteonecrosis of subchondral cancellous bone followed by a reparative process. A misshapen metatarsal head frequently is an incidental radiographic finding, and careful questioning of the patient often reveals a period during adolescence when pain was noted in the forefoot.

Because the second toe frequently is the longest and the second ray the least mobile, excessive pressure on the metatarsal head on weight bearing could cause repetitive microfractures, loss of blood supply to subchondral bone, collapse of this cancellous bone, and cartilage deformation. Synovitis accompanies the process, and if it is prolonged and severe, limitation of motion, especially in extension, results. With this loss of extension of the metatarsophalangeal joint, weight bearing causes abnormal stress to be applied to the metatarsal shaft, which becomes widened from bicortical thickening. In addition to irregular ossification of the primary ossification center of the metatarsal head and widening of the metatarsal shaft, osteochondral fragmentation can occur around the metatarsal head (Fig. 4.61).

The symptoms include pain around the involved metatarsophalangeal joint primarily on weight bearing, local

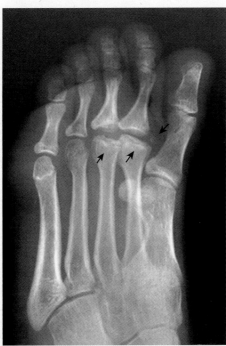

FIGURE 4.61   Freiberg infraction. Note flattening of second and third metatarsal heads and irregularity and separated bone fragment *(arrows)*. (Courtesy of Steve Ikard, MD.)

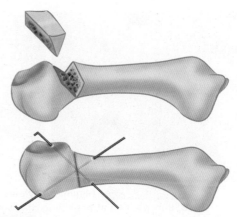

FIGURE 4.62   Dorsal closing wedge osteotomy and cross-pinning. **SEE TECHNIQUE 4.28.**

tenderness around the metatarsophalangeal joint, and limitation of motion. If a synovitis is present, swelling becomes apparent.

Most patients with Freiberg infraction can be treated conservatively with modification of activities, semirigid orthoses, and metatarsal bars. A short leg walking cast with a toe extension may be needed if other nonoperative treatment fails. Occasionally, crutches are needed to rest the painful foot completely.

If conservative management fails, surgical treatments include (1) resection of the metatarsal head (Giannestras), (2) elevation of the depressed fragment of the metatarsal head and bone grafting of the defect (Smillie), (3) resection of the base of the proximal phalanx with syndactylization of the second and third toes (Trott), (4) dorsal closing wedge osteotomy of the metatarsal head (Gauthier and Elbay), and (5) joint debridement and metatarsal head remodeling (Freiberg and Mann). Helix-Giordanino et al. reported good results in 28 of 30 patients treated with the Gauthier dorsal cuneiform osteotomy, and Pereira et al. described excellent or good results in 20 patients evaluated at 23 years after dorsal wedge osteotomy. A systematic review identified a more than 90% resolution of pain and full return to activity in patients treated with joint-sparing procedures.

Kilic et al. compared cheilectomy and microfracture to cheilectomy and dorsal crescentic osteotomy and found no significant differences in outcomes; both techniques obtained significant improvements in pain and range of motion. More recently, transplantation of an osteochondral plug from the ipsilateral knee to the second metatarsal head has been described in a few patients with late-stage Freiberg disease.

We have been pleased with the joint debridement and metatarsal head remodeling and use it most often. We have used MRI to evaluate the metatarsal head. If the lesion is localized to the dorsum of the metatarsal head with the remainder of the metatarsal head not involved, a dorsiflexion closing wedge osteotomy of the metatarsal neck has been used with some success. Rarely we have added resection of the base of the proximal phalanx. This shortens the toe significantly, and because 90% of the patients are in late adolescence or early adulthood, we try to avoid this resection. Joint debridement and remodeling of the metatarsal head should suffice. A number of other treatments have been proposed for the treatment of this condition, but lack numbers or long-term follow-up to give clear guidance that they are superior to current recommendations. The patient must be informed before surgery that some permanent limitation of motion is usual. Because motion in the affected joint frequently is limited anyway, this usually is not a deterrent to surgery. Metatarsal bars or pads should be used for 3 to 6 months after surgery.

DORSAL CLOSING WEDGE OSTEOTOMY FOR FREIBERG DISEASE

TECHNIQUE 4.28

(CHAO ET AL.)

- Use a dorsal approach to expose the metatarsal head. Make a longitudinal incision in the capsule and debride the joint, removing loose fragments. Perform a partial synovectomy.
- Make a dorsal closing wedge osteotomy over the distal normal metaphysis, removing sufficient bone to bring the healthy plantar part of the metatarsal head into articulation with the phalanx (Fig. 4.62).
- Do not remove the lesion, but rotate it proximally and dorsally.
- The angle of the closing wedge should maintain the length of the involved metatarsal bone as much as possible.
- Temporarily fix the osteotomy with crossed percutaneous Kirschner wires. As an alternative, absorbable pins can be used for fixation, avoiding a second procedure for removal of the Kirschner wires.

POSTOPERATIVE CARE A light compressive dressing is applied, and the foot is immobilized in a short leg walking cast for 4 weeks. Pins are removed at 4 weeks, and weight bearing is allowed as tolerated. Patients are not allowed to run or engage in any strenuous physical activity for 8 weeks after surgery.

JOINT DEBRIDEMENT AND METATARSAL HEAD REMODELING FOR FREIBERG DISEASE

TECHNIQUE 4.29

- Through an angled incision, the apex of which is the lateral margin of the metatarsophalangeal joint, expose the extensor hood.
- Ligate any crossing veins returning to the dorsal venous arch.
- Expose the entire extensor expansion over the metatarsophalangeal joint.
- Identify the extensor digitorum brevis as it joins the extensor digitorum longus and section the former at this juncture.
- Incise the extensor hood just lateral to the extensor digitorum longus and retract this tendon medially.
- Through a longitudinal capsulotomy, enter the metatarsophalangeal joint and reflect the capsule medially and laterally by sharp dissection to expose the metatarsal head. The degree of degeneration of the metatarsal head often is striking compared with the radiographic findings.
- Remove all osteochondral fragments. A small 0.045-inch Kirschner wire may be used to microfracture the base of the defect at this point.
- Distract the toe manually, and by flexing it acutely, expose the entire metatarsal head. Both collateral ligaments may require division to allow this.
- At this point, use judgment to determine the degree of arthroplasty needed. At times, the articular surface has remodeled and appears surprisingly good. In this instance, debride the joint of all loose fragments, remove inflamed synovium if necessary, and perform a Z-plasty lengthening (8 to 12 mm) of the extensor digitorum longus to relieve extensor pressure on the joint. The extensor digitorum brevis should be tenotomized.
- If the metatarsal head is pitted, contour it by removing the articular cartilage. When remodeling the metatarsal head with a rongeur, ensure that no osteophytes remain on its plantar aspect.
- The surface of the metatarsal head usually is depressed dorsally and centrally. Round the remainder of the head to this depth; this usually requires 3 to 4 mm of bone removal circumferentially.
- Irrigate the joint while flexing and extending it to flush any remaining cartilage or bony fragments.
- Secure hemostasis by direct pressure. This is an important step.

- Close the capsule with fine absorbable sutures and apply a dressing that holds the joint reduced.

POSTOPERATIVE CARE Continuous elevation of the foot for 48 hours is recommended, followed by walking in a wooden-soled shoe. At 2 weeks, the skin sutures are removed and the forefoot is redressed, holding the toe in the desired position. At 4 weeks, a wide toe box shoe is allowed, and active and gentle active-assisted range of motion of the second metatarsophalangeal joint is encouraged (Fig. 4.63).

BRACHYMETATARSIA

Brachymetatarsia is a condition in which one of the metatarsals is abnormally short. The fourth ray is most commonly involved, followed by the first and fifth rays. The shortening may be congenital or caused by premature physeal closure resulting from trauma, surgery, infection, or pathologic conditions. In children, brachymetatarsia often occurs in association with disease processes such as Down syndrome, Apert syndrome, Albright osteodystrophy, sickle cell anemia, diastrophic dwarfism, and poliomyelitis. Brachymetatarsia disrupts the normal parabolic arc of the metatarsals (Fig. 4.64), but it rarely causes pain or functional impairment, and most patients seek treatment because of the appearance of the foot. Nonoperative measures, such as padding and use of accommodative devices in a shoe, can relieve pain in adjacent joints but do not correct the deformity or improve the appearance of the foot. Surgery usually is indicated for a metatarsal that is 10 mm or more shorter than the adjacent metatarsal. Surgical options include one-stage lengthening with the use of an interpositional bone graft, gradual lengthening by distraction osteogenesis with or without shortening of the adjacent toes, and shortening of the adjacent toes. Generally, metatarsals that need to be lengthened less than 15 mm can be successfully treated with a one-stage lengthening procedure, whereas gradual distraction is necessary for more length gains. Shortening of the adjacent metatarsals can be done with lengthening to restore the normal parabolic arc of the metatarsal heads.

Cited advantages of one-stage lengthening, with or without bone grafting, include the short time required to achieve union, the small surgical scar, and avoidance of neurovascular impairment and excessive soft-tissue stretching. In a systematic review, Jones et al. found that single-stage lengthening with a bone graft was associated with fewer complications and faster healing times than callus distraction, but with lesser gains in length. If an autograft is used, operative times are longer and a second incision is required for graft harvest; donor site morbidity, such as pain and local infection, also may complicate the procedure. Shortening of the adjacent metatarsals reduces the "target length" and can avoid some of the complications of one-stage lengthening. Giannini et al. described a one-stage lengthening with allograft interposition that was successful in 50 metatarsals, gaining an average of 13 mm in length. The procedure consists of a transverse proximal osteotomy of the metatarsal shaft and interposition of a

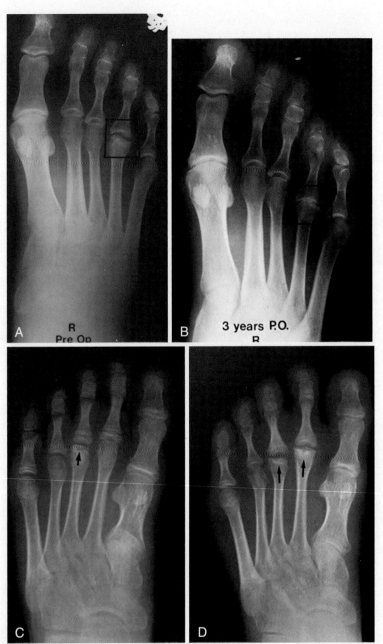

FIGURE 4.63   Freiberg infraction. **A,** Uncommon location. **B,** Three years after joint debridement and remodeling of metatarsal head, motion is limited but patient is active and asymptomatic. **C,** Freiberg infraction of third metatarsal head in teenage girl *(arrow)*. **D,** One year later, second metatarsal head also is involved; *arrows* show Freiberg infractions on second and third metatarsal heads. Patient had hemoglobinopathy. (**C** and **D** courtesy of Steve Ikard, MD.)

metatarsal allograft fixed with an intramedullary Kirschner wire (Fig. 4.65). For patients with multiple-metatarsal involvement, a one-stage combined shortening and lengthening procedure has been described in which intercalary autogenous bone grafts from the shortened metatarsals are used for lengthening. Waizy et al. described a one-stage metatarsal interposition lengthening using autologous fibular grafting in five patients (eight feet). The graft adapted well to the fourth metatarsal, and harvest from the distal fibula caused no functional impairment. They reported high satisfaction and mean extension of 9.01 mm (20.3% extension of the entire metatarsal).

Good or excellent results have been reported in 80% to 100% of patients treated with distraction osteogenesis. Distraction osteogenesis has several reported advantages over one-stage lengthening: no bone grafting is required, tendons are gradually stretched, neurovascular complications are less frequent, weight bearing can be begun sooner, and more length can be gained. Gradual lengthening of 1 mm per day with external fixation and intramedullary nailing was found to be safe and effective in one study of 48 cases of brachymetatarsia. The average length gained was 18.6 ± 6.7 mm (average 38.2% ± 3.1% total metatarsal length). Lee et al. reported patient satisfaction and bone union in

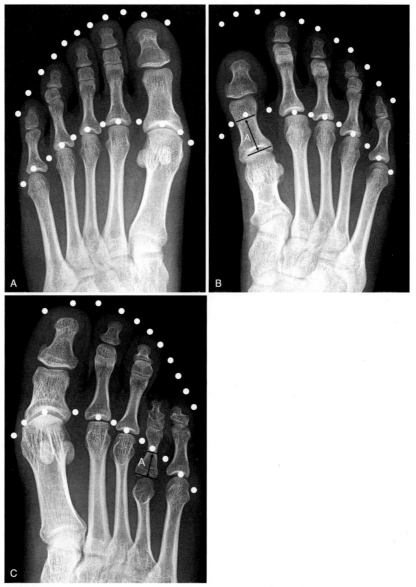

FIGURE 4.64 Brachymetatarsia disrupts normal parabolic arc of metatarsal heads. **A,** Normal toe-tip and metatarsal head parabolas *(dotted lines)*. **B,** Disruption with brachymetatarsia of first metatarsal. **C,** Disruption with brachymetatarsia of fourth metatarsal. Distance marked "A" represents length needed to obtain ideal parabola. (From Lee KB, Park HW, Chung JW, et al: Comparison of the outcomes of distraction osteogenesis for first and fourth brachymetatarsia, J Bone Joint Surg 92A:2709, 2010.)

all 74 metatarsals they treated with distraction osteogenesis for brachymetatarsia of the first and/or fourth metatarsals. The mean gains in length were 17.2 mm in the first metatarsal and 16.3 in the fourth metatarsal. Complications were frequent, however, and there was no improvement in foot function. The most common complication was metatarsophalangeal joint stiffness; others included malalignment of the lengthened metatarsal, fracture through the callus, pin breakage, and pin track infections. Barbier et al. reported a 48% complication rate (26 complications) in 30 patients treated with gradual metatarsal lengthening by a circular external fixator; however, 20 of the complications were considered "benign." Complications have been suggested to be more frequent in metatarsals lengthened more than 40% (Fig. 4.66).

DISTRACTION OSTEOGENESIS FOR LENGTHENING OF THE METATARSAL IN BRACHYMETATARSIA

TECHNIQUE 4.30

(LEE ET AL.)
- Under fluoroscopic guidance, insert two mini-Schanz half-pins (3 mm in diameter) into the proximal metaphysis and two more into the distal metaphysis of the metatarsal.
- For brachymetatarsia of the first metatarsal, direct the distal pins from medial to lateral.

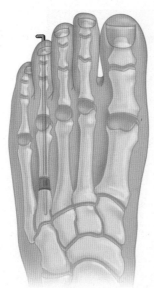

FIGURE 4.65 Lengthening of metatarsal with one-stage allograft interposition (see text). (Redrawn from Giannini S, Faldini C, Pagkrati S, et al: One-stage metatarsal lengthening by allograft interposition: a novel approach for congenital brachymetatarsia, Clin Orthop Relat Res 468:1933, 2010.)

- Apply a unilateral external fixator to the medial aspect of the metatarsal, as parallel to the plantar surface of the foot as possible in the transverse plane to prevent malalignment during lengthening (Fig. 4.67A).
- Make a 1.5-cm medial longitudinal incision at the metatarsal shaft and longitudinally incise and carefully elevate the periosteum.
- With a motorized saw with continuous cooling, make a transverse corticotomy perpendicular to the plantar surface of the foot.
- For fourth brachymetatarsia, insert two mini-Schanz half-pins (2 mm in diameter) into the proximal metaphysis and two more into the distal metaphysis on the dorsolateral aspect of the metatarsal. Take care to ensure that the pins do not entrap the extensor digitorum longus tendon to the fifth toe. Position the proximal two pins lateral to the fifth extensor digitorum longus tendon and the two distal pins medial to it.
- Apply a unilateral external fixator as parallel to the plantar surface of the foot as possible in the sagittal plane (Fig. 4.67B) and parallel to the insertion of the axes of the third and fifth metatarsals in the transverse plane.
- Confirm the proper direction of metatarsal lengthening by distracting the osteotomy approximately 5 mm and assessing the direction of the distraction with fluoroscopy.
- Restore the bone surfaces to apposition.

POSTOPERATIVE CARE Postoperatively, 0.25 mm of distraction is applied three times daily after a 7-day latency period. Distraction rate and rhythm are controlled according to the radiographic findings and the patient's clinical conditions. Radiographs are checked every other week to evaluate the degree of osteogenesis and the condition of the adjacent joint. Distraction is continued until a satisfactory parabola incorporating all five metatarsal heads has been obtained. The external fixator is removed when the callus surrounding the osteotomy has matured. Full weight-bearing, heel-touch ambulation with the use of a postoperative shoe is allowed beginning on the second day after surgery.

ONE-STAGE METATARSAL INTERPOSITION LENGTHENING WITH AUTOLOGOUS FIBULAR GRAFT WITH LOCKING PLATE FIXATION

TECHNIQUE 4.31

(WAIZY ET AL).
- Make a V/Y incision dorsally over the fourth metatarsal (Fig. 4.68A).
- Expose the long extensor tendon and perform a Z-shaped extension. Tenotomize the short extensor tendon (Fig. 4.68B).
- After exposing the metatarsal bone, make a transverse osteotomy cut. Extend and transfix with a Kirschner wire to the third metatarsal bone (Fig. 4.68C).
- Determine the length of interposition graft needed.
- Harvest an appropriate-sized ipsilateral fibular graft approximately 3 cm above the syndesmosis (Fig. 4.68D,E).
- Insert the graft into the gap of the metatarsal bone and fix with a locking plate (Fig. 4.68F).
- Suture the long extensor tendon at the required length. (Waizy et al. performed a distal percutaneous tenotomy of the long flexor tendon in all their patients.)
- Close the wound and use a stabilizing tape dressing to align the toe for 6 weeks (Fig. 4.68G).

POSTOPERATIVE CARE Postoperative care includes 3 weeks of non–weight bearing and 3 weeks of partial weight bearing (15 kg) in a lower extremity walker. Sports are not allowed for a total of 3 months postoperatively.

METATARSAL LENGTHENING BY CIRCULAR EXTERNAL FIXATION

TECHNIQUE 4.32

(BARBIER ET AL.)
- Apply a half-ring as a stable base. Fix the half-ring at the midfoot using two to three Kirschner wires between the tarsometatarsal and transverse tarsal joints and metatarsal bases.

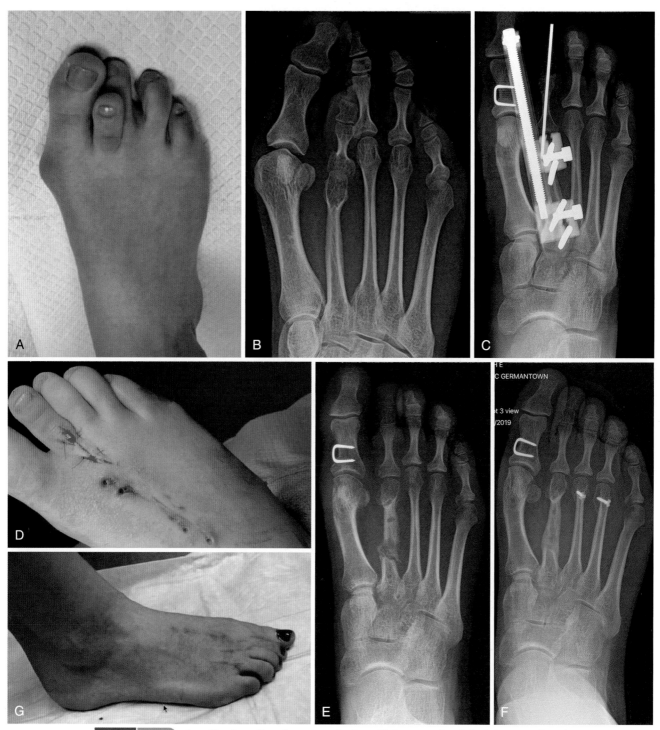

FIGURE 4.66 Lengthening of brachymetatarsia. **A** and **B,** Preoperative clinical photograph and anteroposterior radiograph showing severe brachymetatarsia of second metatarsal. **C,** Application of distraction fixator with osteotomy and cross pinning of second metatarsophalangeal joint. **D** and **E,** After removal of distraction device. **F,** Ultimately, third and fourth distal metatarsal osteotomies were required for final lengthening. **G,** Final postoperative result.

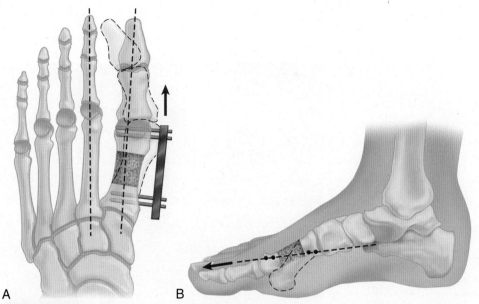

A   B

FIGURE 4.67   Distraction osteogenesis for metatarsal lengthening. External fixator is applied as parallel as possible to axis of second metatarsal in transverse plane **(A)** and to plantar surface of foot in sagittal plane **(B)**. (Redrawn from Lee KB, Park HW, Chung JW, et al: Comparison of the outcomes of distraction osteogenesis for first and fourth brachymetatarsia, J Bone Joint Surg 92A:2709, 2010.) **SEE TECHNIQUE 4.30.**

- Fix one threaded rod per metatarsal to the half-ring and attach it distally to the metatarsal shaft using three or four wires (Fig. 4.69A,B). Take care to not injure the extensor digitorum longus tendon. The rod should be parallel to the plantar foot surface in the sagittal plane and between the two adjacent metatarsal heads in the transverse plane.
- For joint metatarsophalangeal joint immobilization, fix the phalangeal base to the rod by two wires. Place a temporary intramedullary arthrodesis wire between the rod and the interphalangeal joint.
- Place a second rod connecting the first rod and ring to increase construct stability.
- Make a longitudinal incision (0.5 to 1 cm) on the dorsum of the involved metatarsal and perform an extracapsular osteotomy using an osteotome on the base of the metatarsal without performing perforation first to prevent injury of the surrounding structures and thermal damage.

The frame can be extended to the hindfoot if there is additional deformity correction needed.

POSTOPERATIVE CARE The dressing should be changed on the first postoperative day and then every 10 days. Weight bearing and ankle motion are begun from the first postoperative day in a foam sole. Distraction is begun on the sixth postoperative day (±2 days) at a rate of 0.25 mm two to four times a day depending on radiographic and clinical data, with the length assessed every week by radiograph. Once sufficient length is obtained, the arthrodesis wire is removed and the fixation period begun (Fig. 4.69C). The frame is removed after determining the strength of the regenerate and absence of motion after unlocking the frame. Progressive weight bearing is started with crutches. Sports are allowed after 3 months.

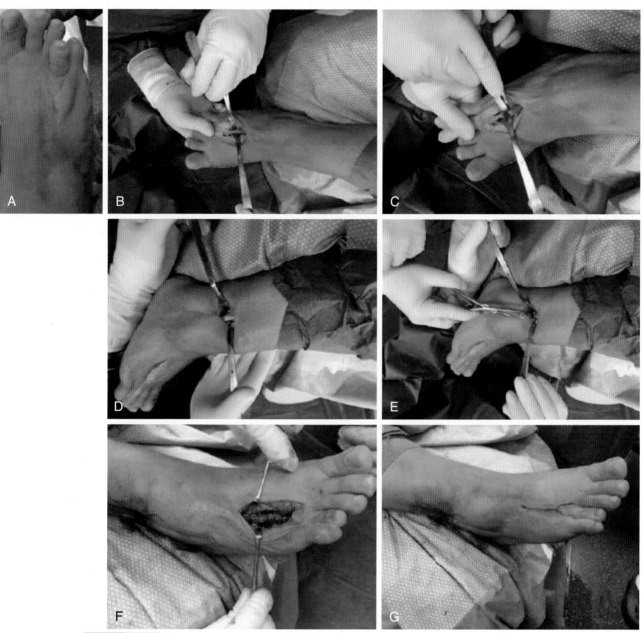

FIGURE 4.68 One-stage metatarsal interposition lengthening with an autologous fibular graft and locking plate fixation. **A,** Incision of fourth metatarsal. **B,** Arthrolysis of fourth metatarsophalangeal joint and Z-shaped extensor tendon lengthening. **C,** Transverse osteotomy of the metatarsal. **D** and **E,** Harvest of the fibular graft. **F,** Graft interposition and locking plate application. **G,** Wound suture and positioning of the fourth toe. (From Waizy H, Polzer H, Schikora N, et al: One-stage metatarsal interposition lengthening with an autologous fibula graft for treatment of brachymetatarsia, Foot Ankle Spec 12(4):330, 2018.) **SEE TECHNIQUE 4.31.**

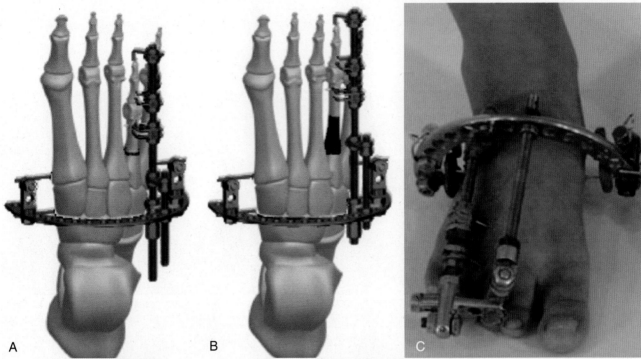

A   B   C

FIGURE 4.69   Circular external fixation for metatarsal lengthening in brachymetatarsia. **A** and **B**, Half-ring fixed at midfoot. Phalanges are temporarily attached to rod with two wires at base of first phalanx and arthrodesis wire bridging interphalangeal joints. **C**, Distraction begins on day six postoperatively.   (From Barbier D, Neretin A, Journeau P, Popkov D: Gradual metatarsal lengthening by external fixation: a new classification of complications and a stable technique to minimize severe complications, Foot Ankle Int 36(11):1369, 2015.) **SEE TECHNIQUE 4.32.**

REFERENCES

METATARSOPHALANGEAL JOINT INSTABILITY

Barg A, Courville XF, Michisch F, et al.: Role of collateral ligaments in metatarsophalangeal stability: a cadaver study, Foot Ankle Int 33:877, 2012.

Bhutta MA, Chauhan D, Zubairy AI, Barrie J: Second metatarsophalangeal joint instability and second metatarsal length association depends on the method of measurement, Foot Ankle Int 31:486, 2010.

Carlson RM, Dux K, Stuck RM: Ultrasound imaging for diagnosis of plantar plate ruptures of the lesser metatarsophalangeal joints: a retrospective case series, J Foot Ankle Surg 52:786, 2013.

Cooper MT, Coughlin MJ: Sequential dissection for exposure of the second metatarsophalangeal joint, Foot Ankle Int 32:294, 2011.

Coughlin MJ, Baumfeld DS, Nery C: Second MTP joint instability: grading of the deformity and description of surgical repair of capsular insufficiency, Phys Sportsmed 39:132, 2011.

Coughlin MJ, Schutt SA, Hirose CB, et al.: Metatarsophalangeal joint pathology in crossover second toe deformity: a cadaveric study, Foot Ankle Int 33:133, 2012.

Doty JF, Coughlin MJ: Metatarsophalangeal joint instability of the lesser toes and plantar plate deficiency, J Am Acad Orthop Surg 22:235, 2014.

Doty JF, Coughlin MJ, Weil Jr L, Nery C: Etiology and management of lesser toe metatarsophalangeal joint instability, Foot Ankle Clin 19:385, 2014.

Ellis SJ, Young E, Endo Y, et al.: Correction of multiplanar deformity of the second toe with metatarsophalangeal release and extensor brevis reconstruction, Foot Ankle Int 34:792, 2013.

Feuerstein CA, Weil Jr L, Weil Sr LS, et al.: Static versus dynamic musculoskeletal ultrasound for detection of plantar plate pathology, Foot Ankle Spec 7:259, 2014.

Finney FT, Cata E, Holmes JR, Talusan PG: Anatomy and physiology of the lesser metatarsophalangeal joints, Foot Ankle Clin 23(1):1, 2018.

Finney FT, Lee S, Scott J, et al.: Biomechanical evaluation of suture configurations in lesser toe plantar plate repairs, Foot Ankle Int 39(7):836, 2018.

Flint WW, Macias DM, Jastifer JR, et al.: Plantar plate repair for lesser metatarsophalangeal joint instability, Foot Ankle Int 38(3):234, 2017.

Haque S, Kakwani R, Chadwick C, et al.: Outcome of minimally invasitve distal metatarsal metaphyseal osteotomy (DMMO) for lesser toe metatarsalgia, Foot Ankle Int 37(1):58, 2016.

Henry J, Besse JL, Fessy MH: Distal osteotomy of the lateral metatarsals: a series of 72 cases comparing the Weil osteotomy and the DMOO percutaneous osteotomy, Orthop Traumatol Surg Res 97(6 Suppl):S57, 2011.

Hsu RY, Barg A, Nickisch F: Lesser metatarsophalangeal joint instability: advancements in plantar plate reconstruction, Foot Ankle Clin 23(1):127, 2018.

Jacison JB, Saltzman CL, Nickisch F: Plantar plate pathology and repair, Tech Foot Ankle Surg 13:121, 2014.

Jastifer JR, Coughlin MJ: Exposure via sequential release of the metatarsophalangeal joint for plantar plate rupture through a dorsal approach without an intraarticular osteotomy, Foot Ankle Int 36:335, 2015.

Joseph R, Schroeder K, Greenberg M: A retrospective analysis of lesser metatarsophalangeal joint fusion as a treatment option for hammertoe pathology associated with metatarsophalangeal joint instability, J Foot Ankle Surg 51:57, 2012.

Klein EE, Weil Jr L, Weil Sr LS, et al.: Positive drawer test combined with radiographic deviation of the third metatarsophalangeal joint suggests high grade tear of the second metatarsophalangeal joint plantar plate, Foot Ankle Spec 7:466, 2014.

Klinge SA, McClure P, Fellars T, DiGiovanni CW: Modification of the Weil/Maceira metatarsal osteotomy for coronal plane malalignment during crossover toe correction: case series, Foot Ankle Int 35:584, 2014.

Magnan B, Bonetti I, Negri S, et al.: Percutaneous distal osteotomy of lesser metatarsals (DMMO) for treatment of metatarsalgia with metatarsophalangeal instability, Foot Ankle Surg 24(5):400, 2018.

Mas NM, van der Grinten M, Bramer WM, Kleinrensink GJ: Metatarsophalangeal joint stability: a systematic review on the plantar plate of the lesser toes, *J Foot Ankle Res* 9:32, 2016.

Nery C, Baumfeld D: Lesser metatarsophalangeal joint instability, treatment with tendon transfers, *Foot Ankle Clin* 23(1):103, 2018.

Nery C, Raduan FC, Catena F, et al.: Plantar plate radiofrequency and Weil osteotomy for subtle metatarsophalangeal joint instability, *J Orthop Surg Res* 10:180, 2015.

Nery C, Coughlin MJ, Baumfeld D, et al.: Prospective evaluation of protocol for surgical treatment of lesser MTP joint plantar plate tears, *Foot Ankle Int* 35:876, 2014.

Nery C, Coughlin MJ, Baumfeld D, Mann TS: Lesser metatarsophalangeal joint instability: prospective evaluation and repair of plantar plate and capsular insufficiency, *Foot Ankle Int* 33:301, 2012.

Peck CN, MacLeod A, Barrie J: Lesser metatarsophalangeal instability: presentation, management, and outcomes, *Foot Ankle Int* 33:565, 2012.

Suero EM, Meyers KN, Bohne WH: Stability of the metatarsophalangeal joint of the lesser toes: a cadaveric study, *J Orthop Res* 30:1995, 2012.

Wang B, Guss A, Chalayon O, et al.: Deep transverse metatarsal ligament and static stability of lesser metatarsophalangeal joints: a cadaveric study, *Foot Ankle Int* 36:573, 2015.

Watson TS, Reid DY, Frerichs TL: Dorsal approach for plantar plate repair with Weil osteotomy: operative technique, *Foot Ankle Int* 35:730, 2014.

Weber JR, Aubin PM, Ledoux WR, Sangeorzan BJ: Second metatarsal length is positively correlated with increased pressure and medial deviation of the second toe in a robotic cadaveric simulation of gait, *Foot Ankle Int* 33:312, 2012.

Wong TC, Kong SW: Minimally invasive distal metatarsal osteotomy in the treatment of primary metatarsalgia, *J Orthop Trauma Rehabil* 17:17, 2013.

Yamada AF, Crema MD, Nery C, et al.: Second and third metatarsophalangeal plantar plate tears: diagnostic performance of direct and indirect MRI features using surgical findings as the reference standard, *AJR Am J Roentgenol* 209(2):100, 2017.

HAMMER TOES

Atinga M, Dodd L, Foote J, Palmer S: Prospective review of medium term outcomes following interpositional arthroplasty for hammer toe deformity correction, *Foot Ankle Surg* 17:256, 2011.

Boffeli TJ, Thompson JC, Tabatt JA: Two-pin fixation of proximal interphalangeal joint fusion for hammertoe correction, *J Foot Ankle Surg* 55(3):480, 2016.

Boyce L, Dhukaram V: Transdermal glyceryl trinitrate in the treatment of ischemia following toe deformity correction: a case series, *Foot Ankle Int* 35:1226, 2014.

Catena F, Doty JF, Jastifer J, et al.: Prospective study of hammertoe correction with an intramedullary implant, *Foot Ankle Int* 35:319, 2014.

Coillard JY, Petri GJ, van Damme G, et al.: Stabilization of proximal interphalangeal joint in lesser toe deformities with an angulated intramedullary implant, *Foot Ankle Int* 35:401, 2014.

Ellington JK, Anderson RB, Davis WH, et al.: Radiographic analysis of proximal interphalangeal joint arthrodesis with an intramedullary fusion device for lesser toe deformities, *Foot Ankle Int* 31:372, 2010.

Guelfi M, Pantalone A, Cambiaso Daniel J, et al.: Arthrodesis of proximal inter-phalangeal joint for hammertoe: intramedullary device options, *J Orthop Traumatol* 16(4):269, 2015.

Harmer JL, Wilkinson A, Maher AJ: A midterm review of lesser toe arthrodesis with an intramedullary implant, *Foot Ankle Spec* 10(5):458, 2017.

Jay RM, Malay DS, Landsman AS, et al.: Interphalangeal joint fusion: a randomized controlled clinical trial, *J Foot Ankle Surg* 55(4):697, 2016.

Joseph R, Schroeder K, Greenberg M: A retrospective analysis of lesser metatarsophalangeal joint fusion as a treatment option for hammertoe pathology associated with metatarsophalangeal joint instability, *J Foot Ankle Surg* 51:57, 2012.

Klammer G, Baumann G, Moor BK, et al.: Early complications and recurrence rates after Kirschner wire transfixion in lesser toe surgery: a prospective randomized study, *Foot Ankle Int* 33:105, 2012.

Konkel KF, Sover ER, Menger AG, Halberg JM: Hammer toe correction using an absorbable pin, *Foot Ankle Int* 32:973, 2011.

Kramer WC, Parman M, Marks RM: Hammertoe correction with K-wire fixation, *Foot Ankle Int* 36:494, 2015.

Lui TH, Chan LK, Chan KB: Modified plantar plate tenodesis for correction of claw toe deformity, *Foot Ankle Int* 31:584, 2010.

Obrador C, Losa-Iglesias M, Becerro-de-Bengoa-Vallejo R, Kabbash CA: Comparative study of intramedullary hammertoe fixation, *Foot Ankle Int* 39(4):415, 2018.

Richman SH, Siqueira MB, McCullough KA, Berkowitz M: Correction of hammertoe deformity with novel intramedullary PIP fusion device versus K-wire fixation, *Foot Ankle Int* 38(2):174, 2017.

Scholl A, McCarty J, Scholl D, Mar A: Smart toe® implant versus buried Kirschner wire for proximal interphalangeal joint arthrodesis: a comparative study, *J Foot Ankle Surg* 552:580, 2013.

Schrier JC, Keijsers NL, Matricali GA, et al.: Lesser toe PIP joint resection versus PIP joint fusion: a randomized clinical trial, *Foot Ankle Int* 37(6):569, 2016.

Wendelstein JA, Goger P, Bock P, Schuh R, et al.: Bioabsorbable fixation screw for proximal interphalangeal arthrodesis of lesser toe deformities, *Foot Ankle Int* 38(9):1020, 2017.

Witt BL, Hyer CF: Treatment of hammertoe deformity using a one-piece intramedullary device: a case series, *J Foot Ankle Surg* 51:450, 2012.

MALLET TOE

Molloy A, Shariff R: Mallet toe deformity, *Foot Ankle Clin* 16:537, 2011.

Myerson MS, Filippi J: Bone block lengthening of the proximal interphalangeal joint for managing the floppy toe deformity, *Foot Ankle Clin* 15:663, 2010.

Salari N, Faro FD, Miller SD: Dorsal opening wedge osteotomy of second proximal phalanx for second MTP dorsiflexion, *Foot Ankle Int* 31:1021, 2010.

CORNS AND CALLUSES
BUNIONETTE

Bertrand T, Parekh SG: Bunionette deformity: etiology, nonsurgical management, and lateral exostectomy, *Foot Ankle Clin* 16:679, 2011.

Cooper MT, Coughlin MJ: Subcapital oblique osteotomy for correction of bunionette deformity: medium-term results, *Foot Ankle Int* 34:1376, 2013.

Cooper MT, Coughlin MR: Subcapital oblique fifth metatarsal osteotomy versus distal chevron osteotomy for correction of bunionette deformity: a cadaveric study, *Foot Ankle Spec* 5:313, 2012.

Hrubina M, Skotak M, Letocha J, Dzupa V: The modified scarf osteotomy in the treatment of tailor's bunion: midterm follow-up, *Acta Orthop Belg* 81(1):57, 2015.

Laffenetre O, Millet-Barbé B, Darcel V, et al.: Percutaneous bunionette correction: results of a 49-case retrospective study at a mean 34 months' followup, *Orthop Traumatol Surg Res* 101(2):179, 2015.

Lee DC, de Cesar Netto C, Staggers JR, et al.: Clinical and radiographic outcomes of the Kramer osteotomy in the treatment of bunionette deformity, *Foot Ankle Surg* 24(6):530, 2018.

Magnan B, Samaila E, Merlini M, et al.: Percutaneous distal osteotomy of the fifth metatarsal for correction of bunionette, *J Bone Joint Surg* 93A:2116, 2011.

Malagelada F, Dalmau-Pastor M, Sahirad C, et al.: Anatomical considerations for minimally invasive osteotomy of the fifth metatarsal for bunionette correction, *A pilot study, Foot (Edinb)* 36:39, 2018.

Molenaers B, Vanlommel J, Deprez P: Percutaneous hardware free corrective osteotomy for bunionnette deformity, *Acta Orthop Belg* 83(2):284, 2017.

Morawe GA, Schmieschek MHT: Minimally invasive bunionette correction, *Oper Orthop Traumatol* 30(3):184, 2018.

Shi GG, Humayun A, Whalen JL, Kitaoka HB: Management of bunionette deformity, *J Am Acad Orthop Surg* 26(19):3396, 2018.

Shimobayashi M, Tanaka Y, Taniguchi A, et al.: Radiographic morphologic characteristics of bunionette deformity, *Foot Ankle Int* 37(3):320, 2016.

Teoh KH, Hariharan K: Minimally invasive distal metatarsal metaphyseal osteotomy (DMMO) of the fifth metatarsal for bunionette correction, *Foot Ankle Int* 39(4):450, 2018.

Waizy H, Jastifer JR, Stukenborg-Colsman C, Claassen L: The reverse Ludloff osteotomy for bunionette deformity, *Foot Ankle Spec* 2016, [Epub ahead of print].

Weil Jr L, Weil Sr LS: Osteotomies for bunionette deformity, *Foot Ankle Clin* 16:689, 2011.

FREIBERG DISEASE

Helix-Giordanino M, Randier E, Frey S, et al.: Treatment of Freiberg's disease by Gauthier's dorsal cuneiform osteotomy: retrospective study of 30 cases, *Orthop Traumatol Surg Res* 101(6 Suppl):S221, 2015.

Kilic A, Cepni KS, Aybar A, et al.: A comparative study between two different surgical techniques in the treatment of late-stage Freiberg's disease, *Foot Ankle Surg* 19:234, 2013.

Pereira BS, Frada T, Freitas D, et al.: Long-term follow-up of dorsal wedge osteotomy for pediatric Freiberg disease, *Foot Ankle Int* 37:90, 2016.

Schade VL: Surgical management of Freiberg's infraction: a systematic review, *Foot Ankle Spec* 8:498, 2015.

BRACHYMETATARSIA

Barbier D, Neretin A, Journeau P, Popkov D: Gradual metatarsal lengthening by external fixation: a new classification of complications and a stable technique to minimize severe complications, *Foot Ankle Int* 36:1369, 2015.

Blakenhorn BD, Kerner PJ, DiGiovanni CW: Clinical tip: one stage lengthening of fourth brachymetatarsia using fibular autograft, *Foot Ankle Int* 31:175, 2010.

Córdoba-Fernández A, Vera-Gómez ML: Literature review of brachymetatarsia, *Orthop Nurs* 37(5):292, 2018.

Fusini F, Langella F, Catani O, et al.: Mini-invasive treatment for brachymetatarsia of the fourth ray in females: percutaneous osteotomy with mini-burr and external fixation. A case series, *J Foot Ankle Surg* 56(2):390, 2017.

Giannini S, Faldini C, Pagkrati S, et al.: One-stage metatarsal lengthening by allograft interposition: a novel approach for congenital brachymetatarsia, *Clin Orthop Relat Res* 468:1933, 2010.

Hosny GA, Ahmed AS: Distraction osteogenesis of fourth brachymetatarsia, *Foot Ankle Surg* 22(1):12, 2016.

Hwang SM, Song JK, Kim HT: Metatarsal lengthening by callotasis in adults with first brachymetatarsia, *Foot Ankle Int* 33:1103, 2012.

Jones MD, Pinegar DM, Rincker SA: Callus distraction versus single-stage lengthening with bone graft for treatment of brachymetatarsia: a systematic review, *J Foot Ankle Surg* 54:927, 2015.

Kumar P, Pillai A, Bate JA, Henry J: Distraction osteogenesis for brachymetatarsia using initial circular fixator and early trans-fixation metatarsal K-wires- a series of three cases, *J Surg Case Rep* 10:269, 2018.

Lamm BM: Percutaneous distraction osteogenesis for treatment of brachymetatarsia, *J Foot Ankle Surg* 49:197, 2010.

Lamm BM, Gourdine-Shaw MC: Problems, obstacles, and complications of metatarsal lengthening for the treatment of brachymetatarsia, *Clin Podiatr Med Surg* 27:561, 2010.

Lee KB, Park HW, Chung JY, et al.: Comparison of distraction osteogenesis for first and fourth brachymetatarsia, *J Bone Joint Surg* 92A:2709, 2010.

Peña-Martínez VM, Palacios-Barajas D, Blanco-Rivera JC, et al.: Results of external fixation and metatarsophalangeal joint fixation with K-wire in brachymetatarsia, *Foot Ankle Int* 39(8):942, 2018.

Scher DM, Blyakher A, Krantzow M: A modified surgical technique for lengthening of a metatarsal using an external fixator, *HSS J* 6:235, 2010.

Waizy H, Polzer H, Schikora N, et al.: One-stage metatarsal interposition lengthening with an autologous fibula graft for treatment of brachymetatarsia, *Foot Ankle Spec*, 2018, [Epub ahead of print].

The complete list of references is available online at ExpertConsult.com.

CHAPTER 5

ARTHRITIS OF THE FOOT

David R. Richardson

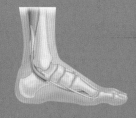

INFLAMMATORY AND DEGENERATIVE ARTHRITIS

Arthritis is a term used broadly to refer to joint pain and subsequent joint destruction, and it often is used to describe several different conditions that have the common characteristic of joint pain and destruction but different histopathology and underlying mechanisms. Because of these differences, the pharmaceutical treatment varies dramatically, but surgical treatment is relatively uniform and depends largely on underlying stability, amount of joint involvement, and patient symptoms.

The inflammatory arthritides include gout, lupus, psoriatic arthritis, and rheumatoid arthritis. For the foot and ankle surgeon, rheumatoid arthritis is one of the most common chronic inflammatory causes of patients seeking care. It is characterized by synovitis, rheumatoid nodules, and vasculitis. In the musculoskeletal system, rheumatoid arthritis manifests as a persistent, symmetric polyarthritis of the hands and feet or any synovial-lined joint. A genetic component is known, but rheumatoid arthritis does not show segregation patterns seen in single and high-penetrance genes, and most studies support the concept that the actual disease-conferring sequence encompasses amino acids 67 through 74 of the *HLA-DRB1* gene. Joint destruction results primarily from T cells and B cells, inciting a cascade that leads to the release of proteases and collagenases from chondrocytes and synovial fibroblasts. At least four of seven criteria must be present for the diagnosis of rheumatoid arthritis: (1) morning stiffness, (2) arthritis of three or more joint areas, (3) arthritis of the hand joints (swelling), (4) symmetric arthritis, (5) rheumatoid nodules, (6) serum rheumatoid factor positive, and (7) radiographic changes of the hand and wrist associated with rheumatoid arthritis (must include erosions and decalcification of involved joints). Episodic pain is more often associated with an inflammatory process, and this history should lead the clinician to further investigate if the diagnosis of osteoarthritis is not certain. No test result is absolutely confirmatory for rheumatoid arthritis; the diagnosis is made based on clinical, laboratory, and imaging features. Certain serologic studies may be helpful and should be included if an inflammatory process is suspected (Box 5.1).

Almost 90% of adult patients with rheumatoid arthritis will have symptomatic arthritis of the feet of varying severity. Approximately 17% of patients with rheumatoid arthritis present initially with symptoms affecting the joints of the feet, and even mild-to-moderate rheumatoid arthritis has a significant negative impact on an individual's mobility and functional capacity. Therefore a high index of suspicion should be maintained.

In contrast to rheumatoid arthritis, *seronegative arthritis* often involves the insertion of tendons into bone (the enthesis). The most common seronegative arthritides include Reiter syndrome, psoriatic arthritis, and ankylosing spondylitis. Unlike rheumatoid arthritis, which has a female predominance, there is a male predominance in each of these except psoriatic arthritis, which has a male to female ratio of 1:1. These diseases have an association with HLA genes, particularly HLA-B27. In young patients with bilateral disease, one should be cognizant of the possibility of a causative inflammatory process.

SIGNS AND SYMPTOMS

Early clinical manifestations are similar for both inflammatory and degenerative arthritis. Pain typically is exacerbated with activity and relieved with rest. Patients, especially those with inflammatory arthropathy, typically consider their ankle rather than forefoot complaints to be more consequential. With more advanced disease, less activity causes pain and many patients describe pain with rest or at night. A typical patient with arthritis in the foot and ankle will describe pain with stair climbing, extremes of motion such as with squatting or toe raises, and rotational movement (e.g., during a golf swing). Weather patterns often have been reported to influence pain in this group of patients, and although the literature is conflicting, it appears that changes in barometric pressure may affect patients with arthritis. Disease and inflammation of the soft tissue often accompany joint disease; however, they may be independent of one another. This is an important distinction because radiographic osteoarthritis or rheumatoid arthritis may in fact be an incidental finding unrelated to the true cause of symptoms, especially in patients with inflammatory arthritis. Treating the extraarticular causes of pain, such as synovitis or bursitis, may significantly relieve symptoms while preserving the joint space.

Serologic Studies Helpful in the Diagnosis of Rheumatoid Arthritis

- Erythrocyte sedimentation rate (ESR)—inflammation.
- C-reactive protein (CRP)—inflammation.
- Complete blood cell count (CBC)—anemia of chronic disease.
- Rheumatoid factor (RF) assay—positive in 60% to 80%, false-positive in 25%, positive in fewer than 40% with early rheumatoid arthritis, not specific for rheumatoid arthritis.
- Antinuclear antibody (ANA) assay—present in 25% to 30% of patients with rheumatoid arthritis, not specific for rheumatoid arthritis (95% of those are positive for systemic lupus erythematosus).
- Anticyclic citrullinated peptide (anti-CCP) assay—98% specific for rheumatoid arthritis.
- Anti-RA33 antibody assay—85% specific for rheumatoid arthritis.

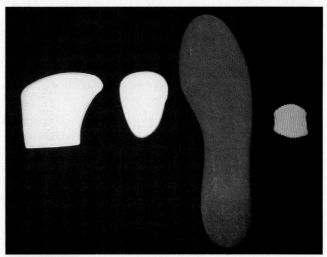

FIGURE 5.1   Orthoses, such as those shown here, can mitigate pain and improve function in some patients with rheumatoid deformities of foot.

NONOPERATIVE TREATMENT

Arthritis in most patients can be managed nonoperatively, and the percentage of patients with inflammatory arthritis requiring surgery has dramatically decreased over time. In fact, currently, patients with rheumatoid arthritis have a relative risk of undergoing surgery that is less than half of that in those treated in the past 2 decades of the 20th century. This is likely due to both improvements in medication targeting new molecular pathways and the increased emphasis on early intensive treatment regimens.

Nonoperative treatment should begin with an honest conversation about activity modification emphasizing low-impact exercises. Exercise is important for the overall health of the patient, and a decrease in activity should be avoided if possible. If the patient is overweight, diet counseling is appropriate. Shoe modification also may benefit the patient significantly. Wide toe-box, rocker-bottom shoes often are very successful for patients with midfoot and forefoot arthritis. Adding a carbon plate insert or built-in steel sole will limit motion by stiffening the shoe, thus preventing painful motion at the midfoot and forefoot. Custom foot orthotics seem to improve pain and relieve plantar forefoot pressure; however, the literature is inconclusive regarding orthotics improving foot function, walking speed, gait, quality of life, or progression of the hallux valgus angle. Braces and orthotics may significantly mitigate pain and improve function (Fig. 5.1).

Antiinflammatory medication can be tried in patients in whom it is not contraindicated. Corticosteroid injections can be used for both diagnosis and therapy. Studies have shown that fluoroscopic or CT-guided intraarticular injections with local anesthetic, with or without corticosteroid, can assist in determining which joints are symptomatic. This is particularly useful when the small joints of the midfoot are involved. Caution is necessary in patients whose pain is unrelieved, even for a brief period, with a local anesthetic intraarticular injection. It is unlikely that surgery on this joint will significantly improve symptoms. For patients with inflammatory arthritis, open communication between the surgeon and rheumatologist will allow optimization of care, especially in the perioperative period.

FOREFOOT

Hallux rigidus refers to arthritis of the first metatarsophalangeal joint. Described by Davies-Colley as a plantarflexed proximal phalanx relative to the metatarsal head, he coined the term *hallux flexus*. Cotterill, in 1887, referred to the limitation of motion in the first metatarsophalangeal joint as hallux rigidus. Understanding of this condition has advanced over time, but the true etiology remains elusive. It is thought to begin with damage to the cartilage by a traumatic event, most often in adolescence, or repetitive stress caused by hyperextension of the first metatarsophalangeal joint in activities involving running, hallux valgus interphalangeus, or an abnormally long first metatarsal. Family history usually is positive in patients with bilateral hallux rigidus. Injury to the soft tissue of the great toe, such as turf toe, also may result in progressive arthritis. Increased stress, whether due to a cartilage lesion or abnormal mechanics of the joint, leads to synovitis, joint destruction, and pain. Treatment of hallux rigidus is described in other chapter, and treatment of arthritis involving the lesser toes is discussed in other chapter.

ETIOLOGY OF JOINT DESTRUCTION

The etiology of joint destruction in rheumatoid arthritis differs from that of the degenerative or traumatic process seen in patients without inflammatory changes. The effect of osteoarthritis is large and seems to be increasing in the general population. The risk of developing osteoarthritis is complex and multifactorial, but several factors have strong evidence supporting their contributions. Increasing age, female sex, lower socioeconomic status, obesity, family history, joint injury and alignment, and occupational joint loading have been associated with osteoarthritis. Many other factors are being investigated, including metabolic pathways (e.g., serum leptin), joint shape, limb-length inequality, bone density, and more. Well-controlled studies are still needed to assess the prevalence of risk factors specific to the foot and ankle.

The frequency of orthopaedic surgery has been decreasing in patients with rheumatoid arthritis. There is also a trend toward improved long-term outcomes. Improvements in medical treatment partially explain this trend. However, drug therapy cannot perfectly suppress disease activity, and therefore many patients progress to more aggressive intervention. The trend toward milder disease because of advances in drug therapy may lead patients to seek treatment for better function as measured by activities of daily living. In rheumatoid arthritis, immune complexes within the synovial membrane lead to an inflammatory cell response that causes synovial hyperplasia and joint destruction. Hallux valgus is the predominant clinical manifestation of rheumatoid arthritis and may not be associated with significant joint destruction. Marginal articular erosions are noted on early radiographs, followed by progressive deformity of the joint. Synovitis resulting in release of inflammatory enzymes causes weakening of the capsular ligaments. This leads to not only valgus of the first

metatarsophalangeal joint but also weakening of the intrinsic muscles of the lesser toes, causing metatarsophalangeal joint hyperextension. Chronic dorsal subluxation of the metatarsophalangeal joints leads to imbalance between the intrinsic (the interossei and lumbricals) and extrinsic (flexor digitorum longus and flexor hallucis longus) muscles. The interossei are pulled dorsal to the axis of rotation, thereby converting them to weak extensors. The deformity is compounded by the loss of excursion of the extensor digitorum brevis and longus, which can no longer extend the middle and distal interphalangeal joints, leading to a claw toe deformity. Over time the proximal phalanx of the lesser toes dislocates completely and comes to lie on the dorsal aspect of the metatarsophalangeal neck while the first metatarsophalangeal joint often deforms into a valgus posture (Fig. 5.2).

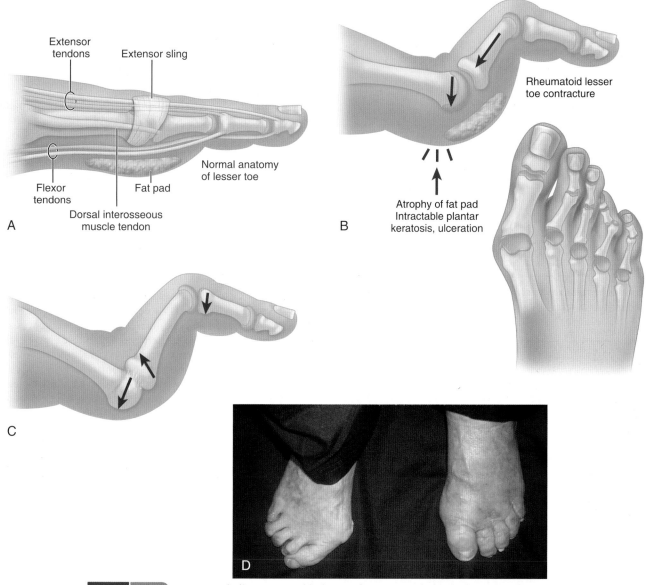

FIGURE 5.2 **A,** Normal alignment and balance of metatarsophalangeal joints and toes. **B,** As rheumatoid deformity progresses, imbalance occurs with progressive dorsal subluxation of metatarsophalangeal joint and deformity of lesser toes. **C,** End-stage deformity with dislocation of metatarsophalangeal joint and proximal phalanx ankylosed to dorsal aspect of metatarsal head. **D,** Severe claw toe deformity in right foot of patient with rheumatoid arthritis; left foot has been surgically corrected.

Several clinically important deformities stem from hyperextension of the metatarsophalangeal joints, including distal migration of the forefoot pad, painful plantar callosities over protruding metatarsal heads (Fig. 5.3), skin ulceration over bony prominences, flexion contracture of the middle and distal digital joints of the lesser toes and interphalangeal joint of the hallux, painful corns over the dorsum of the middle joints, and end corns at the nail-pulp junction (Fig. 5.4). Although hammer toes can occur as isolated deformities unassociated with metatarsophalangeal joint synovitis and deformity, their

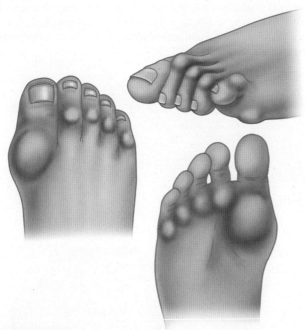

FIGURE 5.3 Rheumatoid foot. Note multiple deformities of rheumatoid arthritis of forefoot with hallux valgus, subluxed and dislocated metatarsophalangeal joints, claw toes, hammer toes, and bursal formation.

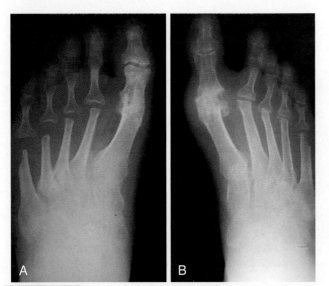

FIGURE 5.4 **A,** Small proliferation of bone at end of fifth metatarsal (right foot). Joint spaces 1 year after surgery are maintained because of adequate bone resection. **B,** Inadequate bone resection with loss of joint space.

isolated occurrence is uncommon in patients with rheumatoid arthritis. In seronegative spondyloarthropathies, such as psoriatic arthropathy, arthritic deformity of the proximal interphalangeal joints and resultant hammer toe deformity are common; however, it may be unassociated with metatarsophalangeal joint involvement. Hallux valgus deformity is present in most patients with inflammatory arthritis and may be due to the lack of a second digit buttress when a claw toe is present. The fifth digit often is in a varus position.

TREATMENT

Conservative options should be offered before surgical treatment. Pain and swelling in the ankle have been correlated with limitation and disability more than pain and swelling of the forefoot. Pain and disease duration, more than radiographic damage, influence disability. Conservative treatment may be more effective for forefoot disease than for hindfoot or ankle pathology. Patients with rheumatoid arthritis have been found to have an altered "plantar pressure pain threshold": decreased plantar foot sensitivity in all regions compared with a control group. Because of this decreased sensitivity, pedobarography may be useful early in the disease process to correct excessive plantar loading before symptoms become significant. Due to the association between rheumatoid arthritis and neuropathy, one should be aware of the possibility of Charcot neuroarthropathy in this population. Medical management should be optimized in all patients. Despite the significant progress made in the treatment of rheumatoid arthritis, foot pain remains common and disabling. After inflammatory disease in the foot is diagnosed, treatment should be coordinated with a rheumatologist.

Initially, patients are treated in extra-deep shoes with a wide, high toe-box and a molded insert that accommodates bony prominences. Several studies have shown that supportive shoes and foot orthoses can produce significant improvement of symptoms in patients with arthritis. Semirigid orthoses appear to be more effective than soft orthoses. Early use is recommended. Rocker soles and steel shanks may help relieve midfoot pain and counteract stiffness. Toe sleeves and spacers, corn pads, and debridement of plantar callosities also may help. These treatments can be used indefinitely, but surgery usually is required because of continued pain, increasing deformity, and patient dissatisfaction with unattractive footwear that needs frequent modifications as old deformities progress or new deformities develop. Additionally, if the tibiotalar joint is involved, the use of a double upright brace with a limited-motion or locked ankle joint and an inside (valgus-correcting) T-strap may aid in the nonoperative management. Before forefoot arthroplasty is recommended, the patient must understand that the disease process is progressive and that surgical correction of deformity should be considered palliative rather than definitive or curative. If the patient and physician enter surgical management of the arthritic rheumatoid forefoot with this perspective, both should be rewarded with the outcome, provided that an uncommon or unexpected complication does not develop.

Many different types of surgery are used for treatment of arthritis of the foot, and it is important to continue to compare the effectiveness of these different interventions. Patient-reported and performance outcomes are critical to evaluate effectiveness. For example, the Foot Function Index has demonstrated reliability and responsiveness in evaluating patients following foot surgery in those with rheumatoid arthritis, and preoperative PROMIS scores have shown the ability to predict postoperative success after foot and ankle surgery.

■ AVOIDING COMPLICATIONS IN FOOT SURGERY

Complications can be reduced to a minimum if the following recommendations are carefully considered:

1. Clean the skin meticulously, especially between the toes and around the nails, for 10 to 15 minutes before surgery, and apply a sterile wrap. This procedure is repeated in the operating room, but less scrub time is needed.
2. Use a prophylactic antibiotic routinely, usually 30 minutes before the incision is made.
3. Pay careful attention to the presence and intensity of the pedal pulses. If there is asymmetry between the pedal pulses of the two feet, ask a peripheral vascular consultant to see the patient before surgery. Alternatively, if it is possible to measure peripheral pressures, request ankle-brachial pressure ratios or toe pressures. In nondiabetic patients, an ankle pressure of 90 mm Hg or more, or an ankle-brachial pressure ratio of 0.7 or more, should allow forefoot wound healing.
4. Carefully inspect the skin of the foot and distal leg for any evidence of vasculitis, which manifests as macules and papules, usually over the anterolateral border of the distal tibia and dorsolateral surface of the foot. They are slightly raised, do not blanch with pressure, and occasionally have a small necrotic preulcerative center. Rheumatoid nodules are caused by vasculitis of the subcutaneous connective tissue and should alert the examiner if found on the foot. Mononeuritis multiplex is the result of immune complex-mediated vasculitis of the peripheral nerves of the lower extremities. A patient with hyperesthesia of the skin of the foot (not simply painful joints from synovitis or painful callosities) should be examined carefully for impaired sensation; the abnormalities may be sensory, motor, or mixed. In patients with inflammatory arthritis, if doubt exists after carefully examining the feet for evidence of vasculitis, a rheumatology consultation or a skin biopsy is warranted before surgery.
5. If a patient is taking an immune suppressive medication, consider removing the sutures at 3 weeks or longer instead of the customary 2 weeks.
6. Elevate the feet to the maximal level for 48 to 72 hours postoperatively.

The use of methotrexate, gold, nonsteroidal antiinflammatory medications, steroids, or hydroxychloroquine in the perioperative period was not found to contribute to postoperative healing or infectious complications in 30 patients with rheumatoid arthritis. Also, age, sex, and the presence of rheumatoid nodules, either alone or in conjunction with medications, did not increase the risk of postoperative healing or infectious complications. The 32% overall complication rate emphasizes, however, the need for patient education and preoperative planning in patients with rheumatoid inflammatory arthritis.

■ FOREFOOT ARTHROPLASTY

Provided adequate bone resection is performed, the clinical results of forefoot arthroplasty, regardless of the specific technique, are rewarding, especially in patients with inflammatory arthritis. Reduced pain, increased ambulatory function,

improved appearance, and the ability to wear a variety of footwear should be the result in 80% to 90% of patients. After 3 to 5 years, this percentage begins to decrease, however, especially if objective measures, such as recurrence of hallux valgus and callosities, dorsal posturing of the toes on metatarsal remnants, and bony proliferation on the distal end of the metatarsals, are considered (Fig. 5.4). In patients with rheumatoid arthritis, plantar pressure improves while gait parameters and disability are not adversely affected after lesser metatarsal arthroplasty. Although the patient's subjective assessment of the arthroplasty may remain good, it is likely that, with enough time, these recurrent deformities will become symptomatic. Preoperative factors predictive of recurrent deformity after arthroplasty include severe hallux valgus and dislocation grades of the lesser metatarsophalangeal joints.

Many patients gradually reduce their level of activity because of the generalized nature of the disease, and this might explain the good subjective results despite poor objective outcomes: the deformity has been reported to recur in more than 50% of patients with rheumatoid arthritis, although up to 97% of patients are satisfied with their results.

In patients with inflammatory arthritis, forefoot arthroplasty is directed primarily at the metatarsophalangeal joint deformity. Although the exact technique varies according to the training of the surgeon and the severity of the deformities, adequate bony resection to allow the phalanges to realign loosely with the metatarsals is mandatory. Resection of all five metatarsal heads (Fig. 5.5), as well as fusion of the first metatarsal and resection of metatarsals two through five, have both been shown to produce adequate results (Fig. 5.6). In addition, all four of the lesser toes must be treated in the same manner, regardless of the varying severity of involvement of each ray. There are occasional exceptions to this axiom, with removal of only one or two of the lesser metatarsal heads required, but the patient must be informed that removal of the remaining lesser metatarsal heads may be necessary. In patients with osteoarthritis of the lesser toes, there has been a trend toward joint preservation. These techniques are described elsewhere (Chapter 2).

The goals of forefoot arthroplasty are to relieve pain, correct deformity with concomitant cosmetic improvement, improve ambulatory function, and, ideally, allow a reasonable variety of footwear. Several reported series confirm these goals as realistic and attainable if patients are carefully selected, operative and postoperative care are meticulously performed, and patients are adequately informed of the progressive nature of this disease. Satisfactory outcomes have been reported in 54% to 96% of patients after resection of all five metatarsal heads, with poor results attributed to insufficient resection of bony elements or an irregular line of resection. A comparison of the various arthroplasty techniques found good pain relief and more normal shoewear in 97% of patients, regardless of the type of arthroplasty, as long as adequate bone was removed and the metatarsal remnant did not protrude into the plantar weight-bearing pad.

Resection, interpositional, and replacement arthroplasties and hemiarthroplasty are discussed in other chapter. Early results of silicone-rubber, single-stem replacement arthroplasty were satisfactory, but concerns about silicone synovitis have made this procedure obsolete. Hemiarthroplasty, resurfacing of the proximal phalangeal or metatarsal joint surface, has been reported to be successful but should be performed with caution because no long-term studies are yet

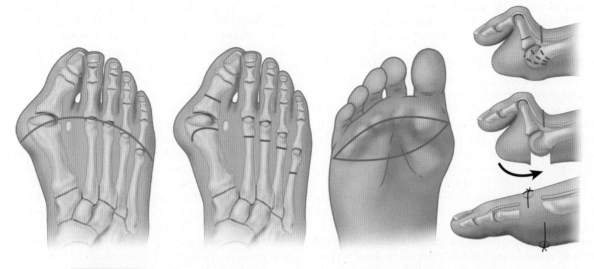

FIGURE 5.5   Forefoot arthroplasty, with resection of metatarsal heads 1 through 5.

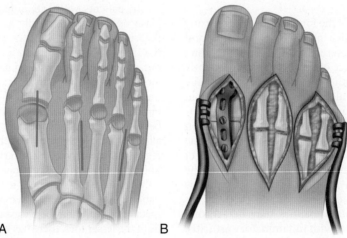

A   B

FIGURE 5.6   **A** and **B**, First metatarsophalangeal joint arthrodesis fixed with plate and one oblique screw.

available. Currently, the long-term survival and outcomes of the newer first metatarsophalangeal prostheses have not been clearly established although there are promising short-term and intermediate-term data involving synthetic cartilage implants. As with all surgery, patient selection and counseling are important.

■ ARTHRODESIS OF THE FIRST METATARSOPHALANGEAL JOINT IN THE RHEUMATOID PATIENT

Arthrodesis of the first metatarsophalangeal joint with varying degrees of bony shortening at the metatarsophalangeal joints of the lesser toes, as needed, has been reported to obtain satisfactory results in 80% to 90% of patients with inflammatory arthropathy. Treatment of hallux rigidus is discussed in chapter 2.

Many recommendations have been made concerning the valgus alignment of the hallux (15 to 30 degrees) and the amount of dorsiflexion (10 to 30 degrees) to be obtained at arthrodesis. We recommend approximately 15 to 20 degrees of valgus and 30 degrees of dorsiflexion from the first

metatarsal axis (approximately 15 degrees of dorsiflexion in reference to the plantar aspect of the foot). The hallux should be placed in neutral rotation also. Excellent gait patterns have been described after first metatarsophalangeal joint arthrodesis, as well as improved first-second intermetatarsal angles. Rarely is a metatarsal osteotomy necessary in conjunction with the arthrodesis. Comparisons of arthrodesis and arthroplasty have found that pain relief, balance, cosmesis, and ability to fit the foot in a normal shoe were better after arthrodesis than after excisional arthroplasty.

From review of published series on rheumatoid forefoot procedures, several conclusions emerge:

1. In 80% to 90% of patients, a satisfactory result can be expected.
2. Inadequate relaxation of the soft tissues around the metatarsophalangeal joints from insufficient bony resection can compromise the result (Fig. 5.7).
3. Unequal lengths of the metatarsal remnants or metatarsals that do not cascade in a gentle curve from metatarsals two through five are likely to compromise the result.

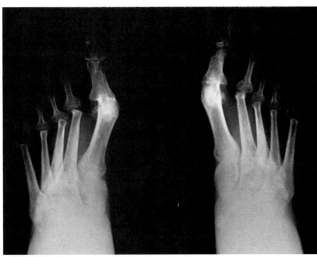

FIGURE 5.7   Ensure adequate resection of lesser metatarsals.

4. Bony fragments remaining in the forefoot weight-bearing pad after removal of the metatarsophalangeal joints may compromise an otherwise good outcome.
5. Dorsal or plantar incisions are reasonable, but delicate care of the soft tissue during dissection and adequate hemostasis is mandatory.
6. Pain relief, walking endurance, and footwear variety should be improved enough to warrant the procedure.
7. A satisfactory result may deteriorate with time.
8. Arthrodesis of the first metatarsophalangeal joint combined with lesser metatarsophalangeal joint resections may reduce the complications of recurrence of deformity, painful callosities beneath the lesser metatarsal remnants, and deterioration of a satisfactory result with time. Joint preservation should usually be limited to patients with mild to moderate deformity.
9. Surgical intervention for the rheumatoid foot should involve a multidisciplinary approach with medical control of the disease and associated disorders and close communication with a knowledgeable orthotist.
10. A precontoured locking or nonlocking low-profile metatarsophalangeal joint fusion plate on the dorsal aspect of the metatarsophalangeal joint in conjunction with an axial-plane oblique interfragmentary screw has shown superior biomechanical strength and rotatory stability compared with other alternatives. The ability of compression staples to control rotational forces is still in question, and these should be used with caution.

ARTHRODESIS OF THE FIRST METATARSOPHALANGEAL JOINT WITH RESECTION OF THE LESSER METATARSOPHALANGEAL JOINTS

Arthrodesis of the first metatarsophalangeal joint with resection of the lesser metatarsal heads reestablishes the fat pad beneath the metatarsal heads and allows a greater variety of footwear. Even though the tips of the toes may not touch the ground when the patient stands,

balance is not impaired. Osteoclasis may be used to try to correct the proximal interphalangeal joint deformity, but tearing of the plantar skin is common, and most surgeons now recommend interphalangeal arthroplasty with removal of the head and neck of the proximal phalanges for fixed deformities.

TECHNIQUE 5.1

(THOMPSON AND MANN)
- Make a dorsal longitudinal incision centered over the first metatarsophalangeal joint and just medial to the extensor hallucis longus tendon. In patients who are at risk for problems with wound healing, a medial approach may be preferable.
- Protect the dorsomedial branch of the superficial peroneal nerve.
- Open the capsule in line with the skin incision, and remove any hypertrophic synovium (Fig. 5.8A).
- Release the joint capsule medially and laterally sufficiently to expose the articular surfaces.
- Prepare the metatarsophalangeal joint using a sagittal saw to create a flat cut (Fig. 5.8B), and remove the distal portion (5 mm) of the first metatarsal head. Make the cut with the toe in about 20 degrees of valgus and approximately 15 degrees of dorsiflexion from the plantar aspect of the foot (Fig. 5.8B).
- Completely free the base of the proximal phalanx of its soft-tissue attachments, and excise the proximal portion (3 to 5 mm) of the proximal phalanx.
- Hold the great toe in 20 degrees of valgus and 15 degrees of dorsiflexion in relation to the plantar aspect of the foot, and make the osteotomy parallel to the one in the metatarsal head (Fig. 5.8C).
- Appose the two flat surfaces, and observe the alignment.
- Alternatively, use commercially available cannulated conical reamers to create a cone arthrodesis (see Technique 5.2). This allows for easier placement of the metatarsophalangeal joint in the correct position and provides excellent bony contact, although it may not be as stable as a congruent flat cut.
- Usually, more bone must be removed for arthrodesis in patients with rheumatoid arthritis than in patients with hallux rigidus to compensate for removal of the other metatarsal heads so that the hallux is not too long.
- Approach the lesser metatarsophalangeal joints through two dorsal longitudinal incisions in the second and fourth web spaces (Fig. 5.8D). Begin each incision in the web space, and continue it proximally for 3 to 4 cm. Identify the extensor tendons (Fig. 5.8E). Trace the tendons distally to the base of the proximal phalanx (the extensor digitorum brevis is slightly lateral and deep to the extensor digitorum longus). Transect or lengthen the extensor digitorum longus if needed. Enter the metatarsophalangeal joint on the medial side of the extensor tendons to joints two and three and lateral to the extensor digitorum in toes four and five.
- After identifying the base of the proximal phalanx beneath the extensor tendons, free contracted soft-tissue attachments to the base of the proximal phalanx with sharp dissection.
- Perform synovectomy if needed; this may be difficult because of the degree of dislocation. Occasionally, the base of the proximal phalanx is ankylosed to the neck of the

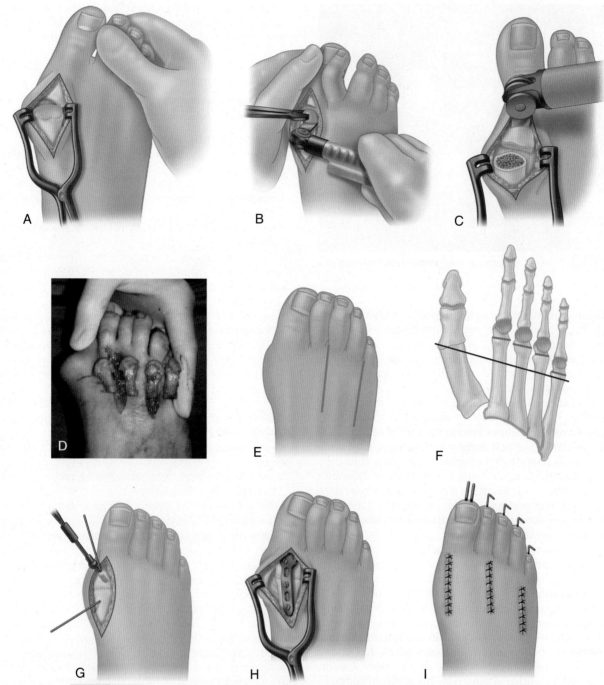

FIGURE 5.8   **A,** Metatarsophalangeal joint is exposed through dorsal approach. **B,** Distal 3 to 5 mm of metatarsal head is removed with sagittal saw. **C,** Base of proximal phalanx is removed. **D,** Incisions for excisional arthroplasty. **E,** Lesser metatarsophalangeal joints are approached through dorsal incisions in second and fourth web spaces. **F,** Diagram showing resection of metatarsal heads. **G,** After fusion site has been stabilized with Kirschner wires, interfragmentary screw is inserted if bone stock is strong enough. **H,** Fixation of arthrodesis site with six-hole, one-quarter tubular AO plate. **I,** Pinning of arthrodesis site with ⅛-inch threaded Steinmann pins. **SEE TECHNIQUE 5.1.**

metatarsal and must be pried off the neck before the soft tissue is detached.

- When the base of the proximal phalanx is free of its soft-tissue attachments, pull the toe distally and make a longitudinal cut along the dorsal aspect of the distal portion of the metatarsal. Strip the soft tissue medially and laterally

off the distal portion of the metatarsal, and with sharp dissection cut any remaining capsular tissue. Strip the soft tissue circumferentially around the distal portion of the metatarsal head and neck.

- Preserve the common digital nerves and arteries in the respective intermetatarsal spaces by limiting dissection to the shafts of the metatarsals. Preserve the dorsal nerves if possible; if not, coagulate them carefully.

- When all the soft tissues around the lesser metatarsophalangeal joints are released, remove the lesser metatarsal heads at the level of the neck of the metatarsal, producing a gentle slope laterally (Fig. 5.8F). A curved McGlamry or Hohmann retractor is often helpful to obtain exposure. If less than the complete metatarsal head is removed, stiffness or plantar callus may result.
- If any significant synovial cysts are present on the plantar aspect of the foot, remove the dorsal half of the cyst and use a rongeur to remove the soft tissues beneath. To ensure adequate plantar padding, do not remove too much tissue and fat.
- Realign the lesser toes and collapse the joint space to see how much more shortening of the first metatarsophalangeal joint is necessary to accommodate the loss of the metatarsal heads. Usually, about 1 cm more shortening is required, and this can be removed from the metatarsal rather than from the base of the proximal phalanx. At this time, make any necessary adjustment in the alignment of the first metatarsophalangeal joint. When this has been done, the first and second toes should be about the same length and the other lesser toes should have a smooth, laterally sloping cascade.
- Stabilize the first metatarsophalangeal joint with guide pins for two 3.5- to 4.5-mm cannulated screws (Fig. 5.8G). If the bone quality is good, two interfragmentary screws across the metatarsophalangeal joint in a crossed fashion to gain interfragmentary compression has shown good results with relatively low cost.
- However, in patients with osteopenia, apply a precontoured, locking or nonlocking low-profile metatarsophalangeal joint fusion plate to the dorsal aspect of the metatarsophalangeal joint, and secure it with a 3.2- or 4.0-mm cancellous screw (Fig. 5.8H). An interfragmentary screw should be used for rotational stability. This construct has shown superior biomechanical strength and rotatory stability compared to other fixation methods.
- If the bone is too soft for screw placement, use two ⅛-inch, double-threaded Steinmann pins. Drill the pins out in a retrograde fashion, starting at the base of the proximal phalanx through the tip of the toe. Position the toe and drive the pins back across the metatarsophalangeal joint into the metatarsal. Although this gives excellent fixation in patients with soft bone, it is not recommended in patients with good bone stock because the pins violate the interphalangeal joint (Fig. 5.8I).
- Stabilize each lesser metatarsophalangeal joint with a 0.054-inch (1.4-mm) Kirschner wire placed through the tip of the toe in a retrograde fashion. Hold the interphalangeal joint previously straightened by osteoclasis (the technique used in mild fixed proximal interphalangeal flexion deformities), or more commonly by proximal interphalangeal joint arthroplasty, in proper alignment while placing the pin across the toe. Advance the wire proximally down the metatarsal shaft. Use a wire that is long enough to allow its tip to become embedded in the base of the metatarsal.
- Close the capsules and wounds with interrupted 2-0 sutures (Monocryl; Ethicon, Piscataway, NJ) placed subcutaneously and simple interrupted nylon sutures on the skin. Apply a sterile compression dressing.

POSTOPERATIVE CARE The circulatory status of the toes should be monitored carefully after surgery, especially after correction of severe deformity. If the toe remains blanched, this may indicate that the arterial circulation has not returned because the toe was stretched too far longitudinally along the Kirschner wire. If the toe is cyanotic, it may have been shortened too much, with multiple folds in the vein. If the color does not normalize within 30 minutes, the postoperative compression dressing should be released. If after 2 hours the color is still unsatisfactory, the pin should be removed. The foot is elevated consistently for 4 days, and the sutures are removed after 10 to 14 days. The wounds are inspected, and a new dressing is applied. Only heel weight bearing is allowed until 4 weeks after surgery. Radiographs are obtained at 4 and 8 weeks. At 4 weeks the arthrodesis has consolidated enough to allow full-weight ambulation in a hard postoperative shoe, and the dressing is discontinued. At 8 weeks, the patient can begin to wear loose sneakers or extra-deep shoes. Ambulation in the postoperative shoe is continued until arthrodesis is complete, usually at 8 to 12 weeks.

CONE ARTHRODESIS OF THE FIRST METATARSOPHALANGEAL JOINT

TECHNIQUE 5.2

- Make a dorsal longitudinal incision centered over the first metatarsophalangeal joint and just medial to the extensor hallucis longus tendon (Fig. 5.9A). Begin the incision just proximal to the interphalangeal joint, and extend it to 3 cm proximal to the metatarsophalangeal joint. If it is expected that the patient will have problems with wound healing, use of a medial approach is reasonable.
- Protect the dorsomedial branch of the superficial peroneal nerve.
- Open the capsule in line with the skin incision, and remove any hypertrophic synovium.
- Release the joint capsule medially and laterally on the phalangeal and metatarsal sides of the joint to expose the articular surfaces sufficiently and to allow for at least 3 to 5 mm of bony resection.
- Displace the proximal phalanx plantarly to expose the metatarsal head. Use a sagittal saw to remove the articular cartilage of the metatarsal head in a circumferential manner to create the shape of a cone.
- Use a sagittal saw to remove the articular cartilage from the base of the proximal phalanx. The cut should be perpendicular to the base of the phalanx and only thick enough to reach subchondral bone at the center of this concave surface.
- With a Freer elevator, gently create a concave surface in this soft cancellous bone. The metatarsal head should be congruent to the surface of the proximal phalanx.

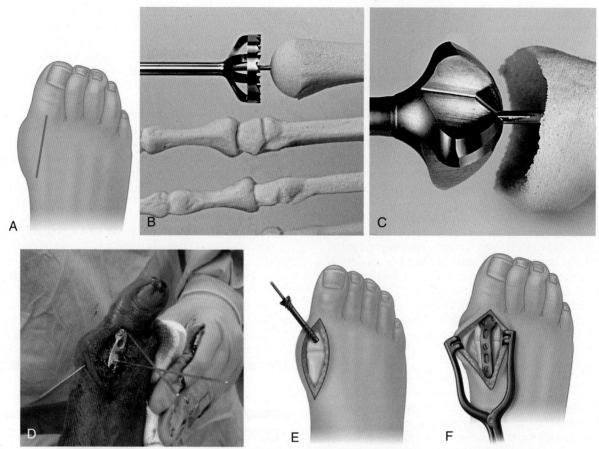

FIGURE 5.9 Cone arthrodesis of first metatarsophalangeal joint. **A,** Metatarsophalangeal joint is exposed through dorsal longitudinal incision just medial to extensor hallucis longus tendon. **B,** First metatarsal is prepared by insertion of guide pin down shaft and use of appropriate-sized female (concave) reamer to remove cartilage and expose subchondral bone. Care must be taken not to leave hallux too long if lesser metatarsal heads are removed. **C,** Proximal phalanx is prepared with different guide pin placed down shaft and corresponding-sized male (convex) reamer. **D,** Dorsal plate is used as guide for alignment of metatarsophalangeal joint arthrodesis and to place provisional Kirschner wire across joint for stability. **E** and **F,** After confirmation of appropriate alignment, contoured plate is secured with multi-use compression screws. **SEE TECHNIQUE 5.2.**

- Alternatively, use a commercially available metatarsophalangeal joint cone-arthrodesis system. First, place a guide pin proximally through the center of the metatarsal head and into the diaphysis using a drill. Use the largest concave reamer over the guide pin to ream the metatarsal head gently (Fig. 5.9B). Use progressively smaller reamers until the appropriate size is used to remove the entire articular surface. Note the size of the final female reamer.
- After removing the guide pin from the metatarsal, place another pin in the center of the proximal phalanx. We recommend using a different guide pin from the one used in the metatarsal because it may have been notched and thus be prone to break. Gently ream the base of the proximal phalanx, starting with the smallest convex reamer. Progress through the reamer sizes until the matching size reamer has been used on the metatarsal and phalangeal sides of the joint (Fig. 5.9C). The articular surfaces should be congruent now and allow significant freedom of motion to place the hallux in the appropriate position.

- After joint preparation by either method, provisionally secure the hallux metatarsophalangeal joint with a Kirschner wire. The method of internal fixation depends on the surgeon's experience and preference. We most often use an obliquely placed headless compression screw with the addition of a precontoured dorsal plate.
- If using a system with precontoured plates, use this plate as a template when positioning the metatarsophalangeal joint (Fig 5.9D). Place the compression screw distal-medial to proximal-lateral to engage the lateral cortex of the metatarsal (Fig. 5.9E). Predrill before placement of the headless screw. Do not countersink the head of the screw past the medial cortex in the proximal phalanx.
- Secure the precontoured, low-profile fusion plate to the dorsal aspect of the metatarsophalangeal joint with 2.7- to 4.0-mm cancellous screws (Fig. 5.9F). In patients with poor bone quality, use the larger screw sizes to gain additional purchase. Locking screws may be necessary.

- Close the capsules and wounds with interrupted 2-0 sutures (Monocryl; Ethicon) placed subcutaneously and simple interrupted nylon sutures on the skin. Apply a sterile compression dressing.

POSTOPERATIVE CARE The foot is elevated for 4 days, and the sutures are removed after 10 to 14 days. The wounds are inspected, and a new dressing is applied. Only heel weight bearing is allowed until postoperative week 4. Radiographs are obtained at 4 and 8 weeks. At 4 weeks after surgery the arthrodesis has consolidated enough to allow full-weight ambulation in a hard postoperative shoe, and the dressing is discontinued. At 8 weeks, the patient can begin to wear loose sneakers or extra-deep shoes. In the rheumatoid foot, swelling may take several months to resolve, and patients often have some initial difficulty with balance because reconstructive surgery changes the forefoot anatomy considerably. First metatarsophalangeal arthrodesis limits heel height and shoe selection, and patients often require new orthoses or shoes after surgery.

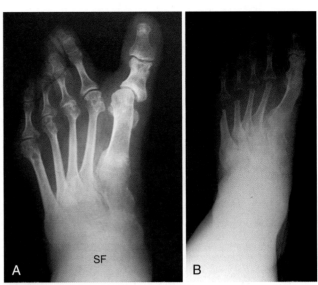

FIGURE 5.10 **A,** Multiple deformities in rheumatoid forefoot with previous basilar metatarsal osteotomy and distal soft-tissue procedure. Hallux varus developed. **B,** One year after arthrodesis of first metatarsophalangeal joint and resection of head and neck of proximal phalanx of digits two through five. Lesser metatarsal heads were removed.

RESECTION OF THE LESSER METATARSAL HEADS THROUGH A PLANTAR APPROACH WITH ARTHRODESIS OF THE FIRST METATARSOPHALANGEAL JOINT

We have found that the degree of deformity can be used to decide whether a dorsal or plantar approach is indicated. In subluxed but passively reducible metatarsophalangeal joints, dorsal longitudinal incisions allow easy access to the metatarsal heads and proximal phalanges without concern for the plantar neurovascular bundles. If the metatarsophalangeal joints are completely dislocated and not passively reducible, however, the metatarsal heads are quite prominent and may be exposed readily on the plantar surface of the foot. In addition, the flexor tendons and neurovascular bundles are out of harm's way in most severe claw deformities, having been brought deeply into the intermetatarsal spaces by the deformity of the metatarsophalangeal joint.

The technique used most frequently at this clinic is resection of *up to* 20% of the entire second, third, and fourth metatarsal, with a generous portion of the fifth metatarsal (30%) removed; arthrodesis of the first metatarsophalangeal joint; excision of both sesamoids; and correction of fixed hammer toes by resection of 30% to 40% of the distal aspect of the proximal phalanx (Fig. 5.10). The phalangeal bases are not resected.

TECHNIQUE 5.3

- Mark the metatarsal heads and outline the proposed skin ellipse as shown in Fig. 5.11A.
- When the skin ellipse has been removed, approach the metatarsal heads longitudinally through the overlying bursa and flexor tendon sheaths. If the flexor tendons are not subluxated into the intermetatarsal spaces, open the

sheaths and retract them to whichever side of the metatarsal head gives the best exposure. Do not injure the flexor tendons, which are now vulnerable in the proximal incision.
- Expose the sides and dorsum of the metatarsal head by sharp dissection, staying close to bone (Fig. 5.11B).
- Remove the metatarsal head, neck, and distal shaft with a bone-biter or power saw and small blade. The osteotomy should proceed in a slightly oblique angle, plantar-proximal to dorsal-distal, to minimize edge loading during the push-off phase of gait.
- Repeat this procedure on each lesser metatarsal, but on the fifth metatarsal remove the entire distal 30% of the metatarsal. A bursa is common on the fifth metatarsal head, and it may recur on the distal remnant after surgery if sufficient bone is not resected. Palpate each metatarsal head to ensure no bony ridge remains and no bony fragments are in the soft tissue. Do not excise the sesamoids through this approach.
- Approach the first metatarsophalangeal joint through a medial incision. Carry the incision to bone, staying directly in the midline of the proximal phalanx, metatarsal head, and distal half of the first metatarsal. Raise the dorsal and plantar flaps at the bone level and not extracapsularly.
- Remove the medial eminence.
- Excise the metatarsal head joint surface and base of the proximal phalanx with an osteotome, saw, or commercial conical reamers at an angle that places the arthrodesis in 10 to 15 degrees of valgus and 15 to 20 degrees of dorsiflexion (Fig. 5.11C).
- The amount of dorsiflexion often is difficult to judge. To avoid malposition, place a Kirschner wire along the joint, and with a large, sterilized goniometer, measure the plane of the heel pad and forefoot pad beneath the first metatarsal head with the pulp pad of the distal phalanx while

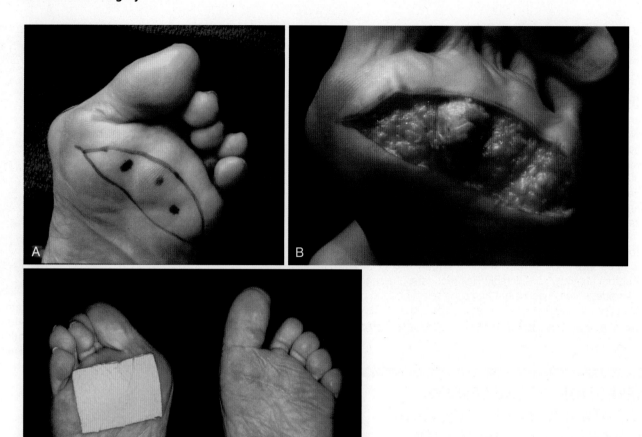

FIGURE 5.11   **A,** Metatarsal heads are dislocated plantarward and are marked; area of skin removed should be no more than 2.5 cm at widest anteroposterior diameter. **B,** Fourth metatarsal head is exposed, and small right-angle retractor is placed plantarward to expose neck and distal shaft. **C,** Articular surfaces of first metatarsophalangeal joint are shaped to allow arthrodesis in 10 to 15 degrees of valgus and 15 to 20 degrees of dorsiflexion. First ray should have been shortened more. **SEE TECHNIQUE 5.3.**

holding the interphalangeal joint in neutral position. This measurement should be no more than 10 degrees, which usually places the dorsiflexion angle at the first metatarsophalangeal joint at 18 to 25 degrees.

■ Removal of the articular surfaces of the first metatarsophalangeal joint makes exposure of the sesamoids easier.

■ Infrequently, the sesamoids need to be removed because of prominence or arthrosis between the sesamoid and first metatarsal head. To help with this often-difficult dissection and excision, place a strong, two-toothed retractor beneath the metatarsal head and lift the first metatarsal.

■ With a small curved elevator, disengage any adhesions of the sesamoids to the metatarsal head. The fibular sesamoid usually is the most adherent.

■ Incise the intersesamoid ligament, and remove the tibial sesamoid. Do not injure the flexor hallucis longus tendon, which is especially vulnerable during this step.

■ Clasp the fibular sesamoid with a Kocher clamp, and pull it medially. Free the soft tissue around the fibular sesamoid by blunt dissection, and excise the sesamoid by sharp dissection. Avoid injury to the neurovascular bundle to the first web, which is vulnerable at the proximal lateral border of the fibular sesamoid.

■ If the sesamoids have been removed, inspect the flexor hallucis longus and cauterize vessels as necessary.

■ The method of internal fixation depends on the surgeon's experience and preference. We most often use an obliquely placed headless compression screw with a precontoured locking or nonlocking dorsal plate. The hallux should not be more than 6 to 8 mm longer than the second toe (Fig. 5.11C).

■ Release the tourniquet or Esmarch wrap, carefully inspect the wound for pulsatile bleeding, and cauterize vessels as needed. Diffuse bleeding is common in these patients because of prolonged use of antiinflammatory agents. Placing the patient in the Trendelenburg position as the wounds are closed usually is sufficient to obtain hemostasis after pulsatile bleeding has been controlled.

- Close the capsule with 2-0 or 3-0 absorbable sutures, and close the skin with 3-0 or 4-0 monofilament nylon. Close the plantar wound with 3-0 monofilament nylon, everting the edges. Use 4-0 nylon for filler stitches if protruding fat is a problem; try to preserve as much fat as possible.
- Apply a conforming but nonconstricting, forefoot dressing.

POSTOPERATIVE CARE The foot is elevated for 4 days, and the sutures are removed after 10 to 14 days, at which time the wounds are inspected and a new dressing is applied. Heel weight bearing is allowed until postoperative week 4. Radiographs are obtained at 4 and 8 weeks. At 4 weeks after surgery the arthrodesis has consolidated and the plantar wound healed enough to allow full weight ambulation in a hard postoperative shoe, and the dressing is discontinued. At 8 weeks, the patient can begin to wear loose sneakers or extra-deep shoes. An extra-deep shoe with a soft upper is recommended for long-term use.

CORRECTION OF FLEXION DEFORMITIES OF THE PROXIMAL INTERPHALANGEAL JOINTS

TECHNIQUE 5.4

- Through a dorsal elliptical or longitudinal incision, incise the extensor tendon, capsule, and collateral ligaments of the proximal interphalangeal joint. It is helpful to incise the capsule just distal to the joint so the collateral ligaments can be released parallel to the plantar surface of the proximal phalanx. Once the soft tissue on the distal aspect of the proximal phalanx has been removed, excise the head and neck of the proximal phalanx (Fig. 5.12). Care must be taken to avoid creating an oblique osteotomy and thus hyperflexing or hyperextending (more problematic) the toe.
- Before closing the dorsal wound over the lesser toe proximal interphalangeal joints, insert 0.054-inch Kirschner wires in a retrograde fashion from the proximal interphalangeal joint distally and through the proximal phalangeal medullary canal and into the lesser metatarsal remnant. Often the Kirschner wires are not necessary if the elliptical incision is used at the proximal interphalangeal joint to provide stability and if a painstakingly applied forefoot dressing is worn for 3 weeks after surgery.
- Remove the tourniquet and obtain hemostasis. Close the wounds with nonabsorbable 4-0 sutures; apply a bulky forefoot compression dressing; and if wires have been used, bend the ends to avoid migration or cover them with commercially supplied protective balls.

POSTOPERATIVE CARE Using a walker or with some assistance, the patient is allowed to walk to the bathroom

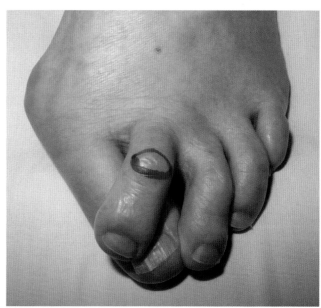

FIGURE 5.12 Dorsal elliptical incision for excision of head and neck of the proximal phalanx for correction of flexion deformity. **SEE TECHNIQUE 5.4.**

or to a bedside commode on the day of surgery. After 72 hours, the patient is allowed to be up and to bear weight to tolerance.

MIDFOOT

Arthritis of the midfoot is not uncommon, yet the literature specific to this entity is limited. Much of the literature relates to treating sequelae of Lisfranc injuries. Arthritis of the midfoot may result not only from trauma but also as a result of osteoarthritis or inflammatory disease. Instability of the tarsometatarsal joint may result in progressive collapse of the midfoot and degenerative changes to the joints. This is most often seen in the first tarsometatarsal joint and may or may not be associated with hallux valgus or posterior tibial pathology. Regardless of the underlying cause, significant disability may result from this condition due to the collapse of the longitudinal arch with weight bearing. This results in pain due to abnormal joint mechanics. Bony prominences, both dorsally and plantarly, make shoewear difficult.

The midfoot is composed of three columns: the first tarsometatarsal joint forms the medial column, the second and third tarsometatarsal joints the middle column, and the fourth and fifth tarsometatarsal joints the lateral column (Fig. 5.13). The midfoot is aligned when the medial border of the first metatarsal joint aligns with the medial border of the medial cuneiform, the medial border of the second metatarsal joint aligns with the medial border of the middle cuneiform, and the medial border of the fourth metatarsal joint is aligned with the medial border of the cuboid (Fig. 5.13). The Lisfranc articulation comprises the tarsometatarsal joints (first through third metatarsocuneiform and the fourth and fifth metatarsocuboid). In the coronal plane, each of the cuneiforms is wedge shaped with the dorsal aspect wider than plantar. This forms a "Roman arch," providing inherent stability due to the bony architecture (Fig. 5.14). The second metatarsal base is recessed between the medial and

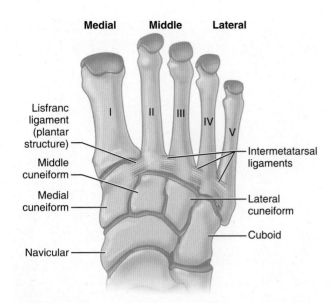

Medial **Middle** **Lateral**

Lisfranc
ligament
(plantar
structure)

Middle
cuneiform

Medial
cuneiform

Navicular

Intermetatarsal
ligaments

Lateral
cuneiform

Cuboid

FIGURE 5.13 Three columns of midfoot. Midfoot is aligned when medial border of second metatarsal base is aligned with medial border of middle cuneiform and medial border of fourth metatarsal is aligned with medial border of cuboid. In addition, space between medial and middle cuneiform should be symmetric when compared to contralateral injured foot.

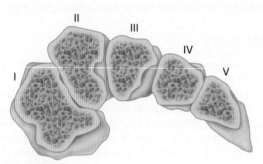

FIGURE 5.14 Coronal section through metatarsal bases illustrating the Roman arch configuration.

lateral cuneiforms, creating stability at the second metatarsal joint. Tight ligamentous attachments, as well as the peroneus longus, adductor hallucis, flexor hallucis brevis, plantar fascia, and tibialis posterior and anterior, contribute to stability. There is no ligamentous attachment from the base of the first metatarsal to the second metatarsal joints. The Lisfranc ligament (three components) courses from the middle cuneiform to the base of the second metatarsal joint and provides significant stability in this region. The fairly rigid midfoot connects the mobile hindfoot to the mobile forefoot.

Despite the relative lack of mobility in the midfoot, arc of motion in the lateral column is approximately 20 degrees and therefore important to proper biomechanics. Preservation of the fourth and fifth tarsometatarsal joints should be considered a priority. Fusion of these joints results in a rigid midfoot, and even severe arthritis often is not symptomatic. In an attempt to avoid arthrodesis of an arthritic painful lateral column, techniques for arthroplasty of these joints have been devised, including tendon arthroplasty and spherical ceramic interpositional arthroplasty.

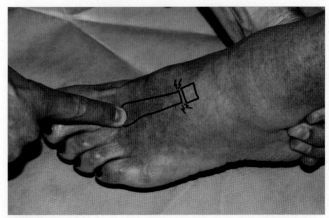

FIGURE 5.15 "Piano key" test for evaluation of midfoot (see text).

Despite reluctance to fuse the lateral midfoot joints, good results have been reported after arthrodesis of the fourth and fifth tarsometatarsal joints. Although most of these patients had neuropathy, pain, function, and American Orthopaedic Foot and Ankle Society scores also improved significantly in those with normal sensation. Multiple methods of fixation have been used for tarsometatarsal arthrodesis, including plantar plating, crossed screws, and external fixation; external fixation is not recommended except in the presence of ulceration. Another area of controversy is whether to reduce midfoot deformity *before* fusion. Midfoot arthritis often leads to an abduction, pronation, and dorsiflexion deformity. Most studies suggest better results with improved alignment and restoration of bony architecture.

Examination of the arthritic midfoot is difficult. Small joints with limited motion make differentiating pain a challenge. Provocative maneuvers about the midfoot often cause diffuse pain. Keiserman et al. described a "piano key" test in which pushing the metatarsal head in a plantar direction causes cantilever stress at the corresponding tarsometatarsal joint (Fig. 5.15). Anteroposterior, lateral, and oblique radiographs should be obtained in a weight-bearing position to assess for joint destruction, instability, and deformity. CT may be useful also, but most centers do not have the ability to obtain these with weight-bearing simulation. Differential injections using an anesthetic also can be helpful and can be done under ultrasound, fluoroscopic, or CT guidance (Fig. 5.16). Adding a steroid to the injection may provide therapeutic as well as diagnostic benefits. Hindfoot deformity often accompanies a midfoot pathologic process and must be carefully evaluated and treated surgically, if needed.

TREATMENT

Conservative treatment of midfoot arthritis includes steroid injections, physiotherapy, shoe modification, use of orthoses, and bracing. Rocker soles on extra-depth stiff shoes with accommodative inserts (Fig. 5.17) may improve pain and ambulation significantly. For more advanced arthritis, an ankle-foot orthosis can be used to support the longitudinal arch (Fig. 5.18). Arthritis of the midfoot often progresses, however, and surgery may become necessary to relieve pain.

■ FIRST METATARSAL-MEDIAL CUNEIFORM ARTHRODESIS

The technique for first metatarsal-medial cuneiform arthrodesis is described in chapter 2.

■ MIDFOOT ARTHRODESIS

Surgery is indicated for patients for whom conservative management fails. Preoperative planning is based on the symptomatic joints as determined by physical examination and differential injections. Although radiographs and CT scans play an important role in planning, especially in patients with posttraumatic deformity, they must be interpreted with care. Arthritic joints may be asymptomatic, especially in the more mobile lateral column. Alternatively, joints with minimal arthritic changes may be quite symptomatic and need to be included in the fusion. Patients with posttraumatic arthritis tend to be younger than those with atraumatic degeneration.

Multiple joints often are included in the fusion, with the medial and middle columns most often involved. If the navicular-medial cuneiform joint is involved, the navicular-middle cuneiform joint usually should be included in the fusion as well. The intercuneiform joint should be included if both tarsometatarsal joints are fused (e.g., if both the first and second tarsometatarsal joints are fused, the medial/middle intercuneiform joint should be included). Preservation of the joints of the lateral column is desirable, but fusion may be needed for stability, especially in the neuropathic foot. Deformity correction is a priority and may be difficult after traumatic collapse. Use of the bone graft has been shown to improve fusion rates in some studies.

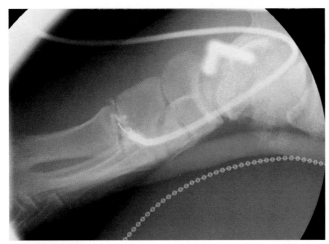

FIGURE 5.16 CT-guided or, more commonly, ultrasound-guided differential injection can be helpful in diagnosis of midfoot arthritis.

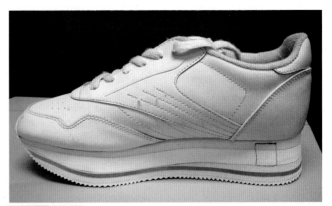

FIGURE 5.17 Extra-depth stiff shoes with rocker soles can be effective nonoperative treatment for midfoot arthritis.

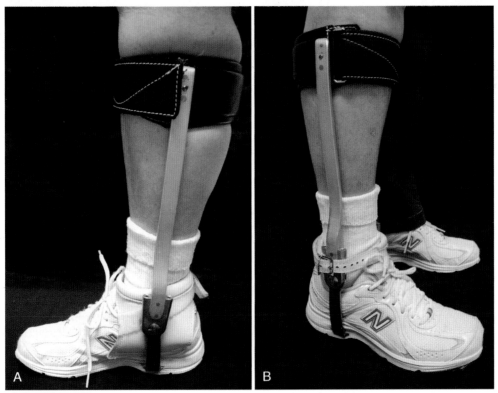

FIGURE 5.18 **A** and **B**, For more advanced arthritis, an ankle-foot orthosis, such as this double-upright brace, can be used for support of the longitudinal arch.

MIDFOOT ARTHRODESIS

TECHNIQUE 5.5

- Place the patient supine on the operating table. Usually a hip bump is not needed because the fusion involves only the medial and middle columns.
- After induction of spinal or general anesthesia and administration of a popliteal block for postoperative pain control, place a well-padded thigh tourniquet.
- Make a dorsal longitudinal incision just medial to the second metatarsal joint (Fig. 5.19A) to allow access to the first and second tarsometatarsal joints and the intercuneiform joints. The incision can be extended if the naviculocuneiform joints are to be included in the fusion.
- If the third tarsometatarsal joint is to be included in the fusion, make a curvilinear incision with the apex laterally. If necessary, make a separate incision centered just medial to the fourth metatarsal joint (Fig. 5.19A).
- If the fourth and fifth tarsometatarsal joints must be approached, a third incision may be needed dorsolaterally, centered over the fifth tarsometatarsal joint (Fig. 5.19A). Take care to avoid damage to branches of the sural or intermediate branch of the superficial peroneal nerves.
- Protect the dorsomedial cutaneous branch of the superficial peroneal nerve.
- Retract the extensor hallucis longus medially, and mobilize the extensor hallucis brevis so that it can be retracted either medially or laterally depending on whether the first or second tarsometatarsal joint needs to be exposed (Fig. 5.19B).
- The dorsalis pedis and deep peroneal nerve lie just plantar to the extensor hallucis brevis and must be mobilized. Place a vessel loop to protect these structures.
- Release the joint capsule in line with the incision and raise full-thickness flaps in a subperiosteal fashion.
- Identify the joints to be fused with fluoroscopy.
- Thoroughly denude the joint to expose subchondral bone. Take care when preparing the tarsometatarsal joints to avoid removing excess bone dorsally, thus hyperextending the metatarsal joint. We routinely use a 2.0-mm bit to drill holes on both sides of the joint and crosshatch the surfaces with a ¼-inch osteotome.
- Once the joints have been prepared and adequately mobilized, place the foot in a plantigrade position and provisionally secure this position with Kirschner wires.
- Begin with reduction of the first tarsometatarsal joint, which usually is in some abduction and dorsiflexion. Then reduce other joints to this now-stable medial column. Pay close attention to the sagittal plane reduction to avoid metatarsalgia.
- Obtain fluoroscopic images in multiple planes to ensure that all deformity has been corrected and there is good bone apposition. Bone graft (autologous or bone substitute) may be needed.
- Multiple forms of fixation are available. We place a 4.0-mm cannulated screw in a lagged technique along with dorsal plates or compression staples. Occasionally, a medial or plantar plate is used. This requires a separate incision, careful dissection, and placement of the plate over the anterior tibial tendon insertion (Fig. 5.20).

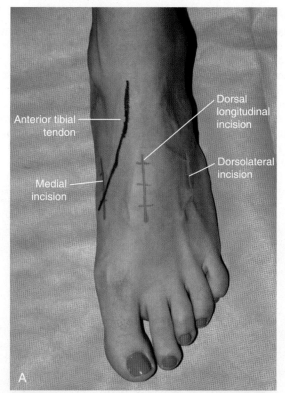

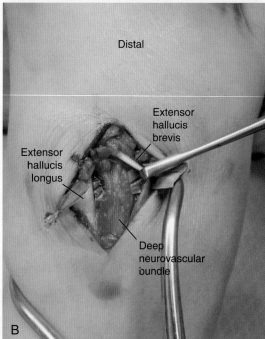

FIGURE 5.19 Midfoot arthrodesis (see text). **A,** Dorsal longitudinal incision is made just medial to second metatarsal. If medial plate is used, separate medial incision is made extending from mid-first metatarsal to navicular tuberosity. If exposure of fourth and fifth tarsometatarsal joints is needed, dorsolateral incision is made over fifth tarsometatarsal joint. **B,** Extensor hallucis longus is retracted medially, and extensor hallucis brevis is retracted medially or laterally depending on exposure needed. **SEE TECHNIQUE 5.5.**

- We prefer to use an oblique screw and a plate or compression staple to secure the first tarsometatarsal joint. The other joints usually require only one staple or small dorsal plate.
- Headed screws placed from the metatarsal into the cuneiform require countersinking into the bone to avoid fracture of the dorsal cortex as the screw head is seated. A burr can be used to facilitate this.
- Usually only one screw is needed across the intercuneiform joint, although a staple can be added if needed.
- Release the tourniquet, obtain hemostasis, and close the subcutaneous tissue with absorbable sutures. Close the skin with nylon sutures in a nontensioned, everted fashion.

POSTOPERATIVE CARE A compressive dressing and well-padded posterior splint are placed. The patient is instructed to elevate the extremity above the level of the heart for several days. Non–weight bearing ambulation with an assistive device is then gradually advanced. If a plantar plate has been used, immediate postoperative full weight bearing is possible. Sutures are removed after 12 to 14 days, and heel weight bearing in a rigid shoe is allowed. At 8 weeks after surgery, the patient can increase to full weight bearing in a wide toe-box shoe with a carbon insert (Fig. 5.21), assuming radiographs show at least partial union. A custom-molded orthotic device also may be beneficial.

HINDFOOT

Primary degenerative arthritis with good alignment may occur in the hindfoot but is usually associated with some instability or deformity. This often is due to imbalance of dynamic stabilizers of the hindfoot (e.g., the posterior tibial or peroneal tendon). However, ankle, midfoot, and forefoot pathologic processes may lead to abnormal alignment of an otherwise normal hindfoot and eventually contribute to insufficiency of the static stabilizers and degeneration of the transverse tarsal and subtalar joints. Subtalar motion is most commonly affected, and most patients being considered for subtalar or triple arthrodesis present with a contracture of the gastrocsoleus complex. Examination with the patient bearing weight is required to determine the structures affected.

The ankle and hindfoot are involved in 30% to 60% of rheumatoid arthritis patients. Hindfoot deformity often is the most limiting aspect to ambulation. The most important clinical problems of the rheumatoid hindfoot are heel valgus with resultant midfoot arch collapse and forefoot rotation in an axial plane. These problems may be caused by synovitis, synovial hypertrophy, or articular destruction of the tibiotalar (ankle), subtalar, and talonavicular joints.

Patients often present with a complaint of aching pain in the sinus tarsi and subfibular region, often activity related and associated with swelling. Any indication of an inflammatory arthropathy such as bilateral or multiple joint complaints or joint degeneration in a young patient with no history of trauma must be investigated. Steroid injections

and bracing often are quite beneficial, especially in early stages. Progressive arthritis often results in increased deformity, causing pain and making shoewear or even bracing difficult.

TREATMENT

Failure of conservative treatment or persistent synovitis and synovial hypertrophy that are unrelieved after 6 months of medical therapy is an indication for surgery. Combined bony and soft-tissue procedures often are beneficial to realign the hindfoot in patients with a flexible deformity. In patients with inflammatory arthropathy, however, tendon transfer, tendon graft, or tendon advancement should be used with caution because of the destructive underlying disease process. Bony stabilization is needed to maintain correction and relieve symptoms (most commonly, pain and tenderness in the sinus tarsi and along the peroneal tendons from calcaneal and fibular abutment). An exception to this is heel valgus with symptoms only along the course of the posterior tibial tendon with obvious tenosynovitis and synovial hypertrophy of this structure. A tenosynovectomy of the posterior tibial tendon may relieve symptoms if no lateral hindfoot pain is present and the deformity of the subtalar and midtarsal joints is completely reducible.

If symptomatic hindfoot valgus is unrelieved by arch supports, appropriate footwear, ankle and hindfoot bracing, and oral antiinflammatory medication, an arthrodesis is indicated, provided that the tibiotalar joint is stable. A subtalar joint arthrodesis is indicated for symptomatic arthrosis and to help correct heel valgus if the midtarsal joint has been spared by the rheumatoid destructive process; if not, a triple arthrodesis is indicated. Isolated subtalar fusion can correct only a mild amount of hindfoot valgus, and a medial displacement calcaneal osteotomy may need to be added. The standard technique for triple arthrodesis is described later in this chapter, and other techniques for triple arthrodesis are described elsewhere. As the effect of fusion on adjacent joints has become better understood, there has been interest in more limited arthrodesis techniques. For patients without involvement of the calcaneocuboid joint, Sammarco et al. described "double" arthrodesis, with fusion of the talonavicular and subtalar joints, and Wachter et al. described arthrodesis of the talonavicular and subtalar joints through a single medial incision. As adjacent joint arthritis occurs after arthrodesis of the ankle and hindfoot, motion-sparing procedures may be useful to help mitigate progression in select patients (Fig. 5.22).

A weight-bearing radiograph of the ankle joint aids in the diagnosis of ankle joint instability. The goal of surgical treatment is to restore hindfoot stability in the appropriate position; 5 to 10 degrees of hindfoot valgus should remain. This may require manually lifting the head and neck of the talus dorsally and laterally and bringing the forefoot medially and plantarward until the position of the hindfoot is corrected. Forefoot supination must be avoided when final fixation is placed across the talonavicular joint. A percutaneous lengthening of the Achilles tendon may be required if reduction places the ankle in equinus. Two incisions are most often used, one anterolateral and one medial, combined with internal fixation of the talonavicular and calcaneocuboid joints with staples, screws, or plates.

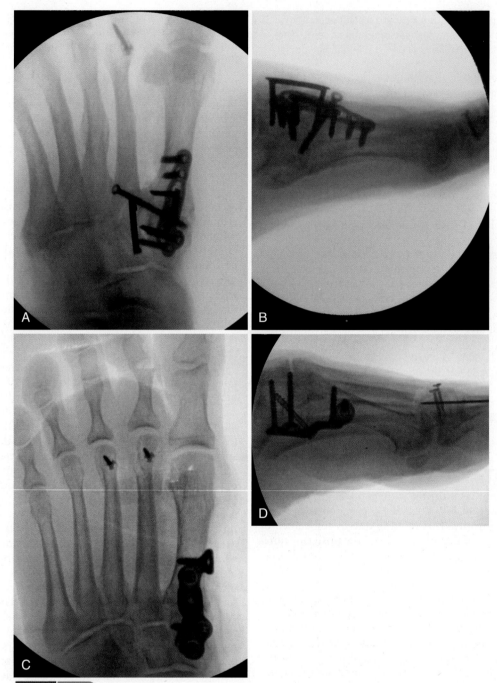

FIGURE **5.20** **A** and **B,** Midfoot arthrodesis with dorsal staple and plate fixation or, **C** and **D,** plantar plate fixation.

SUBTALAR ARTHRODESIS

TECHNIQUE 5.6

- For postoperative pain control, a popliteal block is placed in preoperative holding.
- Begin a straight lateral incision 1 cm inferior to the tip of the fibular malleolus, extending distally over the antero-lateral border of the calcaneus and cuboid (Fig. 5.23A).

Protect the sural nerve and peroneal tendons in the posterior aspect of the wound.
- Abduct and adduct the midfoot to locate the calcaneo-cuboid joint and invert and evert the subtalar joint for location.
- Locate the proximal tendons of origin of the extensor digitorum brevis and extensor hallucis brevis, and with sharp dissection lift them from the sinus tarsi under the lateral border of the muscle belly.
- Extend the dissection, lifting the extensor digitorum brevis from proximal to distal until the calcaneocuboid joint is

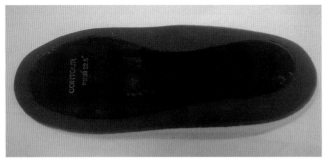

FIGURE 5.21 Carbon inserts used for 12 months postoperatively. A custom-molded orthosis also may be beneficial.

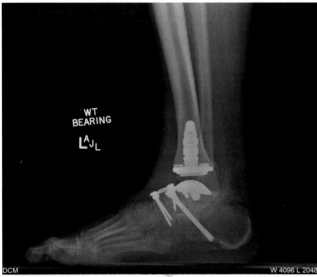

FIGURE 5.22 Total ankle arthroplasty and double hindfoot arthrodesis performed in patient with pantalar arthritis.

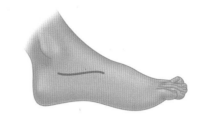

A

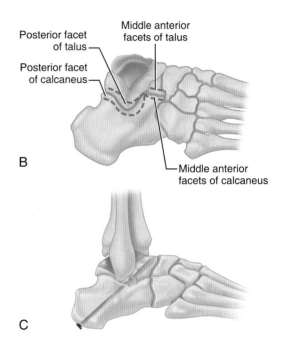

B

Posterior facet of talus

Posterior facet of calcaneus

Middle anterior facets of talus

Middle anterior facets of calcaneus

C

FIGURE 5.23 Subtalar arthrodesis. **A,** Skin incision. **B,** Cannulated screw from neck-body juncture to calcaneal tuberosity. **C,** Fixation with two cannulated screws. **SEE TECHNIQUE 5.6.**

exposed. Do not open the calcaneocuboid joint, but use a small-blade knife to identify the joint. This would not violate the dorsolateral calcaneocuboid ligament or the lateral calcaneocuboid ligament.

- Enter the joint just superior to the lateral calcaneocuboid ligament. These two important ligaments, along with the bifurcate ligament and a portion of the short plantar ligament, are stabilizers of the calcaneocuboid joint.
- Identify the subtalar joint, and remove the deep components of the inferior extensor retinaculum from the floor of the sinus tarsi. Also release the talocalcaneal interosseous ligament that is medial and posterior to the cervical ligament.
- When this area is cleaned of all soft tissue, place a right-angle retractor or a curved Hohmann retractor parallel to the posterior facet to lift the peroneal tendons laterally and posteriorly to allow better exposure of the subtalar joint.
- Place a lamina spreader into the depths of the sinus tarsi so that it rests on the inferior or plantar aspect of the talar neck and just lateral to the middle and anterior facet components of the talocalcaneal articulation.

- Depending on the condition of the joint surfaces, start debridement with a curet or an osteotome and begin anterolaterally over the talar side.
- If the posterior facet cannot be seen, distract further with the lamina spreader to allow joint preparation under direct vision. If the joint is so fibrosed and scarred that this is difficult to do, drill multiple holes on both surfaces to make some room for further debridement of the joint. Posteromedially, as the posterior facet curves downward or plantarward, the flexor hallucis longus tendon is vulnerable.
- Remove all eburnated or subchondral bone down to bleeding, cancellous bony surfaces (Fig. 5.23B). Small, thin osteotomes, both curved and straight, and curets are helpful. We routinely use a 2.0-mm bit to drill holes on both sides of the joint and crosshatch the surfaces with a ¼-inch osteotome.
- When the posterior facet has been prepared for arthrodesis, evaluate the position of the foot with the denuded surfaces apposed. If the subluxation is severe (more than one third of the lateral surface of the calcaneus is exposed and abutting against the fibula), a subtalar arthrodesis alone would not correct this deformity and a medial dis-

placement calcaneal osteotomy will be necessary. If sub-luxation of the joint is not severe (less than one third of the lateral surface of the calcaneus is exposed and abutting against the fibula), adequate dissection, distraction, and manual translation can correct the deformity.

- Place the calcaneus in the proper position of 8 to 10 degrees of valgus and the tibiotalar joint at 90 degrees to the leg.
- Use one or two 0.062-inch Kirschner wires for temporary fixation, or insert a guidewire over which a cannulated screw can be passed.
- At this point, decide if a bone graft is needed. This decision is based on position and apposition. If the heel is in too much valgus when the denuded surfaces are apposed, a bone graft is required to fill the gap laterally to place the heel in the correct position (5 to 10 degrees of valgus).
- Place a cannulated or noncannulated 7.0- or 6.5-mm, partially threaded screw from the posterior aspect of the tuberosity of the calcaneus into the body of the talus in an oblique direction while the subtalar joint is held reduced. The entrance point for the screw is approximately 1 cm lateral to the midline of the tuberosity of the calcaneus near the junction of the heel pad and the skin covering the hindfoot. The best fixation is obtained by having the screw or pin exit the talus just distal to the body-neck junction so that the threads of the screw can grip the superior cortex of the talar neck. This allows some compression and slightly plantarflexes the talar head, thereby improving the talar declination angle. This will decrease the risk of anterior ankle impingement.
- Place a second screw in a slightly divergent manner across the posterior facet of the subtalar joint, taking care not to violate the tibiotalar joint. The threads should rest just distal to the arthrodesis site (Fig. 5.23C). Screw fixation is associated with improved postoperative function compared with fixation with compression staples.
- For more secure fixation in osteopenic bone, use a washer on the head of the screw.
- Look at the position of the arthrodesis from the plantar aspect and also medially and laterally.
- Deflate the tourniquet, obtain hemostasis, and apply a well-padded short leg cast. If significant bleeding is expected, place a ⅛-inch drain with continuous suction for 24 hours.
- If a popliteal block has not been used, perform an ankle block with 0.5% bupivacaine (Marcaine) for pain control in the immediate postoperative period.

POSTOPERATIVE CARE Although patients with co-morbidities may need to be admitted for 1 to 2 days, in most patients this technique can be done as an outpatient procedure. If the patient is frail or has an unstable gait, touch-down weight bearing is allowed or the patient is encouraged to use a wheelchair for the first 4 to 6 weeks. At 14 to 17 days, the sutures are removed and another short leg cast is applied. Full weight bearing without assistance is not allowed for 6 weeks. The arthrodesis usually has progressed to early fusion by 6 weeks postoperatively, at which time a removable walking boot is worn until 9 weeks after surgery, depending on the radiographic appearance of the arthrodesis site.

ARTHROSCOPIC SUBTALAR ARTHRODESIS

Advances in techniques and instrumentation for foot and ankle arthroscopy have allowed the development of arthroscopic techniques for subtalar arthrodesis. In the years since the first reports of arthroscopic subtalar arthrodesis (ASTA) in the mid-1990s, the technique has gained credibility as an acceptable procedure for isolated subtalar arthritis, with reported fusion rates of 91% to 100%. ASTA may result in faster recovery, less pain, and fewer postoperative complications in properly selected patients. Significant deformity correction is not possible with this technique.

Originally, the technique described arthroscopic arthrodesis through anterolateral, posterolateral, and accessory lateral portals with the patient supine or in the lateral decubitus position. More recently, posterior arthroscopic subtalar arthrodesis (PASTA) techniques have used two or three portals with the patient prone. Suggested advantages for prone positioning include better and safer access to the posteromedial corner, better understanding of the shape of the posterior subtalar joint, easier placement of screws from the calcaneus posteriorly toward the neck of the talus, and easier intraoperative fluoroscopic imaging than are provided by the conventional lateral portals. Amendola and others have demonstrated good results when only the posterior facet is fused. Several clinical and cadaver studies have shown that injury to the posterior neurovascular bundles may be avoided with this approach as long as one is familiar with the anatomy and debridement is conducted lateral to the flexor hallucis longus. Distances from the posteromedial portal and the tibial nerve (6.4 mm), posterior tibial artery (9.6 mm), and medial calcaneal nerve (17.1 mm) allow sufficient space for the arthroscopic procedure. We recommend that the surgeon be a skilled arthroscopist and familiar with foot and ankle anatomy before proceeding with this technique. We have modified the positioning to allow anterolateral, posterolateral and posteromedial portals. This allows better visualization and complete debridement of the subtalar joint.

TECHNIQUE 5.7

- Administer a general anesthetic combined with a regional nerve block.
- Place the patient in a lateral or prone position, depending on which portals are chosen, and drape the operative extremity free. We use a modified prone position with the patient on a beanbag or ipsilateral bump to further externally rotate the leg and allow access to the posterior and anterolateral portals. This position also allows the surgical leg to be placed on a lucent bump for easier fluoroscopic imaging (Fig. 5.24).
- After standard preparation and draping, including preoperative antibiotics, mark on the skin the locations of the Achilles tendon and tip of the lateral malleoli. The posterior portals are just proximal to this line.
- Mark the estimated locations of the sural nerve, peroneal tendons, and the posteromedial neurovascular bundle (Fig. 5.25).

- Apply and inflate a thigh tourniquet.
- Soft-tissue distraction may be useful, but placing a blunt cannula through the anterolateral portal into the sinus tarsi usually will allow adequate visualization (Fig. 5.26). Bony distraction is not recommended.
- With the patient in the semiprone position, the most common portals are the anterolateral, posterolateral, and posteromedial portals:

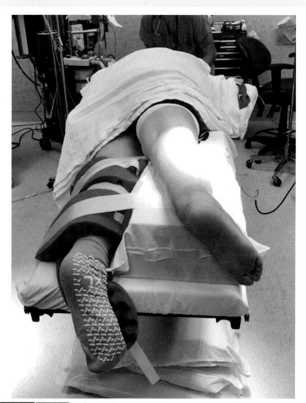

FIGURE 5.24 Modified prone position for arthroscopic subtalar arthrodesis. **SEE TECHNIQUE 5.7.**

- The anterolateral portal is 1 cm anterior to the tip of the fibula, just posterior to the center of the sinus tarsi (Fig. 5.25, *line B*).
- The posterolateral portal is just lateral to the Achilles tendon and 2 cm proximal to the tip of the fibula (Fig. 5.25, *line C*). The sural nerve is at risk with this portal.
- With the patient semiprone, working space must be created by removing part of the posterior fat pad. This is commonly accomplished with 3.5-mm instruments. The flexor hallucis longus should be located using the arthroscopic instruments, and all work should be performed lateral to this anatomic landmark. The posterior ligaments and capsule must be partially debrided to allow access to the talocalcaneal joint.
- This semiprone approach allows better access to both the posterior and anterior facets. If possible, retention of the interosseous ligament may improve blood supply.
- Small 2.7- to 3-mm instruments with a 30-degree scope often are necessary to begin intraarticular debridement, but larger (3.5- to 4-mm) instruments can be used once space is created.
- Identify exact portal position with an 18-gauge spinal needle. Fluoroscopy is helpful in placing instruments in the correct orientation (Fig. 5.27).
- Inflate the joint with 10 to 20 mL of lidocaine with epinephrine. Inversion of the foot indicates successful joint instillation.
- Create the portals by making a small incision in the skin and gently spreading the subcutaneous tissue with a straight hemostat.
- For the anterolateral approach, enter the joint with the clamp and then place a blunt trocar to assist with distraction.
- Create the posterolateral portal first by directing the arthroscope in line with the second metatarsal when the hindfoot is in neutral position.
- Establish the posteromedial portal under endoscopic vision, taking care to direct all instruments lateral to the flexor hallucis longus.

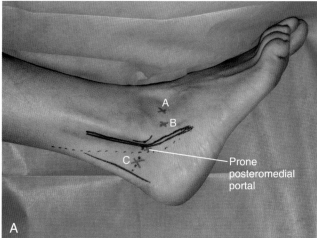

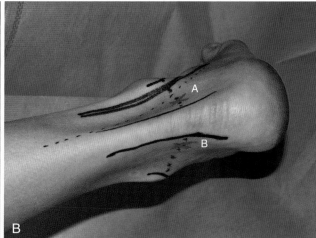

FIGURE 5.25 **A,** Arthroscopic subtalar arthrodesis. Locations of sural nerve, peroneal tendons, and posteromedial neurovascular bundle are marked. Portals are shown with patient in lateral position. *A,* Accessory sinus tarsi portal; *B,* anterolateral portal; *C,* posterolateral portal. **B,** Arthroscopic subtalar arthrodesis with patient prone. *A,* Posteromedial portal; *B,* accessory lateral portal. **SEE TECHNIQUE 5.7.**

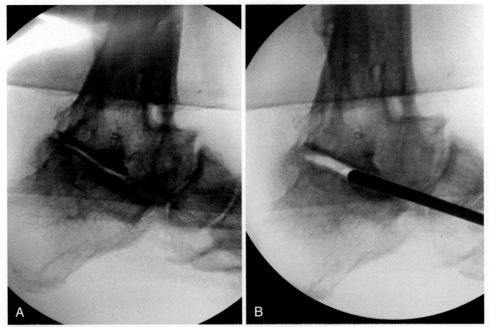

FIGURE 5.26   **A** and **B,** Placing blunt cannula through anterolateral portal into sinus tarsi usually will allow adequate visualization.

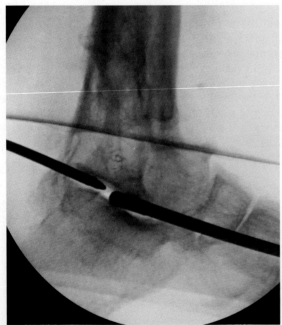

FIGURE 5.27   Fluoroscopy is helpful in placing instruments in correct orientation.

- Use all three portals in an alternating fashion for viewing, distraction, and instrumentation.
- Perform synovectomy and debridement with a 4.0-mm full-radius resector (Fig. 5.28).
- Use an acromioplasty burr, a shaver, and curved curets to remove the articular cartilage from the entire posterior facet (Fig. 5.28).

- Remove 1 to 2 mm of subchondral bone posterior to the interosseous ligament until cancellous bone is visible (Fig. 5.28A), and create multiple holes with a microscopic awl (Fig. 5.28B). Take care not to alter the geometry of the joint.
- If necessary, insert allograft bone. This can be done by harvesting calcaneal autograft with a trephine and inserting it into the anterolateral portal for placement (Fig. 5.28C and D).
- Insert a guide pin at the posterolateral calcaneus and angle it anterosuperiorly toward the talar neck. The best fixation is obtained by having the screw exit the talus just distal to the body-neck junction so that the threads of the screw can grip the superior cortex of the talar neck. Place this pin proximal to the weight-bearing surface of the heel and distal to the initial attachment of the Achilles tendon. Confirm pin placement with fluoroscopy.
- Place a second guide pin just medial and superior to the first.
- Place a 6.5- to 8.0-mm cannulated cancellous screw over each guide pin (Fig. 5.29).
- Examine the arthrodesis clinically for subtalar motion and hindfoot position and fluoroscopically for proper screw placement.
- Close the skin incisions with nylon sutures and apply a bulky dressing and posterior splint.

POSTOPERATIVE CARE Patients are instructed to elevate leg for 5 to 7 days. The splint is removed and a short leg removable cast is applied at this time. The patient is kept non–weight bearing for 6 weeks, followed by gradual weight bearing until radiographs show complete union and the patient has no pain with ambulation.

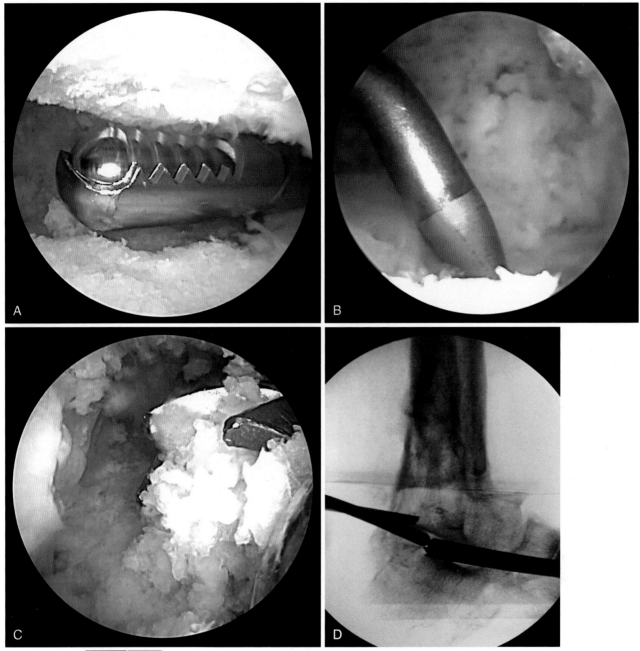

FIGURE 5.28 Arthroscopic subtalar arthrodesis. **A,** 1 to 2 mm of subchondral bone is removed posterior to interosseous ligament. **B,** Microscopic awl use to create multiple holes in cancellous bone. **C and D,** Harvesting and placement of calcaneal autograft. **SEE TECHNIQUE 5.7.**

TALONAVICULAR JOINT ARTHRODESIS

TECHNIQUE 5.8

- Make an incision at the anterior aspect of the medial malleolus just medial to the anterior tibial tendon and ending at the naviculocuneiform joint (Fig. 5.30A). Carry the dissection through subcutaneous tissue and fat to expose the capsule. Protect the anterior tibial tendon beneath the dorsal skin flap.

- Release the capsule medially and dorsally.
- Using a small, curved osteotome or curet, remove the articular cartilage from the talonavicular joint. Use a distractor to increase exposure of the talonavicular joint.
- Remove as much of the articular surface as possible through this incision. Abducting, adducting, plantarflexing, and dorsiflexing the ankle during distraction allows preparation of 90% of the talonavicular articulation. Use a 2.0-mm bit to drill holes on both sides of the joint, and crosshatch the surfaces with a ¼-inch osteotome.
- Place the foot into satisfactory alignment with the calcaneus in 5 to 10 degrees of valgus and the forefoot in neutral

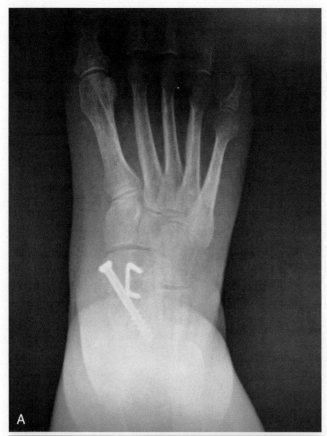

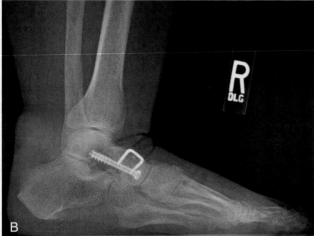

FIGURE 5.29   Fixation with cannulated screw and staple.

abduction and adduction. Do not leave the forefoot supinated. Derotate it when the heel is in the proper position and the talonavicular joint is apposed (Fig. 5.31).

- Make a small trough in the dorsomedial edge of the medial cuneiform where the screw head would rest without levering on the cortex (Fig. 5.31).
- Place a guidewire from medial plantar distally to lateral and dorsal proximally, entering the head and neck portion of the talus.
- Drill parallel to the wire, or ream over it with a partially cannulated screw.

- Measure the length of the screw and tap the screw path (tapping usually is not needed in patients with rheumatoid arthritis but is needed in patients with osteoarthritis).
- Using a partially threaded, 6.5- or 7-mm screw, lag the surfaces together (Fig. 5.30 B, C). Occasionally, the bone is so osteopenic that a washer is needed. The dorsomedial incision will then allow a compression plate or staple to be placed dorsal and lateral to the screw to control rotation and add stability.
- Release the tourniquet, insert a drain if necessary, close the wound in layers, and apply a well-padded splint.

POSTOPERATIVE CARE If placed, the drain is removed the day after surgery. The dressing is changed at 10 to 14 days after surgery, and a short leg, non–weight bearing cast is applied and worn until postoperative week 5, at which time the cast is removed and radiographs are obtained. If early union is evident, the patient is allowed to walk in a walking boot for the next 3 weeks. At 8 weeks after surgery, if union of the arthrodesis site is evident, no further immobilization is required.

TRIPLE ARTHRODESIS

TECHNIQUE 5.9

- Begin a straight lateral incision 1 cm inferior to the tip of the fibular malleolus. Extend it distally over the anterolateral border of the calcaneus and cuboid (Fig. 5.31A).
- Protect the peroneal tendons and the common branch of the sural nerve at the posterior or proximal end of the incision. Also be aware of the dorsal branch of the sural nerve, including the communicating branch to the most lateral branch of the superficial peroneal nerve and the common digital branch to the fourth web space. If necessary for exposure, transect the communicating branch (Fig. 5.31B).
- Abduct and adduct the midfoot to locate the calcaneocuboid joint and invert and evert the subtalar joint for location.
- Locate the proximal tendons of origin of the extensor digitorum brevis and extensor hallucis brevis, and with sharp dissection lift them from the sinus tarsi and dissect along the lateral or inferior border of the muscle belly. The motor nerve to the short extensors enters from the deep peroneal nerve in the medial part of the muscle and is not vulnerable.
- Extend the dissection, lifting the extensor digitorum brevis from proximal to distal until the calcaneocuboid joint is well exposed.
- Expose the calcaneocuboid joint, debriding it with a curet and osteotome, and drill multiple small holes on both sides of the joint. Ensure that the entire surface of the calcaneocuboid joint is debrided, especially medially and inferiorly. Use a lamina spreader or other small bone distractor to help with the deep exposure of this articulation.

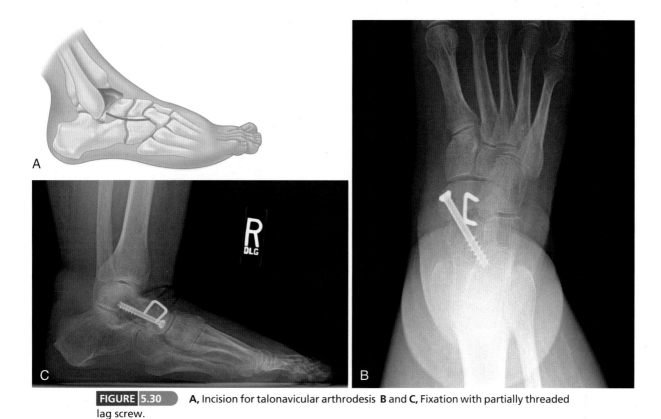

FIGURE 5.30   **A,** Incision for talonavicular arthrodesis **B** and **C,** Fixation with partially threaded lag screw.

- Identify the subtalar joint and remove the deep components of the inferior extensor retinaculum from the floor of the sinus tarsi. Release the talocalcaneal interosseous ligament.
- When this area has been cleaned of all soft tissue, place a right-angle retractor or a curved Hohmann retractor parallel to the posterior facet to lift the peroneal tendons laterally and posteriorly, allowing better exposure of the subtalar joint.
- Place a lamina spreader into the depths of the sinus tarsi so that it rests on the inferior or plantar aspect of the talar neck and just lateral to the middle and anterior facet components of the talocalcaneal articulation (see Fig. 5.25B).
- Depending on the condition of the joint surfaces, start with a curet or an osteotome and begin debridement anterolaterally over the talar side.
- If the posterior facet cannot be seen, distract with a laminar spreader so that the joint preparation is done under direct vision. If the joint is so fibrosed and scarred that this is difficult, use a 2-mm bit to drill multiple holes on both surfaces to make some room for further debridement of the joint. Posteromedially, as the posterior facet curves downward or plantarward, the flexor hallucis longus tendon is vulnerable.
- Remove all eburnated or subchondral bone down to bleeding, cancellous bony surfaces. Small, thin osteotomes, both curved and straight, are helpful. A bur also is useful if cold irrigation is used to prevent thermal necrosis. Use a 2.0-mm bit to drill holes on both sides of the joint, and crosshatch the surfaces with a ¼-inch osteotome.
- When the posterior facet has been prepared for arthrodesis, evaluate the position of the foot with the posterior facet apposed. If the subluxation is severe (more than one

third of the lateral surface of the calcaneus is exposed and abutting against the fibula), the subtalar portion of the triple arthrodesis alone would not correct this deformity. If subluxation of the joint is not severe (less than one third of the lateral surface of the calcaneus is exposed), adequate dissection, distraction, and manual translation can correct the deformity. Place the calcaneus in the proper position of 8 to 10 degrees of valgus.
- To expose the talonavicular joint, make a straight or gently curved anteromedial incision extending from the anterior aspect of the medial malleolus just medial to the anterior tibial tendon to the naviculocuneiform joint (Fig. 5.30C).
- If a branch of the saphenous nerve is identified and compromises exposure, it can be sacrificed. Tie or coagulate the branches of the saphenous vein to the medial tarsus and the communicating veins crossing the wound more or less at right angles.
- Abduct and adduct the foot until the talonavicular joint can be clearly identified. When the medial aspect of the talonavicular joint has been identified, raise a full-thickness flap dorsally and plantarly. The deep peroneal nerve and dorsalis pedis artery would be in the dorsal flap.
- Expose the medial and dorsal aspects of the talonavicular joint and remove all capsular tissue.
- Inspect the joint surfaces and clear them with a curet or an osteotome, depending on the condition of the articular surfaces. A curved osteotome may be helpful.
- Expose the entire articular surface of the navicular and clean it of all eburnated and subchondral bone. Use a 2.0-mm bit to drill holes on both sides of the joint, and crosshatch the surfaces with a ¼-inch osteotome.
- Using a rongeur, mold the surface of the talus until it rests in the depths of the concavity of the navicular. If required,

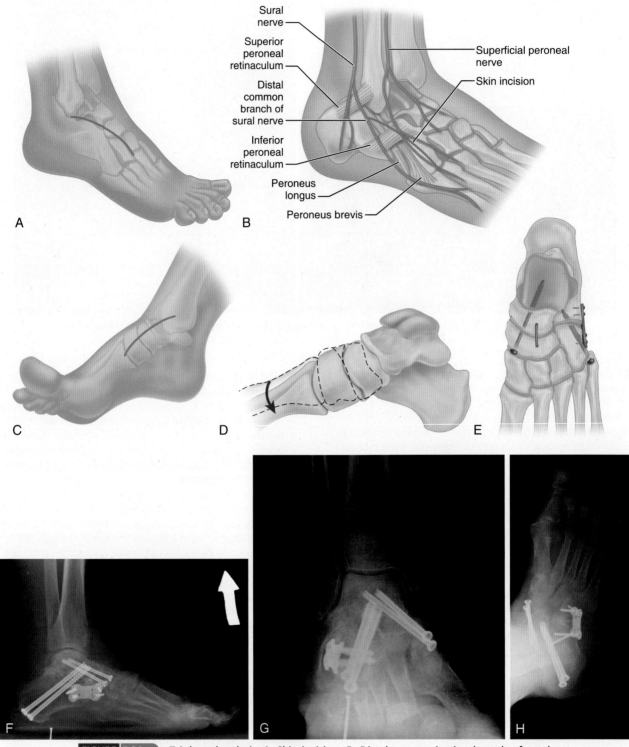

Sural nerve

Superior peroneal retinaculum

Distal common branch of sural nerve

Inferior peroneal retinaculum

Peroneus longus

Peroneus brevis

Superficial peroneal nerve

Skin incision

FIGURE 5.31 Triple arthrodesis. **A,** Skin incision. **B,** Distal communicating branch of sural nerve. **C,** Dorsomedial skin incision. **D,** Correction of forefoot supination after hindfoot reduced. **E,** Calcaneocuboid and talonavicular cannulated screw fixation. Lateral **(F),** anteroposterior **(G),** and oblique **(H)** views of completed arthrodesis. **SEE TECHNIQUE 5.9.**

it is preferable to remove a significant portion of the talar head rather than settle for inadequate reduction of the talonavicular joint.

- Through the lateral incision (for the calcaneocuboid and subtalar approach), place a right-angle retractor under the full-thickness flap to expose the most lateral aspect of the talonavicular joint. Debride as much as possible from the lateral side of the talonavicular joint.
- Reduce all the joints in an anatomic plantigrade position. Be careful to hold the hindfoot in 8 to 10 degrees of valgus and the talonavicular and calcaneocuboid joints in not only proper sagittal and axial planes but also proper rotation. Do not allow the forefoot to be fixed in supination.
- Fix the subtalar joint first so that the forefoot can be properly pronated and adducted at the time of talonavicular fusion. Place a cannulated or noncannulated 7.0- or 6.5-mm, partially threaded screw from the posterior aspect of the tuberosity of the calcaneus into the body of the talus in an oblique direction while the subtalar joint is held reduced. The entrance point for the screw is approximately 1 cm lateral to the midline of the tuberosity of the calcaneus near the junction of the heel pad and the skin covering the hindfoot. The best fixation is obtained by having the screw or pin exit the talus just distal to the body-neck junction so that the threads of the screw can grip the superior cortex of the talar neck. This allows some compression and slightly plantarflexes the talar head, thereby improving the talar declination angle. This will decrease the risk of anterior ankle impingement.
- Place a second screw in a slightly divergent manner across the posterior facet of the subtalar joint, taking care not to violate the tibiotalar joint. The threads should rest just distal to the arthrodesis site (Fig. 5.32C).
- Fix the talonavicular joint second, using a partially threaded, large cancellous screw (6.5 or 7.0 mm) over a guidewire that has been placed under image intensification across the navicular and into the talus. Check the position of the talonavicular arthrodesis site as well as the forefoot position when only one 0.062-inch Kirschner wire or the guidewire for the cannulated screw has been inserted. It is easy to adjust the position at this point but difficult if the final fixation is in place. One screw and a dorsal plate or staple are often used. Removing a small portion of the superomedial articular surface of the medial cuneiform through that hole and drill across the calcaneocuboid joint toward the posterior aspect of the tuberosity of the calcaneus. Drill and tap over the guide pin. Countersink the drill hole. Alternatively, a compression plate or staple can be used (Fig. 5.31E), which has been shown to withstand higher loads until failure; however, this may cause sural nerve irritation in some patients. Before final fixation, ensure that the joint surfaces are opposed.
- Fill any gaps with cancellous bone graft. This usually is taken from the tuberosity of the calcaneus or the anteromedial surface of the distal metaphysis of the tibia, or cancellous bank bone can be used.
- Do not sacrifice proper alignment in any plane because the surfaces are not completely apposed.
- Deflate the tourniquet, and place a suction drain in the lateral wound. Place the extensor digitorum brevis back

into the sinus tarsi and close the wound in layers. Apply a well-padded splint.

POSTOPERATIVE CARE The patient is encouraged to elevate the extremity consistently for 4 days. Non–weight bearing for 6 weeks is encouraged unless the patient is too frail. If the patient cannot stand without touch-down weight bearing, this is allowed. At 2 weeks, the sutures are removed and a short leg cast is applied. Full weight bearing is not allowed until 6 weeks after surgery. A walking boot is worn for another 3 weeks, or until the arthrodesis is solid (Fig. 5.31F-H). At the end of 9 weeks, the boot is removed and the patient is placed in support hose and a large, soft-soled, cushioned shoe. The patient must be informed that swelling may persist for 4 to 6 months and that occasionally it persists indefinitely.

ISOLATED MEDIAL INCISION FOR DOUBLE AND TRIPLE ARTHRODESIS

An all-medial approach to double or triple arthrodesis is indicated for patients at risk for lateral wound complications. This technique may be useful in patients with previous infection or deformity rendering the lateral skin tenuous. Also, patients with systemic disease associated with wound healing problems (e.g., rheumatoid arthritis) may benefit from a single incision around the foot.

TECHNIQUE 5.10

(MYERSON)

- Make a 2-cm longitudinal incision over the peroneal tendons approximately 10 cm proximal to the level of the ankle joint. To avoid wound problems, do not make the incision on the lateral aspect of the foot.
- Use a mosquito clamp to deliver the peroneus longus and brevis tendons out of the incision; divide the peroneus brevis and perform a tenodesis of the peroneus brevis to the longus. We recommend leaving the peroneus longus tendon intact to aid in inversion and first-ray plantarflexion.
- Make a 10-cm medial curvilinear incision extending from the undersurface of the medial malleolus and centered dorsomedially over the talonavicular joint extending to the anterior tibial tendon (Fig. 5.32A).
- Divide the subcutaneous tissue and talonavicular joint capsule longitudinally. If a branch of the saphenous nerve is identified and compromises exposure, it can be sacrificed.
- Tie or coagulate the branches of the saphenous vein to the medial tarsus and the communicating veins crossing the wound more or less at right angles.
- Abduct and adduct the foot until the talonavicular joint can be clearly identified.
- Incise the posterior tibial tendon from its insertion on the navicular, and tag it with a Vicryl suture. This can be repaired to soft tissue if the muscle is adequate.
- Use small bone distractors to expose the talonavicular joint and gain the necessary exposure (Fig. 5.32B). Use a

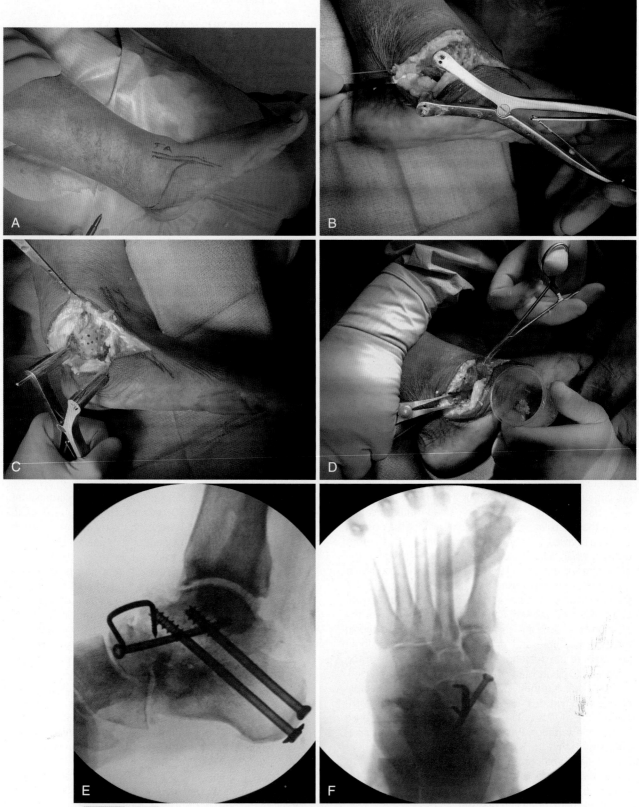

FIGURE 5.32   Triple arthrodesis through single medial incision. **A,** Incision. **B,** Exposure of the talonavicular joint. **C,** Hole drilled on both sides of the joint. **D,** Autograft from proximal tibia or iliac crest is used to augment fusion site. **E** and **F,** Fixation can be done with cannulated screws and compression plate or staple. **SEE TECHNIQUE 5.10.**

retractor to protect the flexor hallucis longus, the flexor digitorum longus, and the neurovascular bundle.

- With the anterior, middle, and posterior facets of the subtalar joint exposed, use a curved osteotome and lamina spreader to expose and debride the talonavicular joint, subtalar joint, and sinus tarsi. Pay special attention to the lateral aspect of the talonavicular joint.

- Remove all eburnated or subchondral bone down to bleeding, cancellous bony surfaces. Small, thin osteotomes, both curved and straight, are helpful.

- Use a 2.0-mm bit to drill holes on both sides of the joint, and crosshatch the surfaces with a ¼-inch osteotome (Fig. 5.32C).

- If triple arthrodesis is necessary, preparation of the calcaneocuboid joint is the most challenging aspect of the medial single-incision triple arthrodesis. Sharply release the capsule of the calcaneocuboid joint and the bifurcate ligament by feel with a knife. Place a lamina spreader in the talonavicular joint for exposure. The relatively flat surface of this joint makes debridement and scaling easier.

- We routinely use autograft from the proximal tibia or iliac crest to augment the fusion site (Fig. 5.32D).

- Reduce the subtalar joint and secure it with two 6.5-mm or larger guide pins for cannulated screws. The first should extend from the posterior calcaneus into the talar neck, and the second is placed across the posterior facet into the body of the talus. Measure and place screws to ensure that the anterior screw grasps the dorsal cortex of the talar neck and the posterior screw has all threads across the posterior facet.

- Paying careful attention to any residual forefoot supination or abduction, realign the transverse tarsal joints, and fix the talonavicular joint with two 4.5- or 5.0-mm cannulated screws or one screw and a compression plate or staple as previously described.

- For a triple arthrodesis, place a posteriorly directed percutaneous 4.5- or 5.0-mm screw across the calcaneocuboid joint beginning at the dorsal anterior cuboid (Fig. 5.32E and F).

POSTOPERATIVE CARE A splint is worn for 14 days, and then the sutures are removed. Touch-down weight bearing may be permitted, but often non–weight bearing is encouraged. Full weight bearing can begin at 6 weeks when the patient is placed in a walking boot to be worn until week 9. At the end of 9 weeks, the boot is removed and the patient is placed in support hose and a large, soft-soled, cushioned shoe. The patient must be informed that swelling may persist for 4 to 6 months and that occasionally it persists indefinitely.

■ TIBIOTALOCALCANEAL AND ANKLE ARTHRODESES

Tibiotalocalcaneal and ankle arthrodeses are described in other chapter.

REFERENCES

Ahmad J, Pedowitz D: Management of the rigid arthritic flatfoot in adults: triple arthrodesis, *Foot Ankle Clin* 17:309, 2012.

Albert A, Deleu PA, Leemrijse T, et al.: Posterior arthroscopic subtalar arthrodesis: ten cases at one-year follow-up, *Orthop Traumatol Surg Res* 97:401, 2011.

Amin A, Cullen N, Singh D: Rheumatoid forefoot reconstruction, *Acta Orthop Belg* 76:289, 2010.

Baan H, Drossaers-Bakker W, Dubbeldam R, van de Laar M: We should not forget the foot: relations between signs and symptoms, damage, and function in rheumatoid arthritis, *Clin Rheumatol* 30:1475, 2011.

Bauer T: Percutaneous hindfoot and midfoot fusion, *Foot Ankle Clin* 21:629, 2016.

Brennan SA, Harney T, Queally JM, et al.: Influence of weather variables on pain severity in end-stage osteoarthritis, *Int Orthop* 36:643, 2012.

Buda M, Hagemeijer NC, Kink S, et al.: Effect of fixation type and bone graft on tarsometatarsal fusion, *Foot Ankle Int* 38:1394, 2018.

Camerer M, Ehrenstein B, Hoffstetter P, et al.: High-resolution ultrasound of the midfoot: sonography is more sensitive than conventional radiography in detection of osteophytes and erosions in inflammatory and non-inflammatory joint disease, *Clin Rheumatol* 36:2145, 2017.

Carro LP, Golano P, Escajadillo NF, et al.: Arthroscopic subtalar arthrodesis: the posterior approach in the prone position, *Tech Foot Ankle Surg* 10:127, 2011.

Chan PS, Kong KO: Natural history and imaging of subtalar and midfoot joint disease in rheumatoid arthritis, *Int J Rheum Dis* 16:14, 2013.

Crevoisier X: The isolated talonavicular arthrodesis, *Foot Ankle Clin* 16:49, 2011.

Ellington JK: Hammertoes and clawtoes: proximal interphalangeal joint correction, *Foot Ankle Clin* 16:547, 2011.

Gentchos CE, Anderson JG, Bohay DR: Management of the rigid arthritic flatfoot in the adults. Alternatives to triple arthrodesis, *Foot Ankle Clin* 17:323, 2012.

Grear BJ, Rabinovich A, Brodsky JW: Charcot arthropathy of the foot and ankle associated with rheumatoid arthritis, *Foot Ankle Int* 34:1541, 2013.

Hennessy K, Woodburn J, Steultjens MPM: Custom foot orthoses for rheumatoid arthritis: a systematic review, *Arthritis Care Res* 64:311, 2012.

Herrera-Pérez M, Andarcia-Banuelos C, Barg A, et al.: Comparison of cannulated screws versus compression staples for subtalar arthrodesis fixation, *Foot Ankle Int* 36:203, 2015.

Herscovici Jr D, Sammarco GJ, Sammarco VJ, Scaduto JM: Pantalar arthrodesis for post-traumatic arthritis and diabetic neuroarthropathy of the ankle and hindfoot, *Foot Ankle Int* 32(6):581, 2011.

Hunt KJ, Ellington JK, Anderson RB, et al.: Locked versus nonlocked plate fixation for hallux MTP arthrodesis, *Foot Ankle Int* 32(7):704, 2011.

Kiewiet NJ, Benirschke SK, Brage ME: Triple arthrodesis: tips and tricks to navigate trouble, *Foot Ankle Clin* 19:483, 2014.

Krause FG, Fehlbaum O, Huebschle LM, Weber M: Preservation of lesser metatarsophalangeal joints in rheumatoid forefoot reconstruction, *Foot Ankle Int* 32:131, 2011.

Latt LD, Glisson RR, Adams Jr SB, et al.: Biomechanical comparison of external fixation and compression screws for transverse tarsal joint arthrodesis, *Foot Ankle Int* 36:1235, 2015.

Lee KB, Park CH, Seon JK, Kim MS: Arthroscopic subtalar arthrodesis using a posterior 2-portal approach in the prone position, *Arthroscopy* 26:230, 2010.

Ling JS, Smyth NA, Fraser EJ, et al.: Investigating the relationship between ankle arthrodesis and adjacent-joint arthritis in the hindfoot. A systematic review, *J Bone Joint Surg* 97A:513, 2015.

Ma S, Jin D: Isolated talonavicular arthrodesis, *Foot Ankle Int* 37:905, 2016.

Mayer SA, Zelenski NA, DeOrio JK, et al.: A comparison of nonlocking semi-tubular plates and precontoured locking plates for first metatarsophalangeal joint arthritis, *Foot Ankle Int* 35:438, 2014.

McKinley JC, Shortt N, Arthur C, et al.: Outcomes following pantalar arthrodesis in rheumatoid arthritis, *Foot Ankle Int* 32:681, 2011.

Michelson JD, Addante RA, Charlson MD: Multimodal analgesia therapy reduces length of hospitalization in patients undergoing fusions of the ankle and hindfoot, *Foot Ankle Int* 34:1526, 2013.

Milshteyn MA, Dwyr M, Andrecovich C, et al.: Comparison of two fixation methods for arthrodesis of the calcaneocuboid joint: a biomechanical study, *Foot Ankle Int* 36:98, 2015.

Miniaci-Coxhead SL, Weisenthal B, Ketz JP, et al.: Incidence and radiographic predictors of valgus tibiotalar tilt after hindfoot fusion, *Foot Ankle Int* 38:519, 2017.

Momohara S, Inoue E, Ikari K, et al.: Recent trends in orthopedic surgery aiming to improve quality of life for those with rheumatoid arthritis: data from a large observational cohort, *J Rheumatol* 41:862, 2014.

Muraro GM, Carvajal PF: Arthroscopic arthrodesis of the subtalar joint, *Foot Ankle Clin* 16:83, 2011.

Nemec SA, Habbu RA, Anderson JG, Bohay DR: Outcomes following midfoot arthrodesis for primary arthritis, *Foot Ankle Int* 32:355, 2011.

Nieuwenhuis WP, van Steenbergen HW, Mangnus L, et al.: Evaluation of the diagnostic accuracy of hand and foot MRI for early rheumatoid arthritis, *Rheumatology (Oxford)* 56:1367, 2017.

Niki H, Hirano T, Okada H, Beppu M: Combination joint-preserving surgery for forefoot deformity in patients with rheumatoid arthritis, *J Bone Joint Surg* 92B:380, 2010.

Ohly NE, Breusch SJ: Additive hindfoot arthrodesis for rheumatoid hindfoot disease: a clinical study of patient outcomes and satisfaction, *Clin Rheumatol* 32:1777, 2013.

Onodera T, Kasahara Y, Kasemura T, et al.: A comparative study with in vitro ultrasonographic and histologic grading of metatarsal head cartilage in rheumatoid arthritis, *Foot Ankle Int* 36:774, 2015.

Patel A, Rao S, Nawoczenski D, et al.: Midfoot arthritis, *J Am Acad Orthop Surg* 18:417, 2010.

Paterson KL, Gates L: Clinical assessment and management of foot and ankle osteoarthritis: a review of current evidence and focus on pharmacological treatment, *Drugs Aging* 36:203, 2019.

Pekarek B, Osher L, Buck S, Bowen M: Intra-articular corticosteroid injections: a critical literature review with up-to-date findings, *Foot (Edinb)* 21:66, 2011.

Reina-Bueno M, Váquez-Bautista MDC, Pérez-García S, et al.: Effectiveness of custom-made foot orthoses in patients with rheumatoid arthritis: a randomized controlled trial, *Clin Rehabil* 33:661, 2019.

Rosenbaum D, Timte B, Schmiegel A, et al.: First ray resection arthroplasty versus arthrodesis in the treatment of the rheumatoid foot, *Foot Ankle Int* 32:589, 2011.

Shirzad K, Kiesau CD, DeOrio JK, Parekh SG: Lesser toe deformities, *J Am Acad Orthop Surg* 19:505, 2011.

Silvagni E, Di Battista M, Bonifacio AF, et al.: One year in review 2019: novelties in the treatment of rheumatoid arthritis, *Clin Exp Rheumatol* 37:519, 2019.

Stegeman M, Louwerens JWK, van der Woude J, et al.: Outcome after operative fusion of the tarsal joints: a systematic review, *J Foot Ankle Surg* 54:636, 2015.

Thelen S, Rütt J, Wild M, et al.: The influence of talonavicular versus double arthrodesis on load dependent motion of the midtarsal joint, *Arch Orthop Trauma Surg* 130:47, 2010.

Thevendran G, Wang C, Pinney SJ, et al.: Nonunion risk assessment in foot and ankle surgery: proposing a predictive risk assessment model, *Foot Ankle Int* 36:901, 2015.

Tiihonen R, Eerik S, Ikävalko M, et al.: Comparison of bioreplaceable interposition arthroplasty with metatarsal head resection of the rheumatoid foot, *Foot Ankle Int* 31:505, 2010.

van der Leeden M, Steultjens MP, van Schaardenburg D, Dekker J: Forefoot disease activity in rheumatoid arthritis patients in remission: results of a cohort study, *Arthritis Res Ther* 12:R3, 2010.

Viens NA, Adams SB, Nunley II JA: Ceramic interpositional arthroplasty for fourth and fifth tarsometatarsal joint arthritis, *J Surg Orthop Adv* 21:126, 2012.

Weinraub GM, Schuberth JM, Lee M, et al.: Isolated medial incisional approach to subtalar and talonavicular arthrodesis, *J Foot Ankle Surg* 49:326, 2010.

Wilkinson VH, Rowbotham EL, Grainger AJ: Imaging in foot and ankle arthritis, *Semin Musculoskelet Radiol* 20:167, 2016.

Zubler V, Agten CA, Pfirrmann CW, et al.: Frequency of arthritis-like MRI findings in the forefeet of healthy volunteers versus patients with symptomatic rheumatoid arthritis or psoriatic arthritis, *AJR Am J Roentgenol* 208:W45, 2017.

The complete list of references is available online at Expert Consult.com.

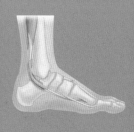

DIABETIC FOOT

EPIDEMIOLOGY

The American Diabetes Association estimates that in 2015, 30.3 million Americans (9.4% of the population) had diabetes, with 4.1 million Americans over the age of 18 with prediabetes. The prevalence of diabetes in Americans aged 65 years and older is 25.2%, and it is the seventh leading cause of death in the United States. The prevalence has been increasing, from 24 million people in 2007 to 25.8 million in 2010. Complications associated with diabetes are numerous and include hypoglycemia, hypertension, dyslipidemia, stroke, heart attack, retinopathy, and kidney disease. In 2010, there were 73,000 nontraumatic lower-limb amputations performed in adults aged 20 years and older with a diagnosis of diabetes. The Global Burden of Disease Study of 2015 estimated that diabetes affects 435 million people worldwide, and its associated disabilities are twice as impactful as chronic kidney disease, ischemic heart disease, and cerebrovascular disease. The number is expected to rise to 642 million people living with diabetes worldwide by 2040.

The often-reported direct costs of diabetes include medications, dressings, and surgical procedures. The indirect costs, however, are more difficult to define and include work time lost due to illness, loss of productivity, patient anxiety, and the effect on family members. In 2017, the total cost of diagnosed diabetes in the US was $327 billion, with $237 billion in direct medical costs and $90 billion in reduced productivity. This represents a 333% increase in spending since 1997. After adjusting for population differences, the average expenditures for medical costs are 2.3 times higher in patients with diabetes than those without. Up to 25% of the annual expenditures on diabetic care are due to directly to foot ulcers and their complications, including infection and amputation. A diabetic patient has a lifetime risk of developing a diabetic foot ulcer of 15%, with an annual incidence of 2%. Medicare patients with a diabetic foot ulcer are seen by a health care provider an average of 14 times per year and have 1.5 hospitalizations each year at a reimbursed cost of $33,000 annually. Those with a lower extremity amputation have over $52,000 in reimbursed costs for Medicare services each year.

Diabetes mellitus impacts numerous body systems, and the orthopaedist must be aware of its manifestations and impact on the entire patient, not just on the treatment of foot and ankle conditions. In 2008, 29% of patients with diabetes aged 40 years and older had diabetic retinopathy, leading to 20,000 new cases of blindness each year. Combined with the loss of tactile sensation from peripheral neuropathy, this loss of vision leads to an increased risk of falls and may make the daily inspection of the foot difficult or impossible.

BASIC SCIENCE

On a basic science level, the increased concentration of glucose in the body has numerous deleterious effects. A histologic examination of the plantar skin of diabetic and nondiabetic patients showed significantly thicker elastic septae and dermal layers in diabetic tissue, which may play a role in the biomechanical changes leading to ulcer formation. Ultrasound examinations of Achilles tendons have shown disorganized tendon fibers and calcification in 75% of diabetic patients without foot problems. A study examining peak midfoot joint pressures in diabetic and nondiabetic cadaver feet during simulated walking showed 46% higher dynamic pressures in the first metatarsocuneiform, medial and middle naviculocuneiform, and the first intercuneiform joints in specimens from diabetic patients.

Studies have estimated that as many as 65% of people with type 1 or 2 diabetes have evidence of peripheral neuropathy and that its presence is the most predictive factor for the development of diabetic foot ulcers. Neuropathy is also an independent predictor of increased complications after foot and ankle surgery. The length of time that a patient has had diabetes and the level of metabolic control are the main predictors for the development, progression, and extent of neuropathy. No consensus exists on the mechanism for the development of peripheral neuropathy in diabetic patients; it likely is multifactorial, with roots in both vascular and metabolic processes. With high levels of blood glucose, hemoglobin and proteins become glycosylated and form end products that precipitate in the walls of small peripheral vessels and nerve tissue. Investigators have demonstrated that diabetic patients have glycation of the arterial vessel walls, thickening of the basement membranes, and reduced endothelial nitric oxide activity. Examination of the nerves has shown multifocal ischemic proximal nerve lesions and epineural vessel atherosclerosis. Metabolic causes include accumulation of sorbitol,

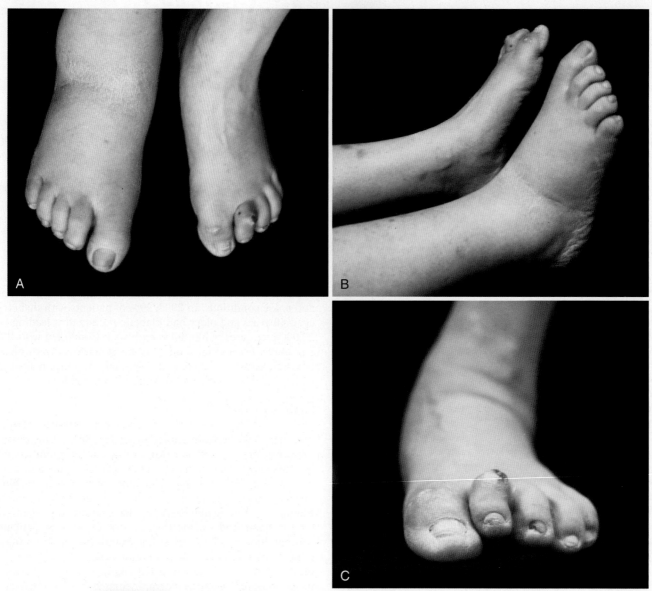

FIGURE 6.1 **A** and **B,** Fixed flexion deformities of interphalangeal joint of hallux and proximal interphalangeal joint of second toe on left foot. **C,** Neither first nor second metatarsophalangeal joint could be passively flexed to neutral.

enzyme deficiencies, and increased oxygen-free radical activity. Chronically elevated glucose levels worsen this process for prolonged time periods, with the end result of motor, sensory, and autonomic nerve dysfunction. The absence of skin oils released by autonomic signals leads to increased susceptibility to fissuring of the skin from mild trauma. Joint contractures develop around the toes due to muscle imbalance from motor neuropathy. Weak intrinsic muscles become overpowered by stronger extrinsic muscles, leading to development of hammer toes, claw toes, and distal migration of the fat pad (Fig. 6.1). Muscle contractures of the gastrocsoleus complex increase the force load transmitted to the forefoot. The loss of protective sensation is pivotal because it blunts the patient's awareness of something being wrong and delays the request for care because of the absence of pain.

The effects of end products of glycosylation deposited into the arterioles also lead to heart disease and hypertension.

Diabetic individuals are four times more likely to suffer a stroke than nondiabetic ones and are twice as likely to develop peripheral arterial disease. Peripheral arterial disease increases susceptibility to ischemic ulcers and compounds the effect of diabetes; diabetic patients with peripheral arterial disease are nine times more likely to develop a foot ulcer. The small vessels in the kidneys are also affected, and diabetes continues to be the leading cause of end-stage renal disease. Diabetes also impairs the immune system because of alterations in the chemotaxis abilities of polymorphonuclear cells and cell wall abnormalities that make patients susceptible to secondary infections.

HISTORY AND PHYSICAL EXAMINATION

A thorough history should be obtained from all patients presenting for treatment of diabetic foot problems. The physician should inquire about any episodes of ulceration, prior amputations, known neuropathic arthropathy, impaired vision, renal history, presence of paresthesias or numbness, and any symptoms of claudication. Because of impaired sensation, patients may deny any history of trauma or pain before the development of a foot ulcer.

The first portion of the physical examination begins with inspection of the patient's footwear. Shoes should be well fitting and in good repair. Undersized shoes increase pressure over bony prominences and lead to ulceration and infection. An adequate toe-box is important to allow room for forefoot deformities, if present. Abnormal wear patterns suggest a structural or dynamic foot deformity. The inside of the shoe should be inspected to evaluate for prominent seams or foreign bodies, which may not be felt due to neuropathy. Next is a careful inspection of the patient's feet. Atrophy of the extensor digitorum brevis, the presence of claw toes or hammer toes, and/or foot drop indicates motor neuropathy. Any corns or calluses should be noted because these are signs of increased pressure, both internal and external, and may be the precursor to later ulcer formation. Any ulcers present should be measured in cross-section and depth. The simplest method is to measure the longest part of the ulcer and multiply this by the widest part to obtain a cross-sectional area. A sterile cotton swab can be used to probe the wound to determine the depth and extent of any exposed structures. The wound bed should be described in terms of granulation, fibrous or necrotic tissue, and the presence or absence of probed bone. In a study of 1666 patients, Lavery et al. found that the ability to probe bone in the ulcer had a 57% positive predictive value for the presence of osteomyelitis and a negative predictive value of 96%. The presence or absence of hair growth and shiny skin should be documented; taut, shiny skin and an absence of hair may be signs of peripheral arterial disease. Autonomic dysfunction leads to dry, scaly skin and should be noted. Any erythema or swelling should be noted, as these may be signs of infection or Charcot neuroarthropathy. The clinical appearance of a foot affected by Charcot neuroarthropathy may be indistinguishable from that of an infected foot: both will have calor, edema, and erythema. Elevation of the leg may assist in the diagnosis because the edema from Charcot neuroarthropathy typically subsides with elevation while that from infection remains localized to the foot. With the patient standing, inspection of the foot reveals any abnormalities in the arch of the foot and hindfoot alignment that will alter plantar pressures. Range of motion of the ankle should be recorded with the knee extended and flexed to assess for contracture of the gastrocnemius (Silfverskiöld test). Contracture of the gastrocnemius is evident when ankle dorsiflexion is less with the knee extended than with the knee flexed because of its insertion proximal to the knee joint. Equal decreases in dorsiflexion with the knee flexed and extended indicate Achilles tendon contracture. Gait should be observed to assess the patient's balance and safety mobilizing.

A difference in skin temperature of the foot may indicate the presence of a vascular disease. The ability or inability to palpate pulses, along with the quality of the pulse, should be documented. Diminished or absent pulses require further testing with a Doppler examination. The ankle-brachial index (ABI) is a useful noninvasive screening tool that is predictive of wound healing. A normal ABI is 0.9 to 1.2, whereas values more than 1.3 suggest noncompressible vessels caused by calcification. An ABI of less than 0.5 suggests that an ulcer is

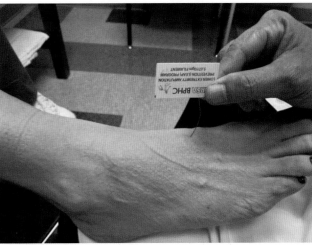

FIGURE 6.2 Measurement of toe systolic pressure with manual photoplethysmography (PPG) unit (Smartdop 45, Hadeco Inc., Kawasaki, Japan) (From Romanos MT, Raspovic A, Perrin BM: The reliability of toe systolic pressure and the toe brachial index in patients with diabetes, *Foot Ankle Res* 3:31, 2010.)

unlikely to heal without vascular intervention because ankle systolic pressures of more than 60 mm Hg and 90 mm Hg have been reported as necessary for healing in diabetic patients. A difference in ABI of more than 0.15 between extremities is a significant finding and should be further investigated. In patients with incompressible vessels, toe pressures may be more reliable because the most distal vessels are often spared (Fig. 6.2). Absolute toe pressures should be higher than 70 mm Hg, and a normal toe/brachial index of more than 0.7 is normal. Toe pressures of more than 40 mm Hg are associated with wound healing.

A neurologic examination evaluates for the presence or absence of peripheral neuropathy. With a thorough physical examination, electrodiagnostic studies are rarely necessary to assist in the diagnosis or treatment of neuropathy. Although the severity of neuropathy is on a spectrum, the threshold of importance to the clinician is the inability to feel the Semmes-Weinstein 5.07 monofilament (Fig. 6.3). The inability to feel the 10 g of pressure from this monofilament is one of the most predictive risk factors for the development of foot morbidity. Typical screening involves 10 g monofilament testing of 10 sites on the foot; however, equivalent results can be obtained more quickly using a 4.5 g monofilament beneath both first metatarsal heads. Decreased perception of the vibration of a 128 Hz tuning fork at the tip of the great toe is also used in clinical practice. Absence of an ankle reflex is one of the earliest signs of neuropathy and has been associated with increased foot ulceration.

ULCER CLASSIFICATION

Determining ulcer size at each visit is useful for evaluating healing progress and for predictive value. In a study of 203 diabetic patients with foot ulcers, Sheehan et al. found that ulcers that showed at least a 50% reduction in size after 4 weeks had significantly higher healing rates at 12 weeks than those that did not. Ince et al. found that of 410 diabetic foot ulcers, 96% of those less than 1 cm^2 in dimension eventually healed without any form of amputation, while only 72% of ulcers larger than 3 cm^2 did so.

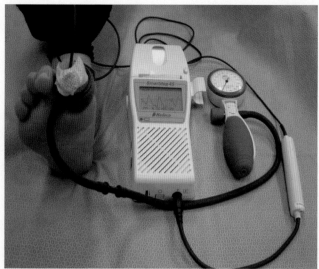

FIGURE 6.3 Evaluating protective sensation with 5.07 Semmes-Weinstein monofilament.

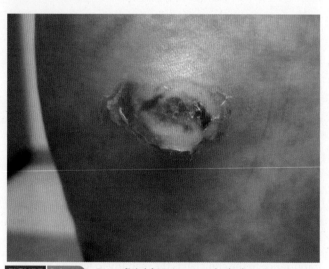

FIGURE 6.4 Superficial (Wagner grade I) ulcer.

TABLE 6.1

Wagner Classification for Foot Ulcers

GRADE	DESCRIPTION
0	Skin at risk
I	Superficial ulcer (Fig. 6.4)
II	Exposed tendon and deep structures (Fig. 6.5)
III	Deep ulcers with abscess or osteomyelitis (Fig. 6.6)
IV	Partial gangrene
V	More extensive gangrene

Classifying the ulcer is useful to guide treatment decisions. The most commonly used classification system was initially described by Meggitt and later expanded by Wagner (Table 6.1 and Figs. 6.4, 6.5, and 6.6). Brodsky noted that Wagner grades IV and V ulcers were ischemic and modified

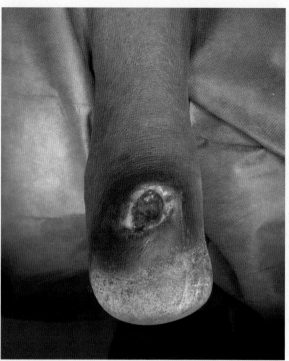

FIGURE 6.5 Deep (Wagner grade II) ulcer with exposed tendon and joint capsule. (From Brodsky JW: The diabetic foot. In: Coughlin MJ, Mann RA, Saltzman CL, editors: *Surgery of the foot and ankle*, ed 8, Philadelphia, 2007, Elsevier.)

this classification by differentiating between ischemic and neuropathic ulcers with the depth-ischemia classification (Table 6.2). Ulcers that are infected and ischemic are 90 times more likely to be treated with an amputation than ulcers without infection or ischemia. The presence of an infected ulcer portends a 40% to 55% chance of some form of amputation.

LABORATORY EVALUATION

If infection is suspected clinically, complete blood count (CBC), erythrocyte sedimentation rate (ESR), and C-reactive protein (CRP) tests are beneficial to establish baseline parameters to which comparisons can be made during treatment. The primary care practitioner or orthopaedist should obtain hemoglobin A1C levels every 3 months. A prospective study of 1285 veterans with diabetes showed that higher hemoglobin A1C levels were an independent risk factor for the development of a diabetic foot ulcer, as were impaired vision, monofilament insensitivity, and history of prior ulcer. Several longitudinal observational investigations have shown that maintenance of a lower hemoglobin A1C level is related to less development of peripheral neuropathy and lower subjective pain scores. Patients with hemoglobin A1C levels higher than 7% or preoperative glucose levels of more than 200 mg/dL before ankle or hindfoot arthrodesis have a higher rate of complications, including nonunion, infection, and wound healing problems.

IMAGING

Diagnostic imaging provides useful information in differentiating soft-tissue infection from osteomyelitis and Charcot arthropathy from infection. Numerous imaging modalities are available, and it is important to understand the advantages

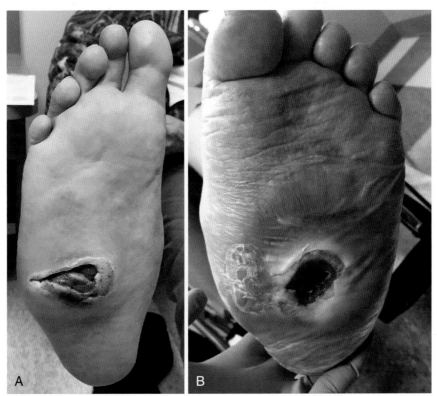

FIGURE 6.6 **A,** Wagner grade II ulcer. **B,** Wagner grade III ulcer.

and drawbacks of each to avoid multiple costly, and perhaps unnecessary, examinations.

Radiographs are generally the first imaging modality used because of their widespread availability. Although many of these findings are not specific to osteoarthropathy or osteomyelitis, radiographic examination should look for demineralization, loss of normal bone trabecular pattern, periosteal reaction, and joint destruction (Fig. 6.7). These findings can also be present in trauma, systemic illness, and oncologic diagnoses. The presence of air in the soft tissues may be a sign of local ulceration or the presence of a gas-producing organism. The early stages of osteomyelitis are not detectable on radiographs, as it often takes weeks to months before changes in the bone are evident. There is insufficient evidence to recommend plain radiographs as the sole imaging modality to diagnose osteomyelitis or distinguish it from neuroarthropathy. Because Charcot arthropathy progresses in radiographically identifiable stages, radiographs are the imaging modality of choice to determine stage and to guide treatment.

CT scanning is useful to provide details about the bone architecture in multiple planes and to show subtle changes, sequestra, and cortical disruptions. Differentiation between inflammation, fibrosis, granulation tissue, and purulence, however, is not possible with this modality. CT scanning, especially weight-bearing CT if available, is useful to guide planning for bony surgery, but is not routinely used in isolation for evaluation of diabetic feet.

Various scintigraphy studies are available with Technetium-99, gallium citrate, indium-tagged white blood cells, sulfur colloid, and human immune globulin. Technetium and gallium scans involve directly injecting a tracer into the bloodstream, whereas tagged scans require a preimage blood draw to label white blood cells with a radioactive tracer before recirculating the blood through the patient. Combinations of these tests have been used to attempt to distinguish osteomyelitis from Charcot arthropathy. Early inflammatory changes in Charcot arthropathy involve accumulation of white blood cells even in the absence of infection, which is why tagged white blood cell scans may show a false positive for infection. A three-phase bone scan involves an initial perfusion phase imaged a few seconds after injection of a tracer, a blood-pool image obtained 5 minutes later, and a static bone image obtained 3 hours later after urinary excretion decreases tracer levels. This test can be significantly impacted by local blood flow and capillary permeability. Classically, cellulitis causes increased uptake in the first two phases but uptake is normal in the third phase, whereas osteomyelitis and Charcot arthropathy often result in abnormal uptake in all three phases. The blood-pool phase shows the amount of hyperemia such as that occurs with trauma and degenerative joint diseases; however, the inflammation, fractures, and chronic infections of a Charcot foot also increase the local hyperemia. Changes caused by infection are visible sooner on scintigraphy than on radiographs, and pooled data have shown scintigraphy to have an 81% sensitivity but only 28% specificity. With all scintigraphy, decreased spatial resolution and bone overlap lead to difficulty in determining which bones are affected rather than broad regions (e.g., hindfoot, midfoot, forefoot).

Positron emission tomography (PET) scanning is a technique in which a radiotracer (fluorine-18 fluorodeoxyglucose) is injected and is taken up by areas of higher metabolic activity. Sites of active inflammation show increased uptake caused by hypercellular marrow, while areas of marrow suppression such as with osteomyelitis show decreased uptake. Several small studies have compared PET combined with

TABLE 6.2

Brodsky Depth-Ischemia Classification for Foot Ulcers

DEPTH

Classification	Description
0	At risk foot, no ulceration
1	Superficial ulceration, no infection
2	Deep ulceration, tendons or joint exposed
3	Extensive ulceration or abscess

ISCHEMIA

A	Not ischemic
B	Ischemia without gangrene
C	Partial forefoot gangrene
D	Complete gangrene

Depth

Grade 0
No break in skin

Grade 1
Superficial ulcer

Grade 2
Exposed tendons, joints

Grade 3
Exposed bone and/or abscess/ osteomyelitis

Ischemia

Grade A
No ischemia

Grade B
Ischemia not gangrenous

Grade C
Partial foot gangrene

Grade D
Complete gangrene

Modified from Brodsky JW: The diabetic foot. In: Coughlin MJ, Mann RA, Saltzman CL, editors: *Surgery of the foot and ankle*, Philadelphia, 2007, Mosby, p 1297.

CT scanning (PET/CT) to MRI for detection or exclusion of osteomyelitis with mixed results; at this time there is insufficient evidence to recommend PET/CT for routine imaging in diabetic feet. Some studies have reported that a hybrid technique—Tc-99m WBC-labeled single photon emission computed tomography (SPECT/CT) imaging—is useful in the diagnosis of osteomyelitis in diabetic feet and in determining the effectiveness of treatment (Fig. 6.8). This is relatively new technology, and research is limited at this time; further research is warranted to determine the role of Tc-99m WBC SPECT/CT in the diabetic foot.

MRI has numerous advantages in that it avoids radiation, can be completed in a relatively short amount of time, differentiates soft-tissue processes in multiple planes, and is widely available. MRI findings of osteomyelitis in the foot are decreased signal intensity on T1-weighted images and increased signal activity on T2-weighted or fat-suppressed images. Localized edema from an ulcer adjacent to bone may be misinterpreted as osteomyelitis, and distinguishing osteomyelitis from Charcot changes is difficult if not impossible. In biopsy-proven osteomyelitis of diabetic feet, MRI has been reported to show 90% sensitivity and 79% specificity in detecting the correct diagnosis; however, in the presence of an ulcer, sensitivity decreases. In a meta-analysis, Dinh et al. found MRI to be the most accurate imaging test for diagnosis of osteomyelitis in a diabetic foot (Table 6.3), whereas Lauri et al., in a meta-analysis, showed highest specificity with tagged WBC scan and PET scan. MRI is useful to determine the extent of osteomyelitis for surgical planning after the diagnosis has already been confirmed. Although both scintigraphy and MRI are sensitive, false positives may exist at sites of active arthropathy. A negative result, however, does suggest

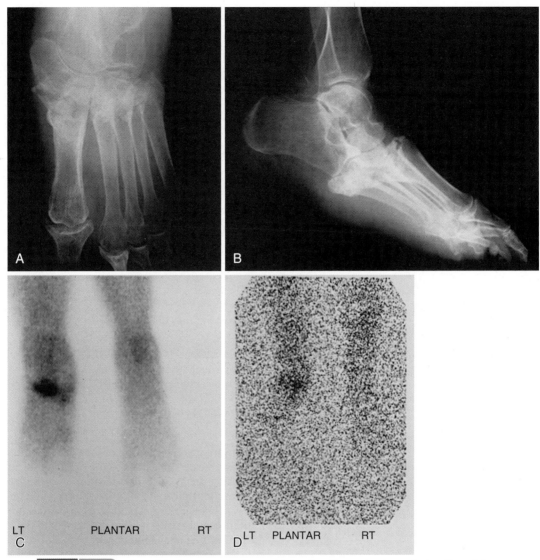

FIGURE 6.7 **A** and **B,** Anteroposterior and lateral radiographs show destruction of tarso-metatarsal joints. Note equinus deformity on lateral view. **C** and **D,** Technetium (R3) and indium scans strongly suggest osteomyelitis in addition to neuropathy.

that osteomyelitis is unlikely to be present. All results must be considered in the context of the clinical findings.

TREATMENT

The primary goals of treatment of diabetic foot ulcers are healing of the ulcer, prevention of secondary infection and recurrence, and avoidance of amputation. Recognizing and conveying the significance of a foot ulcer to the patient are important: a 44% 5-year mortality and mean survival of 50 months after onset of a new diabetic foot ulcer have been reported. Assal demonstrated that the cost savings in avoiding amputation are significant: in 1995, the direct cost of nine below-knee amputations was equivalent to the salaries of three physicians, five nurses, one dietitian, one secretary, and three auxiliary staff combined. In a more recent study from the Veterans Health Administration, the cost associated with a single lower-limb amputation was $60,647.

Existing treatments are numerous and include newer ideas such as bioengineered skin, platelet-derived growth factor, and collagen-calcium alginate dressings. The most

standard treatments are debridement and off-loading of the affected area. Because of the complexities of treating diabetic feet, including impaired blood supply, osteoporotic bone, and neuropathy, a multidisciplinary approach is most beneficial. Multidisciplinary care has been shown to be cost-effective, to decrease the future amputation rate, and to be especially beneficial for patients over the age of 70 years. Expertise is often required from subspecialists in orthopaedics, vascular surgery, orthotics, infectious disease, endocrinology, and wound nursing. Vascular consultation should be considered when rest pain, claudication, or ischemic ulcers are present. Endocrinology may assist if blood glucose levels cannot be controlled by the primary care practitioner or if the patient shows unusual response to standard glycemic control measures. Infectious disease consultation may be helpful when a patient fails to respond to empiric antibiotic therapy or if there is potential for renal or hepatic toxicity with culture-specific antibiotic therapy.

Primary responsibility for the patient remains with the surgeon; however, other office personnel who are

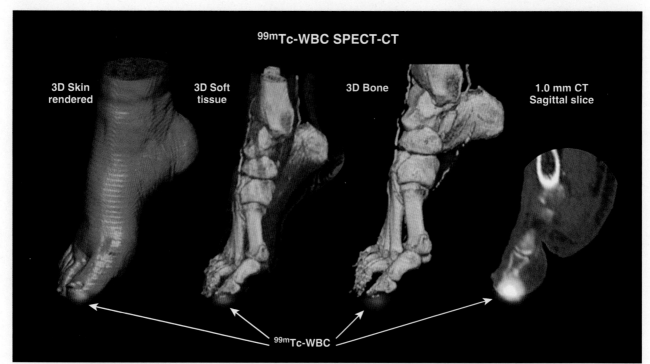

FIGURE 6.8 99m Tc WBC SPECT/CT hybrid imaging of diabetic foot with osteomyelitis of first digit terminal tuft. Extent, depth, severity, and bone involvement of infection were not clinically apparent. (From Erdman WA, Buethe J, Bhore R, et al: Indexing severity of diabetic foot infection with 99m Tc WBC SPECT/CT hybrid imaging, *Diabetes Care* 35:1826, 2012.)

TABLE 6.3

Imaging Modalities for Diagnosis of Osteomyelitis Associated With Diabetic Foot Ulcer

DIAGNOSTIC MODALITY	SENSITIVITY (%)	SPECIFICITY (%)
Probe-to-bone test or exposed bone	60	91
Radiography	54	68
MRI	90	79
Bone scan	81	28
Leukocyte scan	74	68

Modified from Dinh MT, Abad CL, Safdar N: Diagnostic accuracy of the physical examination and imaging tests for osteomyelitis underlying diabetic foot ulcers: meta-analysis, *Clin Infect Dis* 47:519, 2008.

appropriately trained may enhance routine foot care and patient education. A nurse with advanced training in wound care, ostomy, and continence is an asset to both the treating surgeon and the patient.

Evaluation of a foot ulcer begins with identification of any underlying conditions (Fig. 6.9). Any evidence of ischemia, venous stasis, or pressure from shoes must be identified and treated. Systemic factors, including glucose control, smoking, and diet, should be controlled to optimize the wound-healing environment. All areas surrounding the wound should be inspected for periwound callus and necrotic tissue. A thickened callus will increase pressure on the underlying tissue when the patient bears weight on the foot and may prevent the inward epithelialization of the ulcer from the border area. Thickened callus may also be the precursor of an ulcer.

Using the Wagner classification of foot ulcers (see Table 6.1), grade 0 ulcers should be treated with serial examinations, patient education, and accommodative footwear. Grade I ulcers can be treated with debridement in the clinic and off-loading with a total contact cast, walking brace, or other custom footwear. Grade II ulcers require surgical debridement, culture-specific antibiotics, and off-loading with total contact casting. Grade III ulcers (Fig. 6.10) require surgical debridement or partial amputation with off-loading and culture-specific antibiotics. Grade IV and V ulcers require local or larger amputation based on the extent of infection. In the ischemic classification of Brodsky et al. (see Table 6.2), type B ischemia should be considered for noninvasive vascular testing and reconstruction with bypass or angioplasty. Type C involvement may require reconstructive vascular surgery with partial amputation, while type D requires thorough vascular evaluation and likely major extremity amputation.

Debridement, whether done in the clinic or operating room, involves sharply removing all hypertrophic callus and nonviable tissue. The goal is to convert a chronic nonhealing wound into an acute wound capable of progressing through the natural phases of wound healing. All infected tissue, including soft tissue and bone, must be excised. This decreases the bacterial load and the detrimental cellular breakdown products such as matrix metalloproteinases from the wound bed. Wagner grade I ulcers can be debrided in the office, while those with deeper exposed structures warrant operative debridement. The most important aspect in the treatment of grade I ulcers is off-loading of the affected region, rather than the type of dressing used. Any necrotic

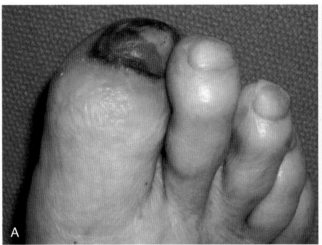
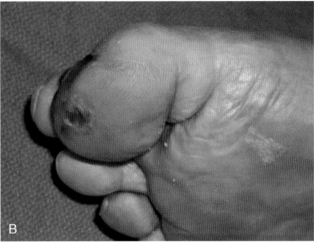

FIGURE 6.9 Plantar ulceration due to fixed interphalangeal joint flexion. **A,** Dorsal view. **B,** Plantar view. (From Brodsky JW: The diabetic foot. In: Coughlin MJ, Mann RA, Saltzman CL, editors: *Surgery of the foot and ankle*, ed 8, Philadelphia, 2007, Elsevier.)

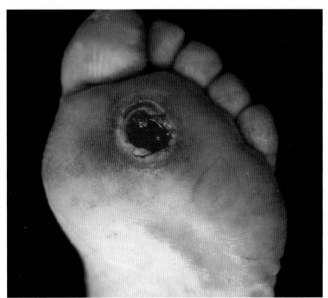

FIGURE 6.10 Grade III ulcer under second metatarsal head extends into metatarsal head with presumptive contiguous osteomyelitis.

tissue present serves as a medium for bacterial growth and should be excised. Ulcers should be probed with a sterile swab; if bone is encountered, osteomyelitis may be presumed. Ulcers with direct communication to bone generally require surgical debridement.

A scalpel can be used in the office to thin thick peri-wound callus, or a pumice stone may suffice if the callus is thin. The scalpel is held with the blade roughly parallel to the callus edge, and thin layers are removed until the entire callus has been excised. In patients with intact plantar sensation, this may be painful and difficult to tolerate without a local anesthetic. Insensate diabetic patients may not require any additional anesthesia for callus thinning in the office.

Numerous products are available to deal with the fluid exudate from chronic ulcers. This exudate has been shown to contain numerous cellular breakdown products, including metalloproteinases that inhibit cellular proliferation. Removal of this fluid is thought to promote wound healing.

Ulcers with fibrinous debris may be best treated by moist-to-dry gauze dressing changes. A moist piece of gauze placed on the wound and allowed to dry provides a mechanical debridement when it is removed. This is a nonselective debridement, however, and healthy viable tissue may also be removed during this process. Wet-to-dry dressings of saline-soaked gauze have shown an aggregate mean healing rate of 24% at 12 weeks and 31% at 20 weeks. Collagenase-based enzymatic cleaners are also an option in the management of foot ulcers. They are selective for nonviable tissue but are ineffective at removing callus. Daily dressing changes with foams, hydrofibers, calcium alginates, hydrocolloids, negative pressure sponges, and crystalline sodium chloride gauze for exudative wounds and hydrogels for dry wounds have been reported. A systematic review of local antibiotic devices used to improve wound healing in diabetic foot infections showed a lack of good-quality evidence to support these treatments. Negative pressure wound therapy (NPWT) devices are another option to assist in ulcer healing. The exact mechanism of action of NPWT is unknown; however, studies have shown that it may increase local blood flow, decrease edema, and increase the concentration of growth factors in the local wound fluid. A 2018 Cochrane review showed low-certainty evidence that NPWT increases the number of wounds healed compared to standard dressings or that it reduces time to wound healing. Although studies exist for each of these that show improvement compared with a control group, no study to date has shown superiority to the healing rates of a total contact cast and no study has directly compared the dressing change protocol to a total contact cast protocol.

Erythema, induration, increased exudate, and pain are symptoms of an infected ulcer. Infection significantly slows the healing process and must be treated with systemic antibiotics in addition to debridement. Cultures of the ulcer are generally not recommended because the sensitivity in isolating the causative organism is low. Most ulcers are colonized with bacteria that has not invaded the deep tissue and do not require antibiotics. When wound cultures are obtained, this should be done after thorough debridement of the wound. The goal is to identify the organism invading the viable tissue rather than that occurring in the necrotic areas; viable tissue should be swabbed, not the tissue to be debrided.

Wounds should be cleansed with saline irrigant using a syringe and needle to increase the pressure applied. This decreases local bacteria levels and removes any local debris. Harsh chemicals such as hydrogen peroxide and betadine should not be applied because these can damage the viable tissue in the ulcer and further delay healing. A dressing applied daily to maintain a moist environment in the ulcer will minimize desiccation and facilitate healing. The dressing used should be based on the characteristics of the ulcer. Ulcers with large quantities of exudate require a more absorptive dressing, while low exudative ulcers should have moisture added (moist-to-dry dressing).

Routine nail care may be provided by the physician or nurse if the patient is unable to do so. A straight nail clipper should be used to transversely cut the nail to avoid any skin overgrowth at the medial and lateral borders, which may increase the chance of developing an ingrown nail.

Hyperbaric oxygen (HBO) has been used as a treatment for diabetic foot ulcers and randomized trials have shown 54% healing using HBO compared with 25% for standard methods. In a study of 25,562 Wagner grade 3 and 4 wounds, Ennis et al. showed that HBO may increase wound healing rates from 56% without HBO to 60% to 75% with HBO, depending on how closely the patient adheres to the prescribed therapy. Several important issues remain to be solved, including the economics, access, and selection criteria for which patients would benefit most from HBO. It currently appears that HBO is an option for patients with difficult-to-heal diabetic foot ulcers.

■ PATIENT EDUCATION

Patient education for diabetic patients has been shown to be cost-effective, improve patient quality of life, and reduce the risk of lower extremity amputation by 50% to 85%. Regular education is important; research has shown that 20% of diabetic patients lack basic knowledge about the risk the disease poses to their feet, with retention of the information decreasing over time. Basic guidelines recommended by the American Orthopaedic Foot and Ankle Society should be reviewed and reinforced at each patient visit. Patients should be reminded to wear shoes at all times and to never use corn or callous removers. Feet should be inspected daily, and any signs of erythema, ulceration, or nail problems should be brought to the attention of the care provider. Feet should be bathed daily with mild soap and a soft brush for the areas around the nails. When drying the feet, attention should be paid to the web spaces because these areas often trap moisture. If the web spaces remain overly moist, lamb's wool may be placed in between the toes to avoid maceration. Lotion of lanolin cream should be applied, and cotton or other natural fiber socks should be worn to absorb perspiration. White socks are helpful to quickly identify any areas of drainage or bleeding. Ideal shoes are those made of soft leather with adjustable lacing or straps over the instep and a wide toe box.

Diabetic patients with normal sensation and minimal to no deformity should be provided basic education and should have an annual examination. Normal footwear can be used with caution, avoiding any shoes with a narrow toe box or that are undersized. Patients with insensate feet but no deformity require a daily self-examination, pressure-relieving custom insoles replaced every 6 months, and an examination twice annually. Oxford leather shoes with laces and adequate size to accommodate a pressure-relieving insole are recommended. Insensate feet with deformity are considered "at risk" and need custom insoles with an Oxford-style shoe and follow-up every 4 months. At-risk patients with any history of ulceration should be evaluated every 2 months and consideration should be given to referral to an orthopaedic foot and ankle specialist.

■ TOTAL CONTACT CASTING

Reducing pressure on plantar ulcers is crucial to aid healing. Forefoot pressures can be reduced with prefabricated shoes more easily than midfoot or hindfoot ulcers. Total contact casting is more effective than prefabricated shoes for the midfoot and hindfoot (Fig. 6.11). A total contact cast redistributes forces from the plantar surface of the foot to the leg, which reduces the force on the foot even with weight-bearing activity. Total contact casting is also beneficial in that it reduces edema in the extremity, which is why the cast must be changed regularly to prevent loosening that can lead to further ulceration. Patients are unable to remove the cast so there is a forced compliance aspect compared with a prefabricated shoe or boot. Nouman et al. showed significant reduction and redistribution of peak plantar pressure at the toes and forefoot compared to other regions of the foot, with the midfoot having increased pressures. Total contact casting for plantar ulcers (Fig. 6.12) showed significantly better healing (89.5%) than removable prefabricated walking boots (65%) or shoes (58%). This is similar to the 88% healing rate reported at 41 days with total contact casting alone in a study comparing casting alone to casting with percutaneous Achilles lengthening. Patients may bear weight in a total contact cast because moderate ambulation has not been shown to increase healing times of foot ulcers in a cast. Patients have been shown to decrease their activity over the course of a day in a total contact cast, which reduces the stress on the foot.

Total contact casting is not a benign treatment, however; it has been shown to have a 6% to 17% occurrence of new ulcer formation and a 0.25% rate of permanent sequelae. Although there are numerous studies reporting success with total contact casting, some centers do not use this technique regularly, opting instead for removable prefabricated boots. These removable boots do provide off-loading in patients with mild deformity, but multiple studies have shown reduced efficacy when compared with total contact casting. One study of patients with mild deformities showed equivalent results between total contact casting and a removable walking boot that was wrapped in fiberglass to force patient compliance, emphasizing the importance of patient compliance on outcome. In patients with moderate to severe deformities, prefabricated boots are unable to provide the same outcomes as a custom-molded total contact cast because of issues with fit and less ability to accommodate the fluid shifts.

TOTAL CONTACT CAST APPLICATION

TECHNIQUE 6.1

(MCBRYDE)
- Place a partial piece of thick foam just distal to the patella if required.

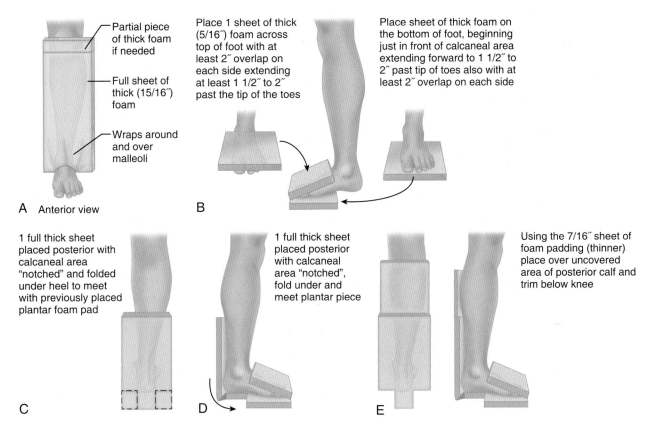

Partial piece of thick foam if needed

Full sheet of thick (15/16″) foam

Wraps around and over malleoli

A Anterior view

Place 1 sheet of thick (5/16″) foam across top of foot with at least 2″ overlap on each side extending at least 1 1/2″ to 2″ past the tip of the toes

Place sheet of thick foam on the bottom of foot, beginning just in front of calcaneal area extending forward to 1 1/2″ to 2″ past tip of toes also with at least 2″ overlap on each side

B

1 full thick sheet placed posterior with calcaneal area "notched" and folded under heel to meet with previously placed plantar foam pad

C

1 full thick sheet placed posterior with calcaneal area "notched", fold under and meet plantar piece

D

Using the 7/16″ sheet of foam padding (thinner) place over uncovered area of posterior calf and trim below knee

E

Turning attention to thick foam pieces placed on top of and under foot

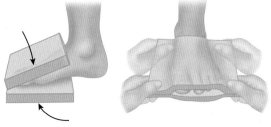

F "Pinch" the foam along inside and outside of forefoot while contouring to forefoot, this "sandwich" type of pinching foam will leave an impression in foam which can now be trimmed away

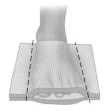

G

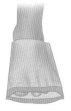

H When molding along inside and outside of foam, do not pinch toe end closed... leave open

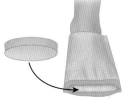

I From thick foam remnant, cut piece to fill in open toe area

Once all areas to be casted have been 100% enclosed by foam padding, Webril cast padding is used to enclose all areas to be casted as well. When wrapping/rolling Webril, every effort should be used to "pull" this padding as much as can be done, right up to its breaking point of tearing while avoiding any wrinkles. The purpose of this technique is to try and compress foam padding as much as possible and maintain "mold" of lower extremity including end of toe area. Depending on circumference of extremity, it may be possible to compress foam with palm of one hand while passing Webril padding around extremity with palm area of opposite hand, thus wrapping area already being somewhat compressed. When applying the fiberglass, do not pull or apply tension while wrapping.

FIGURE 6.11 Technique for application of total contact cast. **SEE TECHNIQUE 6.1.**

- Place a full sheet of thick (15/16 inch) foam around the leg from the knee to the ankle, and wrap it around and over the malleoli (Fig. 6.11A).
- Place a sheet of thick foam across the top of the foot with at least 2 inches of overlap on each side and extending at least 1.5 to 2 inches past the tip of the toes (Fig. 6.11B).

- Place a sheet of thick foam on the bottom of the foot, beginning just in front of the calcaneal area, extending forward to 1.5 to 2 inches past the tip of the toes, also with at least 2 inches of overlap on each side (Fig. 6.11C).
- Place one full thick foam sheet posterior, with the calcaneal area "notched" and folded under the heel to meet the previously placed plantar foam pad (Fig. 6.11D).

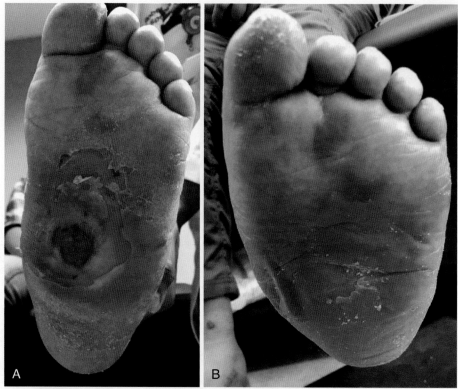

FIGURE 6.12 **(A)** Plantar ulcer healed **(B)** after 2 months in total contact cast.

- Place a ⁷⁄₁₆ inch (thinner) sheet of foam padding over the uncovered area of the posterior calf and trim below the knee (Fig. 6.11E).
- Turning attention to the thick foam pieces placed on top of and under the foot, "pinch" the foam along the inside and outside of the forefoot while contouring to the forefoot (Fig. 6.11F). This "sandwich" type of pinching the foam will leave an impression in the foam that can now be trimmed away (Fig. 6.11G).
- Do not pinch the toe end closed, leave it open (Fig. 6.11H). Cut a piece from a thick foam remnant to fill in the open toe area (Fig. 6.11I).
- Once all areas to be casted have been completely enclosed by foam padding, use Webril cast padding to enclose all areas to be casted. When wrapping the Webril, try to "pull" this padding as much as possible, right up to its breaking point, while avoiding any wrinkles. This is done to try and compress the foam padding as much as possible and maintain the "mold" of the lower extremity. Alternatively, compress the foam with the palm of one hand while passing the Webril padding around the extremity with the palm area of the opposite hand.
- Begin wrapping the fiberglass as usual, keeping in mind that the toe area must be covered. A "flip-flop" or "fan fold" technique may help in covering this area of the cast.
- Once a basic foundation has been completed, place a 4-inch X 38-inch fiberglass splint on top of the forefoot area, bring it out over the toe area and under the foot, extending upward over the calcaneal area.
- Use a layer of fiberglass to secure the splint and toe area; trim out the most proximal area and the remainder of the cast.

TREATMENT OF PERIPHERAL NEUROPATHY

Numerous classes of pharmacologic agents have been developed to treat peripheral neuropathy, including anticonvulsants (gabapentin and pregabalin), tricyclic antidepressants, serotonin reuptake inhibitors, mild analgesics (tramadol), and topical agents (capsaicin). These agents have been shown to perform better than placebo, but head-to-head trials have shown more significant differences in costs than in effectiveness. Nonpharmacologic modalities, such as nerve stimulation and ultrasound, have not shown consistent results. Nerve conduction deficits have been identified in the periphery in this population and surgical release of the entrapment has been suggested to be of benefit, but no outcomes-oriented prospective randomized trials have been reported to date.

■ SURGICAL MANAGEMENT

Indications for surgical management are grossly contaminated wounds, unbraceable deformity, gastrocnemius contracture, underlying bone prominence that impedes wound healing, and failure of conservative management. The goal is to provide a stable, braceable foot with a healed soft-tissue envelope. Prophylactic surgery may be considered in patients who are at risk for wound breakdown caused by joint instability or bony prominence. Hammer toes and clawtoes can be corrected if they cannot be accommodated by shoe wear or if correction will assist in healing of a forefoot ulcer.

Flexor tenotomy as treatment for isolated toe ulcerations showed more than 90% healing rates in a mean of 40 days, with a 12% recurrence rate at 2-year follow-up. Ulcerations at the medial interphalangeal joint of the hallux can be treated by resection of the medial condyles of the proximal and distal phalanges or by a modified Keller procedure (removal of the proximal third of the proximal phalanx).Ulcerations at the tip of the hallux are often caused by flexion deformity of the interphalangeal joint. Plantar metatarsophalangeal joint ulcerations are common, difficult to heal, and associated with a high risk of amputation. Pressure is often caused by sesamoids underlying the joint, and treatment may involve partial or complete resection of the medial sesamoid through a medial incision, dorsiflexion osteotomy of the first metatarsal, and resection of the joint. If the medial sesamoid is resected, the intersesamoidal ligament must be preserved and sutured to the abductor hallucis to prevent postoperative hallux valgus. Resection of both sesamoids is contraindicated because it will lead to dorsal subluxation of the hallux and increase the plantar pressures at the metatarsophalangeal joint. Arthrodesis of the interphalangeal joint should be considered to relieve plantar pressure at the tip of the hallux.

Achilles tendon lengthening and/or gastrocnemius recession should be considered for patients with forefoot ulcers in whom conservative management has failed and contractures have developed. Use of Achilles tendon lengthening procedures as part of the treatment of diabetic foot ulcers in the US increased 143% between 2000 and 2010. Contracture of the Achilles increases forefoot pressure, with subsequent ulceration. In one study, peak plantar pressures and ulcer recurrence rates were decreased by 25% to 50% 2 years after an Achilles lengthening. In a study comparing total contact casting alone to casting with percutaneous Achilles tendon lengthening, similar wound healing rates were reported; however, patients treated surgically had significantly fewer recurrences of ulceration at 2-year follow-up (38% compared with 81%). Gastrocnemius recession has also been reported to increase healing rates in midfoot ulcerations. Lengthening of the Achilles is not without drawbacks because, although the forefoot pressures normalize, plantarflexion strength remains weakened.

Exostectomy may be required in patients with bony deformity and ulceration. A sufficient period of off-loading with total contact casting should be completed before surgery. The bony prominence is excised through a direct plantar approach or a medial or lateral incision parallel to the plantar surface of the foot with full-thickness flaps. After the prominence is excised, the surrounding bone is leveled to avoid creating any new ridges of bone that could cause further ulceration. Evidence of infection on preoperative imaging may necessitate wider surgical excision. Major tendon attachments (anterior and posterior tibial tendons, peroneus longus tendon) may require release to allow complete excision of the exostosis, followed by re-anchoring of the tendons. If stability of the foot is compromised by excision of the exostosis, arthrodesis is indicated. In patients with neuropathic arthropathy, arthrodesis in conjunction with osteotomy may be required to achieve a plantigrade, braceable foot.

For patients in whom other surgical management fails, who have nonreconstructable vascular disease, or in whom infection is uncontrollable, amputation is the last surgical option. The National Diabetes Advisory Board estimates that 5% to 15% of diabetic patients will require a lower-extremity amputation in their lifetime. Query of the Medicare claims database, however, shows a trend in the US over the past decade of more limb-sparing procedures: the total number of amputations decreased by 28% and more amputations were performed distally at limb-preserving locations. Wukich et al. reported that 75% of patients had improved quality-of-life scores 1 year after transtibial amputation for diabetes-related

foot complications, with a strong correlation between lower scores and nonambulatory status.

The level of amputation depends on the location of infection and likelihood of healing of the surgical wound. Salvage of the foot should be attempted whenever possible because transtibial amputation alters the biomechanics of the extremity, which increases oxygen consumption and energy expenditure while decreasing motivation for ambulation secondary to the inconvenience of a prosthesis or psychologic stress. One-year mortality after transtibial amputation is 20%, with a 5-year mortality of 65%. Preservation of a portion of the foot gives the patient an end-bearing limb that facilitates ambulation without a prosthesis and improves functional outcome. In the forefoot, ray resection or transmetatarsal amputation may be sufficient in a patient with palpable pulses; however, the same wound in a patient with vascular pathology may require transtibial amputation. In the midfoot, a talonavicular-calcaneocuboid disarticulation (Chopart) or Syme amputation may allow ambulation without prosthesis. A viable heel pad is required for a Syme amputation. In the hindfoot, other than partial calcanectomy for isolated infection of the posterior calcaneal tubercle, below-knee amputation is generally recommended. Partial calcanectomy has been shown to have an unpredictable postoperative course, questionable durability, and increased mortality rate long term compared with transtibial amputation. A comparison of partial foot amputations to transtibial amputation found transmetatarsal amputation to be associated with a statistically lower mortality rate at 1 and 3 years after surgery, with transmetatarsal and Chopart amputations having high ambulatory levels and the longest durability. The single most important factor predicting success of a partial foot amputation is the hemoglobin A1C level at time of surgery, with some authors recommending no elective or trauma surgery for a diabetic patient with an A1C level of more than 8% unless necessary to save life or limb.

Nerve decompression in the treatment of diabetic peripheral neuropathy is controversial. Proponents of decompression point out that nerves in diabetic patients are more susceptible to compression because of increased water content of the nerve, and that surgical decompression may increase nutrient flow and decrease recurrence of symptoms. One study of 42 patients treated with nerve decompression in addition to standard ulcer treatment showed a 4.8% recurrence rate on the operative leg compared with 21.4% on the contralateral (nonoperative) leg at 3-year follow-up. The procedure may be indicated in a patient with symptoms in a specific dermatome (not a global neuropathy) with a Tinel sign on the nerve for that dermatome. This technique has not gained wide acceptance and should be done only in carefully selected patients. A 2008 Cochrane review demonstrated that evidence to support nerve decompression for diabetic neuropathy is limited. Surgical treatment of diabetic peripheral neuropathy remains a controversial issue at this time and cannot be recommended without further study.

TRAUMA IN DIABETIC PATIENTS

The reported rates of total complications in diabetic patients with traumatic injuries range from 14% to 43%, with diabetic patients three times more likely to develop a complication than nondiabetic patients. These patients often have poor vascularity, tenuous soft-tissue envelopes, and reduced capacity to heal from a surgical insult. Fracture healing in diabetic patients is slowed from impaired vascular proliferation, cellular proliferation, and mineralization of fracture callus. Basic science research using diabetic rat models has demonstrated decreased callus size, stiffness, and tensile strength compared with nondiabetic rats, with severity correlating to the degree of glycemic control. Normalization of glycemic levels in these poorly controlled rat models has also shown normalization of callus mechanical properties, which emphasizes the importance of perioperative glucose control. Complications from treatment are frequent and include nonunion, malunion, loss of fixation, infection, poor wound healing, and secondary Charcot arthropathy. When examining the patient, it is important to note the presence or absence of pulses in addition to the integrity of the skin. If pulses are absent, vascular consultation for possible reconstruction should be undertaken urgently before any operative fixation of the traumatic injury. Surgical fixation of a traumatic injury in an extremity lacking the capacity to heal will most likely end in amputation; however, nonoperative management is not a benign treatment, as complications can occur with prolonged casting as well.

Most stable fractures are treated nonoperatively with prolonged immobilization. A general rule is to double the immobilization time for diabetic patients with fractures.

Unstable ankle fractures in patients without peripheral vascular disease are treated surgically to restore stability and alignment and to provide a stable environment for the soft tissues to heal. Lovy et al. showed a 21-fold increased odds of a complication with nonoperative treatment compared to operative treatment in displaced diabetic ankle fractures (75% vs. 12.5% complication rate). Stable fixation may be difficult to obtain because of poor bone quality. Larger implants are desirable for strength, but this increases the local insult to the soft tissues and may compromise wound healing. Fixation can be supplemented by transarticular screws, additional syndesmotic screws, and/or external fixation (Figs. 6.13 and 6.14). Consideration should be given to the use of 500 to 1000 mg of topically applied vancomycin powder before skin closure; Wukich et al. showed a 73% reduction in surgical site infections in diabetic patients, with an 80% reduction in deep infections. Regardless of the method of fixation chosen, the period of immobilization postoperatively must be increased significantly from that of a nondiabetic patient. Neuropathic patients should be non–weight bearing in a cast for 3 months, followed by weight bearing in a cast for an additional 2 to 3 months, and then braced for 1 year. In patients with failed initial operative management of bimalleolar ankle fractures in diabetic patients, Vaudreuil et al. showed higher rates of limb salvage procedures and decreased number of operations compared to revision by open reduction and internal fixation, with an overall limb salvage rate of 82% in this difficult patient population.

CHARCOT ARTHROPATHY
BACKGROUND
Charcot arthropathy is a neurodegenerative process that occurs in phases that include bony destruction, resorption, and resulting consolidated deformity that can threaten both the function and viability of the limb. Jean-Martin Charcot first described it in 1868 in the setting of tabes dorsalis. Diabetes is the most common cause of Charcot arthropathy today, but other etiologies include syphilis, heavy metal poisoning, alcoholic or congenital neuropathy, leprosy,

rheumatoid arthritis, and idiopathic causes. Diabetic patients with Charcot arthropathy have a lower quality of life than diabetic patients without arthropathy.

NATURAL HISTORY
The natural history of Charcot arthropathy begins with acute inflammation and swelling and progresses to bone resorption. As swelling decreases, the bones begin to consolidate and increase the stability of the foot. Development of Charcot arthropathy in diabetic patients does not appear to be related to body weight, even though mechanical stress plays a significant role in its pathogenesis. Recurrence of Charcot arthropathy has been linked to a higher body mass index. Radiographic parameters such as the Meary angle, cuboid height, calcaneal pitch, and hindfoot-forefoot angle, worsen over time and, generally, the medial column of the foot fails before the lateral column from the pull of the posterior tibial tendon. Sagittal plane deformities are more likely to be associated with ulceration than transverse plane abnormalities. Intervention with immobilization early in the disease process is recommended to avoid future progression to advanced stages that are prone to complications and need for surgical intervention.

PATHOGENESIS
Joints in the body are formed of synovium, tendons, ligaments, cartilage, and bone, all of which are innervated except articular cartilage. Each of these structures contains mechanoreceptors, nociceptors, and free nerve endings that are sensitive to, and respond to, tensile stress. There also exists a reflex arc from these structures to surround muscles that assist in maintaining joint stability. This complex interplay between joint tissue receptors and muscle is disrupted by neuropathy, which forms the basis of joint destruction caused by chronic neuropathy. Many of the free nerve endings in joints contain inflammatory modulators, such as substance P, which have a vasodilatory effect and induce mast cell degranulation. Histologic examination of bone samples from diabetic patients with and without Charcot arthropathy showed inflammatory myxoid infiltration with disorganized trabecular patterns in Charcot bone but not in diabetic controls. A study examining the histologic qualities of trabecular bone in diabetic and nondiabetic patients and those with Charcot arthropathy demonstrated an inflammatory myxoid infiltrate, a statistically significant decrease in the number of trabeculae, and disorganized trabecular patterns in diabetics with Charcot arthropathy. The trabeculae in the Charcot bone had poorer quality than the other groups. These findings reinforce the clinical findings of more fragile bone and more susceptibility to fracture in diabetic patients with Charcot arthropathy.

Although the exact etiology is unknown, Charcot arthropathy is likely multifactorial with cellular, biomechanical, and environmental variables. Increased mechanical forces are created from altered joint morphology resulting from periarticular osteopenia and lack of proprioceptive feedback. These increased forces lead to further joint deterioration in a negative feedback loop. There are two theories regarding the pathogenesis of Charcot arthropathy. The neurovascular, or French, theory was first proposed by Charcot and suggests that neurologic damage precedes and is responsible for the destructive changes. It proposes that damage to the nervous system causes autonomic dysfunction, which increases local

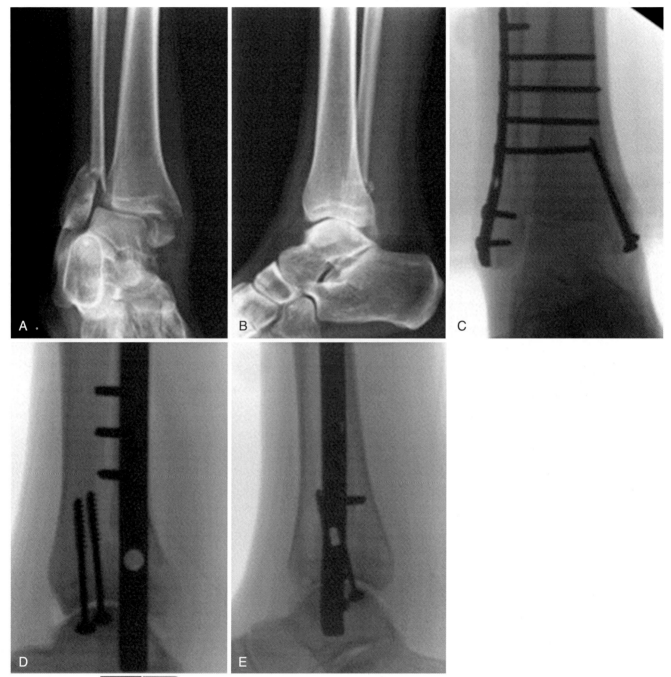

FIGURE 6.13 **A** and **B,** Preoperative radiographs of bimalleolar ankle fracture-subluxation in 19-year-old man with 12-year history of insulin-dependent diabetes mellitus. **C-E,** Fixation with fibular plating, medial malleolar screw fixation, and supplemental syndesmotic screws. (From Gandhi A, Liporace F, Azad V, et al: Diabetic fracture healing, *Foot Ankle Clin North Am* 11:805, 2006.)

blood flow due to arteriovenous shunting and leads to bone resorption. The neurotraumatic, or German, theory supported by Virchow and Volkman suggests that repetitive microtrauma causes the bony changes due to absent protective mechanisms. It proposes that the body does not respond to these microtraumatic stresses because the joint is insensitive from neuropathy and the stress is not perceived. The true pathogenesis is likely a combination of these theories. An early animal study in which sectioning of the posterior nerve roots was followed by activity showed bony changes

consistent with Charcot arthropathy in 71%. A later similar study of denervation of animal limbs followed by casting of the limbs noted a difference in response to immobilization between the denervated and nondenervated groups. This suggests that trauma, although important, is not primarily responsible for the changes seen in Charcot arthropathy.

CLASSIFICATION

Charcot arthropathy can be classified by the anatomic site of involvement (Fig. 6.15). Type 1 involving the tarsometatarsal

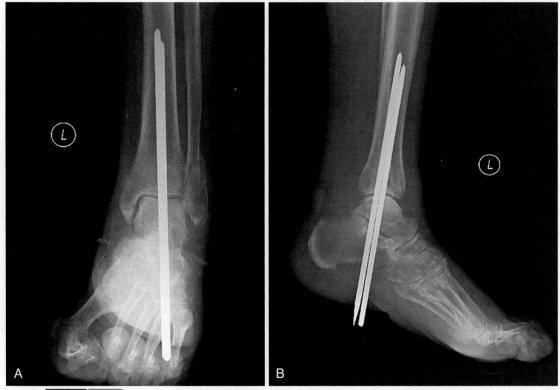

FIGURE 6.14   **A** and **B,** Percutaneous fixation of ankle fracture in diabetic patient.

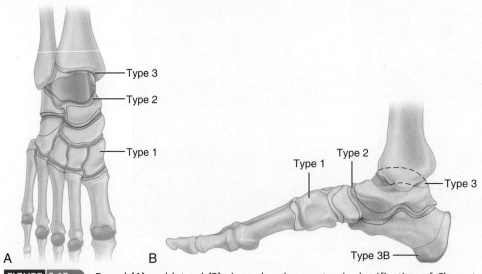

FIGURE 6.15   Dorsal **(A)** and lateral **(B)** views showing anatomic classification of Charcot arthropathy (see text). (Redrawn from Brodsky JW: The diabetic foot. In: Coughlin MJ, Mann RA, Saltzman CL, editors: *Surgery of the foot and ankle*, ed 8, Philadelphia, 2007, Elsevier.)

and naviculocuneiform joints is most common (60%). Midfoot involvement, specifically the tarsometatarsal joints, is most frequent and is characterized by hindfoot valgus caused by forefoot abduction with a contracted gastrocsoleus complex (Fig. 6.16). This combined pathoanatomy may lead to a stable rocker-bottom deformity with possible secondary plantar ulcerations in this area. Type 2 is the second most common type (25%) and primarily involves the hindfoot, including the subtalar, talonavicular, and calcaneocuboid joints, and may also progress to a rocker-bottom deformity from plantar

flexion of the talar head, but typically develops marked varus or valgus alignment of the hindfoot. Type 3A (10%) involves the ankle and often results in ulcerations over the prominent malleoli. Ankle involvement generally requires operative intervention because of marked instability. Type 3B (5%) presents as a pathologic fracture of the calcaneal tuberosity from avulsion. Primary hindfoot and ankle involvement are not well tolerated and conservative management often fails.

Pinzur and Schiff suggested a new classification system for midtarsal Charcot arthropathy based on their experience

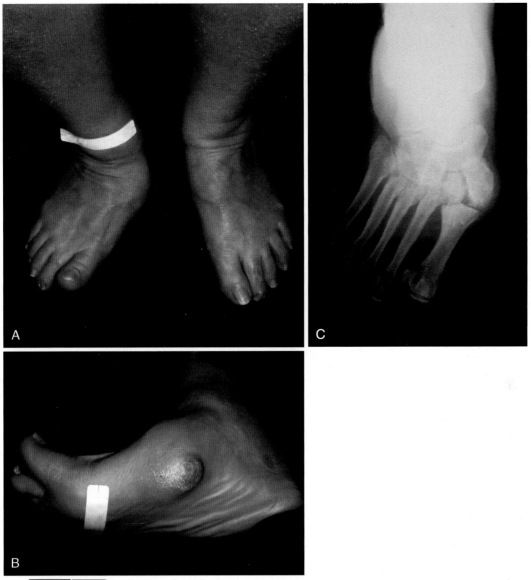

FIGURE 6.16 **A** and **B,** Collapse at Lisfranc joints, valgus posturing of forefoot, and shortening of first ray. Prominence medially is medial cuneiform. **C,** Same foot with subluxations at tarsometatarsal joints, fragmentation of bone, shortening and angulation of first ray, and new bone formation.

with 214 patients over a 12-year period; the classification is based on the relationship of the forefoot to the hindfoot and the integrity of the talocalcaneal joint on weight-bearing radiographs. A valgus deformity is present when the heel is in valgus and the forefoot is normal or abducted (Fig. 6.17A-C), a varus deformity is present if the heel is in varus and the forefoot is adducted (Fig. 6.18A-C), and a dislocation is present if there is loss of integrity of the talocalcaneal articulation with the heel in valgus and an abducted forefoot (Fig. 6.19A-F). All patients were treated with a single-stage Achilles tendon lengthening, resection of infection, wedge resection at the apex of the deformity, and application of a three-level static ring external fixator. Overall, 77% achieved a favorable outcome, with significant differences noted based on the classification system. Valgus deformities had 87% favorable outcomes, dislocations had 70.3% favorable outcomes, and varus deformities had the lowest rate (56%) of favorable outcomes.

Eichenholtz developed a commonly used classification system based on the stage of healing as assessed by radiographs and clinical signs of inflammation (Table 6.4). Some authors have questioned the validity of the Eichenholtz classification system and prefer an MRI or PET/CT-based classification to detect earlier changes that may be missed on initial radiographs.

TREATMENT

Combined, the anatomic and Eichenholtz staging systems are useful in guiding treatment decisions for patients with Charcot arthropathy. Immobilization remains the primary treatment method, with the goal of maintaining a plantigrade foot with a closed soft-tissue envelope that is able to withstand weight-bearing forces. Stage 1 disease is treated with a total contact cast, which offloads the involved region and provides stability and alignment through the healing phases. As radiographic and clinical signs of healing become evident (stage 2), patients

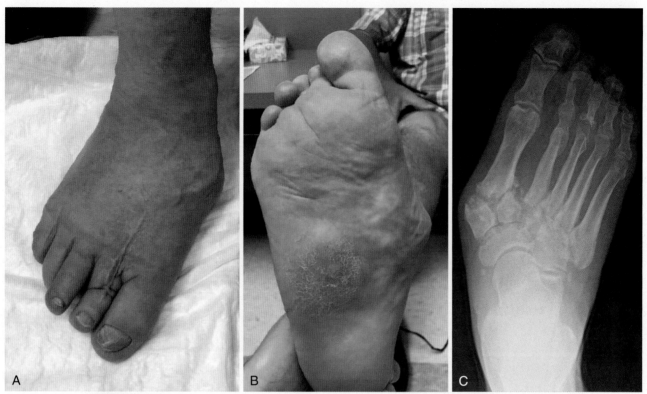

FIGURE 6.17 Midtarsal Charcot arthropathy with valgus deformity (Pinzur and Schiff classification, see text).

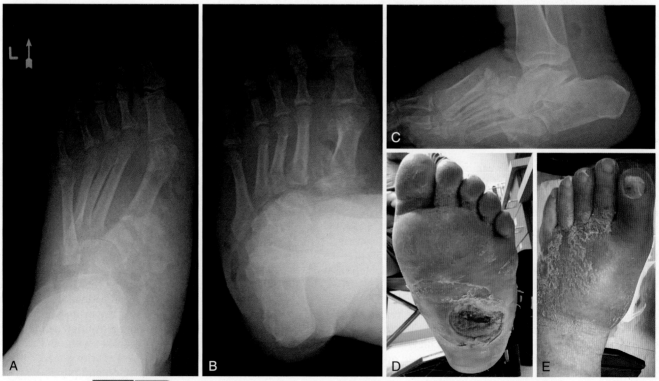

FIGURE 6.18 Midtarsal Charcot arthropathy with varus deformity (Pinzur and Schiff classification, see text).

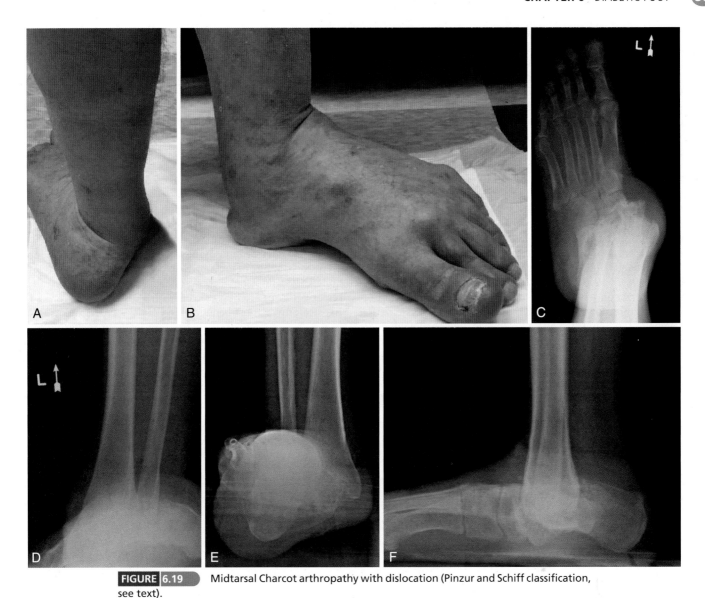

FIGURE 6.19 Midtarsal Charcot arthropathy with dislocation (Pinzur and Schiff classification, see text).

TABLE 6.4

Eichenholtz Classification of Charcot Arthropathy in the Diabetic Foot

STAGE	RADIOGRAPHIC SIGNS	CLINICAL SIGNS
0	No osteoporosis noted	Unilateral edema, erythema; warm, intact skin
1 Fragmentation	Osseous destruction, joint subluxation/dislocation	Similar to stage 0
2 Coalescence	Absorption of bone debris with coalescence of small fracture fragments	Decreased erythema, warmth, edema
3 Consolidation	Consolidation and remodeling fracture fragments	No edema, warmth, or erythema

can be transitioned into a prefabricated boot or a custom-molded ankle-foot-orthosis. When consolidation is complete and swelling resolves completely (stage 3), an accommodative shoe with molded orthosis is sufficient. Patients should be counseled from the outset that even with intensive treatment, up to 50% may require surgical intervention. Vitamin D supplementation should be considered for all patients because research has shown frequent hypovitaminosis D in diabetic patients and clarified its role in the pathogenesis and treatment of Charcot arthropathy. Studies on the use of calcitonin and bisphosphonates have shown limited effectiveness, and these medications are currently not considered standard of care.

Traditionally, elective surgery was avoided in this high-risk group because of increased rates of infection, nonunion, and delayed wound healing. Over the past decade, however, operative management has become more frequent due to improvements in glycemic control and methods of fixation. Surgical management of Charcot arthropathy may be considered for instability with resulting soft-tissue compromise. An observational study by members of the American Orthopaedic Foot and Ankle Society Charcot Study Group showed that individuals with Charcot arthropathy have a significantly impaired quality of life and that this impairment does not improve with traditional accommodative bracing. Many surgeons prefer to delay surgery until the inflammatory phase has resolved for fear that the bone in this phase has poor healing and osteoclastic resorption, making it insufficient to hold fixation; however, delaying surgical intervention for unstable deformities may lead to an ulceration that could preclude internal fixation. A retrospective study by Simon et al. of 14 patients with Eichenholtz stage I Charcot arthropathy treated with arthrodesis for midfoot deformity showed that all patients healed without complications and were able to return to full weight bearing 15 weeks after surgery, with no ulcerations at 41 months of follow-up. There are no studies currently directly comparing early operative intervention to immobilization therapy in early-stage Charcot deformity.

The decision to operate is made only after consideration of each individual patient's situation, including comorbidities, severity and location of deformity, compliance, stability, and condition of the soft-tissue envelope. A systematic review of the literature showed primarily low-level evidence, with no studies comparing different techniques, methods of fixation, or outcomes between surgically and nonsurgically treated patients. The review concluded that the evidence for acute phase surgical intervention is inconclusive, and there is insufficient evidence to recommend one form of fixation over another. In our experience, patients with unstable deformities and well-controlled diabetes (A1C less than 8 mg/dL) are encouraged to consider early surgical intervention with internal fixation, whereas those with poorly controlled diabetes are immobilized in a total contact cast while optimized for surgical intervention. Ulceration does not preclude the use of internal fixation if infected bone is fully resected at the time of surgical correction. External fixation is used in appropriately selected patients for severely infected deformity or when the soft tissues are not suitable for internal fixation.

The primary goals of surgical intervention are to allow the patient to eventually ambulate on a stable, plantigrade foot while preventing ulceration, infection, and amputation by decreasing sites of underlying pressure and improving alignment and stability of the foot. Sites of pressure from underlying bone that cannot be accommodated or relieved by prostheses or orthoses are best treated with exostectomy (Fig. 6.20). Exostectomy is most beneficial in Brodsky type 1 deformities in which tarsometatarsal destruction leads to rocker-bottom deformity and increased midfoot plantar pressures. Care must be taken to remove enough bone to relieve the underlying pressure without further disrupting the stability of the foot.

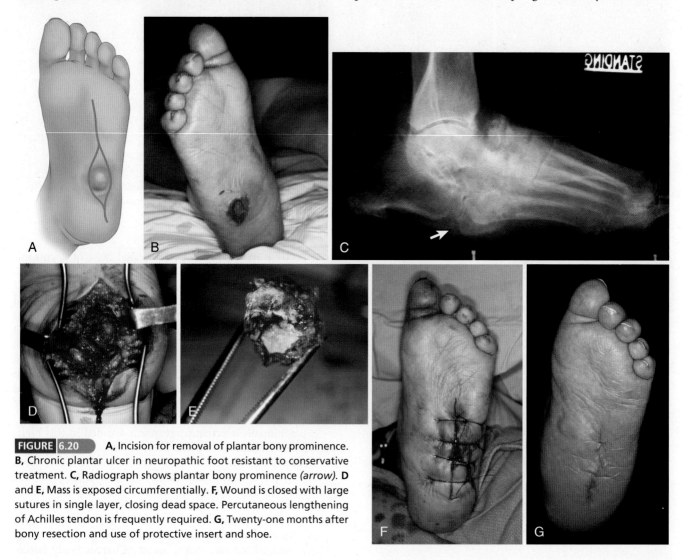

FIGURE 6.20   **A,** Incision for removal of plantar bony prominence. **B,** Chronic plantar ulcer in neuropathic foot resistant to conservative treatment. **C,** Radiograph shows plantar bony prominence *(arrow).* **D** and **E,** Mass is exposed circumferentially. **F,** Wound is closed with large sutures in single layer, closing dead space. Percutaneous lengthening of Achilles tendon is frequently required. **G,** Twenty-one months after bony resection and use of protective insert and shoe.

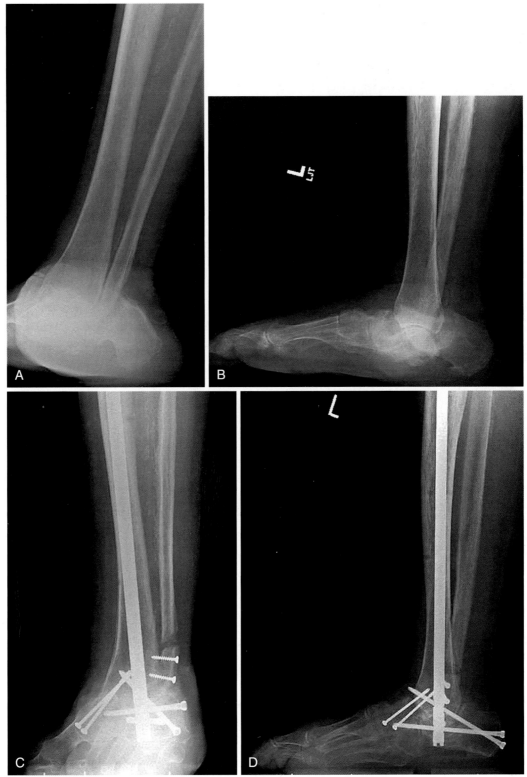

FIGURE 6.21   A and B, Charcot arthropathy. C and D, After tibiotalocalcaneal arthrodesis with intramedullary nail.

Patients with instability and resultant pain or ulceration may be best treated with arthrodesis (Fig. 6.21). Despite a high rate of partial unions (24%), the literature does demonstrate success with arthrodesis in patients in whom conservative management fails. Many patients with diabetic Charcot arthropathy are unable to follow protected weight-bearing regimens after surgery, which may explain both the increased nonunion rate and the relatively high rate of asymptomatic fibrous unions (Fig. 6.22). The procedure chosen depends on the location and severity of disease, in addition to surgeon preference. Type 1

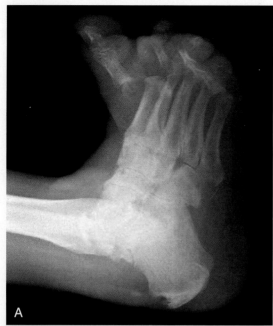

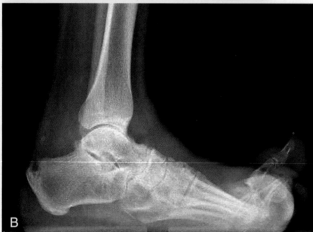

FIGURE 6.22   **A** and **B,** Charcot arthropathy of forefoot.

arthrodesis (Fig. 6.24). Intramedullary fixation of the midfoot can also be done with or without additional medial plating for enhanced stability (Fig. 6.25).

Operative correction of Charcot ankle deformities are associated with high complication rates and high risks of failure; Harkin et al. showed a 50% excellent or good clinical outcome in 56 consecutive patients treated with single-stage external fixation or retrograde locked intramedullary nail. Tomczak described a technique using an antibiotic cement-coated intramedullary nail with external fixation for limb salvage in eight severely deformed and infected neuropathic ankles, with an 87% limb preservation rate at an average of 3-year follow-up.

In patients with uncontrollable infection or failed operative treatment, amputation preserving as much length as possible may be the best option (Fig. 6.26). An estimated 2% to 3% of patients with Charcot arthropathy have amputations each year, whereas nearly a third of patients with arthropathy and an ulcer require major amputations. Although amputation is often incorrectly viewed as a failure, studies have shown improved quality of life and satisfaction in this difficult patient population.

MIDFOOT RECONSTRUCTION WITH INTRAMEDULLARY BEAMING

For this procedure, it is important to remember that the goal of the operation is to restore a stable plantigrade foot. The anatomy in a Charcot foot is not normal and cannot be restored to a normal state. Significant biplanar osteotomies and bone resections are typically performed rather than individual joint reductions, as would be done for traumatic injuries.

TECHNIQUE 6.2

(BETTIN)
- After administration of a regional block and general anesthesia, place the patient on the operating table with a bump under the ipsilateral hip and the leg elevated onto an elevated ramp or blankets.
- Typically, the ankle and hindfoot are in significant equinus compared to the forefoot. Perform an aggressive percutaneous Achilles tendon lengthening; in some cases, complete tenotomy is required.
- Make an extensile medial approach. A longitudinal incision can be made in line with the first ray; however, we often use a curvilinear incision through the skin to better access the dorsally subluxated tarsometatarsal joints as well as the plantarly translated talar head.
- Develop full-thickness flaps. Typically, the anterior tibial tendon is released off its insertion and tagged for repair at the completion of the procedure. Depending on the deformity, the posterior tibial tendon may need to be released as well.
- Expose the deformity dorsally and plantarly so that Hohmann retractors can be placed to protect neurovascular structures.
- Make a lateral incision from the anterior process of the calcaneus onto the base of the fourth and fifth metatarsals. Release the peroneus brevis tendon off the base of the fifth metatarsal.

deformities generally require midfoot arthrodesis, whereas type 2 deformities require triple arthrodesis. Osteotomies and wedge resections may be required to improve alignment before arthrodesis and can be done in a single procedure or staged procedures. Kroin et al. showed significantly improved quality of life in 25 consecutive patients after surgical reconstruction of midfoot Charcot deformities with single-stage external fixation compared to traditional accommodative treatment.

Intramedullary beams can be used alone or in conjunction with additional internal or external fixation. Ford et al. were able to obtain an ulcer-free plantigrade foot in 84% of 25 patients using this technique, with a 46% radiographic union rate, 24% deep infection rate, and 16% amputation rate. In general, internal fixation methods are used in the absence of infection, whereas multiplanar external fixation is useful in the presence of infection or a poor soft-tissue envelope (Fig. 6.23). Stronger fixation with thicker plates combined with larger screws is required in patients with Charcot arthropathy because of their osteopenic bone. In the midfoot, a plate applied on the plantar surface takes advantage of the tension-band principle to increase compressive forces at the site of

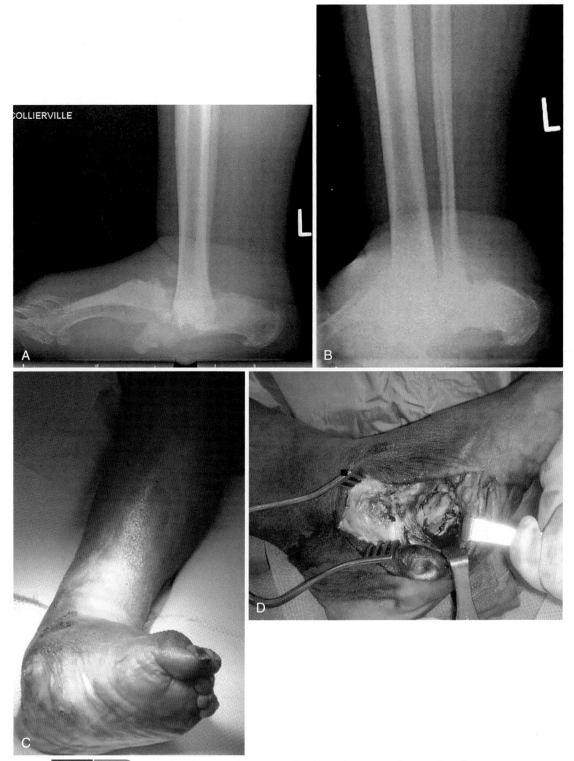

FIGURE 6.23   **A** and **B,** Charcot arthropathy of ankle with osteomyelitis. **C,** Clinical appearance of foot with medial ulcer. **D** and **E,** Removal of infected talus.

Continued

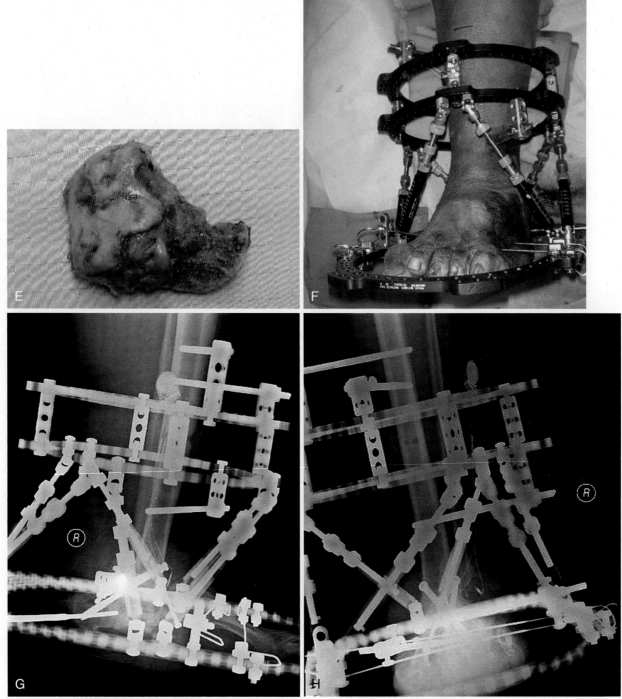

FIGURE 6.23, Cont'd   **F,** Application of hybrid external fixator. **G** and **H,** Postoperative radiographs showing hybrid fixator in place.

- Once the deformity can be accessed from medial and lateral, begin correction of the deformity. With a mature deformity, a biplanar osteotomy can be completed with a sagittal saw. In many situations, individual bones can be excised in their entirety and the foot reconstructed into a plantigrade position.
- With midfoot Charcot deformities, completely excise the medial, middle, and lateral cuneiforms, along with most

or all of the cuboid, and morcellize it into bone graft. Send cultures of tissue and bone for laboratory analysis to guide postoperative antibiotic therapy if indicated.
- Remove any residual cartilage in the remaining joints of the medial and lateral column and prepare the joint surfaces for fusion.
- Place the foot into a plantigrade position and insert Kirschner wires for provisional fixation. Place the hindfoot

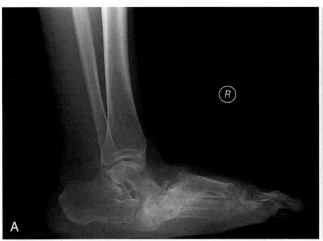
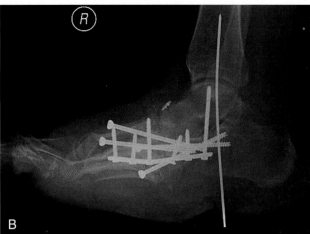

FIGURE 6.24 **A,** Charcot arthropathy of midfoot. **B,** Use of plate on plantar surface takes advantage of tension band principle to provide stronger fixation.

into neutral dorsiflexion and pin it to the tibia. A Schantz pin can be inserted into the posterior calcaneus and a T-handled chuck placed overtop and used as a handle to correct the hindfoot equinus before pinning the hindfoot to the tibia in neutral position. Now the midfoot and forefoot are pinned to the corrected hindfoot in a plantigrade position.

- At this point, determine the method of fixation. In cases of chronic ulceration with osteomyelitis, we tend to apply a static Ilizarov external fixator (Fig. 6.27). If no osteomyelitis is present or suspected, we prefer internal fixation.
- For internal fixation, we prefer intramedullary fusion bolts (solid) and/or beams (cannulated), with an additional medial locking plate with screws above and below the bolts/beams.
- Make a dorsal incision over the first metatarsophalangeal joint and retract the extensor tendon laterally. Plantarflex the joint and insert a guide pin for the fusion bolt retrograde into the first metatarsal. Confirm with fluoroscopy that the starting point is aiming into the talar head on the AP and lateral radiographs, and then advance the guide pin a short distance into the metatarsal.
- Tap the wire with a mallet so that it will find the canal of the metatarsal until it exits the base of the first metatarsal. Use fluoroscopy to confirm that the trajectory is still appropriately aimed into the talus and then advance the guide pin under power into the center of the talar head and body.
- Measure the guide pin and select the appropriately sized fusion bolt. Insert a cannulated reamer over the guide wire from the first metatarsal into the talus. With the reamer still in place, place additional Kirschner wires around the reamer in multiple planes to hold the position of the foot while the reamer and guide wire are removed.
- Insert the appropriately sized solid fusion bolt into position. Alternatively, a cannulated beam can be placed over the guide wire so that the guide wire can remain in place until fixation is fully achieved. The increased bending strength of a solid fusion bolt over a cannulated beam is attractive.

- Use AP and oblique fluoroscopy to determine if a fusion beam can be placed through the fourth or third metatarsal into the calcaneus to stabilize the lateral column. If the anatomy is suitable, place a retrograde beam through the fourth metatarsal into the calcaneus. Pack additional bone graft between the fourth metatarsal and calcaneus around the beam; the cuboid has typically been excised.
- Contour a medial locking plate to the medial column of the foot. If required, use a saw to resect additional bone to allow the stout plates to sit flush on the medial bone surface. Place variable angle locking screws in the plate above and below the bolts and beams from the medial side to capture as much bone as possible.
- Pack additional bone graft into any other bone voids. If the bases of the fifth metatarsal, calcaneus, or cuboid are prominent, excise them with a saw.
- Release the tourniquet and obtain hemostasis.
- Vancomycin powder is routinely placed into the wounds before closure with thick monofilament suture in the released tendons and deep structures. Use thin monofilament suture for the subcutaneous layer and nylon for the skin. If significant hindfoot equinus was corrected, the provisional Kirschner wire from the calcaneus to the tibia can be left in place and clipped external to the skin so that it can be removed in the clinic, typically approximately 6 weeks after surgery.

POSTOPERATIVE CARE

- The patient is placed into a posterior slab plaster splint with a stirrup. Postoperatively, sutures are removed approximately 3 to 4 weeks after surgery. The patient remains in a total contact cast with biweekly cast changes for 10 to 12 weeks. The patient is told to be non–weight bearing, but most Charcot patients have difficulty following these instructions. Weight bearing is advanced at 10 to 12 weeks after surgery in a diabetic walking boot, while accommodative inserts, a wide toe box, and an extra-depth shoe with a full-length steel shank are manufactured. This can be made into a double upright brace if required for any ankle pathology.

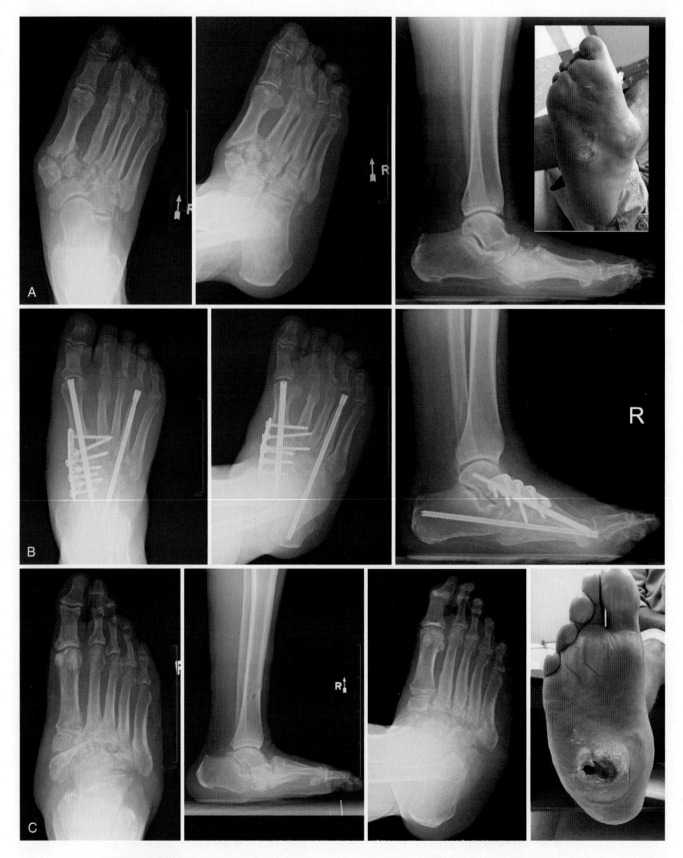

FIGURE 6.25 **A-G,** Midfoot arthrodesis with "bolts and beams" fixation for added stability.
SEE TECHNIQUE 6.2.

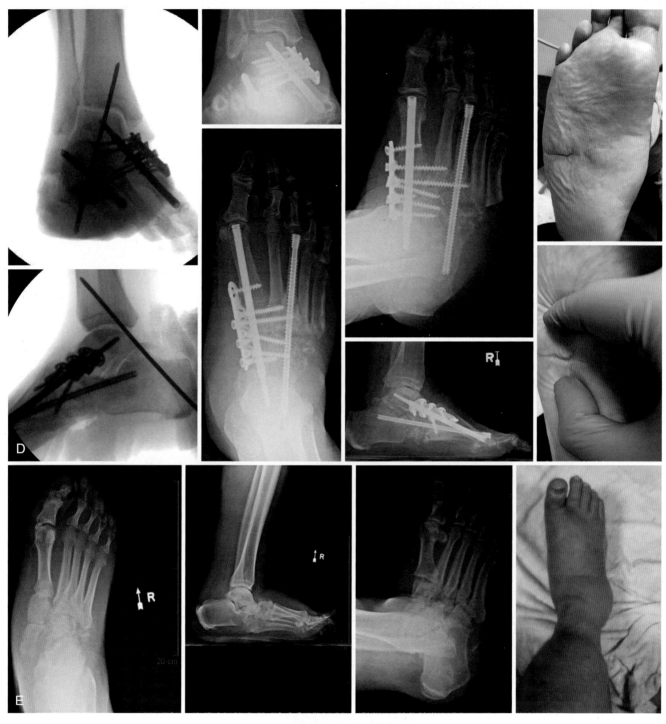

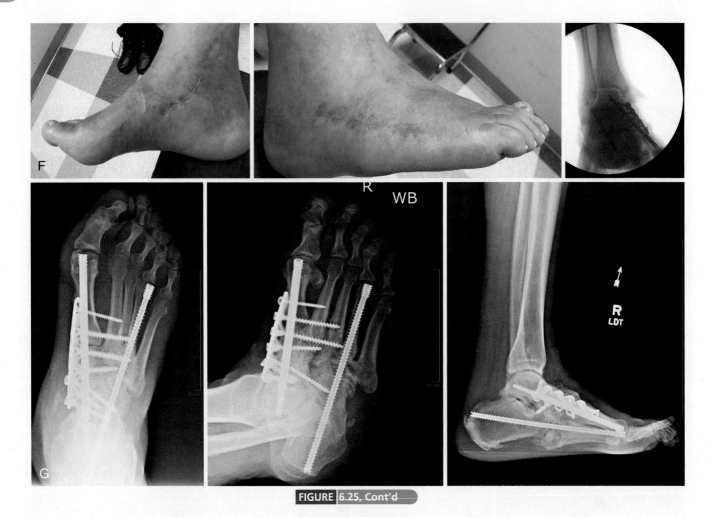

FIGURE 6.25, Cont'd

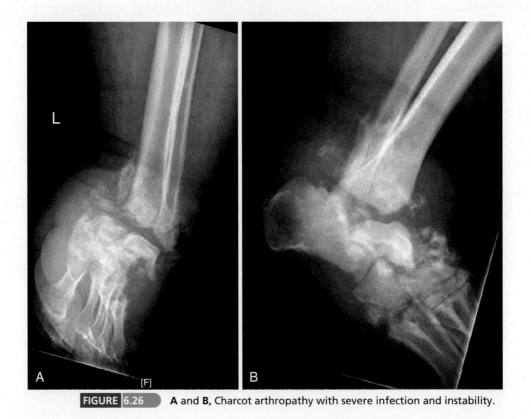

FIGURE 6.26   **A** and **B,** Charcot arthropathy with severe infection and instability.

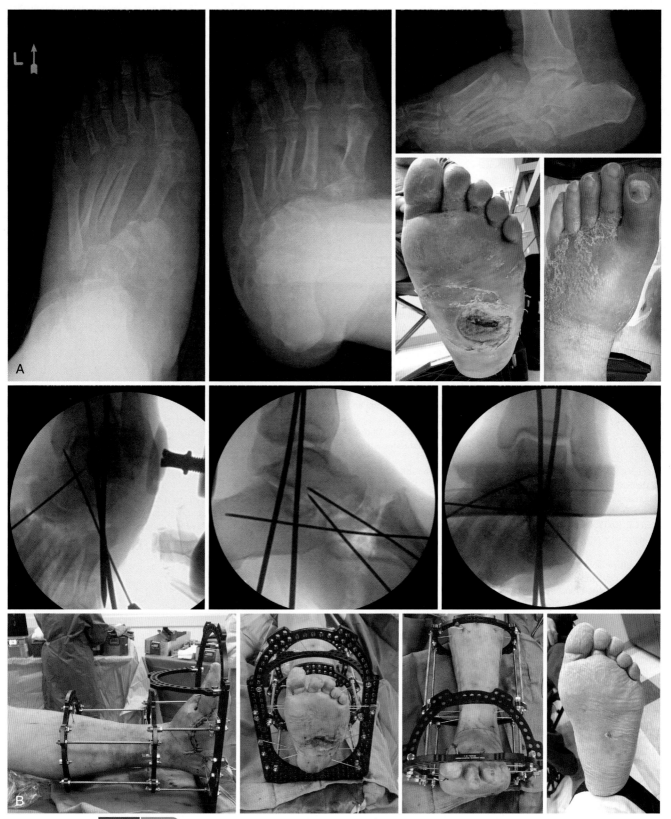

FIGURE 6.27 Static Ilizarov fixator can be used for chronic ulceration with osteomyelitis. **SEE TECHNIQUE 6.2.**

REFERENCES

Anderson JG, Bohay DR, Eller EB, Witt BL: Gastrocnemius recession, *Foot Ankle Clin* 19:767, 2014.

Anderson LB, DiPreta J: Charcot of the calcaneus, *Foot Ankle Clin North Am* 11:824, 2006.

Assal M, Ray A, Stern R: Realignment and extended fusion with use of a medial column screw for midfoot deformities secondary to diabetic neuropathy: surgical technique, *J Bone Joint Surg* 92A(Suppl 1 Pt 2):20, 2010.

Aulivola B, Craig RM: Decision making in the dysvascular lower extremity, *Foot Ankle Clin North Am* 15:391, 2010.

Baglioni P, Malik M, Okosieme OE: Acute Charcot foot, *BMJ* 344:e1397, 2012.

Bariteau J, Tenebaum S, Rabinovich A, Brodsky J: Charcot arthropathy of the foot and ankle in patients with idiopathic neuropathy, *Foot Ankle Int* 35:996, 2014.

Belatti D, Phisitkul P: Declines in lower extremity amputation in the US Medicare population, 2000-2010, *Foot Ankle Int* 34:923, 2013.

Besse JL, Leemrijse T, Deleu PA: Diabetic foot: the orthopedic surgery angle, *Orthop Traumatol Surg Res* 97:314, 2011.

Brodsky J, Bratjbord J, Coleman S: Effect of heating on the mechanical properties of insole materials, *Foot Ankle Int* 33:772, 2012.

Brown M, Tang W, Patel A, Baumhauer J: Partial foot amputation in patients with diabetic foot ulcers, *Foot Ankle Int* 33:707, 2012.

Callaghan BC, Feldman EL: Painful diabetic neuropathy: many similarly effective therapies with widely dissimilar costs, *Ann Intern Med* 161:674, 2014.

Capobianco CM, Stapleton JJ, Zgonis T: Soft tissue reconstruction pyramid in the diabetic foot, *Foot Ankle Spec* 3:241, 2010.

Cavanagh PR, Bus SA: Off-loading the diabetic foot for ulcer prevention and healing, *Plast Reconstr Surg* 127(Suppl 1):248S, 2011.

Centers for Disease Control and Prevention: *National Diabetes Statistics Report: Estimates of Diabetes and Its Burden in the United States*, Atlanta, 2014, US Department of Health and Human Services.

Chantelau EA, Grützner G: Is the Eichenholtz classification still valid for the diabetic Charcot foot? *Swiss Med Wkly* 24:144, 2014.

Chapman Z, Shuttleworth CM, Huber JW: High levels of anxiety and depression in diabetic patients with Charcot foot, *J Foot Ankle Res* 7:22, 2014.

Chen CE, Ko JY, Fong CY, Juhn RJ: Treatment of diabetic foot infection with hyperbaric oxygen therapy, *Foot Ankle Surg* 10:91, 2010.

Crawford F, Cezard G, Chappell FM: The development and validation of a multivariable prognostic model to predict foot ulceration in diabetes using a systematic review and individual patient data meta-analyses, *Diabet Med* 35:1480, 2018.

Cuttica DJ, Philbin TM: Surgery for diabetic foot infections, *Foot Ankle Clin North Am* 15:465, 2010.

Dissanayake SU, Bowling FL, Jude EB: The diabetic Charcot foot, *Curr Diabetes Rev* 8:195, 2012.

Edwards J, Stapley S: Debridement of diabetic foot ulcers, *Cochrane Database Syst Rev* 20:CD003556, 2010.

Ennis WJ, Huang ET, Gordon H: Impact of hyperbaric oxygen on more advanced Wagner grades 3 and 4 diabetic foot ulcers: matching therapy to specific wound conditions, *Adv Wound Care (New Rochelle)* 7:397, 2018.

Erdman WA, Buethe J, Bhore R, et al.: Indexing severity of diabetic foot infection with 99m Tc-WBC SPECT/CT hybrid imaging, *Diabetes Care* 35:1826, 2012.

Estess A, Marquand N, Charlton TP, Thordarson DB: Navicular subluxation as a radiographic finding in Charcot neuroarthropathy, *Foot Ankle Int* 34:1548, 2013.

Fablia E, Caravaggi C, Clerici G, et al.: Effectiveness of removable walker cast versus nonremovable fibreglass off-bearing cast in the healing of diabetic plantar foot ulcer, *Diabetes Care* 33:1419, 2010.

Ford SE, Cohen BE, Davis WH, et al.: Clinical outcomes and complications of midfoot Charcot reconstruction with intramedullary beaming, *Foot Ankle Int* 40:18, 2019.

Franklin H, Rajan M, Tseng CL, et al.: Cost of lower-limb amputation in U.S. veterans with diabetes using health services data in fiscal years 2004 and 2010, *J Rehabil Res Dev* 51:1325, 2014.

Game FL, Hinchliffe RJ, Apelqvist J, et al.: A systematic review of interventions to enhance the healing of chronic ulcers of the foot in diabetes, *Diabetes Metab Res Rev* 28(Suppl 1):119, 2012.

Grear BJ, Rabinovich A, Brodsky JW: Charcot arthropathy of the foot and ankle associated with rheumatoid arthritis, *Foot Ankle Int* 34:1541, 2013.

Gutekunst DJ, Hastings MK, Bohnert KL, et al.: Removable cast walker boots yield greater forefoot off-loading than total contact casts, *Clin Biomech (Bristol, Avon)* 26:649, 2011.

Harkin EA, Schneider AM, Murphy M, et al.: Deformity and clinical outcomes following operative correction of Charcot ankle, *Foot Ankle Int* 40:145, 2019.

Hastings MK, Johnson JE, Strube MJ, et al.: Progression of foot deformity in Charcot neuropathic osteoarthropathy, *J Bone Joint Surg Am* 95:1206, 2013.

Hastings MK, Sinacore DR, Mercer-Bolton N, et al.: Precision of foot alignment measures in Charcot arthropathy, *Foot Ankle Int* 32:867, 2011.

Johnson JE, Anderson SA: One-stage resection and pin stabilization of first metatarsophalangeal joint for chronic plantar ulcer with osteomyelitis, *Foot Ankle Int* 31:973, 2010.

Karatepe O, Eken I, Acet E, et al.: Vacuum assisted closure improves the quality of life in patients with diabetic foot, *Acta Chir Belg* 111:298, 2011.

Kearney TP, Hunt NA, Lavery LA: Safety and effectiveness of flexor tenotomies to heal toe ulcers in persons with diabetes, *Diabetes Res Clin Pract* 89:224, 2010.

Kim BS, Choi WJ, Baek MK, et al.: Limb salvage in severe diabetic foot infection, *Foot Ankle Int* 32:31, 2011.

Kranke P, Bennett MH, Martyn-St James M, et al.: Hyperbaric oxygen therapy for chronic wounds, *Cochrane Database Syst Rev* 4:CD004123, 2012.

Kroin E, Chaharbakhshi EO, Schiff A, et al.: Improvement in quality of life following operative correction of midtarsal charcot foot deformity, *Foot Ankle Int* 39:808, 2018.

Kroin E, Schiff A, Pinzur MS, et al.: Functional impairment of patients undergoing surgical correction for Charcot foot arthropathy, *Foot Ankle Int* 38:705, 2017.

La Fontaine J, Shibuya N, Sampson HW, Valderrama P: Trabecular quality and cellular characteristics of normal, diabetic, and charcot bone, *J Foot Ankle Surg* 50:648, 2011.

Lauri C, Tamminga M, Glaudemans AWJM, et al.: Detection of osteomyelitis in the diabetic foot by imaging techniques: a systematic review and meta-analysis comparing MRI, white blood cell scintigraphy, and FDG-PET, *Diabetes Care* 40:1111, 2017.

Lazaga F, Van Asten SA, Nichols A, et al.: Hybrid imaging with 99m Tc-WBC SPECT/CT to monitor the effect of therapy in diabetic foot osteomyelitis, *Int Wound J* 13:1158, 2016.

Lipsky BAS, Peters EJG, Berendt AR, et al.: Specific guidelines for the treatment of diabetic foot infections 2011, *Diabetes Metab Res Rev* 28(Suppl 1):234, 2012.

Liu Z, Dumville JC, Hinchliffe RJ, et al.: Negative pressure wound therapy for treating foot wounds in people with diabetes mellitus, *Cochrane Database Syst Rev* 10:CD010318.

Löndahl M: Hyperbaric oxygen therapy as adjunctive treatment of diabetic foot ulcers, *Med Clin North Am* 97:957, 2013.

Lovy AJ, Dowdell J, Keswani A, et al.: Nonoperative versus operative treatment of displaced ankle fractures in diabetics, *Foot Ankle Int* 38:255, 2017.

Lowery NJ, Woods JB, Armstrong DG, Wukich DK: Surgical management of Charcot neuroarthropathy of the foot and ankle: a systematic review, *Foot Ankle Int* 33:113, 2012.

Mabilleau G, Edmonds ME: Role of neuropathy on fracture healing in Charcot neuro-osteoarthropathy, *J Musculoskelet Neuronal Interact* 10:84, 2010.

Margolis DJ, Malay DS, Hoffstad OJ, et al.: *Economic burden of diabetic foot ulcers and amputations: data points #3*, Rockville MD, Agency for Healthcare Research and Quality, 2011, Available at: http://www.ncbi.nlm.nih.gov/books/NBK65152/. Accessed 5 March 2019.

Marson BA, Deshmukh SR, Grindlay DJC, et al.: A systematic review of local antibiotic devices used to improve wound healing following the surgical management of foot infections in diabetics, *Bone Joint J* 100-B:1409, 2018.

Marx RC, Mizel MS: What's new in foot and ankle surgery, *J Bone Joint Surg* 92A:512, 2010.

Mehta SK, Breitbart EA, Berberian WS, et al.: Bone and wound healing in the diabetic patients, *Foot Ankle Clin* 15:411, 2010.

Mittlmeier T, Klaue K, Haar P, Beck M: Should one consider primary surgical reconstruction in charcot arthropathy of the feet? *Clin Orthop Relat Res* 468:1002, 2010.

Myers TG, Lowery NJ, Frykberg RG, Wukich DK: Ankle and hindfoot fusions: comparison of outcomes in patients with and without diabetes, *Foot Ankle Int* 33:20, 2012.

Nickerson DS, Rader AJ: Nerve decompression after diabetic foot ulceration may protect against recurrence: a 3-year controlled, prospective analysis, *J Am Podiatr Med Assoc* 104:66, 2014.

Nouman M, Leelasamran W, Chatpun S: Effectiveness of total contact orthosis for plantar pressure redistribution in neuropathic diabetic patients during different walking activities, *Foot Ankle Int* 38:901, 2017.

Osterhoff G, Böni T, Berli M: Recurrence of acute Charcot neuropathic osteoarthropathy after conservative treatment, *Foot Ankle Int* 34:359, 2013.

Petrova NL, Dew TK, Musto RL, et al.: Inflammatory and bone turnover markers in a cross-sectional and prospective study of acute Charcot osteoarthropathy, *Diabet Med* 32:267, 2015.

Pino AE, Taghva S, Chapman C, Bowker JH: Lower-limb amputations in patients with diabetes mellitus, *Orthopedics* 34:e885, 2011.

Pinzur MS: Diabetic peripheral neuropathy, *Foot Ankle Clin* 16:345, 2011.

Pinzur MS, Gil J, Belmares J: Treatment of osteomyelitis in charcot foot with single-stage resection of infection, correction of deformity, and maintenance with ring fixation, *Foot Ankle Int* 33:1069, 2012.

Pinzur MS, Schiff AP: Deformity and clinical outcomes following operative correction of Charcot foot: a new classification with implications for treatment, *Foot Ankle Int* 39:265, 2018.

Przybylski MM, Holloway S, Vyce SD, Obando A: Diagnosing osteomyelitis in the diabetic foot: a pilot study to examine the sensitivity and specificity of Tc99m white blood cell-labelled single photon emission computed tomography/computed tomography, *Int Wound J* 13:382, 2016.

Ramanujam CL, Stepleton JJ, Zgonis T: Negative-pressure wound therapy in the management of diabetic Charcot foot and ankle wounds, *Diabet Foot Ankle* 4, 2013.

Raspovic KM, Wukich DK: Self-reported quality of life in patients with diabetes: a comparison of patients with and without Charcot neuroarthropathy, *Foot Ankle Int* 35:195, 2014.

Romanos MT, Raspovic A, Perrin BM: The reliability of toe systolic pressure and the toe brachial index in patients with diabetes, *Foot Ankle Res* 3:31, 2010.

Ross AJ, Mendicino RW, Catanzariti AR: Role of body mass index in acute charcot neuroarthropathy, *J Foot Ankle Surg* 52:6, 2013.

Ruotolo V, Di Pietro B, Giurato L, et al.: A new natural history of Charcot foot: clinical evolution and final outcome of stage O Charcot neuroarthropathy in a tertiary referral diabetic foot clinic, *Clin Nucl Med* 38:506, 2013.

Shen W, Wukich D: Orthopaedic surgery and the diabetic Charcot foot, *Med Clin North Am* 97:873, 2013.

Sohn MW, Stuck RM, Pinzur M, et al.: Lower-extremity amputation risk after charcot arthropathy and diabetic foot ulcer, *Diabetes Care* 33:98, 2010.

Stone C, Smith N: Resection arthroplasty, external fixation, and negative pressure dressing for first metatarsophalangeal joint ulcers, *Foot Ankle Int* 32:272, 2011.

Tamir E, Tamir J, Beer Y, et al.: Resection arthroplasty for resistant ulcers underlying the hallux in insensate diabetics, *Foot Ankle Int* 36:969, 2015.

Taylor SM, Johnson BL, Samies NL, et al.: Contemporary management of diabetic neuropathic foot ulceration: a study of 917 consecutively treated limbs, *J Am Coll Surg* 212:532, 2011.

Tomczak C, Beaman D, Perkins S: Combined intramedullary nail coated with antibiotic-containing cement and ring fixation for limb salvage in the severely deformed, infected, neuroarthropathic ankle, *Foot Ankle Int* 40:48, 2019.

Vaudreuil NJ, Fourman MS, Wukich DK: Limb salvage after failed initial operative management of bimalleolar ankle fractures in diabetic neuropathy, *Foot Ankle Int* 38:248, 2017.

Vouillarmet J, Morelec I, Thivolet C: Assessing diabetic foot osteomyelitis remission with white blood cell SPECT/CT imaging, *Diabet Med* 31:1093, 2014.

Wang YN, Lee K, Ledloux WR: Histomorphological evaluation of diabetic and non-diabetic plantar soft tissue, *Foot Ankle Int* 32:802, 2011.

Wukich DK: Current concepts review: diabetic foot ulcers, *Foot Ankle Int* 31:460, 2010.

Wukich K, Ahn J, Raspovic KM, et al.: Improved quality of life after trans-tibial amputation in patients with diabetes-related foot complications, *Int J Low Extrem Wounds* 16:114, 2017.

Wukich DK, Crim BE, Frykberg RG, Rosario BL: Neuropathy and poorly controlled diabetes increase the rate of surgical site infection after foot and ankle surgery, *J Bone Joint Surg Am* 96:832, 2014.

Wukich DK, Dikis JW, Monaco SJ, et al.: Topically applied vancomycin powder reduces the rate of surgical site infection in diabetic patients undergoing foot and ankle surgery, *Foot Ankle Int* 36:1017, 2015.

Wukich DK, Hobizal KB, Brooks MM: Severity of diabetic foot infection and rate of limb salvage, *Foot Ankle Int* 34:351, 2013.

Wukich DK, Joseph A, Ryan M, et al.: Outcomes of ankle fractures in patients with uncomplicated versus complicated diabetes, *Foot Ankle Int* 32:120, 2011.

Wukich DK, McMillen RL, Lowery NJ, Frykberg RG: Surgical site infections after foot and ankle surgery: a comparison of patients with and without diabetes, *Diabetes Care* 34:2211, 2011.

Wukich DK, Pearson KT: Self-reported outcomes of trans-tibial amputations for non-reconstructable Charcot neuroarthropathy in patients with diabetes: a preliminary report, *Diabet Med* 30:e87, 2013.

Wukich DK, Raspovic KM, Hobizal KB, Rosario B: Radiographic analysis of diabetic midfoot charcot neuropathy with and without midfoot ulceration, *Foot Ankle Int* 35:1108, 2014.

Wukich DK, Sung W, Wipf SA, Armstrong DG: The consequences of complacency: managing the effects of unrecognized Charcot feet, *Diabet Med* 28:195, 2011.

The complete list of references is available online at Expert Consult.com.

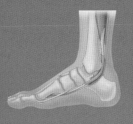

TARSAL TUNNEL SYNDROME

ANATOMY AND ETIOLOGY

The tarsal tunnel is a fibroosseous tunnel within the posteromedial ankle and hindfoot in which the tibial nerve, posterior tibial artery, accompanying veins, posterior tibial tendon, flexor digitorum longus, and flexor hallucis longus tendons pass into the foot. The flexor retinaculum acts as the roof of this tunnel and extends from the medial malleolus to the medial side of the calcaneal tuberosity. The medial distal tibia, talus, and calcaneus make up the tunnel's floor. Septa, which separate the posterior tibial, flexor digitorum longus, and flexor hallucis longus tendons, project from the fibrous roof to the calcaneus. Between the flexor digitorum longus and flexor hallucis longus tendons, the tibial nerve, posterior tibial artery, and accompanying veins pass to enter the foot.

Before reaching the foot, the tibial nerve divides into three terminal branches: the medial calcaneal nerve (MCN), lateral plantar nerve (LPN), and medial plantar nerve (MPN). Tibial nerve branch morphology varies, but typically the tibial nerve branches within the tunnel just proximal and deep to the upper edge of the abductor hallucis muscle. The MCN branches first, traveling posteriorly to the subcutaneous tissue. Coming off posteriorly, the first branch of the LPN passes under the abductor, over the medial fascia of the quadrates plantae, deep to the plantar fascia, and under the heel to the flexor digitorum brevis, where it sends a sensory branch to the central heel skin, and terminates in the abductor digiti quinti. The first branch of the LPN may branch from the main tibial nerve but still travels under the abductor with the LPN. Anterior to its first branch, the LPN passes deep to the abductor fascia and plantar fascia and over the quadrates plantae. Then it continues distally under the flexor digitorum brevis, terminating in the fourth web space and supplying a branch to the third web space. The LPN also supplies motor branches to the intrinsic muscles. Finally, the MPN innervates the abductor and continues under the abductor and the plantar fascia to form the common digital nerves, which terminate to the first, second, and third web spaces and motor branches to the interossei and lumbricals.

Historically, the term *tarsal tunnel syndrome* referred to tibial nerve entrapment beneath the flexor retinaculum. In 1987 Heimkes and colleagues first described distal tarsal tunnel syndrome, in which the distal tibial nerve branches are entrapped as they enter the foot. Together, proximal and distal tarsal tunnel syndromes encompass a spectrum of tibial nerve entrapment within the tarsal canal.

Sources of constriction beneath and adjacent to the tarsal tunnel include bone fragments, tenosynovitis, ganglia, soft-tissue encroachment in inflammatory arthritis, varicosities, neural tumors (neurilemmoma; Fig. 7.1), perineural fibrosis, tarsal coalition, and calcaneal osteotomies. Furthermore, a fixed valgus hindfoot can predispose to chronic traction neuropathy of the posterior tibial nerve or one of its branches.

CLINICAL FINDINGS AND DIAGNOSIS

Clinical symptoms of tarsal tunnel syndrome vary, and this disorder should be kept in mind whenever unexplained dysesthesias are present in the plantar aspect of the foot, in the

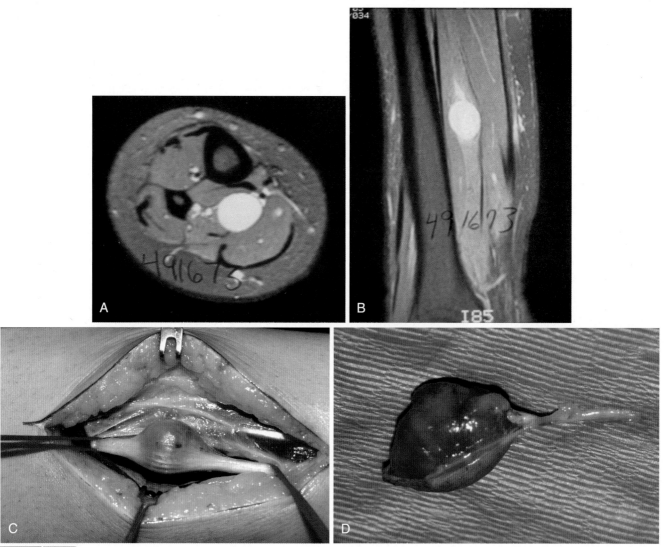

FIGURE 7.1 CT scan **(A)** and MRI **(B)** clearly identify neurilemmoma in a 40-year-old man with positive Tinel sign. Note fullness in posterior soft tissues. Gross specimen: unsectioned **(C)** and sectioned **(D)**. Microscopically, mass was neurilemmoma. Although they are nerve sheath tumors, some neurilemmomas cannot be removed without excision of nerve branch.

toes, or over the medial distal calf (Valleix phenomenon). Symptoms may be similar to those of plantar fasciitis, but unlike plantar fasciitis, nerve entrapment symptoms do not resolve quickly. Making the diagnosis difficult, typical neurogenic symptoms are not always present and symptoms may be present at night, during exercise, or at rest. Symptoms can be confined to the lateral plantar nerve, medial plantar nerve, or medial calcaneal nerve.

A thorough, detailed examination, aided with a good patient history, improves diagnostic accuracy. Careful examination for subtle sensory abnormalities or differences in temperature, sweating pattern, and skin abnormalities may lead to the correct diagnosis. Although a common complaint, sensory abnormalities often are difficult to detect. Dryness and scaliness of the skin may be present over *only* the lateral or medial plantar nerve distribution. Atrophy of the abductor hallucis, abductor digiti minimi, or both, often a difficult finding to detect, may be obvious compared with the asymptomatic foot. Point tenderness of the medial heel in the soft spot at the lower edge of the abductor hallucis may indicate distal entrapment of the tibial branches, and a Tinel sign over the flexor retinaculum may indicate proximal entrapment.

Abouelela and Zohiery described a "triple compression test" for diagnosing tarsal tunnel syndrome: the ankle is plantarflexed and the foot is inverted (increasing the tarsal tunnel compartment pressures), then digital compression is applied over the tibial nerve. Fifty patients with symptoms suggestive of tarsal tunnel syndrome and 40 asymptomatic patients were tested, and the tarsal tunnel diagnosis was confirmed with electrophysiologic testing. Test sensitivity was 86% and specificity was 100%.

Kinoshita et al. described another provocative maneuver to elicit symptoms suggesting tarsal tunnel syndrome. The dorsiflexion-eversion test is done by maximally everting and dorsiflexing the ankle passively, while all the metatarsophalangeal joints also are maximally dorsiflexed. This position is held for 5 to 10 seconds. In a comparison of 100 feet in asymptomatic volunteers with 44 feet in symptomatic patients, the authors found that the patients' symptoms were exacerbated in 36 of the 44 feet. None of the feet in the control group exhibited symptoms with this maneuver. After release of the tarsal tunnel, the dorsiflexion-eversion test elicited tarsal tunnel symptoms in only three feet, all of which had calcaneal fractures.

Imaging modalities can assist the evaluation of tarsal tunnel syndrome. Plain radiographs demonstrate osseous abnormalities (e.g., fractures or talocalcaneal coalitions) that may contribute to tarsal tunnel symptoms. The use of ultrasound in the evaluation of tarsal tunnel has been reported; however, we prefer MRI because of the improved detail of the tarsal contents. MRI has been shown to identify the cause of the tarsal tunnel syndrome in up to 88% of patients. More important, MRI aids with surgical planning by providing detailed characteristics and location of space-occupying lesions.

Electrodiagnostic testing is indicated for any patient suspected of having compression of the tibial nerve beneath the flexor retinaculum. In an evidence-based review of the usefulness of electrodiagnostic testing in suspected tarsal tunnel syndrome, Patel et al. recommended the use of nerve conduction studies but found insufficient data to recommend the use of electromyography. Electrical studies also are useful in identifying an unsuspected peripheral neuropathy suggestive of a systemic, rather than localized, nerve injury. Despite evidence demonstrating their usefulness, electrodiagnostic studies can be normal in patients with tarsal tunnel syndrome, and negative electrodiagnostic testing does not provide a contraindication for surgery.

TREATMENT

Initially, 6 to 12 weeks of ankle immobilization in a night splint, antiinflammatory agents, and a wide, cushioned, comfortable shoe are recommended. If distal tarsal tunnel syndrome is suspected, an orthosis with a relief channel within the medial arch may be effective; a standard orthosis with a longitudinal arch may worsen symptoms. Caution is recommended in advising surgical treatment of tarsal tunnel syndrome in patients who are older (60 to 80 years old), have posttraumatic scarring within the tarsal canal, have no objective cause for symptoms (idiopathic), and those with protracted psychiatric illness. Symptoms caused by space-occupying lesions should be treated surgically. When conservative treatment fails, surgical treatment is indicated.

If surgical treatment is indicated, the tibial nerve and its branches must be meticulously exposed and unroofed. The release must include incision of 1 to 2 cm of the deep fascia above the proximal edge of the flexor retinaculum and following the medial and lateral plantar nerves beneath the abductor hallucis because one or both of these branches may pass through fascial slings as they enter the plantar surface of the foot. The dissection is refined by the use of magnification, a tourniquet, small dissecting scissors, and nontoothed forceps. Space-occupying lesions should be excised and alignment disorders corrected.

Patients with definite lesions generally respond better to surgical decompression than those with idiopathic or traumatic etiologies. With no identifiable cause, however, the relief of symptoms is less predictable, with approximately 25% of patients achieving little or no relief. Rarely, symptoms may even worsen after surgical release. Symptom duration of less than 1 year also has been cited as a predictor of better outcomes. There are few outcome studies of tarsal tunnel release, and the evidence generally is level IV or V.

Even closer scrutiny of the clinical factors that can influence a surgical decision is required for revision tarsal tunnel release because diagnosing an "inadequate release" often is difficult, even with knowledge of the original procedure. Failures can occur from incorrect diagnosis, inadequate release, poor technique, or a combination of any of these. To minimize the probability of inadequate release, a complete release of the tibial nerve and its branches is recommended, except in the case of a space-occupying lesion, for which a smaller, lesion-specific release is acceptable. Nerve scarring is likely in patients who had relief after their initial surgery but then experienced a slow return of symptoms. Neurolysis with saphenous vein or collagen wrapping to prevent nerve adherence has been recommended in this situation. Worsening symptoms immediately after surgery may indicate an iatrogenic nerve injury, from which a painful neuroma may develop. Despite careful attention to patient history and physical examination findings, combined with meticulous surgical technique, the outcomes of revision tarsal tunnel release are unpredictable, and appropriate counseling and caution are recommended before treatment.

TARSAL TUNNEL RELEASE

TECHNIQUE 7.1

- Extend the incision from 1 cm plantar to the navicular tuberosity in a proximal direction, bisecting the area between the medial malleolus and the medial aspect of the tuberosity of the calcaneus, and ending 1 cm anterior to the Achilles tendon. With the foot in the gravity equinus position, this is almost a straight line (Fig. 7.2A). Do not undermine the incision.
- Coagulate or tie the superficial veins connecting the plantar and saphenous systems and deepen the incision through the investing fascia of the calf proximally and the medial side of the foot distally. This allows identification of the proximal and distal (posterior and anterior) borders of the flexor retinaculum and the neurovascular bundle before the bundle disappears beneath the retinaculum.
- Occasionally, the nerve is enlarged at the upper border of the retinaculum. Release the retinaculum from a proximal to a distal direction until the muscle fibers of the abductor hallucis are reached.
- Sometimes a medial calcaneal branch penetrates the retinaculum, and care must be taken to avoid severing one or more branches of this nerve (medial calcaneal) to prevent a painful neuroma (Fig. 7.2B).

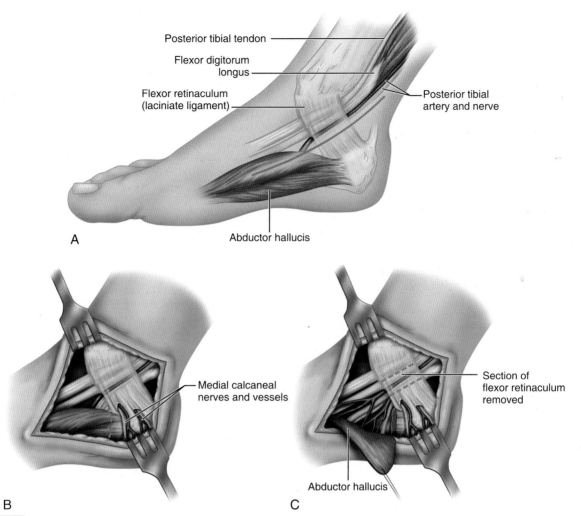

Posterior tibial tendon

Flexor digitorum longus

Flexor retinaculum (laciniate ligament)

Posterior tibial artery and nerve

Abductor hallucis

A

Medial calcaneal nerves and vessels

Section of flexor retinaculum removed

Abductor hallucis

B

C

FIGURE 7.2 Tarsal tunnel release. **A,** Skin incision. **B,** Note branches of medial calcaneal nerve and artery penetrating retinaculum. *Dashed line* indicates incision for reflecting abductor hallucis muscle. **C,** Abductor hallucis is reflected plantarward, and section of flexor retinaculum to be removed is outlined. **SEE TECHNIQUE 7.1.**

■ The tibial nerve divides beneath the flexor retinaculum into the medial and lateral plantar branches. The medial calcaneal branch may arise from the main tibial nerve or its lateral plantar branch (Fig. 7.3A and B). The tibial nerve bifurcates into its medial and lateral components beneath the laciniate ligament in most individuals. When the medial and lateral plantar nerves reach the medial border of the abductor hallucis, they turn plantarward and lateral deep to this muscle.

■ Trace each nerve well distal to the inferior edge of the flexor retinaculum until it is certain that no tethering by the fascial origin of the abductor hallucis exists. This is made easier by releasing part of the origin of the abductor hallucis.

■ If the epineurium appears unequally thickened, it should be incised.

■ Remove a section of the flexor retinaculum over the neurovascular bundle (Fig. 7.2C).

■ Remove the tourniquet and secure hemostasis before closing the wound (skin and subcutaneous tissue only). Apply a sterile compression dressing.

■ Apply a short leg posterior splint to "rest" the wound while the incision is in the initial stages of healing (10 to 14 days).

POSTOPERATIVE CARE A bulky compression dressing and a short leg plaster splint are applied with the foot in mild equinovarus for 10 to 14 days. After sutures are removed, a walking boot for 2 to 4 weeks allows the patient to bear weight to tolerance. Ankle edema persisting for many weeks is common if the dissection has been extensive, and complete recovery may require 6 to 12 months.

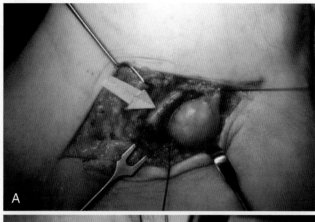

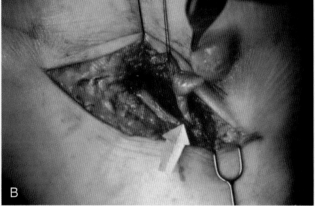

FIGURE 7.3 **A and B,** *Arrow* points to lateral plantar nerve. Tumor involves medial calcaneal branch of nerve. Tumor was resectable, leaving most of this branch intact. **SEE TECHNIQUE 7.1.**

ANTERIOR TARSAL TUNNEL SYNDROME (DEEP PERONEAL NERVE ENTRAPMENT)

The anterior tarsal tunnel syndrome, denoting entrapment of the deep peroneal nerve beneath the inferior extensor retinaculum, also has been described (Fig. 7.4). The symptoms include pain and dysesthesias over the dorsum of the foot and first web space. Examination demonstrates decreased touch and pinprick in the first web space, a possible Tinel sign over the deep peroneal nerve beneath the inferior extensor retinaculum, and rarely, atrophy of the extensor digitorum brevis muscle if the motor branch of the deep peroneal nerve arises more distally than normal (i.e., distal and deep to the inferior extensor retinaculum). Proximally radiating dysesthesias into the anterior compartment of the leg also may occur. The examination should include the assessment of extensor digitorum brevis and extensor hallucis brevis muscles, and sensation should be compared with that of the opposite, asymptomatic foot. If bilateral anterior tarsal tunnel syndrome is present, a diffuse peripheral neuropathy must be suspected.

Mann and Baxter stated that this syndrome most commonly occurs in runners or in patients with dorsal osteophytes at the ankle, midtarsal, or metatarsocuneiform articulation. The most common areas of nerve entrapment are shown in Fig. 7.5. Extensor hallucis brevis hypertrophy in ballet dancers, tight-fitting shoes, hooking the feet under a bar when doing sit-ups, and ganglion cysts, with or without the presence of traumatic osteophytes, also have been reported as causes.

Electrical studies may confirm the diagnosis with fibrillations, positive sharp waves, and reduced motor action potentials in the extensor digitorum brevis and increased distal motor and sensory latencies in the presence of a normal nerve conduction velocity in the deep peroneal nerve from the fibular neck to the ankle. The entrapment often occurs distal to the motor branch to the extensor digitorum brevis.

Successful outcomes have been reported with both operative and nonoperative treatments. Similar to tarsal tunnel syndrome, nonoperative management is the first line of therapy, with the exception that space-occupying lesions can be removed before an extensive course of nonoperative management. Conservative treatment consists of immobilization, identification and removal of external pressure etiologies (e.g., overly tightened shoelaces), neurologics (e.g., gabapentin), and occasional corticosteroid injections. If conservative treatment fails, surgical management is indicated; several small studies have reported good results in 80% to 100% of patients after surgical decompression for anterior tarsal tunnel syndrome. Surgical management includes removing the offending structures, such as resecting impinging osteophytes, excising ganglion cysts, and partial release of the extensor retinaculum or extensor hallucis brevis tendon as needed for decompression. Surgical release most commonly includes an open approach, but authors have described success with endoscopic techniques as well.

ANTERIOR TARSAL TUNNEL RELEASE

TECHNIQUE 7.2

(MANN)

- Before surgery, locate the area of compression at the anterior ankle joint or the dorsal talonavicular joint.
- Make a longitudinal incision 5 to 7 cm long over the dorsum of the foot from the talonavicular joint to the first intermetatarsal space.
- Identify the deep peroneal nerve and dorsalis pedis artery. Identify the deep peroneal nerve as it courses beneath the extensor hallucis brevis and release the constricting portion of the inferior extensor retinaculum.
- Mann and Baxter recommend releasing only the portion of the retinaculum that seems to be constricting the nerve.
- Remove any underlying lesion, such as a ganglion cyst or osteophyte.

POSTOPERATIVE CARE The patient is placed in a cast or removable walking boot and begins weight bearing to tolerance. Once the incision has healed and sutures are removed after 2 weeks, then the patient can resume noncompressive footwear and physical activity as pain and swelling allow.

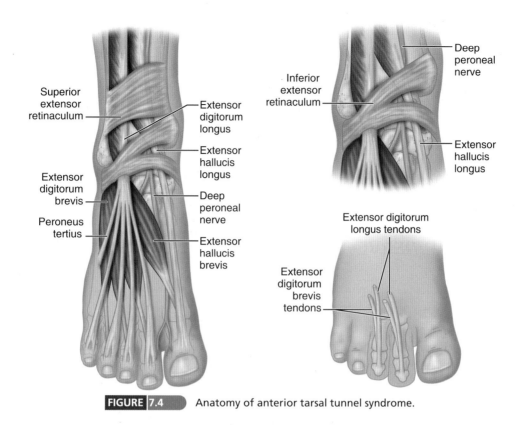

Superior extensor retinaculum

Extensor digitorum longus

Extensor hallucis longus

Extensor digitorum brevis

Peroneus tertius

Deep peroneal nerve

Extensor hallucis brevis

Inferior extensor retinaculum

Deep peroneal nerve

Extensor hallucis longus

Extensor digitorum longus tendons

Extensor digitorum brevis tendons

FIGURE 7.4 Anatomy of anterior tarsal tunnel syndrome.

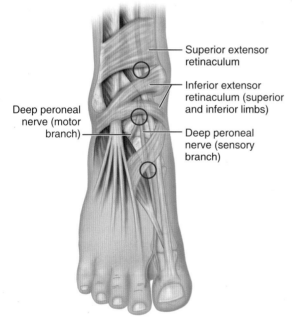

Deep peroneal nerve (motor branch)

Superior extensor retinaculum

Inferior extensor retinaculum (superior and inferior limbs)

Deep peroneal nerve (sensory branch)

FIGURE 7.5 Deep peroneal nerve entrapment. *Circles* denote areas of impingement.

FIRST BRANCH OF LATERAL PLANTAR NERVE ENTRAPMENT

Arising posteriorly off the LPN, the first branch of the LPN passes deep to the abductor hallucis, over the medial fascia of the quadratus plantae, deep to the plantar fascia, and under the calcaneus to the flexor digitorum brevis, terminating in the abductor digiti quinti (ADQ). Entrapment occurs between the lateral border of the abductor hallucis and the medial border of the quadratus

plantae, producing chronic heel pain symptoms. Distinguishing this pathologic process from plantar fasciitis can be difficult, and the two entities may coexist. Electrodiagnostic studies can help with the diagnosis. Advanced imaging may show atrophy of the ADQ, but this atrophy commonly occurs in asymptomatic patients, rendering this finding nonspecific. Patients will have tenderness over the first branch of LPN deep to the abductor hallucis, which is in close proximity to plantar fascia origin. Unlike proximal tarsal tunnel symptoms, patients do not typically complain of numbness. Most patients improve with nonoperative treatment, consisting of heel cups, nonsteroidal antiinflammatory drugs, rest, ice, physical therapy, or steroid injections. However, for those with persistent symptoms, an open or endoscopic release is described, with 83% to 88% good to excellent results.

FIRST BRANCH OF LATERAL PLANTAR NERVE RELEASE AND PARTIAL PLANTAR FASCIA RELEASE

TECHNIQUE 7.3

(BAXTER, PFEFFER, WATSON ET AL.)

- Starting distal to the medial malleolus but in line with its posterior border, extend a 4-cm oblique incision distally over the proximal abductor hallucis muscle.
- Carry the dissection down to the superficial fascia overlying the abductor hallucis muscle. Divide this superficial fascia and retract the muscle belly distally to allow exposure of the deep abductor fascia.
- Decompressing the nerve, release the deep fascia from proximal to plantar to the level of the plantar fascia.

- Identify the plantar fascia and transect the medial half of its width under direct vision.
- Close the wound with interrupted nylon sutures and apply a short leg splint.

POSTOPERATIVE CARE To minimize incisional complications, patients should remain non–weight bearing for 2 weeks. Once the sutures are removed, patients can weight bear as tolerated with a walking boot for another 4 weeks. After weaning out of the boot, supportive footwear is recommended.

MEDIAL PLANTAR NERVE ENTRAPMENT

The MPN typically arises within the tarsal tunnel as the anterior division of the tibial nerve. Within the tarsal tunnel, the MPN runs between the tunnels for the flexor hallucis longus laterally and flexor digitorum longus anteromedially. Passing deep to the abductor hallucis, it enters the plantar foot posterior and plantar to the flexor digitorum longus tendon, continuing superficial (plantar) to that tendon but deep to an interfascicular septum, and connecting the deep abductor fascia to the upper border of the flexor accessorious immediately plantar to the flexor hallucis longus tunnel. At the knot of Henry, the nerve passes plantar (superficial) to the flexor digitorum longus and flexor hallucis longus. At the base of the first metatarsal, the nerve divides into its terminal medial and lateral branches. The MPN provides sensation to the medial plantar foot, plantar first through third toes, and plantar medial half of the fourth toe, and provides motor innervation to the abductor hallucis, flexor hallucis brevis, flexor digitorum brevis, and first lumbrical muscles. Limited literature and reports describe injury to the MPN. Historically, entrapment of this nerve was reported in runners, hence the term *jogger's foot*. Stenosis typically occurs within the knot of Henry. Symptoms consist of medial arch pain and dysesthesias that radiate distally into the medial three toes. Excessive valgus and firm orthotics that apply pressure into the arch may exacerbate symptoms. Treatment consists of eliminating the offending shoes or orthotics, rest, ice, nonsteroidal antiinflammatory drugs, and steroid injection. Only after failure of conservative treatment is surgical release indicated.

SURAL NERVE ENTRAPMENT

The sural nerve is most commonly formed by the medial sural nerve only, a branch of the tibial nerve; but many variations frequently occur, as the nerve is composed of the medial sural and an anastomotic branch from the lateral sural or common peroneal nerve. Knowledge of these anatomic variations is important when evaluating and treating sural nerve pathology. The nerve provides sensory input to the posterior lateral leg and hindfoot, with variable extension to the lateral forefoot. Injury can occur from inversion of the ankle, instability of the ankle, fractures, ganglion cysts, and, most commonly, iatrogenic trauma. Treatment includes identifying and removing (if possible) the source of injury. Medications, including nonsteroidal antiinflammatories, steroid dose packs, or antiepileptic medications, such as gabapentin or pregabalin, can improve symptoms. Nerve blocks also may be diagnostic and therapeutic. If symptoms persist despite conservative treatment, then successful treatment with surgical decompression or excision has been described. Recently, Lans et al. retrospectively reviewed 49 patients with surgically excised sural neuromas. Consistent with previous reports, 63% of patients had pain improvement, and an additional 8% had improvement after a second surgery. Hence, surgical treatment is beneficial, but patients must be warned of the 20% to 30% risk for persistent neuropathic pain.

SUPERFICIAL PERONEAL NERVE ENTRAPMENT

Branching from the common peroneal nerve is the superficial peroneal nerve, which runs within the anterolateral leg compartment, innervating the peroneal longus and peroneal brevis. It exits through deep fascia at the distal third of the leg, where it divides into the medial and intermediate dorsal cutaneous nerve branches, supplying sensation to the dorsal foot. The path of the nerve varies significantly, traveling through the lateral leg compartment only, the anterior leg compartment only, or both compartments. Passing through the fascia creates a site for entrapment. This site of stenosis is further exacerbated by muscle hypertrophy, displaced fractures, direct trauma, mass effect, edema, and inversion injuries. Patients describe vague pain or paresthesia that is worsened by activity over the dorsum of distal third of the leg and foot. At the site of entrapment, examination often reveals a positive Tinel sign associated with a fascial defect. To prevent placing the nerve under tension, conservative treatment involves immobilization and limiting inversion and plantar flexion. Corticosteroid injections can be diagnostic and therapeutic. If conservative treatment fails, then surgical treatment involves release of the stenosing fascia.

INTERDIGITAL NEUROMA

Commonly known by its eponym, Morton's neuroma, the interdigital neuroma is an entrapment of the interdigital nerve near the distal edge of the transverse metatarsal ligament. It occurs most commonly in the third web space, followed by the second web space. Rarely does it involve other web spaces. Metatarsophalangeal joint instability and metatarsalgia must be carefully considered in the working diagnosis.

The true etiology of this entrapment remains controversial. The unique anatomy of the third web space has been cited as a factor contributing to the entrapment. Unique to the third web space, a communicating branch from the common digital branch of the LPN joins the common digital branch from the MPN to innervate the third web space (Fig. 7.6). Because of this communicating branch, the common digital nerve to the third web space has been suggested to be thicker and more likely to be compressed against the unyielding transverse intermetatarsal ligament dorsal to it. Levitsky et al., however, found this communicating branch to be absent in 73% of cadaver feet, and neuromas were identified in almost equal distribution between the second and third web. Other anatomic theories include increased mobility of the fourth tarsometatarsal joint, but this mobility would

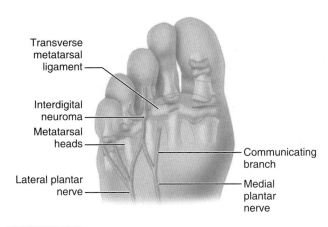

FIGURE 7.6 Most common anatomic location of interdigital neuroma.

Labels: Transverse metatarsal ligament; Interdigital neuroma; Metatarsal heads; Lateral plantar nerve; Communicating branch; Medial plantar nerve

not explain the incidence in the second web space. Thus the etiology remains debatable, and opinions even differ in regard to the cellular pathologic processes in neuroma specimens.

In a strict sense, the term *neuroma* is incorrect because the proliferation of axons seen in a traumatic neuroma is absent. Instead, the enlargement results from the deposition of hyaline and collagenous material, making this pathologic process most likely degenerative rather than proliferative. The repetitive trauma against the deep transverse intermetatarsal ligament is the most likely source for the degenerative process, but even this is uncertain. Repetitive microtrauma, perineural fibrosis, ischemia from vasa nervorum occlusion, and endoneural edema are likely responsible for the symptoms of interdigital neuroma. Because this is not a proliferative process, the term *interdigital neuritis* or *neuralgia,* rather than *interdigital neuroma,* has been suggested.

PATHOLOGIC FINDINGS

The following list summarizes reported pathologic findings:
- Perineural fibrosis (Fig. 7.7A)
- Increased number of intrafascicular arterioles with thickened and hyalinized walls caused by multiple layers of basement membranes (Fig. 7.7B). Demyelinization and degeneration of nerve fibers with a decrease in the number of axis cylinders (Fig. 7.7C)
- Endoneural edema
- Absence of inflammatory changes
- Frequent presence of bursal tissue accompanying the specimen (Fig. 7.7D)

SIGNS AND SYMPTOMS

The primary symptom of interdigital neuroma is pain, which is most often located in the region of the third metatarsal head, and frequently described as burning, aching, or cramping. Trauma may initiate the symptoms, and the duration of pain varies from a few weeks to many years. It is increased with walking and relieved by rest, removing the shoe, or massaging the forefoot. In exploring other possible pain sources, careful examination should include a Lachman test of the metatarsophalangeal joint, dorsal palpation, and palpation under the metatarsal head versus the web space to discern pain etiology. If the tenderness is mostly in the web space and not under the plantar aspect of the proximal phalangeal base or the dorsolateral aspect of the second metatarsophalangeal joint, a

neuroma is likely. The palpable and audible click associated with reproducing the patient's pain is helpful for diagnosis (Mulder's click). This click frequently is present without pain on the opposite asymptomatic foot. Hence, the click alone is not diagnostic. Simulating weight bearing in narrow shoes can reproduce symptoms. Pressure is placed under the web space with the thumb dorsal followed by gentle medial-to-lateral squeezing of the forefoot by the examiner's other hand. Repeating this maneuver followed by relaxation will reproduce painful clicking of the neuroma (Fig. 7.8). Subjective numbness of the toes of the involved interspace is common, but objective signs of decreased sensibility are less common. Women are more commonly affected than men (8:1), and the condition usually is unilateral. The use of sensory action potentials to confirm the diagnosis objectively has yielded variable results. Diagnostic injections have been shown to extravasate into the adjacent web space, making them less sensitive for accurate diagnosis. Although MRI and sonography have been reported for diagnosing interdigital neuroma, they have been shown to be of limited value, so the diagnosis of interdigital neuroma is still a clinical one.

TREATMENT

Numerous reports have confirmed the efficacy of neuroma excision in the third web space. The results of nonoperative treatment, consisting of metatarsal bars or pads, local injection of a steroid preparation into the affected web space, and wide toe box shoes, have been unpredictable but successful often enough to warrant at least a trial period.

In a level 1 prospective, randomized study, Thomson et al. found that at 3-month follow-up, corticosteroid injections produced significantly improved visual analog scale (VAS) scores compared to the control group. However, Lizano-Díez et al. found no difference between corticosteroid with anesthetic injections and anesthetic injection alone at 3 and 6 months. Roughly half of the patients still requested surgical excision. Furthermore, caution is advised with the repetitive use of steroids, which can cause atrophy of the plantar fat pad or disruption of the adjacent joint capsule with resultant toe deviation.

Through nerve sclerosis, alcohol injections have been reported to improve symptoms in short-term follow-up, but Gurdezi et al. found no improvement at long-term follow-up (average, 61 months) in a study of 45 patients: only 29% reported improvement and 36% proceeded with surgical excision. Furthermore, 12 of the 45 patients had minor complications. Epinosa et al. found similar results: only 22% of their 32 patients reported improvement after alcohol-sclerosing injections. A recent systematic review found insufficient high-quality evidence supporting the use of alcohol injections for interdigital neuromas. Because of these poor or inconclusive results, we do not use sclerosing agents for neuroma treatment.

Other than corticosteroid and alcohol injections, less common nonsurgical treatments also have been described through small series. Reported treatments include extracorporeal shockwave therapy (ECSWT), radiofrequency ablation, cryoneurolysis, hyaluronic acid injections, and capsaicin injections. The sparse literature has not validated the safety and efficacy of these alternative modalities.

Surgical excision remains the most predictable management for successful treatment of an interdigital neuroma;

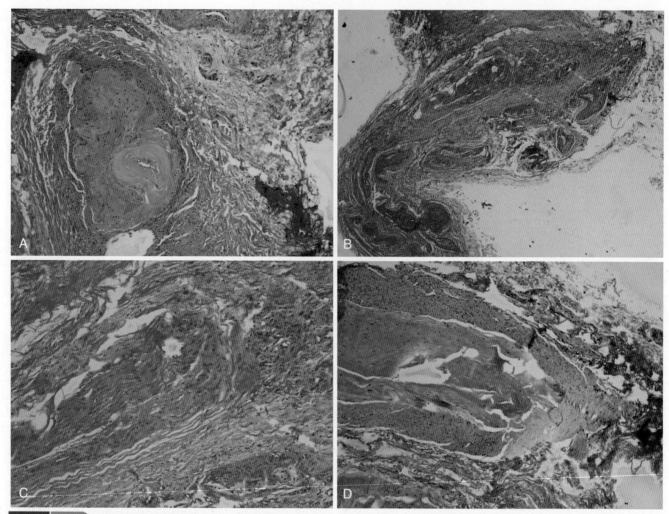

FIGURE 7.7 Pathologic findings of interdigital neuroma. **A,** Interdigital nerve is greatly thickened by perineural fibrous tissue (hematoxylin and eosin stain). **B,** Vessels in region often show degenerative changes such as fraying and duplication of internal elastic lamina (Verhoeff-van Gieson stain). **C,** Some axons are missing, and others show degenerative changes (Bielschowsky stain). **D,** Small bursa may be found in region (hematoxylin and eosin stain). (Courtesy of Bruce Webber, MD.)

however, an accurate diagnosis and patient counseling are critical to ensure optimal outcomes. In most of the series reported, 80% to 95% of the patients are completely asymptomatic and pleased with the result of surgery. However, Mann and Reynolds reported that 65% of patients still noted some local plantar tenderness after surgery, and 20% subjectively rated their result as less than a 50% improvement in symptoms. Another study reported limitation in footwear in 70% of patients, and Womack et al. found that the long-term outcomes of neuroma excision were not as successful as previously reported. More recently, Kasparek and Schneider reported that 76% of 98 feet had an excellent or good result an average of 15 years after neuroma excision. Detailed preoperative examination and careful patient selection for surgery are recommended. In addition, the patient must be informed before surgery that some symptoms may remain after surgery. The surgeon should look carefully for other causes of metatarsalgia that might coexist in a patient with an interdigital neuroma and should explain that any symptoms other than those caused by the interdigital neuroma would not be improved by its excision.

Opinions vary as to whether excision is the operative treatment of choice for interdigital neuroma. Gauthier performed epineural neurolysis using a longitudinal dorsal approach. The deep transverse intermetatarsal ligament was released to facilitate neurolysis. Overall, 28% of the patients either were unimproved or had enough continued symptoms to warrant further treatment. We have had no experience with this technique. Furthermore, the division of the deep transverse intermetatarsal ligament during this procedure is controversial. Whether its division results in a "dropped" metatarsal or splaying of the forefoot remains uncertain. Through the dorsal approach, the nerve is better exposed in its proximal portion if the ligament is divided. Through the plantar approach, the ligament does not impair exposure of the neuroma in its proximal portion and usually is left intact.

The choice of a dorsal or plantar incision for removing a neuroma probably is determined by the surgeon's training. Either approach can be satisfactory, but patients with a plantar incision complain of soreness around the wound for many weeks, which gradually resolves. Each approach has advantages and disadvantages. For a recurrent interdigital neuroma, a plantar approach is recommended because the exposure is excellent. With a dorsal approach, identifying the stump of the neuroma amid the scar tissue can be difficult.

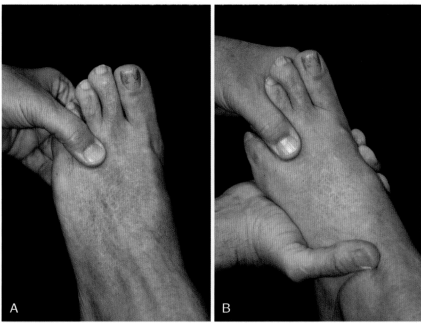

FIGURE 7.8 **A,** Digital manipulation with pressure applied just proximal to metatarsal heads by squeezing forefoot between index finger and thumb. **B,** Simultaneous compression of forefoot with one hand and compression of web space with two fingers of opposite hand.

The plantar approach allows the surgeon to identify the nerve in normal tissue and dissect it out to the involved tissue. Dorsal and plantar longitudinal approaches were compared in one study that assessed sensory loss, number of sick leave weeks, and further treatments. The overall patient satisfaction was not significantly different between the two approaches. Infection, missed nerves, and nerve stump neuroma occurred in the dorsal group, and three minor (2 × 3 mm) intraincisional keratoses occurred in the plantar group. More recently, Nery et al. reported 89% good results, 7% fair results, and 4% poor results at 7-year follow-up of 168 patients who had neuroma excision through a plantar incision.

Regardless of the approach, the nerve is transected as far proximally as the incision allows, but care must be taken not to injure the common digital branches to the second or fourth web spaces. Several plantarly directed nerve branches run from the common digital nerve into the forefoot pad. They are found in the highest concentration in the distal aspect of the common digital nerve, just proximal to its bifurcation into the proper branches. If the nerve is not transected well proximal to the deep transverse intermetatarsal ligament, these plantarly directed nerve fibers can tether or prevent retraction of the common digital nerve, leading to its adherence near the metatarsal head and causing recurring symptoms. Careful localization of the most tender area, and presumably the neuroma stump, before surgery helps the surgeon to locate the nerve during the dissection. Mann recommended the dorsal approach for a recurrent neuroma and for the original excision.

The results of surgery for "recurrent" interdigital neuroma or resection of a neuroma stump are not as predictably satisfactory as the results of primary resection. Forty-three percent of patients in one study were dissatisfied with their clinical outcome or had major reservations about the efficacy of the procedure. Revision surgery for neuroma excision should be approached cautiously, and the patient should be counseled regarding the possibility of an unsatisfactory result after revision surgery for interdigital neuroma.

We currently do not use endoscopy for decompression (release of the transverse metatarsal ligament) or excision of an interdigital neuroma because of the lack of evidence regarding its efficacy and safety. However, Kubota et al. and Lui have reported encouraging case reports and techniques.

INTERDIGITAL NEUROMA EXCISION (DORSAL)

TECHNIQUE 7.4

(AMIS)
- Make a dorsal longitudinal incision 3 to 4 cm proximal to the web and extend it distally, ending just proximal to the web space. It is important not to follow the extensor tendons because they take a more lateral direction. The incision, when properly made, is slightly oblique and medial in relation to the course of the extensor tendons.
- Deepen the dissection and retract the dorsal sensory nerves to the side of least resistance.
- Proximally identify the dorsal interosseous fascia. Follow the dorsal interosseous fascia and muscle distally directly to the bursa overlying the intermetatarsal ligament. Open the bursa and identify the intermetatarsal ligament.
- Bluntly dissect proximally between the third and fourth metatarsals, retracting the corresponding dorsal interosseous muscle medially and opening the web space for better exposure proximally.

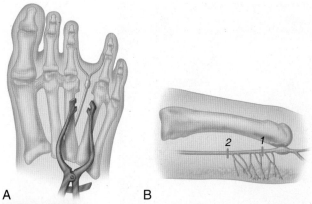

A   **B**

FIGURE 7.9 **A,** Lamina spreader used to expose neuroma. **B,** Lateral view of plantar branches of digital nerve. *1,* Previously recommended level of neurectomy; *2,* currently recommended level of neurectomy (3 cm proximal to ligament) to avoid plantarly directed nerve branches. **SEE TECHNIQUE 7.4.**

- Place a small lamina spreader between the metatarsal necks and spread them apart (Fig. 7.9A).
- Retract the web space fat pad distally with the deep blade of a Senn retractor.
- Sometimes a larger interdigital neuroma can be seen at this point (Fig. 7.10). Do not press up beneath the foot to extrude the neuroma distal to the intermetatarsal ligament because this gives a false sense of exposure and probably is one reason why recurrence or incomplete resection occurs.
- Dissect the intermetatarsal ligament at its distal portion and divide along the entire length longitudinally.
- While protecting the underlying structures, release the intermetatarsal ligament using scissors or a No. 15 blade. Be careful not to damage the lumbrical tendon beneath.
- When the distal portion of the intermetatarsal ligament is identified, free the neurovascular bundle, using scissors to spread under the intermetatarsal ligament from a distal to proximal direction.
- Release the intermetatarsal ligament and remove it proximally with digital manipulation to identify any remaining intermetatarsal ligament that may not have been released. A complete release of the intermetatarsal ligament is essential to the success of this surgery.
- Although the intermetatarsal nerve may not be enlarged to a great degree, the nerve should be dissected and resected as planned regardless of its size. Structures that could be mistaken for the nerve in the web space include the lumbrical tendon, which passes medially to the base of the fourth proximal phalanx, and the common digital artery, which usually crosses proximal medial to distal lateral lying dorsally over the nerve. Often the artery comes out from under the medial metatarsal neck. If identified, dissect the artery away from the nerve and preserve it.
- Dissect the nerve more distally, but not to the two proper digital branches (Fig. 7.11).
- The neuroma usually is at or just distal to the intermetatarsal ligament. Extend the dissection to the distal aspect of the neuroma, dividing it at that point.
- Dissect the nerve circumferentially to 3.0 to 3.5 cm proximal to the neuroma (Fig. 7.9B).

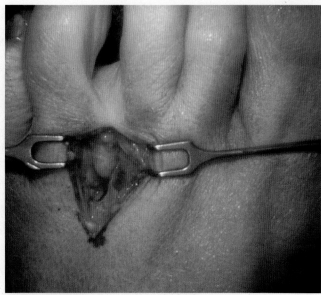

FIGURE 7.10 Interdigital neuroma (dorsal approach). **SEE TECHNIQUE 7.4.**

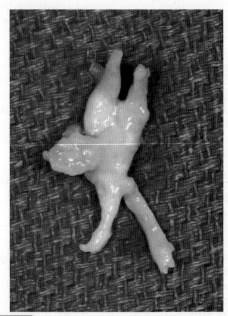

FIGURE 7.11 Common digital nerve with two proper digital branches and neuroma at their junction. **SEE TECHNIQUE 7.4.**

- If the dissection is carried through to the adductor hallucis muscle, partially divide or retract it dorsally with a small right-angle (Ragnell) retractor.
- Divide the plantar-directed branches of the intermetatarsal nerve to the forefoot pad so that the nerve is easily traced proximally. Ensure that the area of transection corresponds to the region of the non–weight-bearing part of the foot, 1 to 2 cm proximal to the weight-bearing pad of the forefoot, by placing a blunt instrument in the same location where the nerve will be transected and palpating it in the plantar aspect of the foot. Dissect more proximally if this non–weight-bearing area is not achieved.

- Divide the nerve at its proximal resting place and remove the nerve that was circumferentially dissected and the neuroma.
- Cauterize the neuroma stump and use a small hemostat to place the nerve stump well proximally and dorsally into the interosseous muscles, preventing it from reaching a weight-bearing area. Send the specimen to the pathology department for biopsy.
- With the lamina spreader still in place, release the tourniquet to determine whether arteries or larger vessels have been transected during the procedure.
- Remove the lamina spreader and place light compression on the forefoot for 5 to 10 minutes while the reactive hyperemia time passes. As an alternative, close the wound under tourniquet control and release the tourniquet after placement of sterile dressings.
- Close the skin loosely using 4-0 nylon sutures in a vertical mattress suture fashion. Place a slightly bulky "sandwich" dressing over a petroleum jelly-impregnated gauze pad and wrap with an elastic bandage with only mild compression.

POSTOPERATIVE CARE For the first few days, the patient rests with maximal elevation of the extremity but may bear weight as tolerated in a postoperative shoe as needed. After the first few days, the patient may increase walking as pain allows. Sutures are removed at 2 to 3 weeks, and plastic strips are placed across the wound for another week. A postoperative shoe usually is needed for 2 to 4 weeks, followed by a wide toe box, soft-vamp shoe for an additional 3 to 4 weeks.

the web space and continue in a proximal direction (Fig. 7.12A). A small, self-retaining retractor is an excellent aid at this point because of fat overlying the plantar aponeurosis.
- Make a longitudinal incision in line with the skin incision through the plantar aponeurosis.
- Using blunt dissection in a longitudinal plane, identify the common digital nerve proximally; dissect it distally to the neuromatous enlargement just proximal to the emergence of the proper digital branches to the adjacent sides of the toes.
- Excise the neuroma, being careful to resect the nerve 2 to 3 cm proximal to the deep transverse intermetatarsal ligament. Incising the deep transverse intermetatarsal ligament that lies dorsal to the neuroma is unnecessary.
- Remove the tourniquet, achieve hemostasis, and close the skin with interrupted nonabsorbable sutures only (Fig. 7.12B).

POSTOPERATIVE CARE A bulky compression dressing is applied to the forefoot, and the extremity is elevated for 24 hours before beginning ambulation in a wooden-soled shoe. We have not seen wound complications as a result of early weight bearing when a postoperative wooden-soled shoe has been used and the patient has been instructed to walk on the heel of the affected foot. If the patient cannot cooperate, however, crutch walking is encouraged until the sutures are removed 2 weeks later, at which time adhesive strips are applied to the wound for another week. The remaining management is the same as described for the dorsal incision.

INTERDIGITAL NEUROMA EXCISION (LONGITUDINAL PLANTAR INCISION)

TECHNIQUE 7.5

- Under tourniquet control with the patient supine and an assistant dorsiflexing the ankle to neutral position, begin a 3- to 4-cm plantar longitudinal incision just proximal to

CAVUS FOOT

In its simplest form, a cavus foot is one with an abnormally high arch. This high arch usually accompanies a spectrum of deformities, including hyperextension of the toes at the metatarsophalangeal joints and hyperflexion at the interphalangeal joints, pronation and adduction of the forefoot (forefoot valgus), a "bony" dorsum of the midfoot with wrinkled skin folds on the medial plantar aspect, lengthened

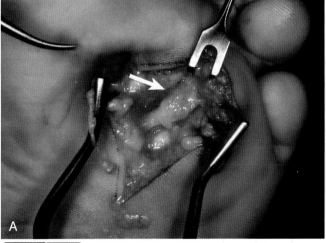
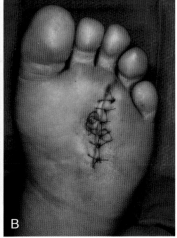

FIGURE 7.12 Interdigital neuroma. **A,** Plantar incision for "recurrent" interdigital neuroma with communicating nerve entering neuroma *(arrow)*. **B,** Closure after neuroma excision. **SEE TECHNIQUE 7.5.**

lateral border of the foot and shortened medial border, calluses beneath the metatarsal heads and lateral column, varied stiffness of the Chopart joint, fixed or flexible heel varus, and tightness of the Achilles tendon with or without an equinus contracture. Although pes cavus with multiple deformities is difficult to define, it is easily recognized (Fig. 7.13); however, it is definitely not easy to treat operatively or nonoperatively.

ETIOLOGY

A cavus foot may result from many different processes, all of which create muscle imbalances that result in deformity. The imbalance may occur from a progressive or static process, leading to variable severities and treatments. Underlying neuromuscular disease, such as Charcot-Marie-Tooth (CMT) or ataxia, leads to more progressive deformities. Other processes (postpoliomyelitis, cerebral palsy, club foot, etc.) are more static, but worsening contractures can still lead to varying cavus deformities. Spinal cord disorders (spinal cord tumors, spinal cord dysraphism, syrinx, etc.) lead to muscle imbalance causing cavus deformity. Even traumatic injuries, resulting in varus malunions or postcompartment syndrome imbalances, can lead to cavus deformity.

Charcot-Marie-Tooth disease is the most common neuromuscular disease causing pes cavus. This disease is actually a heterogeneous group of hereditary sensory and motor neuropathies (HSMN) caused by neural protein mutations affecting peripheral nerve conduction through axon or myelin irregularities. Our understanding and classification of this disease continues to advance. All types are inheritable, but nearly half of the cases result from a new mutation. Characterized by axon demyelination, CMT-1 is the most common type, occurring in over 50% of CMT patients. CMT-1 can be further subdivided into CMT-1A, CMT-1B, and CMT-1C. CMT-2 is the second most common type and may have near-normal nerve conduction velocities. There is striking variability of penetration and clinical expression of this autosomal-dominant disease, even in immediate family members and extended family. CMT-X is found in 10% to 20% and demonstrates an X-linked inheritance pattern. CMT-4 exhibits an autosomal recessive inheritance pattern and is very rare.

PHYSICAL FINDINGS

Regardless of the specific type, all types result in muscle imbalance affecting the lateral and anterior muscle compartments. The clinical expression varies from individual to individual, but the classic muscle imbalances involve weakness of the tibialis anterior while sparing the peroneus longus, resulting in a plantar flexed first metatarsal (Fig. 7.14). To accommodate this forefoot pronation, the hindfoot assumes a varus posture (Fig. 7.15). Additionally, peroneus brevis weakness countered by the near-normal tibialis posterior strength leads to worsening inversion of the midtarsal joints and hindfoot varus deformity. Developing contractures of the plantar fascia and the varus-oriented Achilles tendon further contribute to the deformity. Last, imbalance of the intrinsic-extrinsic muscles enhances the deformity. The intrinsic muscles in the plantar aspect of the foot generally flex the metatarsophalangeal joints and extend the interphalangeal joints. Any weakness of these muscles relative to their antagonists causes plantar

flexion of the metatarsals, hyperextension of the metatarsophalangeal joints, and hyperflexion at the interphalangeal joints (toe clawing).

Patients with cavus deformity as a residual of poliomyelitis usually have different physical findings from patients with CMT disease. Fortunately, with the success of vaccination in the 1950s, postpoliomyelitis cavus is less commonly encountered. Depending on the level of injury and inconsistent recovery, poliomyelitis can cause differing patterns of muscle imbalance and subsequent deformity (Fig. 7.16C). Unlike CMT disease, a weak gastrocnemius-soleus muscle opposite a strong anterior tibial muscle may cause a calcaneal deformity of the hindfoot, with or without hindfoot varus or valgus, depending on which muscle groups have preserved strength. Because of intact sensation and the nonprogressive nature of the deformities, patients with postpoliomyelitis cavus feet typically have a better prognosis than patients with CMT disease.

Traumatic cavus deformity can be caused by deep posterior compartment syndrome or by malunion of midfoot and hindfoot fractures. The deformity may not appear for several months after the local ischemia and muscle fibrosis of the deep posterior compartment, or it may appear as a mild, barely perceptible abnormality that progresses relentlessly to a rigid cavovarus, claw toe deformity. Soft-tissue injuries from crush mechanisms or severe burns can lead to contractures and muscle imbalances that result in cavus deformity. Through altered bony anatomy and joint mechanics, hindfoot malunions (i.e., calcaneal and talar neck malunions) also can create posttraumatic cavus deformities.

In some patients with symptomatic cavus deformities, no definite cause is discovered (Fig. 7.17). In patients with idiopathic deformities, the underlying pathologic mechanism of the cavus deformity is believed to be an imbalance of the extrinsic-intrinsic muscles. As previously discussed, the intrinsic minus foot demonstrates metatarsal plantar flexion and toe clawing in which the hindfoot assumes a varus posture to accommodate the rigid plantar flexed first ray (see Fig. 7.14). Furthermore, patients may display mild, subtle cavovarus as a normal variation within the bell curve for arch height and foot posture. Despite this "normal" variation, patient symptoms still require recognition and appropriate treatment.

RADIOGRAPHIC FINDINGS

Standard radiographic workup involves a standing series of the foot and ankle. Many angles and measurements have been described to help classify foot posture. These specific angles and values are likely most useful in research data collection rather than daily application, but the overall concept in recognizing these abnormal relationships is critical for understanding deformities and formulating treatment plans.

The standing lateral radiograph allows estimation of the contribution of the hindfoot (talus and calcaneus), midfoot (navicular and cuboid-cuneiform), and forefoot (Lisfranc) to the cavus deformity. The standing lateral view allows assessment of calcaneal pitch (see Fig. 7.16A), talo–first metatarsal (Meary's) angle, lateral talocalcaneal angle, and medial-cuneiform height. The extension deformity of the phalanges on the metatarsal heads during weight bearing helps determine the severity of the fixed forefoot deformity (Figs. 7.18 and 7.19). The standing hindfoot alignment view displays the

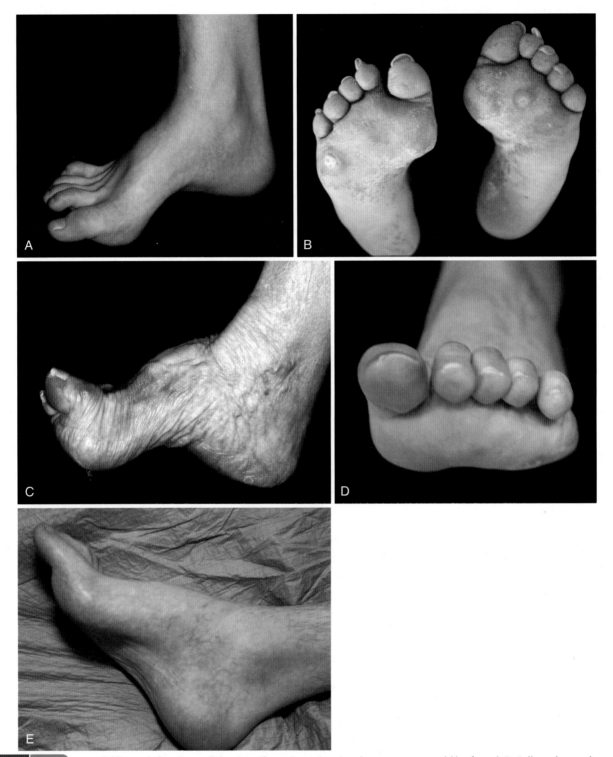

FIGURE 7.13 **A,** Mild cavus deformity and clawing of toes in patient in whom no cause could be found. **B,** Calluses beneath metatarsal heads are most common symptom prompting orthopaedic consultation. **C,** Marked forefoot equinus and resulting dorsal prominence of tarsus in patient with residual poliomyelitis deformity. **D,** Forefoot is pronated in relation to hindfoot during weight bearing; note clawing of toes. **E,** Shortening of medial column of foot.

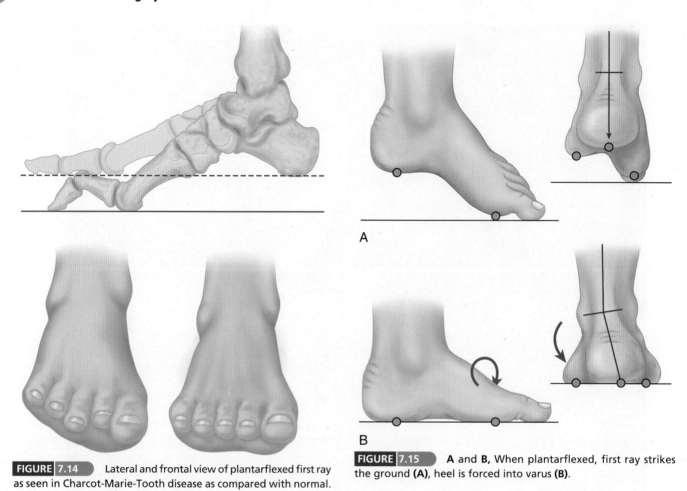

FIGURE 7.14 Lateral and frontal view of plantarflexed first ray as seen in Charcot-Marie-Tooth disease as compared with normal.

FIGURE 7.15 A and B, When plantarflexed, first ray strikes the ground (A), heel is forced into varus (B).

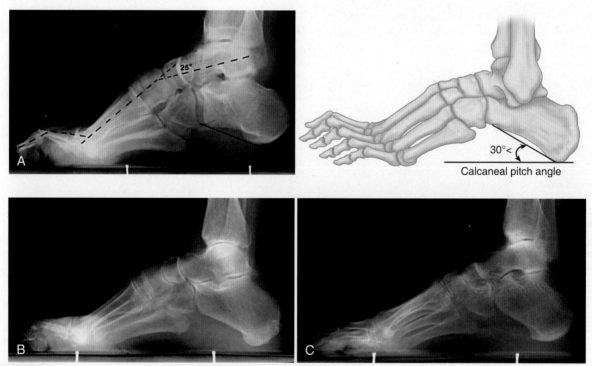

Calcaneal pitch angle

FIGURE 7.16 A, Normal calcaneal pitch, but forefoot equinus in patient with Charcot-Marie-Tooth disease (left). Calcaneal pitch angle measures degree of calcaneus deformity (right). B and C, Calcaneal pitch in idiopathic (B) and postpoliomyelitis (C) deformities.

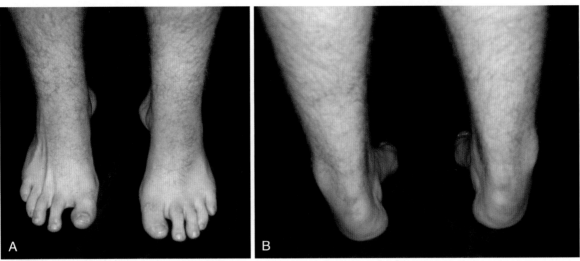

FIGURE 7.17 A and B, Fifteen-year-old boy with "idiopathic" pes cavus diagnosed after extensive neurologic evaluation.

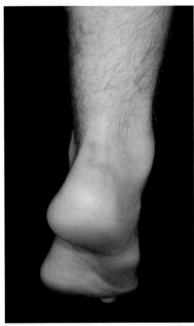

FIGURE 7.18 Eighteen-year-old man with Charcot-Marie-Tooth disease with fixed hindfoot varus, marked forefoot equinus, plantarflexed first ray, forefoot pronation during weight bearing, tight plantar fascia, and contracted Achilles tendon but no palpable contraction of peroneus longus.

relationship of the calcaneus to the tibia, demonstrating varying degrees of hindfoot varus.

Similarly, the standing anteroposterior view allows estimation of the contribution from the hindfoot, midfoot, and forefoot. This view shows talar head overcoverage, metatarsus adductus, talocalcaneal angle, and the talo–first metatarsal angle. In flexible deformities, obtaining a standing anteroposterior foot radiograph with the hindfoot corrected (via Coleman block; see Fig. 7.22) helps corroborate any metatarsus adductus component suspected clinically (Fig. 7.20). The talocalcaneal angle (Kite angle) is determined on this view. The closer the talocalcaneal angle approaches zero, the more parallel the talus is in relation to the calcaneus, indicating hindfoot varus.

Other radiographic findings that may be helpful include (1) degenerative changes in the tibiotalar, subtalar, or midtarsal joints; (2) rotation of the talus in the ankle mortise exhibited by a posterior fibula; and (3) dystrophic ossification in soft tissue suggesting tendon or ligament injury (Fig. 7.21).

Although of questionable benefit for initial conservative treatment, CT scans are invaluable for surgical planning. The advancements in weight-bearing CT and three-dimensional reconstructions help surgeons conceptualize the deformity and localize the apex of the deformity for surgical correction.

TREATMENT

A thorough physical examination is mandatory to understand the deforming forces because not all cavovarus deformities can be treated the same. Determining the apex or cause of deformity and distinguishing flexible from rigid deformities are critical steps in employing appropriate treatment. The Coleman block tests help differentiate flexible, forefoot-driven deformities from stiffer, hindfoot-driven deformities (see Figs. 7.15 and 7.22). Mild metatarsalgia symptoms related to subtle cavus can be alleviated with good callus care, proper footwear, and metatarsal bars or pads. Larger but flexible forefoot-driven deformities may be treated with orthotics with lateral heel posting and first metatarsal head relief, while rigid deformities require more aggressive bracing, such as a double-upright brace with lateral t-strap and lateral sole flare.

Surgically, flexible deformities can be treated with joint-saving procedures, such as tendon transfers and osteotomies, while more rigid deformities may require arthrodesis. Rarely, however, does the cavus deformity cleanly fit the "forefoot-driven" or "hindfoot-driven" classification. Instead, a blend of forefoot-driven and hindfoot-driven deformity with varied stiffness exists, making surgical treatment highly variable. Because of this variable presentation and highly variable surgical treatment in addition to differing etiologies and progression, no standard surgical algorithm exists within the published literature. Therefore surgeons must approach each patient individually.

Generally, mild, flexible forefoot-driven deformities can be corrected by elevating the first ray, releasing the plantar

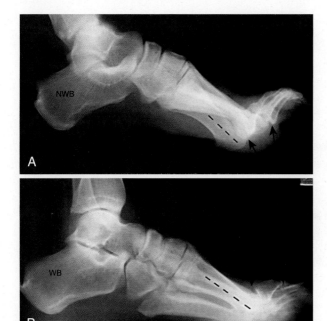

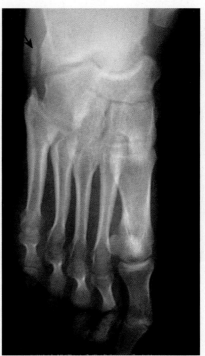

FIGURE **7.19**   **A,** Non–weight-bearing view of cavus and claw toe deformities in patient with Charcot-Marie-Tooth disease. **B,** On weight-bearing view, plantarflexion of first ray is less noticeable but clawed hallux remains, indicating fixed extension contracture at first metatarsophalangeal joint.

FIGURE **7.21**   Dystrophic ossification in patient with Charcot-Marie-Tooth disease. No peroneus longus function was palpable. Ossification was believed to be caused by repetitive small tears in peroneal tendons.

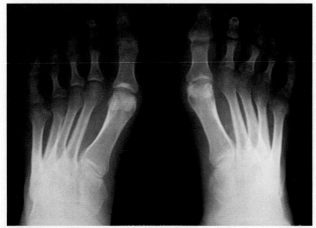

FIGURE **7.20**   Weight-bearing anteroposterior view of cavus foot in patient with Charcot-Marie-Tooth disease; note forefoot adduction and supination. Radiographic metatarsus adductus is partially positional and partially true adductus.

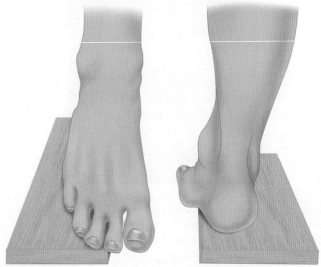

FIGURE **7.22**   Lateral block test. Plantarflexed first metatarsal is allowed to hang free from block; supple hind part of foot then corrects.

fascia (Fig. 7.23), performing a calcaneal osteotomy, and removing the motor imbalances. Elevating the first ray can be achieved through a dorsal closing-wedge osteotomy, vertical osteotomy, first tarsometatarsal arthrodesis, or modified Jones procedure (see Technique 7.7 and Fig. 7.24), in which the extensor hallucis longus is transferred to the first metatarsal neck. Because of the plantar hinge, dorsal closing-wedge osteotomies are stable osteotomies, but an aggressive wedge can produce significant shortening and malunion. Releasing the plantar fascia aids in correcting forefoot pronation and may limit the need for aggressive osseous resections.

The calcaneal osteotomy aids in correcting mild hindfoot deformity. Calcaneal osteotomies include a combination of closing-wedge osteotomies (Dwyer, see Technique 7.11 and Fig. 7.27), lateralizing osteotomies (Saxby and Myerson, see Technique 7.12 and Fig. 7.28), or Z-osteotomies (Knupp, see Technique 7.13 and Fig. 7.29). Cadaver studies have indicated that lateralization, combined with Dwyer osteotomy, and coronal plane internal rotation achieved the greatest correction of

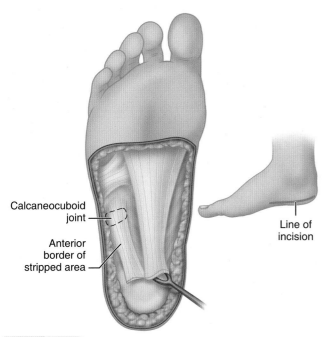

Calcaneocuboid joint

Anterior border of stripped area

Line of incision

FIGURE 7.23 Technique of plantar fascia release. **SEE TECH-NIQUE 7.6.**

heel varus. However, authors have reported that lateralizing the calcaneus reduces the tarsal tunnel volume, raising concern for iatrogenic nerve injury. VanValkenburg et al. reported a 34% incidence of neurologic deficit after laterally approached calcaneal osteotomies, but no difference in neurologic deficit was detected between a traditional Dwyer (no translation) procedure compared with those that added translation. Instead, osteotomy location rather than translation was associated with nerve injury. Osteotomies based more anteriorly (middle third of the calcaneal body) demonstrated higher neurologic deficits than osteotomies that were more posterior (posterior third of the calcaneal body). Jaffe el al. retrospectively reported a cohort undergoing lateralizing calcaneal osteotomies through a medial approach. None of 24 patients developed postoperative tarsal tunnel symptoms. A Z-osteotomy with lateral closing-wedge (Knupp) osteotomy corrects coronal plane rotation without the shortening found in the Dwyer technique.

Despite selected surgical procedures, removing the deforming forces is critical in preventing reoccurrence. As previously discussed, the forces typically consist of the peroneal longus overpowering the tibialis anterior and the tibialis posterior overpowering the peroneal brevis. Therefore, releasing the peroneal longus followed by tenodesis to the peroneal brevis and releasing the posterior tibial tendon followed by transfer to the dorsum of the foot improves motor imbalances.

More moderate, stiffer deformities centered over the midfoot or hindfoot may require additional midfoot osteotomies. Multiple midfoot osteotomies are described in this chapter. Dorsal closing-wedge metatarsal osteotomy (Gould, see Technique 7.14 and Fig. 7.32), V-osteotomy (Japas, see Technique 7.16 and Fig. 7.34), anterior tarsal wedge osteotomy (Cole, see Technique 7.15 and Fig. 7.33), tarsometatarsal truncated-wedge arthrodesis (Jahss, see Technique 7.17 and Fig. 7.35), and several others have described powerful yet

technically demanding osteotomies that should be reserved for significant, stiff deformities centered over the midfoot.

Severe or arthritic deformities typically require arthrodesis procedures. The apex of deformity should determine the appropriate location and type of arthrodesis procedure. Similar to the milder deformities, tendon transfers are still needed in arthrodesis procedures to remove the deforming forces. Even with arthrodesis procedures, surgeons must be vigilant to recognize multiplanar deformities and be prepared to balance the midfoot or forefoot with additional osteotomies after correcting the hindfoot.

In milder, flexible deformities, the lesser toe clawing may passively improve after correcting the hindfoot and midfoot. If the claw deformity is more rigid, then the forefoot should also be treated with hammertoe-like procedures as described below.

◼ FLEXIBLE FOREFOOT-DRIVEN (PLANTAR-FLEXED FIRST RAY) CAVOVARUS DEFORMITY

Occasionally in an adolescent foot, even in mild CMT penetration, if the peroneus longus is transferred to the peroneus brevis accompanied by plantar fascia release, soft-tissue procedures alone correct the forefoot equinus sufficiently to avoid osteotomy or arthrodesis; however, usually one of the osseous procedures described here is also indicated.

◼ PROXIMAL FIRST METATARSAL OSTEOTOMY AND PLANTAR FASCIOTOMY

In flexible, forefoot-driven CMT deformity, the correction of the forefoot equinus should proceed in an orderly fashion, beginning with plantar fascia release (see Technique 7.6) and transfer of the peroneus longus to the peroneus brevis (see section of Technique 7.9). While holding the ankle in neutral, if the plantar flexed first ray is not corrected by these two procedures, a basilar closing-wedge osteotomy of the first metatarsal is done (see section of Technique 7.9). If the hallux is still in a clawed position, then transfer of the extensor hallucis longus to the neck of the first metatarsal with an arthrodesis of the interphalangeal joint of the hallux completes the procedure (Jones, see Technique 7.7 and Fig. 7.24).

PLANTAR FASCIA RELEASE

TECHNIQUE 7.6

- Beginning at medial calcaneal tubercle, make a short longitudinal incision along the medial side of the calcaneus near the glabrous skin border (see Fig. 7.23).
- Dissect through the adipose tissue, visualizing the plantar fascia and abductor hallucis fascia.
- Separate the superficial and deep surfaces of the plantar fascia from the muscle and fat. Incise the fascia transversely close to where it blends into the plantar surface of the calcaneus. Tension through the windlass mechanism (extension of the metatarsophalangeal joints) will place the plantar fascia under tension, allowing easier cutting and separation.
- In severe cases, the abductor fascia may also need to be released.

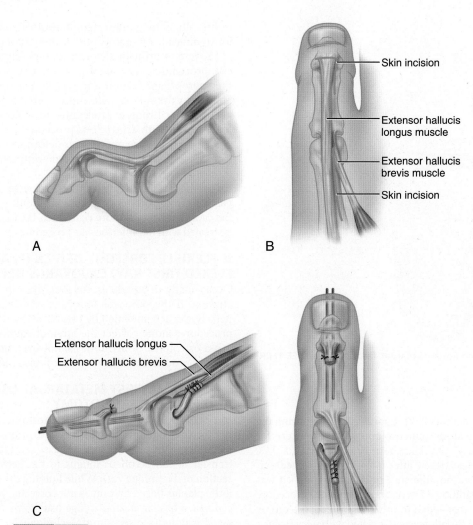

A

B

— Skin incision

— Extensor hallucis longus muscle

— Extensor hallucis brevis muscle

— Skin incision

Extensor hallucis longus —

Extensor hallucis brevis —

C

FIGURE 7.24 Modified Jones procedure for clawing of great toe. **A,** Clawing of great toe. **B,** Skin incisions. **C,** Extensor hallucis longus tendon is attached to neck of first metatarsal; interphalangeal joint is arthrodesed and fixed by medullary wire and by suturing distal end of extensor hallucis longus tendon to soft tissues over proximal phalanx. **SEE TECHNIQUE 7.7.**

- Secure hemostasis and close the wound with nonabsorbable sutures in adult patients.

POSTOPERATIVE CARE Release of the plantar fascia seldom is performed as an isolated procedure. If it is, however, a short leg cast is applied and molded gently into the arch, and the patient is kept non–weight bearing for 3 weeks. A weight-bearing cast or walking boot is worn for another 3 weeks.

TENDON SUSPENSION OF THE FIRST METATARSAL AND INTERPHALANGEAL JOINT ARTHRODESIS

The Jones procedure, which is basically a tendon suspension of the first metatarsal combined with arthrodesis of the interphalangeal joint, has proved

valuable in elevating the plantar flexed first metatarsal. The distal end of the extensor hallucis longus is placed through a hole in the first metatarsal neck (see Fig. 7.24).

TECHNIQUE 7.7

(JONES)

- Expose the interphalangeal joint of the great toe through an L-shaped incision (Fig. 7.24A and B).
- Retract the flap of skin and subcutaneous tissue medially and proximally and expose the tendon of the extensor hallucis longus.
- Cut the tendon transversely 1 cm proximal to the joint and expose the joint.
- Excise the cartilage, approximate the joint surface, and insert two retrograde medullary 0.062-inch Kirschner wires or screws for fixation. Clip the wire off just beneath the skin.
- Expose the neck of the first metatarsal through a 2.5-cm dorsomedial incision extending distally to the proximal extensor skin crease (see Fig. 7.24B).

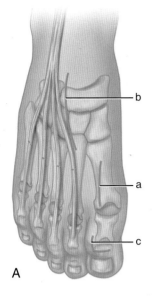

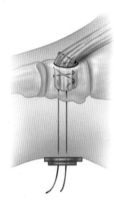

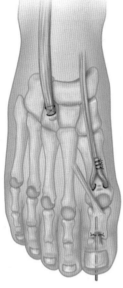

FIGURE 7.25 Transfer of extensor tendons to lateral cuneiform for claw toe deformity (Hibbs procedure). **A,** Incisions. *a* and *c,* Incisions for Jones procedure. *b,* Incision for Hibbs procedure. **B,** Completed procedure combined with Jones procedure. **SEE TECHNIQUE 7.8.**

- Dissect free the extensor hallucis longus tendon but protect the short extensor tendon.
- Cleanly and carefully excise the sheath of the extensor hallucis longus tendon throughout the length of the proximal incision.
- Beginning at the inferomedial aspect of the first metatarsal neck, drill a hole transverse to the long axis of the bone to emerge on the dorsolateral aspect of the neck.
- Pass the tendon through the hole and suture it to itself with interrupted sutures (Fig. 7.24C). The same procedure can be performed on adjacent toes with clawing.
- Close the wounds and apply a short leg walking cast with the ankle in neutral position.

POSTOPERATIVE CARE At 3 weeks, the cast and skin sutures are removed, and a short leg walking cast is reapplied. At 6 weeks, the walking cast and Kirschner wires are removed, and active exercises are started.

EXTENSOR TENDON TRANSFER

The Hibbs technique is a soft-tissue adjuvant procedure in which the extensor digitorum longus is transferred to the lateral cuneiform, providing added dorsiflexion and eversion strength to the hindfoot while removing the deforming forces contributing to metatarsophalangeal joint hyperextension. This procedure is particularly helpful in flexible forefoot deformities with marked intrinsic-extrinsic imbalance, but the overpowering flexor digitorum longus is likely to need release by tenotomy to correct the flexible toe clawing. Claw-toe correction is further discussed later in this chapter and in other chapter.

TECHNIQUE 7.8

(HIBBS)
- Make a curved incision 7.5 to 10 cm long on the dorsum of the foot lateral to the midline and expose the common extensor tendons (Fig. 7.25A).
- Divide the tendons as far distally as feasible, draw their proximal ends through a tunnel in the third cuneiform, and fix them with a nonabsorbable suture (Fig. 7.25B).
- As an alternative, use a plantar button and felt with a Bunnell pull-out stitch.
- Close the wounds and apply a plaster boot cast with the foot in the corrected position.

POSTOPERATIVE CARE Protecting the transfer with cast immobilization is continued for 6 weeks. If utilized, the plantar button is removed at 6 weeks. A walking cast is worn for another 3 weeks.

COMBINED PROXIMAL FIRST METATARSAL OSTEOTOMY, PLANTAR FASCIOTOMY, AND TRANSFER OF THE ANTERIOR TIBIAL TENDON

Ward et al., in treatment for cavus deformity secondary to CMT, also included transfer of the anterior tibial tendon to the lateral cuneiform if grade 4 or 5 strength was present. Later in the study, this transfer was done for a tenodesis to negate any residual deforming force that the anterior tibial muscle may have on the varus component of the cavovarus deformity.

TECHNIQUE 7.9

(WARD ET AL.)

PLANTAR FASCIOTOMY
- Make a 1-cm incision on the medial side of the midfoot over the palpable plantar fascia.
- Bluntly dissect above and below the fascia with a hemostat and release the plantar fascia with a No. 11 blade, while protecting the skin and adjacent structures with small- to medium-sized right-angle retractors.

PERONEUS LONGUS TO PERONEUS BREVIS TENDON TRANSFER

- Make a curvilinear incision laterally over the peroneal tendons from 2 cm proximal to 2 cm distal to the distal tip of the fibular malleolus.
- Identify and gently retract the sural nerve.
- Using a scalpel, open the sheaths of the peroneus longus and brevis tendons.
- Transect the peroneus longus tendon as distally as possible through this same incision at its entrance into the cuboid groove while holding the ankle and foot in equinus and valgus.
- Weave the peroneus longus tendon through the peroneus brevis tendon with a Pulvertaft weave and suture it with multiple No. 0 Vicryl sutures under moderate tension.

PROXIMAL FIRST METATARSAL OSTEOTOMY

- Make a longitudinal incision over the dorsum of the first ray from 2 cm proximal to the first metatarsophalangeal joint to 1 cm proximal to the tarsometatarsal joint.
- Create a 3- to 5-mm dorsal closing wedge osteotomy in the proximal third of the metatarsal shaft. Remove more bone dorsally if needed to level with the adjacent second metatarsal head while closing the osteotomy by dorsiflexing the distal fragment.
- If clawing of the hallux exists, then add the following Jones procedure.

JONES PROCEDURE

- Extend the incision distally to the neck of the proximal phalanx of the hallux.
- Divide the extensor hallucis longus tendon near its insertion.
- Drill a hole through the neck of the first metatarsal with serial sized drill bits to avoid fracturing the metatarsal.
- Pass the extensor hallucis longus tendon from medial to lateral through the metatarsal neck.
- Suture the extensor hallucis longus tendon to itself with an absorbable suture so that it holds the metatarsal in the proper position while placing tension on the basilar osteotomy.
- A small Steinmann pin or screw is usually needed to stabilize the osteotomy.

TRANSFER OF THE ANTERIOR TIBIAL TENDON

- Make a dorsomedial incision over the insertion of the anterior tibial tendon on the navicular.
- Carry the dissection distally to obtain as much length as possible on the tendon stump.
- Divide the anterior tibial tendon at its insertion.
- Pass a No. 2 nonresorbable suture through the tendon stump in a Bunnell fashion.
- Under fluoroscopic control, make a 2-cm longitudinal incision over the lateral cuneiform.
- Pass an 8- or 9-mm drill bit through both cortices of the cuneiform from dorsal to plantar.
- With the use of Keith needles (or a suture anchor), pass the suture ends through this hole. Hold the hindfoot in neutral in the varus/valgus plane and neutral dorsiflexion and tie the sutures over a padded button on the plantar

surface of the foot. A suture anchor can be used in lieu of a padded button; however, the tendon transfer *must* hold the ankle in neutral dorsiflexion with either technique.

POSTOPERATIVE CARE A short leg cast is applied. Weight bearing is not allowed for 6 weeks. If utilized, remove the button after 6 weeks and apply a short leg walking cast for another month.

■ COMBINED MILD FOREFOOT-DRIVEN AND HINDFOOT-DRIVEN VARUS DEFORMITY

As mentioned, it is rare to have a forefoot-driven deformity without any hindfoot varus. Therefore most surgical treatment for mild cavus will involve treatment of the hindfoot varus. This is typically corrected through a valgus-producing calcaneal osteotomy. Rarely, in postpoliomyelitis patients, calcaneocavus deformity may exist without varus. For this rare deformity, a crescentic calcaneal osteotomy, with or without midtarsal osteotomy, has been recommended. Most often there is an associated varus of the heel, requiring a valgus-producing osteotomy (Dwyer, lateralizing, or Z-osteotomy). Only a certain amount of hindfoot varus and midfoot-forefoot cavus can be corrected by calcaneal osteotomies. Thus more severe deformities may require additional midfoot osteotomies and/or hindfoot arthrodesis.

■ OSTEOTOMY OF THE CALCANEUS

CRESCENTIC CALCANEAL OSTEOTOMY

Samilson recommended crescentic calcaneal osteotomy for ambulatory patients with symptomatic calcaneocavus feet. On a lateral radiograph, the calcaneus must be relatively vertical, and the apex of the cavus must be posterior to the midtarsus. The operation does not correct midtarsal or forefoot cavus but does correct hindfoot calcaneocavus.

TECHNIQUE 7.10

(SAMILSON)

- Under tourniquet control, after preparation and draping in the usual manner, make an obliquely placed lateral incision over the posterior tuberosity of the calcaneus, posterior to the subtalar joint. The peroneal tendons should be anterior to the posterior portion of the incision.
- Carry the dissection down to the lateral aspect of the calcaneus.
- Identify and protect the peroneal tendons.
- Perform a plantar fasciotomy.
- Make a crescentic osteotomy in the calcaneus, posterior to the subtalar joint with a curved blade on a Stryker saw or by joining multiple drill holes in the calcaneus with a large curved osteotome (Fig. 7.26).
- Shift the freed posterior tuberosity posterosuperiorly along the osteotomy line to correct the calcaneocavus (Fig. 7.26).

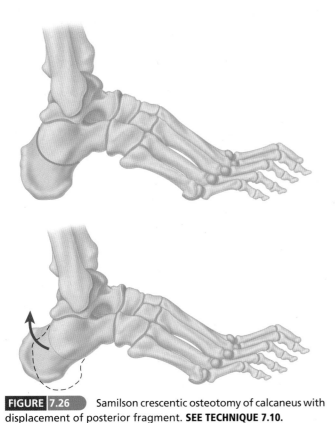

FIGURE 7.26 Samilson crescentic osteotomy of calcaneus with displacement of posterior fragment. **SEE TECHNIQUE 7.10.**

- Secure the fragment with staples or Kirschner wires.
- Close the wound in the usual manner and apply a non–weight-bearing short leg cast.

POSTOPERATIVE CARE Weight bearing should not be allowed for 6 weeks. At that time, a short leg walking boot is worn for another 4 weeks until the osteotomy site has healed.

TECHNIQUE 7.11

(DWYER)
- Divide the plantar fascia subcutaneously to reduce the drop of the forefoot.
- Expose the lateral aspect of the calcaneus through a curved incision paralleling the peroneus longus tendon but 1 cm posterior and inferior to it.
- Turn the entire flap anteriorly until the tendon of the peroneus longus muscle is exposed.
- Strip the periosteum from the superior, lateral, and inferior surfaces of the calcaneus.
- Remove a wedge of bone from the calcaneus just inferior and posterior to the peroneus longus tendon and parallel with it (Fig. 7.27A); make the base of the wedge 8 to 12 mm wide, and taper the wedge to, but not through, the medial cortex.
- Break the medial cortex and close the gap; bring the bony surfaces snugly together by pressing the forefoot into dorsiflexion against the pull of the Achilles tendon (Fig. 7.27B).

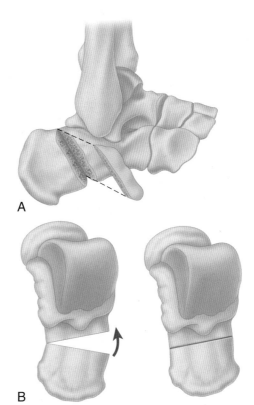

FIGURE 7.27 Dwyer osteotomy of calcaneus for cavus deformity. **A,** Wedge of bone with its base lateral *(colored area)* is resected just inferior and posterior to peroneus longus tendon and parallel to it. **B,** Medial cortex of calcaneus is not divided but is broken manually to close gap. **SEE TECHNIQUE 7.11.**

Failure to obtain closure of the gap is caused by a small piece of bone left behind at the apex of the wedge.
- Ensure that the varus deformity has been corrected and that the heel is in a neutral or even slightly valgus position; failure to correct the varus deformity completely would lead to an increase in the deformity.
- Close the wound and immobilize the foot in a cast from the tibial tuberosity to the toes until the osteotomy is solid.

TRIPLANAR OSTEOTOMY AND LATERAL LIGAMENT RECONSTRUCTION

The triplanar osteotomy corrects all three planes of the cavovarus deformity by lateral translation of the tuberosity fragment, a closing wedge osteotomy laterally to correct the varus, and a proximal sliding of the tuberosity fragment to correct the calcaneal posture of the hindfoot. In addition to the triplanar calcaneal osteotomy, Saxby and Myerson emphasized that the peroneus brevis is not functioning in hereditary sensorimotor neuropathy (CMT disease), and the entire tendon can be used to help stabilize the ankle joint that tilts into varus.

TECHNIQUE 7.12

(SAXBY AND MYERSON)

- Place the patient in the lateral decubitus position. The foot should remain internally rotated but preferably should be perfectly lateral so that the position of the foot is not greatly distorted.
- Make an incision 3 to 4 cm anterior to the insertion of the Achilles tendon and 1 cm inferior to the tip of the fibula (Fig. 7.28A) so that the sural nerve and peroneal tendons are superior or anterior to the incision.
- Extend the oblique incision plantarward from the superior border of the calcaneus to the plantar aspect of the foot so that the inferior aspect meets the margin between the normal and plantar skin. At this point, the incision should be in line with the fibula.
- Carry the dissection through subcutaneous tissue and identify the sural nerve, which may be running in an aberrant course, and retract it superiorly.
- Deepen the incision to the periosteum and calcaneus. Identify the periosteum and divide it with sharp dissection. The entire calcaneus should now be visible from its superior to plantar edges.
- Insert a small, spiked Hohmann retractor into the dorsal and inferior margins of the wound and retract the soft tissue.
- Use a periosteal elevator to strip the periosteum 1 cm on either side to expose the calcaneus further. It is important to expose the calcaneus from its superior to inferior margins.
- Using an oscillating saw, perform the osteotomy in line with the skin incision. Divide the calcaneus, beginning superiorly and moving toward the inferior margin. Do not extend the saw cut into the medial soft tissues. Either the saw can be used and careful attention paid to the exact point at which the saw exits medially, or the medial cortex can be perforated with a large blunt osteotome. Preferably, the triangular wedge of bone laterally should be removed with an oscillating saw before completion of the osteotomy medially (Fig. 7.28B and C). The size of the wedge varies but is approximately 6 mm in width from its superior to inferior margins, tapering to its apical surface medially.
- When a wedge of bone has been removed, remove all remaining cancellous bone chips or fragments, using a curet or rongeur, and complete the osteotomy as described earlier. It is important to divide the medial periosteum to allow translation of the osteotomy.
- In severe deformities, the medial soft tissues are extremely taut, and the osteotomy does not close laterally unless this is completely released. To release the medial soft tissue from the lateral side, insert a large lamina spreader into the lateral aspect of the osteotomy and, with distraction, gradually stretch and divide the periosteum. It should be possible to open the medial surfaces approximately 1 cm using this distraction.
- If the periosteum is divided medially, the osteotomy should close and translate correctly; if not, the contour of the wedge probably is too angulated and more bone should be removed medially.
- Remove any small bone fragments because these prevent apposition of the osteotomy.

- Grasp the posterior portion of the tuberosity and translate it laterally several millimeters and superiorly several millimeters (Fig. 7.28D). The superior translation is important because it changes the calcaneal pitch angle and decreases tension on the Achilles tendon. It is easy to palpate this dorsal overhang, and the lateral translation is done under direct vision.
- While holding the osteotomy in the desired position, have an assistant insert one or two guide pins to determine the correct position for insertion of one or two cannulated cancellous screws. Check the position of the osteotomy fluoroscopically after insertion of the guide pins and evaluate pin position. The screw or screws should cross at a right angle to the osteotomy and start slightly posteriorly and laterally on the tuberosity segment, angled anteriorly and slightly medially.
- When this position has been determined, fix the osteotomy with 6.5- or 7-mm cancellous screws with a 16-mm thread length so that the shanks and not the threads of the screw traverse the osteotomy (Fig. 7.28E). These screws are typically 60 mm long. Excellent compression usually is obtained with one screw, but if sufficient compression is not achieved, a second parallel screw can be inserted easily.
- Close the wound with interrupted Vicryl sutures in the subcutaneous tissue and 4-0 nylon sutures in the skin.
- Apply a posterior plaster splint with the foot in a neutral position.

POSTOPERATIVE CARE Weight bearing is not allowed for 10 days until the sutures are removed. A short leg walking cast is then applied and is worn for 4 weeks.

TECHNIQUE 7.13

(KNUPP ET AL.)

- Place the patient supine on the operating table with a sandbag under the buttock of the affected side to bring the lateral aspect of the hindfoot forward. Exsanguinate the limb.
- To expose the lateral aspect of the calcaneus, make a slightly curved incision, parallel and about 1 cm posterior to the peroneus longus tendon (Fig. 7.29A). Take care not to damage the lateral dorsal cutaneous branch of the sural nerve.
- Strip the periosteum from the lateral wall.
- Make a 2-cm long horizontal osteotomy cut parallel to the plantar fascia (Fig. 7.29B) and then make a vertical cut slightly anterior to the tuberosity (Fig. 7.29C). Use a Hohmann retractor to protect the plantar structures. Make another vertical cut in the posterior half of the concavity of the tuberosity (Fig. 7.29D). Take care not to carry the cut too posteriorly to avoid injuring the Achilles tendon, which should be protected with a second Hohmann retractor.
- Place four Kirschner wires to mark the corners of the bony wedge to be removed.
- Complete the osteotomy using an oscillating saw or an osteotome (Fig. 7.29E) and remove the bone wedge (Fig. 7.29F).
- Displace the tuberosity laterally and close the gap in the desired position (Fig. 7.30). If needed, the calcaneus can be lengthened by displacing the tuberosity posteriorly.

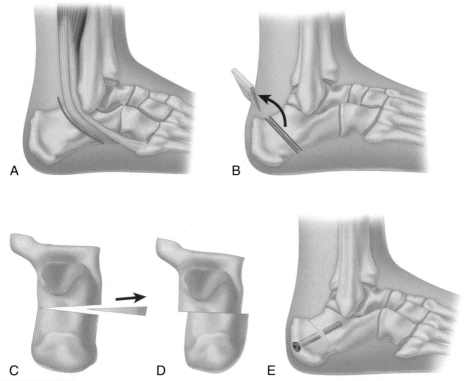

FIGURE 7.28 Saxby and Myerson triplanar osteotomy and lateral ligament reconstruction. **A,** Skin incision beneath both peroneal tendons and sural nerve and in line with peroneal tendons. **B,** Wedge is removed with apex lateral. **C and D,** Calcaneal tuberosity is translated laterally, simultaneously closing wedge. **E,** Tuberosity is secured with a cannulated 7-mm screw. Note dorsal translation of tuberosity. **SEE TECHNIQUE 7.12.**

- Remove the Hohmann retractors and secure the osteotomy with one or two Kirschner wires.
- Check the reduction fluoroscopically before inserting one or two cannulated screws over the Kirschner wires for fixation.
- Close the subcutaneous tissue and the skin with interrupted sutures.

POSTOPERATIVE CARE Apply a compressive dressing and splint to decrease swelling for 2 to 4 days, and then apply a short leg walking cast to be worn for a total of 6 weeks. After the cast is removed, the patient can gradually return to full activity as tolerated.

STIFF, MODERATE MIDFOOT CAVOVARUS DEFORMITY

Stiff, moderate cavus deformity centered over the midtarsal joints (talonavicular-calcaneocuboid, naviculocuneiform joints) can be difficult to correct with the aforementioned procedures (soft-tissue procedures combined with calcaneal osteotomies). For mild-to-moderate fixed cavus deformity at the midfoot, the following osteotomies have been described. Any of these midfoot osteotomies can be technically difficult and may produce a short, wide, unattractive foot, depending on how much bone is removed.

PLANTAR FASCIOTOMIES AND CLOSING WEDGE OSTEOTOMIES

TECHNIQUE 7.14

(GOULD)

DOUBLE PLANTAR FASCIOTOMIES
- Through a lateral heel approach, identify the plantar aponeurosis in a line with the tubercle of the calcaneus (Fig. 7.31). With the points of curved scissors, cut across the aponeurosis near the tuberosity of the calcaneus to avoid damage to the neurovascular bundle on the medial side.
- Make an incision along the medial border of the longitudinal arch and identify the aponeurosis.
- Identify the medial plantar nerve and retract it upward. Under direct vision, transect the aponeurosis with scissors, which may open only sufficiently to receive the fascia.

CLOSING WEDGE GREENSTICK DORSAL PROXIMAL METATARSAL OSTEOTOMIES
- Make three incisions on the dorsum of the foot: one between the bases of the fourth and fifth metatarsals, one between the bases of the second and third metatarsals, and one over the base of the first metatarsal.

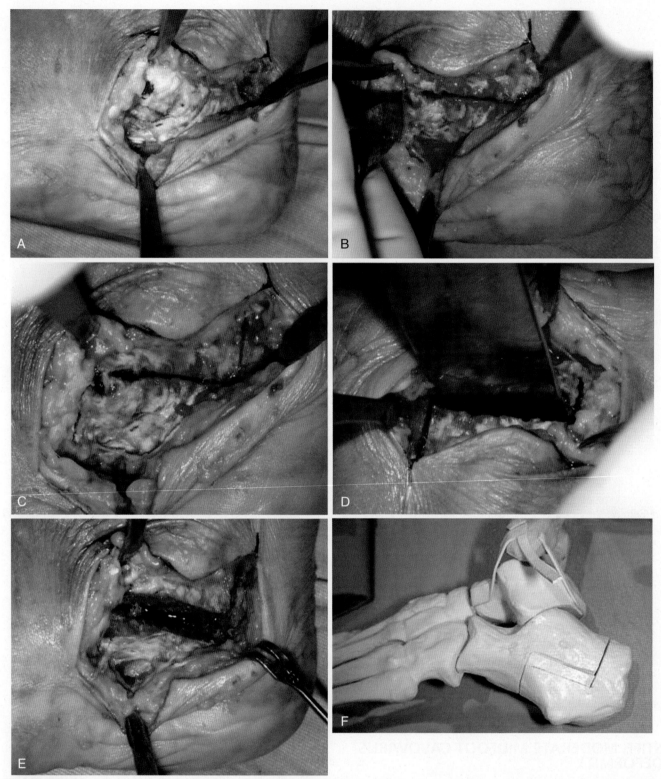

FIGURE 7.29 Knupp et al. Z-shaped calcaneal osteotomy. **A,** Exposure of lateral wall of calcaneus. **B and C,** First horizontal cut. **D,** Two vertical cuts. **E,** Completion of osteotomy with chisel. **F,** After wedge removal and before closing of osteotomy and lateralization of tuberosity. (From Knupp M, Horisberger M, Hintermann B: A new Z-shaped calcaneal osteotomy for 3-plane correction of severe varus deformity of the hindfoot, *Tech Foot Ankle Surg* 7:90, 2008.) **SEE TECHNIQUE 7.13.**

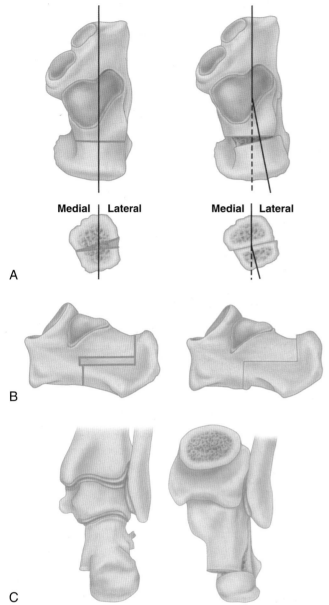

A

B

C

FIGURE 7.30 Knupp et al. Z-shaped calcaneal osteotomy. **A,** Lateralization and valgus placement of tuberosity after Z-osteotomy and translation of calcaneus. **B,** Site of osteotomy and removal of bone wedge. **C,** Lateral translation of calcaneal tuberosity from posterior and from proximal. (Redrawn from Knupp M, Horisberger M, Hintermann B: A new Z-shaped calcaneal osteotomy for 3-plane correction of severe varus deformity of the hindfoot, *Tech Foot Ankle Surg* 7:90, 2008.)

- Continue soft-tissue dissection to about 1 cm distal to the tarsometatarsal joints.
- Retract the tendons medially or laterally, make a sharp longitudinal cut into the periosteum, strip the periosteum medially and laterally, leaving it attached in the plantar region, and insert curved retractors.
- With a thin-bladed power saw, make the proximal cut vertical, two thirds to three fourths of the way through the bone (Fig. 7.32A). Make the distal cut about 4 mm from and angled toward the first cut, cutting about two thirds of the way through and joining the first cut. With a thin-bladed osteotome, carefully remove the intervening wafer of bone.

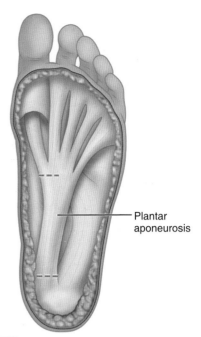

Plantar aponeurosis

FIGURE 7.31 Gould technique for double plantar fasciotomies. **SEE TECHNIQUE 7.14.** (Redrawn from Gould N: Surgery in advanced Charcot-Marie-Tooth disease, *Foot Ankle* 4:267, 1984.) **SEE TECHNIQUE 7.14.**

- Several additional precautions must be taken. When making the distal cut in the first metatarsal, angle it obliquely to correct the metatarsus primus varus that usually exists, creating a biplane osteotomy. Make the osteotomy of the fifth metatarsal near the base so that a plantar ridge does not develop on the weight-bearing surface. After all the osteotomies have been made, each metatarsal is "cracked up" dorsally in turn (Fig. 7.32B), closing the gaps.
- When the foot is plantigrade and no adjustments to the osteotomies are necessary, close the wounds in the usual manner, and apply a short leg walking cast with the ankle in neutral position.

Gould added the Jones procedure (see Technique 7.7) to increase and maintain correction of the first ray. His technique for this does not vary appreciably from the description given.

Equinus of the forefoot also may require the Hibbs procedure (Technique 7.8), which involves transfer of the extensor digitorum longus to the middle cuneiform. In skeletally mature feet, however, plantar fascial release, appropriate osteotomies, and arthrodeses, with or without the Jones procedure, usually correct the forefoot equinus; the claw toe deformity also must be corrected.

ANTERIOR TARSAL WEDGE OSTEOTOMY

TECHNIQUE 7.15

(COLE)
- Make a dorsal longitudinal incision in the midline of the foot beginning just proximal to the midtarsal joints and

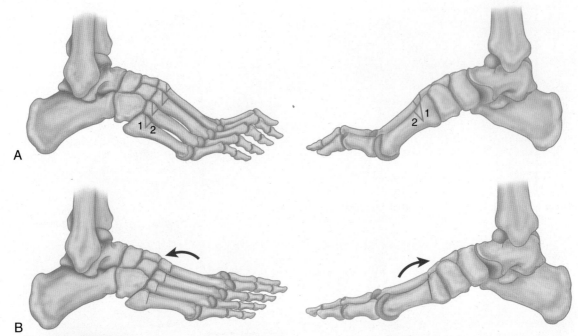

A

B

FIGURE 7.32   Gould closing wedge greenstick dorsal proximal metatarsal osteotomies. **A,** Osteotomies. **B,** Closure of gaps in bone. (Redrawn from Gould N: Surgery in advanced Charcot-Marie-Tooth disease, *Foot Ankle* 4:267, 1984.) **SEE TECHNIQUE 7.14.**

extending distally to the level of the middle of the metatarsal shafts.

- Separate the extensor tendons, usually between those of the third and fourth toes. Incise the periosteum longitudinally and elevate it medially and laterally.
- Identify the tarsal bones with certainty.
- Make an almost vertical transverse osteotomy cut from near the center of the navicular and cuboid to the inferior surface of the tarsus; make a second osteotomy cut, beginning distal to the first and connecting with it at the inferior surface of the tarsus. The distance from the proximal to the distal osteotomy (the width of the wedge) is determined by the severity of the deformity to be corrected (Fig. 7.33).
- Elevate the forefoot and close the defect made by removal of the wedge.
- Close the periosteum with interrupted sutures.
- Apply a plaster cast from the toes to the knee.

POSTOPERATIVE CARE The sutures are removed, and the cast is changed at 2 weeks. The patient remains non–weight bearing for 6 to 8 weeks. With a walking cast or boot, full weight bearing is allowed at 2 months. As swelling and discomfort allows, the cast or boot is discontinued around 2.5 months.

V-OSTEOTOMY OF THE TARSUS

The disadvantage of the anterior tarsal wedge osteotomy is that the deformity is corrected by shortening the convex dorsal surface of the foot, rather than by lengthening the concave plantar surface; consequently, the foot is shortened, widened, and thickened. Japas described a technique to produce a more normal-appearing foot. It consists of a V-osteotomy in which the apex of the V is proximal and at the highest point of the cavus, usually within the navicular. One limb of the V extends laterally and the other medially through the first cuneiform to the medial border. No bone is excised; instead, the proximal border of the distal fragment of the osteotomy is depressed plantarward while the metatarsal heads are elevated, correcting the deformity and lengthening the plantar surface of the foot. The technique is recommended for moderate deformity in children 6 years old or older. Deformities of the hindfoot or midtarsal joint are not corrected by this osteotomy and may require later correction by calcaneal osteotomy or arthrodesis.

TECHNIQUE 7.16

(JAPAS)

- Perform a Steindler plantar fasciotomy through a medial incision on the heel.
- On the dorsum of the foot, make a longitudinal incision 6 to 8 cm long (Fig. 7.34A).
- Carry the dissection between the long extensor tendons of the second and third toes.
- Retract laterally the extensor digitorum brevis and expose extraperiosteally the dorsum of the foot from the talonavicular joint to the tarsometatarsal joints.
- Using a power saw or chisel and osteotome, make the V-osteotomy as follows (Fig. 7.34B). Begin the medial limb of the osteotomy in the first cuneiform immediately proximal to the first metatarsal cuneiform joint and the lateral limb in the cuboid immediately proximal to the

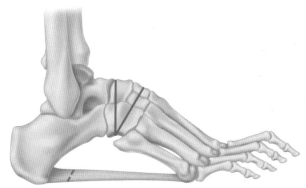

FIGURE 7.33 Cole anterior tarsal wedge osteotomy for cavus deformity. *Colored area* is where wedge is removed. Midtarsal joints are preserved. Plantar fascial release may be required. **SEE TECHNIQUE 7.15.**

joint between this bone and the fifth metatarsal; carry these limbs proximally to join in the midline of the foot at the apex of the cavus deformity, usually within the substance of the navicular. Do not enter the midtarsal joint (Fig. 7.34B and C).

- After the osteotomy has been completed, apply traction to the distal fragment and, using a periosteal elevator, depress its proximal margin plantarward, while elevating the metatarsal heads. If the first metatarsal is in marked equinus, carry the medial limb of the osteotomy through the base of this bone to correct the deformity. Correct any abduction or adduction deformity of the forefoot by simple manipulation.
- When proper alignment has been obtained, fix the osteotomy with one or two Steinmann pins inserted in a posterior direction.
- Remove the tourniquet, obtain hemostasis, and close the incisions.
- If lengthening of the Achilles tendon is necessary, perform this procedure after the tarsal osteotomy.
- Apply a cast from the base of the toes to the tibial tuberosity.

POSTOPERATIVE CARE The sutures are removed, and the cast is changed at 2 weeks. The patient remains non–weight bearing for 2 months. After 2 months, full weight bearing is allowed with a walking cast or boot. As swelling and discomfort allow, the cast or boot is discontinued around 3 months.

TARSOMETATARSAL TRUNCATED-WEDGE ARTHRODESIS

To correct forefoot equinus through the midfoot, Jahss recommended arthrodesis of all tarsometatarsal joints. Jahss did not release the plantar fascia. Instead, he used the shortened plantar fascia to add stability to the osteotomies when the forefoot was dorsiflexed rather than internal fixation.

Jahss performed this procedure in 34 feet in 25 patients with varied diagnoses; none had cerebral palsy. Complications included rotatory valgus deformity of

the forefoot that required compensatory dorsal wedge osteotomy of the first metatarsal (one foot), incomplete correction (one foot), rocker-bottom deformity (two feet), nonunion (two feet), and fifth metatarsal–cuboid arthrodesis (one foot). Jahss did not recommend this procedure for significant cavus deformity at the midtarsal articulation because so much bone must be removed that a rocker-bottom deformity, especially on the lateral side, would result.

TECHNIQUE 7.17

(JAHSS)

- Prepare and drape the lower extremity in the usual manner; do not use a tourniquet.
- With the tip of a finger, palpate the indentation of the first metatarsal–medial cuneiform joint and make a 3.8 cm vertical skin incision on the dorsum of the foot 0.6 cm medial to the extensor hallucis longus (Fig. 7.35A). Center the incision over the joint and, if necessary, extend it slightly proximally and medially.
- Using a thin, sharp, curved 4.8-mm chisel, expose subperiosteally the area to be resected, staying deep to the dorsalis pedis artery.
- With a thin, flat, sharp 2.5-cm osteotome, make the distal osteotomy through the base of the first metatarsal. The osteotome should be as wide as the bone to be cut to avoid piecemeal resection and step-cutting; flush apposition of the osteotomized surfaces increases stability and promotes rapid union.
- Make the proximal osteotomy of the medial cuneiform so that a dorsal truncated wedge can be removed (Fig. 7.35B and C). Avoid any medial wedge that would increase any adductus. It is safer to be conservative, removing 6 to 7 mm as a dorsal wedge; the size can always be increased. Excise truncated rather than triangular wedges of bone, or the plantar fascia will be too tight when the osteotomy is closed, or it may not even permit closure (a truncated wedge does not shorten the overall length of the foot but only lowers the height of the foot to make shoe wear more comfortable).
- Make a second vertical skin incision the same length as the first between the bases of the second and third metatarsals, slightly closer to the third, and their cuneiforms. The base of the second metatarsal tends to extend more proximally than the others.
- Expose the second metatarsal–middle cuneiform joint by similar subperiosteal stripping extending to the first incision to produce a medial longitudinal skin flap. Handle this skin flap and the subsequently developed lateral skin flap with care. Do not retract them or exert more than gentle pressure with a finger to insert the osteotomes.
- Remove a dorsal truncated wedge from the second metatarsal–middle cuneiform joint.
- Working laterally through the same incision, expose and resect the third metatarsal–lateral cuneiform joint.
- Make a third vertical incision just medial to the base of the fifth metatarsal and, in a similar fashion, take wedges from the fourth and fifth metatarsocuboid joints, leaving a second lateral skin flap between the second and third incisions. If the third incision must be extended, lengthen

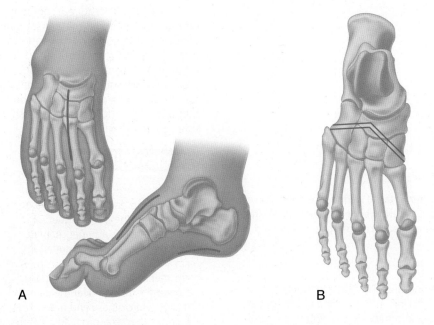

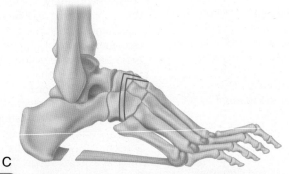

FIGURE 7.34 Japas V-osteotomy of tarsus for cavus deformity. **A,** Skin incisions. **B,** Anterior view of osteotomy. **C,** Lateral view of osteotomy. **SEE TECHNIQUE 7.16.**

the wound proximally and laterally to permit a better blood supply to the second flap; however, the longer the skin incision, the less blood supply to the flaps.

- Dorsiflex the forefoot to close the dorsal wedges (Fig. 7.35D and E).
- Use a finger to palpate in all the wounds and under the flaps to check for any small bone fragments that may block reduction; confirm this by visual inspection.
- Close the osteotomy sites again and palpate the plantar surface of each metatarsal head, feeling for residual depression while keeping the ankle in maximal dorsiflexion. More bone may need to be removed proximally to permit the forefoot to form a right angle with the tibia, while ensuring that all metatarsal heads remain absolutely level (Fig. 7.35F).
- Correct any rotation and adduction deformity.
- The amount of bone removed does not depend on the degree of pes cavus alone, traditionally measured by the angle between the calcaneus and the shaft of the first metatarsal. It is equally dependent on the amount of equinus angulation of the forefoot and any compensatory laxity of the hindfoot, plus the amount of relative fixed depression of each metatarsal head. In general, about 19 mm

of bone usually is removed from the second and third metatarsotarsal joints, slightly less from the first metatarsal–medial cuneiform, and progressively less from the fourth and fifth joints.

- To determine if the foot is plantigrade, measure functional correction by the angle of the plantar surface of the foot to the tibia with the knee in extension and the foot in maximal dorsiflexion. Ideally, this should measure 90 degrees; 5 degrees may be lost after surgery when relaxation of the ankle from general anesthesia has disappeared.
- In severe cavus deformities, do not remove too large a wedge to bring up the forefoot completely; this would result in a rocker-bottom laterally when the wedge is closed. Avoid this by gradually increasing the size of the wedges and repeatedly checking by closing the osteotomy sites.
- If a prominence occurs at the base of the fifth metatarsal when the wedge is closed, excise it with a rongeur through the third skin incision. Removal of the plantar lateral portion of the base of the fifth metatarsal does not disturb peroneus brevis function. Because the dorsal wedge is taken distal to the apex of the longitudinal arch, the tendency for creation of a rocker-bottom is increased. This complication also has been noted after triple arthrodesis.

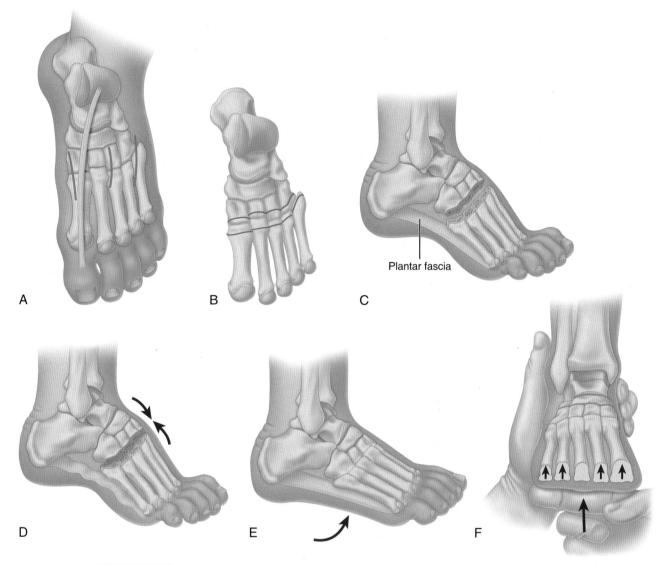

Plantar fascia

A

B

C

D

E

F

FIGURE 7.35 Jahss technique for tarsometatarsal truncated wedge arthrodesis. **A,** Skin incision. **B,** Amount of bone resected. **C–E,** Truncated wedge principle permitting ready closure. Plantar fascia tightens up when wedge is closed, adding stability and eliminating need for internal fixation. **F,** Checking level of metatarsal heads. **SEE TECHNIQUE 7.17.**

- Do not attempt to correct adduction of the forefoot completely and definitely do not overcorrect it because this would cause an annoying prominence medially just proximal to the osteotomy over the medial aspect of the medial cuneiform that is not obvious at surgery.
- Irrigate the wounds and close the skin without subcutaneous sutures.
- Hold the foot in the corrected position and apply a short leg cast with the foot held at a right angle to the tibia. Keep the metatarsals equally plantigrade and without excess abduction or rotation. Ensure the base of the fifth metatarsal does not slip plantarward, which would cause a lateral rocker-bottom deformity.

POSTOPERATIVE CARE The sutures are removed, and the cast is changed at 2 to 3 weeks. Minor adjustment of the forefoot can be made at this time, especially of re-

sidual adductus angulation. At 10 to 12 weeks, full weight bearing is allowed with a walking cast or boot. As swelling and discomfort allows, the cast or boot is discontinued.

STIFF, SEVERE CAVOVARUS DEFORMITY ASSOCIATED WITH ARTHROSIS

TRIPLE ARTHRODESIS

TECHNIQUE 7.18

(SIFFERT, FORSTER, AND NACHAMIE)
- Expose the calcaneocuboid, talonavicular, and subtalar joints through the incision used for ordinary triple arthrodesis.

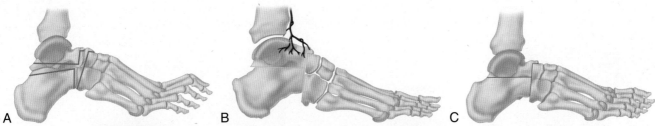

FIGURE 7.36 Siffert, Forster, and Nachamie triple arthrodesis for severe cavus deformity. **A,** Wedge of bone to be removed by osteotomy. Superior part of talar head is retained to form "beak." Bone to be resected from region of midtarsal and subtalar joints is indicated by *colored areas.* Dorsal cortex of navicular is included. **B,** Soft-tissue structures anterior to ankle joint are left undisturbed. **C,** Final position of foot; forefoot has been displaced plantarward, and navicular has been locked beneath remaining part of talar head. **SEE TECHNIQUE 7.18.**

- Denude the calcaneocuboid and subtalar joints of cartilage.
- Excise the dorsal cortex of the navicular.
- Plan the wedge of bone to be removed by osteotomy of the anterior aspect of the calcaneus, the posterior aspect of the navicular, and the inferior aspect of the talar head and neck (Fig. 7.36A); start the osteotomy inferiorly and carry it superiorly to the inferior surface of the talus.
- Resect the inferior part of the talar head and neck to form a beak, leaving undisturbed the soft-tissue structures on the superior aspect of the talus anterior to the ankle joint (Fig. 7.36B).
- Displace the forefoot plantarward and lock the navicular beneath the remaining part of the talar head and neck (Fig. 7.36C).
- When the bones fit together snugly, maintain the position manually by applying slight pressure beneath the forefoot while the cast is being applied; when the fit is not so snug, fix the navicular in proper relationship to the talus by a staple if desired; occasionally, fixing the talus to the calcaneus may be wise.

POSTOPERATIVE CARE A cast is applied with the foot in moderate equinus position and the knee in slight flexion. Firm pressure is exerted on the sole of the foot while the plaster is setting to stretch the plantar structures as much as possible.

An alternative method is shown in Figure 7.37. Occasionally, the deformity is so severe (Fig. 7.38) that the entire navicular is removed (Dunn technique; Fig. 7.39).

TRIPLE ARTHRODESIS

TECHNIQUE 7.19

(LAMBRINUDI)
- With the foot and ankle in extreme plantarflexion, make a lateral radiograph and trace the film. Cut the tracing into three pieces along the outlines of the subtalar and midtarsal joints; from these pieces, the exact amount of bone to

be removed from the talus can be determined accurately before operation. In the tracing, the line representing the articulation of the talus with the tibia is left undisturbed; however, the line corresponding to its plantar and distal parts is to be cut so that, when the navicular and the calcaneocuboid joint are later fitted to it, the foot is in slight equinus in relation to the leg (Fig. 7.40A). Five to 10 degrees is best; if the extremity has shortened, more may be desirable.
- Expose the tarsus through a long lateral curved incision.
- Section the peroneal tendons by a Z-shaped cut, open the talonavicular and calcaneocuboid joints, and divide the interosseous and fibular collateral ligaments of the ankle to permit complete medial dislocation of the tarsus at the subtalar joint.
- With a small power saw (more accurate than a chisel or osteotome), remove the predetermined wedge of bone from the plantar and distal parts of the neck and body of the talus.
- Remove the cartilage and bone from the superior surface of the calcaneus to form a plane parallel with the longitudinal axis of the foot.
- Make a V-shaped trough transversely in the inferior part of the proximal navicular and denude the calcaneocuboid joint of enough bone to correct any lateral deformity.
- Firmly wedge the sharp distal margin of the remaining part of the talus into the prepared trough in the navicular and appose the calcaneus and talus (Fig. 7.40B). Place the distal margin of the talus well medially in the trough; otherwise, the position of the foot would not be satisfactory. (No attempt should be made to compensate in the foot for any tibial torsion.) The talus is now locked in the ankle joint in complete equinus, and the foot cannot be plantarflexed farther.
- Suture the peroneal tendons and close the wound in the routine manner.

POSTOPERATIVE CARE The cast is suspended by slings to an overhead frame for 48 to 72 hours. After 10 to 14 days, the cast is changed, sutures are removed, and non–weight-bearing ambulation on crutches is allowed. This cast is worn for a further 4 weeks, and radiographs are made out of the cast. Weight bearing to tolerance is allowed in a short leg walking cast. This cast is worn until solid bony union is shown clinically and radiographically, usually 12 weeks after surgery.

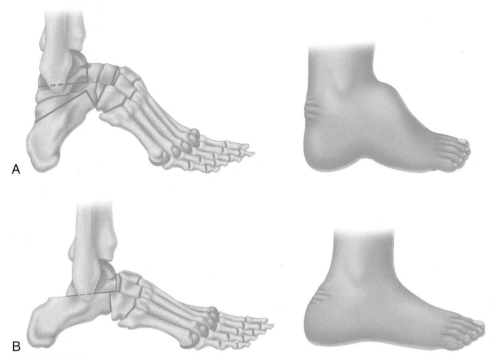

FIGURE 7.37 Triple arthrodesis for calcaneocavus deformity. **A,** Amount of bone resected *(colored area)*. **B,** Position of bones after surgery; foot has been displaced posteriorly at subtalar joint.

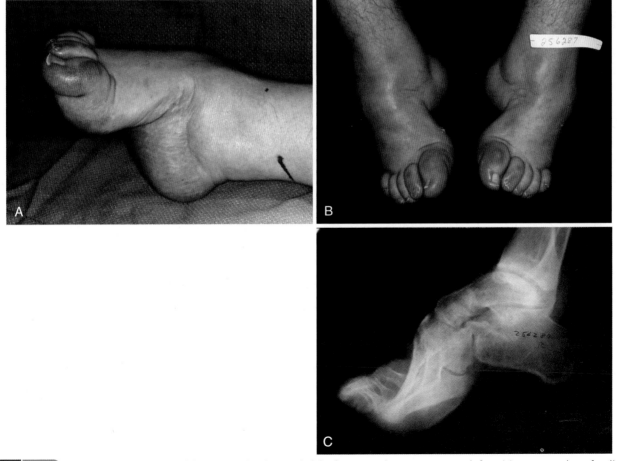

FIGURE 7.38 Medial **(A)** and frontal **(B)** views and radiograph **(C)** of severe calcaneocavovarus deformities as sequelae of poliomyelitis. Entire navicular must be excised to correct cavus deformity.

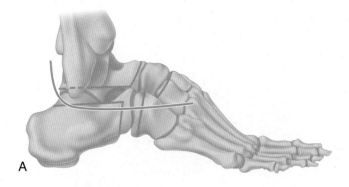

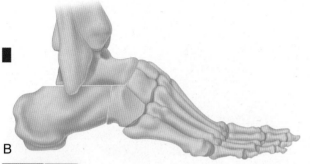

FIGURE 7.39 Dunn arthrodesis. **A,** Position of skin incision *(dashed line)* and amount of bone resected *(colored area)*. **B,** Position of bones after surgery. Foot (except for talus) has been displaced posteriorly at subtalar joint so that head of talus is apposed to cuneiform.

▪ CLAW TOES

In patients with postcompartment syndrome pes cavus, only the claw toe deformities and tight plantar fascia may require surgical treatment, leaving the mild midfoot deformity to appropriate conservative management. For fixed contractures at the metatarsophalangeal and interphalangeal joints, the following are recommended:

1. Lengthening of the extensor hallucis longus and extensor digitorum longus (Fig. 7.41F)
2. Tenotomy of the extensor digitorum brevis and the extensor hallucis brevis (Fig. 7.41B)
3. Dorsal capsulotomy of the metatarsophalangeal joints (Figs. 7.41C and 7.41F)
4. Resection of the head and neck of the proximal phalanges (Fig. 7.41F)
5. Arthrodesis of the hallux interphalangeal joint or plantar plate release with sectioning of the collateral ligaments at the hallux interphalangeal joint with temporary Kirschner wire fixation (Fig. 7.41E)

CORRECTION OF CLAWING OF THE GREAT AND LESSER TOES

TECHNIQUE 7.20

- Through a dorsal, longitudinal incision in the first intermetatarsal space (Fig. 7.41A), expose the extensor tendons to the great and second toes. The terminal branch of the deep peroneal nerve and accompanying first dorsal intermetatarsal artery occupy a slightly deeper plane than the tendons.
- By minimal undermining of each side of the incision, expose the extensor hallucis longus and brevis tendons and the extensor digitorum longus and brevis tendons.
- Lengthen the extensor hallucis longus with a 3-cm coronal (preferred) or sagittal Z-plasty (Fig. 7.41B). Keep in mind that overlapping the tendons during repair is much easier than having insufficient length for the repair when the metatarsophalangeal joint is in neutral position.
- Release the extensor digitorum brevis and extensor hallucis brevis tendons. These tendons are immediately lateral and deep to the extensor digitorum longus and extensor hallucis longus as they approach the metatarsophalangeal joints.
- The correction of the extension posture by tendon lengthening alone can be remarkable. If the deformity is not corrected to neutral position at the metatarsophalangeal joint, proceed with dorsal capsulotomy.
- With the extensor hallucis longus and extensor digitorum longus resting beneath the skin edges, incise the dorsal capsule and both collateral ligaments at the metatarsophalangeal joint (Fig. 7.41C).
- Forcefully flex the metatarsophalangeal joint past neutral, dorsiflex the ankle to neutral, and observe the resting posture of the toes at the metatarsophalangeal joint level. The fixed contracture of the proximal interphalangeal joints is corrected later.
- If the metatarsophalangeal joint can be flexed past neutral, turn attention to the interphalangeal joint of the hallux and the proximal interphalangeal joint of the second toe.
- Approach the interphalangeal joint of the hallux through an L-shaped incision (Fig. 7.41D), with the transverse limb at the joint. The usual error is to place the transverse incision too far proximally; however, if placed too far distally, the germinal matrix of the nail may be damaged. Incise the dorsal capsule (including the extensor hallucis longus terminal tendon) and both collateral ligaments and acutely flex the distal phalanx.
- With a Freer elevator, release the plantar plate from its proximal attachment and dorsiflex the interphalangeal joint.
- If the neutral position can be attained, hold the interphalangeal joint straight with two longitudinal transarticular Kirschner wires or one obliquely placed wire.
- If the neutral position cannot be attained, arthrodese the interphalangeal joint by removing enough bone to allow the joint to assume a neutral position.
- Drive the Kirschner wires retrograde through the distal phalanx so that they emerge 2 to 3 mm plantar to the nail and drive them proximally across the joint into the subchondral bone of the proximal phalanx. Occasionally, the wires must cross the first metatarsophalangeal joint, but usually the bulky forefoot dressing holds that joint in the proper position (Fig. 7.41E).
- Return to the first intermetatarsal space incision and lengthen the extensor digitorum longus, tenotomize the extensor digitorum brevis, and incise the dorsal capsule and collateral ligaments at the metatarsophalangeal joint.

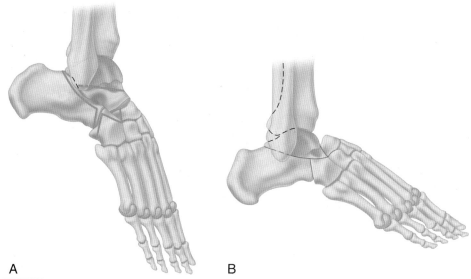

FIGURE 7.40 Lambrinudi arthrodesis. **A,** Part of talus to be resected *(colored area).* **B,** Sharp distal margin of remaining part of talus has been wedged into prepared trough in navicular, and raw osseous surfaces of talus, calcaneus, and cuboid have been apposed. **SEE TECHNIQUE 7.19.**

- Approach the second toe proximal interphalangeal joint through a dorsal elliptical incision (Fig. 7.41F).
- Incise the dorsal capsule and collateral ligaments.
- Raise the extensor tendon proximally and remove the distal third of the proximal phalanx. Remove enough bone so that the toe can be held in neutral position at the proximal interphalangeal joint without bony impingement. This joint can be held in the proper position (0 to 15 degrees of flexion) with a suture passed through the skin and tendon and back through the tendon and skin, and then reverse skin-to-skin in a mattress configuration (Fig. 7.41G).
- Perform the procedure at the third and fourth toes in a similar manner, approaching them through a similar longitudinal incision in the third intermetatarsal space.
- Approach the fifth toe through a straight lateral incision. The fifth toe has no extensor digitorum brevis tendon. If the callosity beneath the fifth metatarsal head is more prominent than beneath the other metatarsal heads, remove the plantar projection of the head flush with the shaft. Suture the tendon of the abductor digiti minimi at the metatarsophalangeal joint to avoid medial subluxation of the fifth toe.
- Approach the proximal interphalangeal joints of the lateral three toes through the same type of dorsal elliptical incision described for the second toe. Straight incisions over these joints may be used if preferred, but the dermodesis effect after removal of the dorsal skin bridge helps hold the proximal interphalangeal joint in good alignment.
- Repair the extensor digitorum longus and extensor hallucis longus tendons with 4-0 nonabsorbable sutures on a small, curved needle while the metatarsophalangeal joint is held in 0 to 10 degrees of extension and the ankle joint is held in neutral.
- Close the skin with 4-0 or 5-0 nonabsorbable sutures and apply a compressive, but not constricting, bulky forefoot dressing to the tips of the toes to hold the toes in the desired position at the metatarsophalangeal and interphalangeal joints.
- Alternatively, use longitudinal Kirschner wires to maintain position, but this usually is unnecessary if the dressing is carefully applied and left in place for 3 weeks.

POSTOPERATIVE CARE With an isolated forefoot procedure, the patient may weight bear in a postoperative shoe. The use of a walker or crutches depends on whether both feet were operated on and the balance of the patient. The dressing is left in place for 2 to 3 weeks. If Kirschner wires were not used to maintain the forefoot reduction, then another forefoot dressing to hold the toes in the proper position is applied and remains for another 10 to 14 days. At 4 to 6 weeks, the Kirschner wires are removed in the clinic or the dressing is discontinued, allowing toe exercises to begin. Discomfort and swelling typically limit closed-toe footwear for 8 to 10 weeks.

SUMMARY OF CAVUS FOOT EVALUATION AND TREATMENT

The important determinants of prognosis and treatment of the cavus foot are as follows:

1. Is the deformity multiplanar or single planar?
2. Is the deformity primarily forefoot, midfoot, hindfoot, or a combination of these?
3. Is one or more of the components fixed?
4. Is the underlying cause one of a progressive course with or without treatment?
5. Are tendon transfers required to maintain the correction gained by arthrodesis or osteotomy?
6. Is there a sensory deficit?

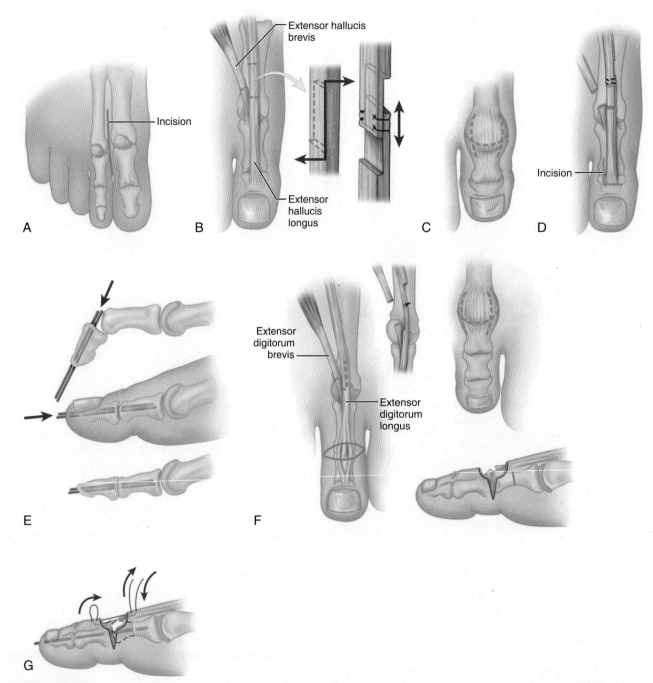

FIGURE 7.41 Surgical technique for clawing of great and second toes. **A,** Incision. **B,** Extensor hallucis longus is lengthened in coronal or sagittal plane, and extensor hallucis brevis is tenotomized. **C,** Dorsal capsulotomy and collateral ligament release. **D,** Approach to interphalangeal joint through separate dorsal incision. **E,** Corrected position on lateral view; arthrodesis of interphalangeal joint of great toe with longitudinal wire down to base of proximal phalanx. **F,** Correction of second toe by excision of head and neck of proximal phalanx, dorsal capsulotomy at metatarsophalangeal joint, lengthening of extensor digitorum longus, and tenotomy of extensor digitorum brevis. **G,** Correction at metatarsophalangeal and proximal interphalangeal joints. **SEE TECHNIQUE 7.20.**

REFERENCES

TARSAL TUNNEL SYNDROME

Abouelela AA, Zohiery AK: The triple compression stress test for diagnosis of tarsal tunnel syndrome, *Foot* 22:146, 2012.

De Bruijn JA, et al.: Superficial peroneal nerve injury risk during a semiblind fasciotomy for anterior chronic exertional compartment syndrome of the leg: an anatomical and clinical study, *Foot Ankle Int* 40(3):343, 2019.

Donovan A, Rosenberg ZS, Cavalcanti CF: MR imaging of entrapment neuropathies of the lower extremity: II. The knee, leg, ankle, and foot, *Radiographics* 30:1001, 2010.

Ferkel E, Davis WH, Ellington JK: Entrapment neuropathies of the foot and ankle, *Clin Sports Med* 34:791, 2015.

Flanigan RM, DiGiovanni BF: Peripheral nerve entrapments of the lower leg, ankle, and foot, *Foot Ankle Clin* 16(2):255, 2011.

Franco MJ, Phillips BZ, Lalchandani GR, Mackinnon SE: Decompression of the superficial peroneal nerve: clinical outcomes and anatomical study, *J Neurosurg* 126:1, 2016.

Gkotsoulias EN, Simonson DC, Roukis TS: Outcomes and safety of endoscopic tarsal tunnel decompression: a systematic review, *Foot Ankle Spec* 7:57, 2014.

Gould JS: Tarsal tunnel syndrome, *Foot Ankle Clin* 16:275, 2011.

Gould JS: Recurrent tarsal tunnel syndrome, *Foot Ankle Clin* 19:451, 2014.

Lans J, Gamo L, DiGiovanni CW, et al.: Etiology and treatment outcomes for sural neuroma, *Foot Ankle Int* 40(5):545, 2019.

Lui TH: Endoscopic anterior tarsal tunnel release: a case repot, *J Foot Ankle Surg* 53:186, 2014.

Luz J, Johnson H, Kohler MJ: Point-of-care ultrasonography in the diagnosis and management of superficial peroneal nerve entrapment: case series, *Foot Ankle Int* 35(12):1362, 2014.

Manske MC, McKeon KE, McCormick JJ, et al.: Arterial anatomy of the posterior tibial nerve in the tarsal tunnel, *J Bone Joint Surg Am* 98(6):499, 2016.

Matsumoto J, Isu T, Kim K, et al.: Clinical features and surgical treatment of superficial peroneal nerve entrapment neuropathy, *Neurol Med -Chir* 58:320, 2018.

Mazzella NL, McMillan AM: Contribution of the sural nerve to postural stability and cutaneous sensation of the lower limb, *Foot Ankle Int* 36(4):450, 2015.

Peck E, Finnoff JT, Smith J: Neuropathies in runners, *Clin Sports Med* 29(3):437, 2010.

Pomeroy G, Wilton J, Anthony S: Entrapment neuropathy about the foot and ankle: an update, *J Am Acad Orthop Surg* 23(1):58, 2015.

Reichert P, Zimmer K, Wnukiewicz W, et al.: Results of surgical treatment of tarsal tunnel syndrome, *Foot Ankle Surg* 21:26, 2015.

Sarrafian SK, Kelikian AS: Nerves. In Kelikian, editor: *Sarrafian's anatomy of the foot and ankle*, ed 3, Philadelphia, 2011, Kluwer/Lippincott, p 381.

Shon LC, Reed MA: Disorders of the nerves. In Coughlin MJ, Saltzman CL, Anderson RB, editors: *Mann's surgery of the foot and ankle*, ed 9, Philadelphia, 2014, WB Saunders/Elsevier, p 612.

Singh G, Kumar VP: Neuroanatomical basis for the tarsal tunnel syndrome, *Foot Ankle Int* 33:513, 2012.

Tennant JN, Rungprai C, Phisitkul P: Bilateral anterior tarsal tunnel syndrome variant secondary to extensor hallucis brevis muscle hypertrophy in a ballet dancer: a case report, *Foot Ankle Surg* 20:e56, 2014.

Thordarson DB: Burial of sural neuroma: technique tip, *Foot Ankle Int* 31:351, 2010.

Yassin M, Garti A, Weissbrot M, Heller E, Robinson D: Treatment of anterior tarsal tunnel syndrome through an endoscopic or open technique, *Foot* 25(3):148, 2015.

INTERDIGITAL NEUROMA

Adams Jr SB, Peters PG, Schon LC: Persistent or recurrent interdigital neuroma, *Foot Ankle Clin* 16:317, 2011.

Campbell CM, Diamond E, Schmit WK, et al.: A randomized, double-blind, placebo-controlled trial of injected capsaicin for pain in Morton's neuroma, *Pain* 157(6):1297, 2016.

Cazzato RL, Garnon J, Ramamurthy N, et al.: Percutaneous MR-guided cryoablation of Morton's neuroma: rationale and technical details after the first 20 patients, *Cardiovasc Intervent Radiol* 39(10):491, 2016.

Chuter GS, Chua YP, Connell DA, Blackney MC: Ultrasound-guided radiofrequency ablation in the management of interdigital (Morton's) neuroma, *Skel Radiol* 42(1):107, 2013.

Claassen L, Bock K, Ettinger M, et al.: Role of MRI in detection of Morton's neuroma, *Foot Ankle Int* 35(10):1002, 2014.

Espinosa N, Seybold JD, Jankauskas L, Erschbamer M: Alcohol sclerosing therapy is not an effective treatment for interdigital neuroma, *Foot Ankle Int* 32:576, 2011.

Gurdezi S, White T, Ramesh P: Alcohol injection for Morton's neuroma: a five-year follow-up, *Foot Ankle Int* 34:1064, 2013.

Hembree CW, Groth AT, Schon LC, Guyton GP: Computed tomography analysis of third webspace injections for interdigital neuroma, *Foot Ankle Int* 34(4):575, 2013.

Kasparek M, Schneider W: Surgical treatment of Morton's neuroma: clinical results after open excision, *Int Orthop* 37:1857, 2013.

Kubota M, Ohno R, Ishijima M, et al.: Minimally invasive endoscopic decompression of the intermetatarsal nerve for Morton's neuroma, *J Orthop* 12(Suppl 1):S101, 2015.

Lee KT, Kim JB, Young KW, et al.: Long-term results of neurectomy in the treatment of Morton's neuroma: more than 10 years' follow-up, *Foot Ankle Spec* 4:349, 2011.

Lui TH: Endoscopic interdigital neurectomy of the foot, *Arth Tech* 6(4):959, 2017.

Mahadevan D, Venkatesan M, Bhatt R, Bhatia M: Diagnostic accuracy of clinical tests for Morton's neuroma compared with ultrasonography, *J Foot Ankle Surg* 54:549, 2015.

Nery C, Raduan F, Del Bouno A, et al.: Plantar approach for excision of a Morton neuroma: a long-term follow-up study, *J Bone Joint Surg Am* 94:654, 2012.

Pace A, Scammell B, Dhar S: The outcome of Morton's neurectomy in the treatment of metatarsalgia, *Int Orthop* 34:51, 2010.

Pasquali C, Vulcano E, Novario R, et al.: Ultrasound-guided alcohol injections for Morton's neuroma, *Foot Ankle Int* 36(1):55, 2015.

Richardson DR, Dean EM: The recurrent Morton neuroma: what now? *Foot Ankle Clin* 19:437, 2014.

Rungprai C, Cychosz CC, Phruetthiphat O, et al.: Simple neurectomy versus neurectomy with intramuscular implantation for interdigital neuroma: a comparative stuy, *Foot Ankle Int* 36(12):1412, 2015.

Santos D, Morrison G, Coda A: Sclerosing alcohol injections for the management of intermetatarsal neuromas: a systematic review, *Foot* 35:36, 2018.

Seok H, Kim SH, Lee SY, Park SW: Extracorpeal shockwave therapy in patients with Morton's neuroma a randomized, placebo-controlled trial, *J Am Podiatr Med Assoc* 106(2):93, 2016.

Thomson CE, Beggs I, Martin DJ, et al.: An injection of corticosteroid plus anesthetic was more effective than anesthetic alone for Morton neuroma, *J Bone Joint Surg Am* 96:334, 2014.

Thomson CE, Beggs I, Martin DJ, et al.: Methylprednisolone injections for the treatment of Morton neuroma: a patient-blinded randomized trial, *J Bone Joint Surg Am* 95:790, 2013.

Valisena S, Petri GF, Ferrero A: Treatment of Morton's neuroma: a systematic review, *Foot Ankle Surg* 24:271, 2018.

CAVUS FOOT

Akoh CC, Phisitkul P: Clinical examination and radiographic assessment of the cavus foot, *Foot Ankle Clin* 24(2):183, 2019.

An TW, Michalski M, Jansson K, Pfeffer G: Comparison of lateralizing calcaneal osteotomies for varus hindfoot correction, *Foot Ankle Int* 39(10):1229, 2018.

Cody EA, Kraszewski AP, Conti MS, et al.: Lateralizing calcaneal osteotomies and their effect on calcaneal alignment: a three-dimensional digital model analysis, *Foot Ankle Int* 39(8):970, 2018.

Dreher T, Beckmann NA, Wenz W: Surgical treatment of severe cavovarus foot deformity in Charcot-Marie-Tooth disease, *J Bone Joint Essent Surg Tech* 5(2):311, 2015.

Dreher T, Wolf SI, Heitzmann D, et al.: Tibialis posterior tendon transfer corrects the foot drop component of cavovarus foot deformity in Charcot-Marie-tooth disease, *Bone Joint Surg Am* 96(6):456, 2014.

Faldini C, Traina F, Nanni M, et al.: Surgical treatment of cavus foot in Charcot-Marie-tooth disease. A review of twenty-four cases: AAOS exhibit selection, *J Bone Joint Surg Am* 97(6):e30, 2015.

Jaffe D, Vier D, Kane J, et al.: Rate of neurologic injury following lateralizing calcaneal osteotomy performed through a medial approach, *Foot Ankle Int* 38(12):1367, 2017.

Jung HG, Park JT, Lee SH: Joint-sparing correction for idiopathic cavus foot: correlation of clinical and radiographic results, *Foot Ankle Clin* 18:659, 2013.

Kaplan JRM, Aiyer A, Derrato RA, et al.: Operative treatment of the cavovarus foot, *Foot Ankle Int* 39(11):1370, 2018.

Krähenbühl N, Weinberg MW: Anatomy and biomechanics of cavovarus deformity, *Foot Ankle Clin* 24(2):173, 2019.

Leeuwesteijn AE, de Visser E, Louwerens JW: Flexible cavovarus feet in Charcot-Marie-Tooth disease treated with first ray proximal dorsiflexion osteotomy combined with soft tissue surgery: a short-term to mid-term outcome study, *Foot Ankle Surg* 16:142, 2010.

Li S, Myerson MS: Failure of surgical treatment in patients with cavovarus deformity: why does this happen and how do we approach treatment? *Foot Ankle Clin* 24(2):361, 2019.

Myerson MS, Myerson CL: Cavus foot: deciding between osteotomy and arthrodesis, *Foot Ankle Clin* 24(2):347, 2019.

Neumann JA, Nickisch F: Neurologic disorders and cavovarus deformity, *Foot Ankle Clin* 24(2):195, 2019.

Pfeffer GB, Michalski MP, Basak T, et al.: Use of 3D prints to compare the efficacy of three different calcaneal osteotomies for the correction of heel varus, *Foot Ankle Int* 39(5):591, 2018.

VanValkenburg S, Hsu RY, Palmer DS, et al.: Neurologic deficit associated with lateralizing calcaneal osteotomy for cavovarus foot correction, *Foot Ankle Int* 37(10):1106, 2016.

The complete list of references is available online at ExpertConsult.com.

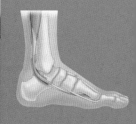

DISORDERS OF NAILS

Benjamin J. Grear

Deformities and diseases of the toenails are some of the most common and most disabling foot problems. They range from minor annoyances to severe life- or limb-threatening conditions, and abnormalities of the toenails can be a sign of a systemic disease process. Often the pain associated with nail disorders has a marked effect on individuals' daily lives. A study of 55 patients with nail disorders found that they were significantly correlated with dysfunction of the lower extremities and, in elderly patients, were likely to increase the risk of falling. Many of the specific nail pathologies and associated systemic disorders are outside the scope of orthopaedic medicine, but awareness and basic understanding are important for any clinician encountering foot and ankle conditions. This chapter briefly highlights nail pathology associated with systemic diseases, tumors, acquired disorders, and surgical techniques.

ANATOMY

The normal nail complex consists of the nail plate, the nail bed, and the surrounding skin. The *nail plate* is the nail proper and consists of two components: the *root,* the portion of the nail plate that is beneath the skin, and the *body,* the exposed portion of the nail plate. The nail plate is made up of overlapping layers of keratinized cells. Beneath the nail plate, the *nail bed* has two components, the *sterile matrix* and the *germinal matrix.* This distal margin of the germinal matrix can be seen through the nail plate as pale, crescent-shaped tissue at the base of the nail plate. This visible portion of the germinal matrix is termed the *lunula.* From the distal margin of the lunula, the germinal matrix extends 5to 8 mm proximally and deep to the proximal nail fold. The germinal matrix is smoother and paler than the adjacent sterile matrix, and it contributes to longitudinal nail plate growth (Fig. 8.1A). Distal to the germinal matrix, the sterile matrix supplies a vascular bed for the nail plate. The margins of skin that overhang the lateral borders of the nail are termed *lateral nail folds.* The proximal nail fold is termed the *eponychium,* and its distal extension that covers the nail root and adheres to the nail plate is the *cuticle.* Finally, the *hyponychium* is the thickened skin located at the distal margin of the nail.

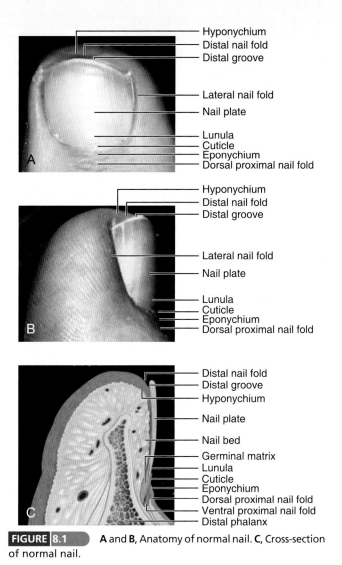

FIGURE 8.1 A and B, Anatomy of normal nail. C, Cross-section of normal nail.

BOX 8.1

Glossary of Terms Describing Pathologic Conditions of the Nail

Acral: Of or belonging to the extremities of peripheral body parts.

Anonychia: Absence of nails. When anonychia is congenital, all the nails are usually absent and the condition is permanent. It can occur temporarily from trauma, systemic or local disease. Also seen in nail-patella syndrome.

Beau lines: Transverse lines or ridges marking repeated disturbances of nail growth. May be associated with trauma or a systemic disease process.

Clubbing: Hypertrophied, curved nail with flattened angle between the nail plate and proximal fold. Associated with chronic pulmonary and cardiac disease.

Hapalonychia: Extremely soft nails that may be prone to splitting; associated with endocrine disturbances, malnutrition, and contact with strong alkali solutions.

Hemorrhage: Bleeding. Beneath toenail, bleeding may be associated with vitamin C deficiency, subacute bacterial endocarditis, and dermatologic disorders. *Subungual hematoma* occurs after trauma to toenail bed.

Hutchinson sign: Hyperpigmentation spreading from nail to surrounding soft tissue. Pathognomonic for melanoma.

Hyperkeratosis: Thickening of the stratum corneum layer of the epidermis.

Hyperkeratosis subungualis: Hypertrophy of the nail bed. May be associated with onychomycosis, psoriasis, and other dermatologic disorders.

Koilonychia: Concavity of the nail plate in both longitudinal and transverse axes. Associated with nutritional disorders, iron deficiency anemia, and endocrine disorders.

Lentigo: A small melanotic spot without pigment, which is potentially malignant and is unrelated to sun exposure.

Leukonychia: White spots or striations in the nail resulting from trauma and systemic diseases, such as nutritional and endocrine deficiencies.

Mees lines: Horizontal striations 1 to 3 mm wide associated with growth arrest.

Melanonychia: A longitudinal streak of pigment visible in or beneath the nail.

Onychauxis: Greatly thickened nail plate caused by persistent mild trauma and onychomycosis.

Onychia: Inflammation of the nail matrix, causing deformity of the nail plate and resulting from trauma, infection, and systemic diseases, such as exanthemas.

Onychitis: Inflammation of the nail.

Onychoclasis: Breakage of the nail plate.

Onychocryptosis: Ingrowing of nails or, more specifically, hypertrophy of the nail lateral fold; also referred to as *hypertrophied ungual labia* or *unguis incarnatus*; one of the most common pathologic conditions of the toenail.

Onychogryphosis: "Claw nail" or "ram's horn nail"; extreme hypertrophy of the nail gives the appearance of a claw or horn. May be congenital or a symptom of many chronic systemic diseases, such as tinea infections. See *onychauxis.*

Onycholysis: Loosening of the nail plate, beginning along the distal or free edge when trauma, injury by chemical agents, or diseases loosen the nail plate. Associated with psoriasis, onychomycosis, acute fevers, and syphilis.

Onychoma: Tumor of the nail unit.

Onychomadesis: Complete loss of the nail plate.

Onychomalacia: Softening of the nail.

Onychomycosis: Fungal infection of the nail associated with fungal disease of the foot.

Onychophosis: Accumulation of callus within the lateral groove, involving the great toe more often than the lesser toes.

Onychoptosis defluvium: Nail shedding.

Onychorrhexis: Longitudinal ridging and splitting of nails caused by dermatoses, nail infections, systemic diseases, senility, or injury by chemical agents.

Onychoschizia: Lamination and scaling away of nails in thin layers caused by dermatoses, syphilis, or chemical agents.

Onychosis: Disease or deformity of the nail plate. Also called *onychopathy.*

Onychotrophia: Atrophy or failure of development of a nail caused by trauma, infection, endocrine dysfunction, or systemic disease.

Orthonyx: Mechanical bracing of nails to correct curvature.

Pachyonychia: Extreme thickening of all the nails. Thickening is more solid and more regular than in onychogryphosis. Usually, a congenital condition associated with hyperkeratosis of the palms and soles.

Paronychia: Inflammation of soft tissues around the nail margin, which can occur after trauma or infection (bacterial or fungal).

Parrot beak nail: Hooked nail deformity where nail curves palmarward. May be caused by tight closure of a digit tip amputation.

Pincer nail: Ingrown toenail with both sides of the nail turned in, nearly forming a complete circle.

Pitting: Tiny depressions in the nail surface; associated with psoriasis and alopecia areata. Also known as "stippling."

Pterygium: Growth of cuticle distal to the nail plate, splitting the nail into two or more portions that gradually decrease in size as the growth widens. Can result from trauma and decreased circulation in the toes.

Stratum corneum: The most superficial layer of the epidermis.

Subungual hematoma: Blood that has collected beneath the nail plate, usually secondary to trauma. Also known as "tennis toe" or "jogger's toe."

Trachyonychia: "Rough nails." A reaction or morphologic pattern, with various clinical appearances and causes.

Yellow nail syndrome: Keratohyalin granules within the nail plate seen only with electron microscopy.

Many descriptive terms and definitions communicate nail pathologies (Box 8.1). Although not always realized, nail pathology may be a sign of other underlying pathology. Many systemic diseases are associated with nail abnormalities (Table 8.1).

TRAUMA

The dropping of heavy objects or activities performed without wearing shoes can cause traumatic injuries that can easily damage the nail plate, nail bed, and underlying phalanx.

TABLE 8.1

Cardiovascular Disorders and Associated Toenail Conditions

DISEASE	PATHOLOGIC CHANGES
Arterial emboli	Splinter hemorrhages
Arteriosclerosis obliterans	Leukonychia partialis
Bacterial endocarditis	Clubbing, splinter hemorrhages
Hypertension	Splinter hemorrhages
Ischemia	Onycholysis, pterygium
Mitral stenosis	Splinter hemorrhages
Myocardial infarction	Mees lines, yellow nail syndrome
Vasculitis	Splinter hemorrhages

These injuries can cause long-term nail plate abnormalities and even nail plate loss. Abnormalities can include ridging, splitting, thickening, and discoloration. Treatment goals for nail bed and plate injuries include repairing the nail bed and maintenance of the eponychial fold to minimize future nail deformity. The sterile matrix is very vascular; hence, subungual hematomas frequently occur with trauma. Treatment of subungual hematomas remains controversial. Past recommendations have included nail plate removal for nail bed exploration and repair for subungual hematomas larger than 50% of the size of the nail or larger than 25% with an underlying fracture. More recently, others have suggested trephination alone is adequate treatment when nail margins are intact.

When nail margins are intact, we typically treat subungual hematomas with trephination or observation depending on the patient's pain and acuity. Trephination can be done by using a heated paperclip to perforate the nail plate. The hematoma cools the paper clip, preventing nail bed injury. Other methods include ophthalmic cautery or needle perforation. Occasionally, more than one opening is required to adequately maintain hematoma decompression.

Despite the controversy, most authors agree that if a subungual hematoma is associated with unstable nail margins, then nail plate removal, exploration, and nail bed repair is indicated to prevent future aesthetic and functional problems. Laceration repairs should be completed with small absorbable suture (7-0 chromic) or medical adhesives (2-octyl cyanoacrylate). After repairing the nail bed, the nail or an alternative material (acrylic nail, aluminum foil, silicon sheeting, or other nonadherent material) should be secured over the nail bed and under the eponychium, preventing adhesions between the eponychium and the germinal matrix. Creating small perforations in the replaced nail or other material is important to prevent fluid accumulation beneath the nail. The nail can be secured with a figure-of-eight stitch or medical adhesive (Fig. 8.2).

DYSTROPHIC NAILS (ONYCHOGRYPOSIS, ONYCHOMYCOSIS)

Deformed nails in elderly and diabetic patients can be difficult to manage at best and catastrophic at worst, especially when associated with an insensitive foot. Having a small

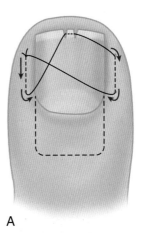

A

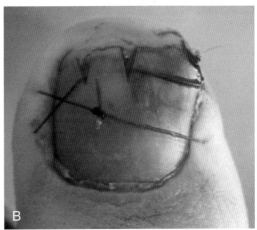

B

FIGURE 8.2   Transverse figure-of-eight suture for securing the nail. (From Bristol SG, Verchere CG: The transverse figure-of-eight suture for securing the nail, J Hand Surg 32:124, 2007.)

double-action rongeur and nail splitter-cutter in the office is recommended. These nails can be reduced quickly and safely with these instruments (Fig. 8.3).

Other than reduction of the nail mass, onychomycosis, or fungal infection of the nails, can often be treated with benign neglect because its main effect is a cosmetic one. If treatment is desired to eradicate the fungal infection, referral to a dermatologist may be warranted for confirmatory testing through appropriate cultures followed by cost-effective medical treatment, either by topical or oral agents. Most treatment regimens are prolonged because it is difficult for various medications to penetrate the nail. Many of the oral medications have serious side effects, and patients should be appropriately monitored for these side effects.

The efficacy of laser therapy for onychomycosis remains controversial. Lasers are approved by the US Food and Drug Administration (FDA) for "temporary increase of clear nail in patients with onychomycosis," but laser treatment has resulted in lower cure rates than oral and topical therapies. Hence, laser treatment is not regarded as a first line treatment for onychomycosis.

OTHER LESIONS OF THE NAILS
SUBUNGUAL EXOSTOSIS

This entity is not a primary nail abnormality; however, it is usually presented as a painful and deformed nail, leaving the

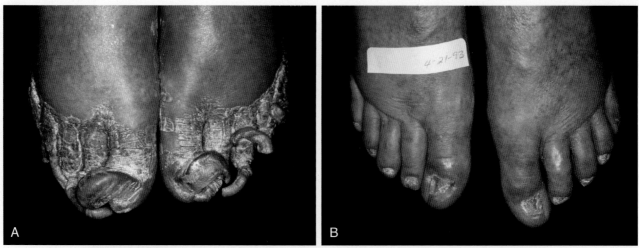

FIGURE 8.3   **A,** Onychomycosis. Ram's horn nails in 90-year-old man. **B,** After nail reduction.

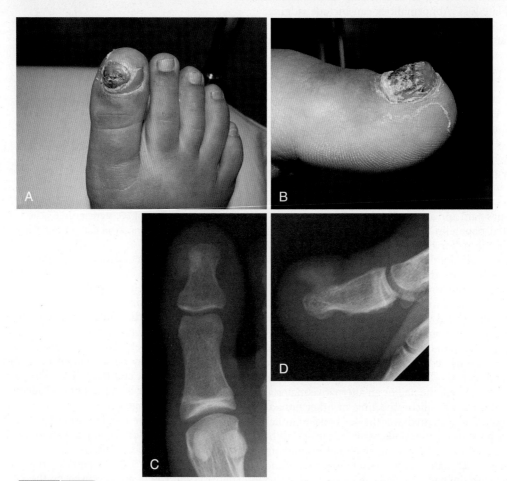

FIGURE 8.4   Subungual exostosis in right hallux of 15-year-old girl who presented with 3-month history of pain and enlarging mass. **A** and **B,** Clinical photographs. **C** and **D,** Radiographs. (From DaCambra MP, Gupta SK, Ferri-de-Barros F: Subungualexostosis of the toes: a systematic review, *Clin Orthop Relat Res* 472:1251–1259, 2014.)

examiner perplexed as to the cause of the pain and deformity (Fig. 8.4). The exostosis of the distal phalanx is formed from fibrous tissue and has a fibrocartilage cap, as opposed to an osteochondroma, which is formed from enchondral ossification and has a hyaline cartilage cap. The chromosomal translocation t(X:6)(q22;q13-14) is linked to this entity, suggesting a neoplastic origin. Routine radiographs of the feet may not show the exostosis because the technique does not emphasize the distal phalanx. Radiographs taken at oblique angles and magnified are helpful. Conservative treatment is not usually successful as this lesion is progressive, and surgical excision is the treatment of choice. If the exostosis has not disrupted the

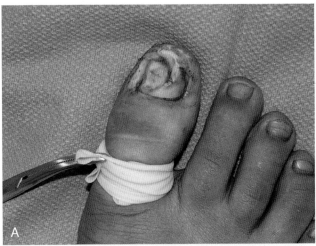

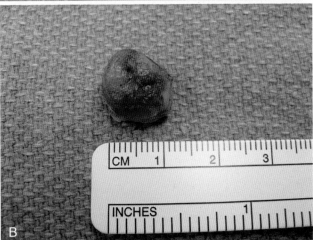

FIGURE 8.5 Marginal excision of subungual exostosis. **A,** Because lesion had invaded nail bed, making it unsalvageable, direct dorsal exostectomy was done. **B,** Osteocartilaginous lesion was marginally resected, and base of stalk was curetted, ronguered, and burred down to create "saucer-like" defect. (From DaCambra MP, Gupta SK, Ferri-de-Barros F: Subungual exostosis of the toes: a systematic review, *Clin Orthop Relat Res* 472:1251–1259, 2014.)

nail bed, the incision should be made lateral or medial to the nail bed, elevating it off the exostosis to remove it to preserve the nail bed (Fig. 8.4). If, however, the nail bed is disrupted, a dorsal incision to remove the exostosis should be used (Fig. 8.5). The most common complication from surgical excision is nail deformity. Recurrence has been reported at 4%.

TECHNIQUE FOR SUBUNGUAL EXOSTOSIS

TECHNIQUE 8.1

(LOKIEC ET AL.)
- After the administration of general anesthesia (young children) or ankle block (adolescents), apply a toe or ankle tourniquet.

- Remove a narrow strip of nail (less than one fourth of the nail width) on the medial side of the toe (Fig. 8.6A) to expose the exostosis.
- Carefully dislodge part of the remaining nail from its proximal attachments at the larger side of the exostosis, leaving the remainder of the nail in place, to fully expose the exostosis abutting and penetrating the nail bed.
- Make a small osteotomy paralleling the distal phalanx to remove the exostosis in one piece (Fig. 8.6B).
- Use a fine rongeur or a burr to produce a smooth surface and remove any residual osteochondroma tissue.
- Irrigate the wound with saline, relocate the elevated nail and suture the nail fold with two small absorbable stitches (Fig. 8.6C) to cover the raw bone of the phalanx.

POSTOPERATIVE CARE The nonadhesive dressings are changed every 3 days during the next 3 weeks. At 3 weeks, the sutures are removed and gradual return to normal-width shoes is allowed.

TECHNIQUE FOR SUBUNGUAL EXOSTOSIS

TECHNIQUE 8.2

(MULTHOPP-STEPHENS AND WALLING)
- Expose the lesion by removing a portion of the nail, or the entire nail if necessary (Fig. 8.7A and B).
- Ellipse the exostosis and carry dissection down to the phalanx where the stalk or base is attached. Do not try to preserve the overlying nail bed (Fig. 8.7C).
- Remove the exostosis, including the cartilaginous cap and the overlying nail bed at its base from the distal phalanx.
- Use a small burr to remove 1 to 2 mm of normal bone at the base of the lesion and smooth the contour of the distal phalanx (Fig. 8.7D).
- Place an Adaptic, nonstick dressing beneath the nail fold.
- Allow the defect to granulate and heal secondarily.

POSTOPERATIVE CARE Patients are placed in a postoperative shoe and allowed to bear weight as tolerated.

SUBUNGUAL AND PERIUNGUAL FIBROMAS
Subungual and periungual fibromas can be most difficult to diagnose preoperatively. A history of long-standing symptoms, several physicians having seen the patient, local tenderness beneath a particular portion of the nail, and a frustrated patient all reinforce the suspicion of this diagnosis. If the mass is readily seen, as it occasionally is, the diagnosis is straightforward. A high index of suspicion for this rare tumor is warranted in patients with tuberous sclerosis because up to 80% may have ungual fibromas (Fig. 8.8).

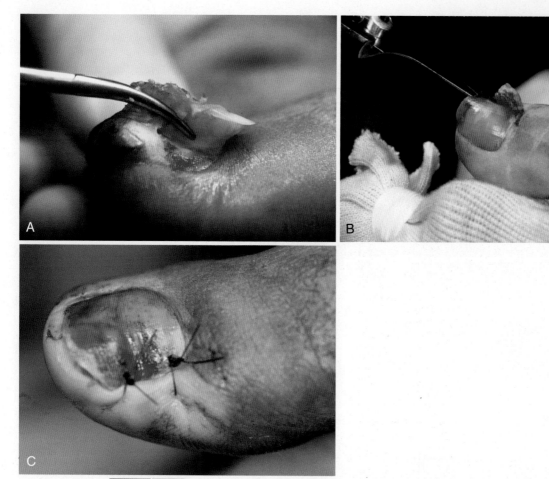

FIGURE 8.6   **A,** Narrow strip of nail over medial side of exostosis is removed, and nail is dislodged to expose exostosis. **B,** Small osteotome paralleling distal phalanx removes exostosis in one piece. **C,** Nail is relocated to cover raw phalanx bone and stitched in place. (From Lokiec F, Ezra E, Krasin E, et al: A simple and efficient surgical technique for subungual exostosis, *J Pediatr Orthop* 21:76–79, 2001.) **SEE TECHNIQUE 8.1.**

TECHNIQUE FOR SUBUNGUAL AND PERIUNGUAL FIBROMAS

TECHNIQUE 8.3

- If the mass is beneath the nail, remove the portion overlying the area of tenderness.
- Magnification and high-intensity lighting are helpful for locating a small, pearly whitish change in color compared with the surrounding matrix. Excise this portion down to the phalanx with a small margin of what appears as normal matrix and then section the tissue. It has a gritty feel when sectioned.
- Send the specimens to pathology with the suspected diagnosis.

POSTOPERATIVE CARE The postoperative care is the same as after incomplete matrixectomy, and permanent deformity of the nail may occur. This is less likely, however, than after removal of a large subungual exostosis.

GLOMUS TUMOR

The glomus tumor is an enigmatic, painful tumor that is rarely seen and represents a proliferation of the normal capsular-neural glomus apparatus. Patients commonly present with a painful, exquisitely tender mass beneath the nail that is accompanied by a faint bluish hue. Except for the slight change in color of the nail overlying the tumor, the nail may appear normal. The nail is normal, and the mass seen through the nail plate is abnormal. Radiographs may reveal a semispherical cortical lesion that, when present, is pathognomonic for a glomus tumor (Fig. 8.9).

Removal of the portion of the nail plate over the area of tenderness and excision of the matrix that appears involved, along with a margin of normal-appearing matrix, is the treatment of choice. The nail that returns should have a normal appearance, but the patient must be warned that this is unpredictable. Magnification and high-intensity lighting facilitate excision of these periungual and subungual masses.

Horst and Nunley described a technique for removal of glomus tumors that uses a full-thickness vascular skin flap to expose the tumor while preserving the nail and nail matrix. They reported complete relief of pain, no wound healing problems, and no recurrences in seven patients in whom this technique was used.

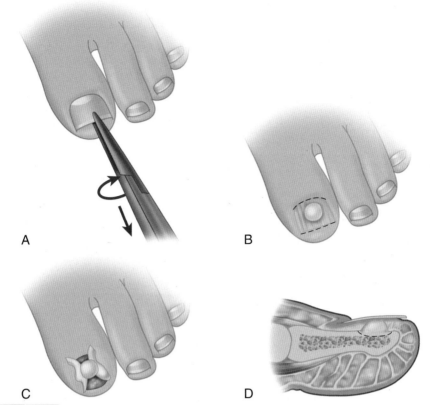

FIGURE 8.7 Surgical excision of subungual exostosis. **A,** Toenail is completely avulsed to expose exostosis. **B,** Longitudinal incision is made in nail bed, avoiding injury to nail matrix. **C,** Nail bed is reflected. **D,** Exostosis is excised with wide margins and nail bed is repaired. (From Walling AK: Soft tissue and bone tumors. In Coughlin MJ, Mann RA, Saltzman CL, editors: *Surgery of the foot and ankle,* ed 8, Philadelphia, 2007, Elsevier.) **SEE TECHNIQUE 8.2.**

TECHNIQUE FOR GLOMUS TUMOR

TECHNIQUE 8.4

(HORST AND NUNLEY)

- Make an inverted L-shaped incision around the nail with the short leg of the L parallel to and 5 mm distal to the distal end of the nail and the long leg of the L 5 mm medial or lateral to the nail, extending proximal to the nail matrix, usually all the way to the joint (Fig. 8.10A).
- Create a full-thickness flap down to bone and sharply elevate it without injuring the nail matrix (Fig. 8.10B).
- Reflect the skin and matrix flap and inspect the interior side. Usually, the glomus tumor is obvious within the tissue or nail matrix as a ball-shaped or egg-shaped opaque, semi-elastic structure (Fig. 4.10C). Occasionally, the tumor has eroded into the distal phalanx.
- Excise the tumor (which is usually well encapsulated) with a small knife or curet.
- Release the tourniquet, control bleeding with bipolar electrocautery, and close the wound in one layer with nylon-interrupted suture.

POSTOPERATIVE CARE The patient is given a hard-soled shoe to wear until the wound heals. Regular shoes can generally be worn at 4 to 6 weeks.

BOX 8.2

ABCDE Acronym for Diagnosis of Melanoma

A: Asymmetry: one half of the lesion is not identical to the other
B: Border: irregular, ragged, or indistinct border
C: Color: more than one color present within the lesion
D: Diameter: larger than 6 mm in diameter
E: Evolution: any change in the lesion in size, shape, or color

MALIGNANT MELANOMA

The orthopaedist seldom makes the initial diagnosis of malignant melanoma (Fig. 8.11). To overlook this diagnosis, however, or not have this diagnosis in the differential could lead to a poor prognosis because a delay in treatment leads to worse outcomes. The standard ABCDE acronym (Box 8.2) is useful for the diagnosis of melanoma but may not be adequate for the foot. Some have suggested the CUBED acronym to aid in the diagnosis in the foot (Box 8.3) because presentation in the foot may be atypical.

Only 2% to 3% of melanomas occur in the nail apparatus, and the occurrence is more common in individuals of Asian or African descent, groups that have a lower incidence of melanoma at other sites. Subungual melanomas are usually painless black discolorations under the nail, but they can also be

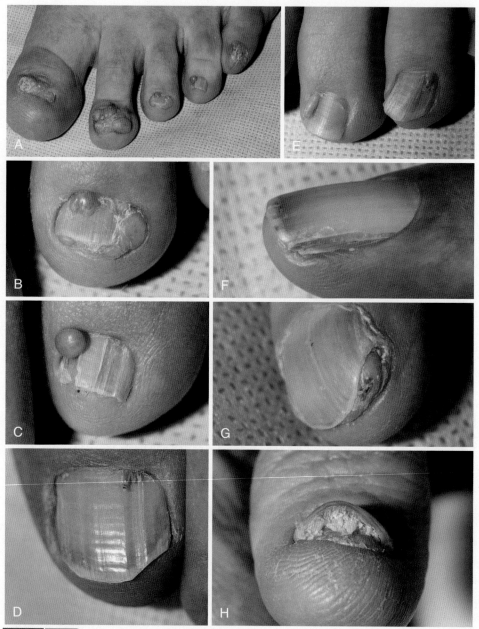

FIGURE 8.8   Periungual fibroma and subungual fibroma in tuberous sclerosis complex. **A,** Ungual fibromas involving all nails. **B,** Third toe shows clove-like periungual fibroma, nail-like periungual fibroma, and subungual fibroma. **C,** Fourth toe shows globoid periungual fibroma and longitudinal groove without visible fibroma. **D,** Three fusiform periungual fibromas filling one longitudinal groove. **E,** Vermiform periungual fibromas. **F,** Longitudinal groove without visible fibroma. **G,** Subungual fibroma protruding from under nail plate. **H,** Elevation of nail plate from subungual fibroma. (From Aldrich CS, Hong CH, Groves L, et al: Acral lesions in tuberous sclerosis complex: insights into pathogenesis, *J Am Acad Dermatol* 63:244–251, 2010.)

amelanotic, and they may or may not involve nail plate changes (Fig. 8.12). Warning signs that may indicate a subungual melanoma include the Hutchinson sign (Fig. 8.12) in which the periungual skin is pigmented around a hyperpigmented nail plate. Differing from melanoma, discoloration from a subungual hematoma dissipates and migrates distally with time. Likewise, any traumatic discoloration of the periungual skin resolves with time as the hematoma subsides (Fig. 8.13).

Longitudinal melanonychia is another benign process that may mimic melanoma. Longitudinal or linear melanonychia is present in 70% to 100% of African-Americans and 10% to 20% of Japanese patients (Fig. 8.14). To further complicate an accurate diagnosis, a pseudo-Hutchinson sign also mimics melanoma. The visualization of nail plate hyperpigmentation through the clear cuticle is termed a pseudo-Hutchinson sign, which is distinctly different than true hyperpigmentation of the periungual skin. To distinguish a pseudo-Hutchinson sign and longitudinal melanonychia from a true Hutchinson sign or melanoma, dermatologists employ dermoscopy and pathology to confirm diagnosis. When diagnosis and staging are finalized, the surgical treatment is a proximal amputation at the metatarsophalangeal joint or proximal metatarsal. For those techniques, see other chapter.

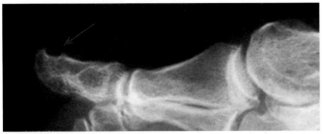

FIGURE 8.9 Lateral radiograph of erosion in distal hallux caused by glomus tumor. (From Polo C, Borda D, Poggio D, et al: Glomus tumor of the hallux. Review of the literature and report of two cases, *Foot Ankle Surg* 18:89–93, 2012.)

INGROWN TOENAIL (ONYCHOCRYPTOSIS, UNGUIS INCARNATUS)

ETIOLOGY

The term *ingrown toenail* is misleading. If used to designate a hook of nail caused by improper nail care growing into

---

BOX 8.3

CUBED Acronym for Diagnosis of Melanoma of the Feet

C: Color: lesions where any part is not skin color
U: Uncertain diagnosis; any lesion that does not have a definitive diagnosis
B: Bleeding lesions on the foot or under the nail, whether direct bleeding or oozing of fluid; includes chronic "granulation tissue"
E: Enlargement or deterioration of a lesion or ulcer despite therapy
D: Delay in healing of any lesion beyond 2 months

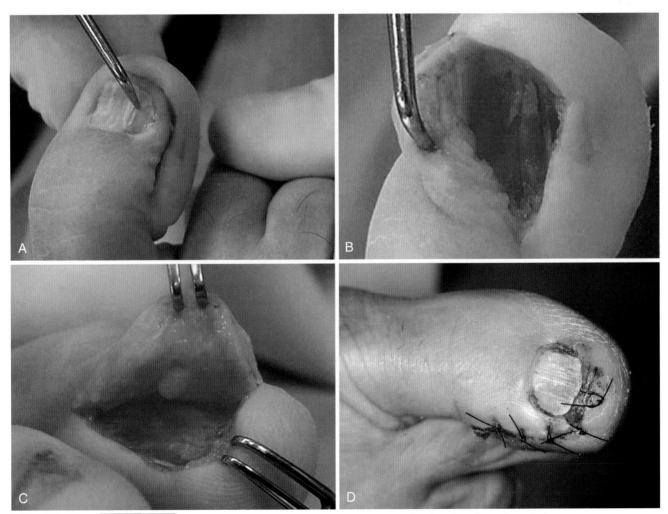

FIGURE 8.10 **A,** L-shaped full-thickness flap. **B,** Elevation of nail with nail matrix and glomus tumor. **C,** Glomus tumor in epithelial bed underneath flap. **D,** Postoperative photograph. (**A-C** from Horst F, Nunley JA: Technique tip: glomus tumors in the foot: a new surgical technique for removal, *Foot Ankle Int* 24:949–951, 2003.) **SEE TECHNIQUE 8.4.**

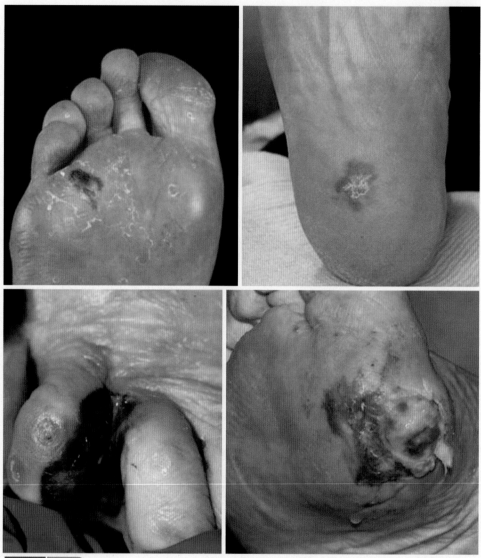

FIGURE 8.11   Various presentations of melanoma on the skin of the foot. (From Bristow IR, de Berker DA, Acland KM, et al: Clinical guidelines for the recognition of melanoma of the foot and nail unit, *J Foot Ankle Res* 3:25, 2010.)

an overlapping nail fold that has obliterated the lateral nail groove, the term is acceptable (see Fig. 8.1B). The most probable cause of the symptom complex is a combination of factors; however, only one of these may be an improperly trimmed nail. The condition is rare in people who do not wear shoes, likely explained by the absence of extrinsic pressure. Within the confines of the shoe toe box, the great toe is pushed toward the second toe, resulting in pressure against the lateral border of the nail, while the shoe itself exerts pressure on the medial side of the nail. This extrinsic pressure causes the nail fold to push into the sharp edge of an improperly cut nail, breaking the skin. The bacterial and fungal flora on the skin enter the open wound, albeit a small one, and inflammation results. A bottlenecked, poorly draining abscess follows, causing erythema, edema, hyperhidrosis, and tenderness. Finally, hypertrophic granulation tissue completes the clinical picture of the familiar infected ingrown toenail (see Fig. 8.1C). The hypertrophic granulation tissue is slowly covered by epithelium, further inhibiting drainage and promoting edema. This

process makes the nail even more vulnerable to injury by extrinsic pressure, and the cycle repeats itself.

NONOPERATIVE MANAGEMENT
■ STAGE I (INFLAMMATORY STAGE)

In stage I, the patient has mild erythema, swelling, and tenderness along the lateral nail fold (Fig. 8.15A). The treatment involves lifting the lateral edge of the nail plate from its embedded position in the dermis of the lateral nail fold. This is easier to perform if done after soaking the foot, which makes the nail softer and more pliable. Nonabsorbent cotton, wool, or acrylic mesh is passed beneath the corner of the nail (Fig. 8.16). This is done gently because it is frequently painful. The patient may need a few days of intermittent warm soaks, a cutout shoe, and modification of activity before the local inflammation is reduced enough to allow this treatment. Once begun, however, the patient can usually introduce more material beneath the nail corner than the physician. The patient repeats the treatment daily until the nail grows out and can then be

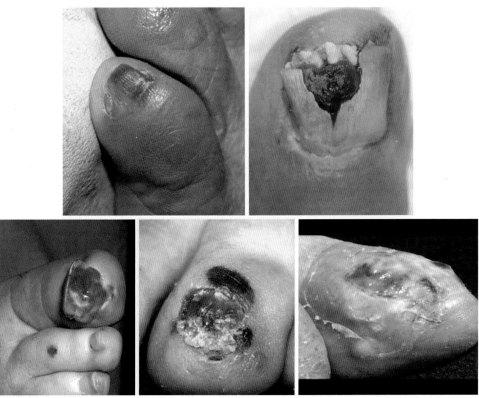

FIGURE 8.12 Various presentations of nail unit melanoma. (From Bristow IR, de Berker DAR, Acland KM, et al: Clinical guidelines for the recognition of melanoma of the foot and nail unit, *J Foot Ankle Res* 3:25, 2010.)

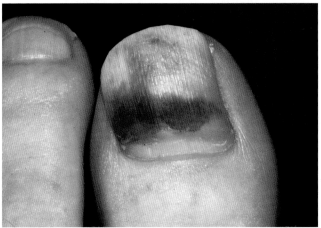

FIGURE 8.13 Subungual hematoma. (From Bristow IR, de Berker DA, Acland KM, et al: Clinical guidelines for the recognition of melanoma of the foot and nail unit, *J Foot Ankle Res* 3:25, 2010.)

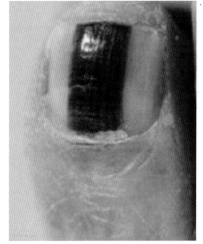

FIGURE 8.14 Longitudinal melanonychia. (From Bristow IR, de Berker DA, Acland KM, et al: Clinical guidelines for the recognition of melanoma of the foot and nail unit, *J Foot Ankle Res* 3:25, 2010.)

trimmed properly. Proper trimming of the nail at right angles to the distal edge of the nail plate is shown in Figure 8.17, with the goal being a squared nail with corners protruding distal to the hyponychium. This treatment is usually successful in 2 to 3 weeks if as much material as is comfortable to the patient is placed beneath the nail edge each day.

Another conservative treatment option is nail splinting, which separates the nail plate from the soft tissue to provide a channel in which the nail can grow. A "gutter splint" that is

affixed to the ingrown nail edge with adhesive tape or a formable acrylic resin such as cyanoacrylate can be fashioned from a sterilized vinyl intravenous drip infusion tube slit from top to bottom, with one end cut diagonally for smooth insertion (Fig. 8.18). Gutter splints can be used with or without the application of an acrylic nail. The use of a resin splint has also been reported as successful, although the duration of application was lengthy (9 months). Reported recurrence rates with various splinting techniques range from 8% to 48%.

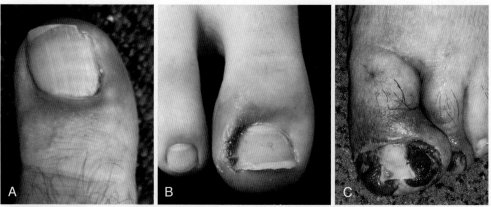

FIGURE 8.15 Different stages of presentation of ingrown toenail. **A,** Stage I: pain, swelling, erythema. **B,** Stage II: signs of inflammation with active or acute infection. **C,** Stage III: chronic infection leading to granulation tissue formation at nail folds. (From Park DH, Singh D: The management of ingrowing toenails, *BMJ* 344:e2089, 2012.)

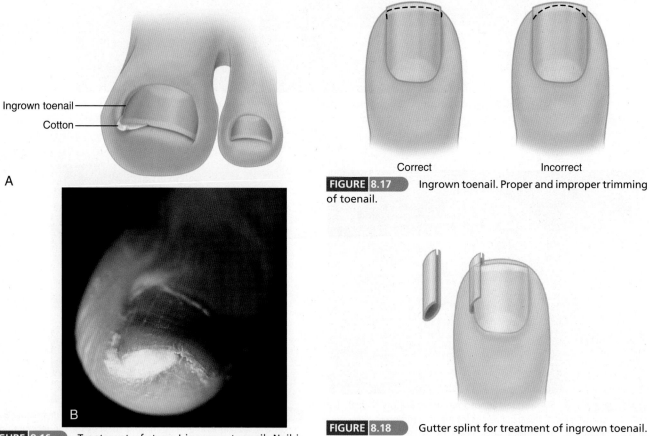

Ingrown toenail

Cotton

A

B

FIGURE 8.16 Treatment of stage I ingrown toenail. Nail is lifted from embedded position with cotton.

Correct   Incorrect

FIGURE 8.17 Ingrown toenail. Proper and improper trimming of toenail.

FIGURE 8.18 Gutter splint for treatment of ingrown toenail. (From Eekhof JA, Van Wijk B, Knuistingh Neven A, et al: Interventions for ingrowing toenails, *Cochrane Database Syst Rev* 4:CD001541, 2012.)

A dynamic correction technique, orthonyxia, uses direct force to lift the nail from the nail fold and releases the pressure exerted on the inflamed soft tissue. Generally, orthonyxia devices consist of two hooks placed on the sides of the nail and connected under tension by wire (Fig. 8.19), "super-elastic" wire, or shape-memory segments. Correction of the nail deformity has been reported to occur within 3 weeks in most patients. Cited advantages of splinting and orthonyxia techniques over operative treatment are less postoperative morbidity, shorter time to recovery, and better cosmetic results.

The "band-aid" method (Fig. 8.20) pulls the nail fold away from the nail to relieve pressure.

■ STAGE II (ABSCESS STAGE)

Stage II is an advancement of stage I. The erythema, edema, hyperhidrosis, and tenderness increase; the nail fold bulges over the nail plate edge; and drainage begins (see Fig. 8.15B). At first, the drainage is a thin, sticky, serous secretion. Because of the abundance of microorganisms normally present on the skin, infection rapidly follows, and the drainage becomes purulent and has a fetid odor. Walking becomes difficult, and shoe wear is almost impossible. It is possible to treat this stage nonoperatively by removing all pressure from the toe, including that from hosiery, and soaking the foot 10 to 15 minutes in warm water four or five times a day. The drainage is cultured, and sensitivities are determined, and a broad-spectrum antibiotic is begun. When the swelling recedes, tenderness should decrease, and the use of material beneath the distal nail corner as described in stage I can be started. This must not be used, however, if the drainage has not stopped and inflammation has not significantly decreased.

■ STAGE III (GRANULATION STAGE)

In stage III, granulation tissue covers the lateral nail fold and inhibits free drainage (see Fig. 8.15C). If this stage is left untreated, epithelium creeps over the edge of the granulations, further inhibiting drainage and precluding any chance of elevating the nail edge from the dermis of the lateral nail fold. This stage can progress into a chronic, relatively asymptomatic condition over several weeks, usually followed by recurrent, acute inflammatory episodes. It is doubtful that this stage can be treated nonoperatively with lasting beneficial results. In stage III and in many patients in stage II, surgical management is preferred. Nonsurgical management of late stage II and stage III lesions is time consuming for the

patient and the physician, and patient compliance is unpredictable. Recurrence is also likely after nonsurgical (and some surgical) treatment when the lesion has progressed this far. The surgical treatment choices are many, but only a few of the most commonly used are described. The recommended anesthetic is local (lidocaine or mepivacaine), without epinephrine, introduced with a small-gauge needle 1cm distal to the first web space, and ensuring that plantar digital nerves and the dorsal sensory branches of the superficial peroneal nerve are well anesthetized.

OPERATIVE MANAGEMENT

The operative treatment of ingrown toenails is based on two viewpoints of etiology. First, the nail is the primary offender causing an inflammatory soft-tissue response. Procedures focus on removing the offending nail plate with or without germinal matrix ablation. In the opposing viewpoint, the nail fold is the primary source, and operative procedures focus on removing or debulking the nail fold.

TOTAL NAIL PLATE REMOVAL

Total nail plate removal without concomitant matrix removal is rarely indicated, unless the abscess has circumducted the nail on both sides and beneath the eponychium so that partial nail plate removal would not provide adequate drainage.

TECHNIQUE 8.5

- When the great toe has been anesthetized, pass a straight, thin hemostat or small, flat nasal elevator beneath the nail in the midline from the hyponychium several millimeters proximal to the nail fold adjacent to the lunula (Fig. 8.21).
- Do not shift the hemostat or elevator back and forth; withdraw and insert it in a similar longitudinal manner beneath each lateral margin of the nail adjacent to the lateral nail fold.
- The nail should become loose enough to extract with a distal pull, unless the nail root still adheres to the eponychium. In this instance, instead of forcefully jerking the nail root loose, sharp dissection with a small blade between the nail plate and eponychium will allow the former to be gently lifted from its bed with little chance of

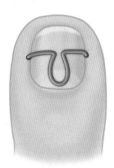

FIGURE 8.19 Orthonyxia uses hooks placed on sides of the nail connected under tension. (From Eekhof JA, Van Wijk B, Knuistingh Neven A, et al: Interventions for ingrowing toenails, *Cochrane Database Syst Rev* 4:CD001541, 2012.)

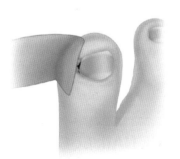
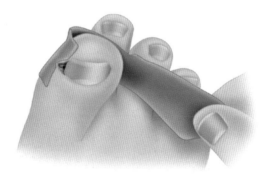
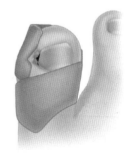

FIGURE 8.20 "Band-aid" method pulls the nail fold away from the nail to relieve pressure. (From Eekhof JA, Van Wijk B, Knuistingh Neven A, et al: Interventions for ingrowing toenails, *Cochrane Database Syst Rev* 4:CD001541, 2012.)

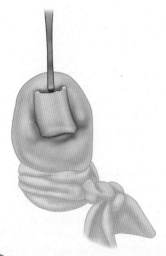

FIGURE 8.21 Total nail plate removal. **SEE TECHNIQUE 8.5.**

damage to the germinal matrix and will reduce bleeding from the nail bed.
- Another choice to remove the last moorings of the nail is with the use of a wide, flat, nasal elevator.

POSTOPERATIVE CARE A nonadherent, single-layer dressing is applied to the nail bed followed by a gently wrapped compression bandage. The foot is elevated for 24 hours, and then the dressing is removed and warm soaks are begun. No constricting hosiery or shoes should be worn for 1 week. The nail takes 4 to 6 months to reform completely, depending on the patient's age. The patient must be informed of this before surgery and forewarned that an upward-turned deformity of the distal nail bed and pulp may develop. This deformity is more likely to occur if the patient has had multiple nail avulsions (Fig. 8.22).

The recurrence rate of ingrown toenail after total nail removal ranges from 32% to 78% in published reports; the recurrence rate after a second avulsion is 70% to 80%. The benefits of total nail avulsion are uniformly rapid relief of symptoms and resolution of infection.

PARTIAL NAIL PLATE REMOVAL

Partial nail plate removal differs little from total nail plate removal.

TECHNIQUE 8.6

- Lift the lateral fourth of the nail from its bed with a small, angled probe or one arm of a narrow, smooth, straight hemostat, and remove it. Do not lift too firmly to avoid detaching the nail from its bed in a lateral direction.
- Using straight scissors, cut the nail plate longitudinally while lifting the lateral fourth off its bed. A curved tip on the scissors is less likely to damage the matrix.

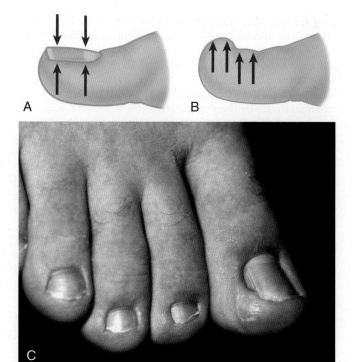

FIGURE 8.22 **A** and **B,** Turned up pulp deformity after multiple nail avulsions for treatment of ingrown toenail. **C,** Turned up deformity after several nail avulsions. **SEE TECHNIQUE 8.5.**

- The nail must be incised to its proximal end beneath the eponychium.
- Remove the granulation tissue by gently scraping with a scalpel or by removing it totally by elliptically excising part of the nail fold.

POSTOPERATIVE CARE Postoperative care is the same as after complete nail plate removal except that the patient can wear a closed, wide toe box shoe by the third or fourth day.

After partial nail plate removal without matrix ablation, the recurrence rate is even higher than after complete nail plate removal. In adolescents, however, this minor procedure, even if it must be repeated, is an attractive alternative to changing the appearance of the nail permanently. The patient, and especially the parents of an adolescent, must be told recurrent nail spicules may form, the nail-forming matrix may be injured, and some permanent deformity, even if minor, may result (Figs. 8.23 and 8.24).

REMOVAL OF THE NAIL EDGE AND ABLATION OF THE NAIL MATRIX

Phenol ablation of nail matrix of ingrown toenails is probably the most common procedure for onychocryptosis and can be done in the office setting.

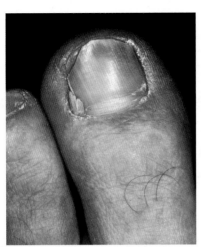

FIGURE 8.23 Inadequate partial nail plate removal. Lateral fourth of nail plate should be removed beneath eponychium. **SEE TECHNIQUE 8.6.**

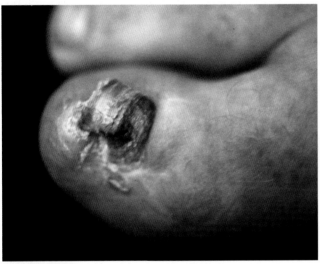

FIGURE 8.24 Deformity of nail bed after laceration of nail matrix.

TECHNIQUE 8.7

- All personnel involved in the procedure should wear gloves to avoid direct contact with phenol, which is corrosive.
- Place a tourniquet (Tourni-cot; Mar-Med Company, Grand Rapids, Michigan), Penrose drain, or a gloved finger at the base of the great toe to ensure a relatively dry dissecting area after the placement of local anesthesia. Elevate the lateral fourth to fifth of the nail edge longitudinally from distal to proximal, including the few millimeters of nail that are beneath the eponychium (Fig. 8.25A).
- When the nail plate has been removed, place antibiotic gel around the nail fold to protect the skin from the effects of the phenol. Place a cotton swab that has been dipped in 80% to 89% phenol solution into the nail groove, extending beneath the eponychium to ensure that the pocket of germinal matrix is exposed to the phenol (Fig. 8.25B). The field should be bloodless, or the phenol will

coagulate the blood instead of affecting the nail tissue. Phenol is useful because it is necrotizing, disinfecting, and anesthetic.

- Rotate the cotton applicator for 30 to 40 seconds, and repeat three more times for a total of 2 to 3 minutes, which is the optimal application time. This is followed by application of 70% isopropyl alcohol to dilute the phenol (Fig. 8.25C).

POSTOPERATIVE CARE The nail edge is covered with nonadherent gauze and a toe dressing (Fig. 8.25D), followed by release of the tourniquet. The patient is placed in a postoperative shoe and instructed to elevate the foot. The patient should be warned about the charred appearance of the skin that is evident when they remove their dressing after 2 to 3 days. Warm Epsom salt soaks are started once the dressing is removed, until the tissues have healed. Nonconstricting shoes are worn until all tenderness and drainage have ceased. Some oozing may occur for 3 to 6 weeks.

A systematic review of the literature determined that recurrence of the ingrown nail is less frequent after phenolization with simple avulsion of the nail than after more invasive excisional surgical procedures, and reported success rates with this technique have been as high as 98%. When comparing surgical and phenol matricectomy, phenol matricectomy had a significantly higher recurrence rate (18% to 32%) than in those with surgical matricectomy (7% to 8%). However, surgical matricectomy is associated with a higher risk of infection, higher pain scores, and lower cosmetic satisfaction. Trichloroacetic acid and sodium hydroxide have also been used for ablation of the nail matrix instead of phenol. Trichloroacetic acid and sodium hydroxide have similar efficacies to phenol but without significant advantages.

Other methods used for ablation of the nail matrix include electrocoagulation, cryotherapy, and carbon dioxide laser vaporization. Laser ablation was reported to significantly reduce operative time and duration of postoperative pain, and to allow a quicker return to daily activities.

The following procedures are more invasive and probably better performed in the operating room, as opposed to the office setting.

PARTIAL NAIL PLATE AND MATRIX REMOVAL

Probably the most frequently done operative procedure for ingrown toenail is that described by Winograd. Although his report involved only five patients, numerous subsequent reports have affirmed the usefulness of the technique. The Winograd technique is useful in late stage II or stage III disorders, especially after a previous, unsuccessful partial or complete nail removal. We have not found it necessary to treat the wound for several days before the procedure to reduce local infection, but have no objection to this being done.

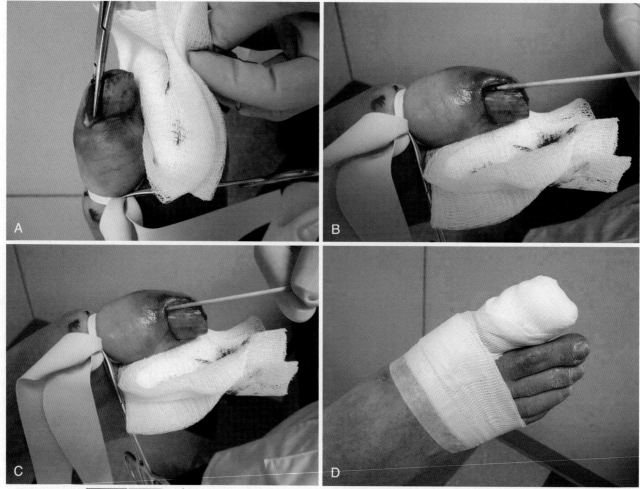

FIGURE 8.25 Removal of nail edge and ablation of nail matrix. **A,** After elevating and cutting, nail edge is removed. **B,** Phenol is applied to nail fold with narrow cotton swab.**C,** Alcohol is applied to neutralize phenol. **D,** Appearance of dressing after procedure. **SEE TECHNIQUE 8.7.**

TECHNIQUE 8.8

(WINOGRAD)

- Beginning 5 to 8 mm proximal to the lunula, make a longitudinal incision in the eponychium extending distally (Fig. 8.26A) while scoring, but not penetrating, the nail plate until its distal edge is reached (Fig. 8.26B).
- Lift the eponychial flap by sharp dissection to reveal the nail root overlying the lateral margin of the germinal matrix. The remainder of the eponychium should be left undisturbed.
- Using a small nasal elevator or small, straight hemostat, lift the lateral border of the nail out of the nail fold by passing the instrument beneath the lateral fourth of the exposed nail.
- Incise this nail margin with a nail splitter (Fig. 8.26C) along the previously scored mark, being sure to reach the most proximal edge of the nail plate.
- With its eponychial cover already reflected and the undersurface of the nail plate lifted off its bed (Fig. 8.26D),

gently remove this segment of nail, exposing the underlying matrix (Fig. 8.26E).
- Remove the exposed matrix by sharp dissection using the scalpel.
- Retract the lateral nail fold to expose the lateral margin of the matrix. Remove the entire matrix and the sterile and germinal portions; take special care to remove the proximal portion of the germinal matrix to reduce the likelihood of recurrent nail formation (Fig. 8.26F).

Even after great care, the patient occasionally develops a tiny nail remnant that may or may not be symptomatic. An attempt to bring the lateral margin of the nail fold to the remaining nail is optional; Heifetz recommended excision of part of the nail fold. The surgeon should be certain that the periosteum of the phalanx has been removed with the matrix (Fig. 8.26G) because this is the most certain means of matrix ablation.

- Return the proximal eponychial flap to its original location; sutures to hold it there are optional (Fig. 8.26H).

- Apply a nonadherent dressing over the exposed phalanx, followed by a nonconstricting gauze wrap (Fig. 8.26I).

POSTOPERATIVE CARE The extremity is elevated for 48 hours, at which time the dressing is removed. Soaks are begun for 10 minutes several times a day, and the wound is covered with only an adhesive bandage. No shoe or hosiery is worn for 5 to 7 days except a postoperative wooden-soled shoe that has no toe box. Later, a wide toe box shoe can usually be worn without discomfort.

Recurrence rates for the Winograd technique vary in the literature from 0% to 86%. This rate can be lowered by full exposure of the germinal matrix, followed by its complete removal. Recurrence rates are higher in patients with previous nail ablations, likely secondary to scarring and, therefore, incomplete exposure of the germinal matrix. Nail deformity may also result from this procedure (Fig. 8.27).

NAIL-FOLD REDUCTION

Nail-fold reduction procedures excise a wedge of normal tissue at a distance from the involved nail fold. By closing the wedge, the nail fold is pulled away from the lateral border of the nail plate, allowing free drainage and reducing inflammation. In the technique described in this chapter, Persichetti et al. removed the nail plate, but others have described a similar technique without nail plate removal (Fig. 8.28).

TECHNIQUE 8.9

(PERSICHETTI ET AL.)
- Mark an ellipse of skin beginning 4 mm lateral to the nail fold (Fig. 8.28A) to maintain viability of the nail fold.
- Completely remove the nail fold and all granulation tissue.
- Remove the outlined wedge-shaped ellipse of skin and subcutaneous tissue, with the apex of the wedge deep in the subcutaneous layer (Fig. 8.28B).

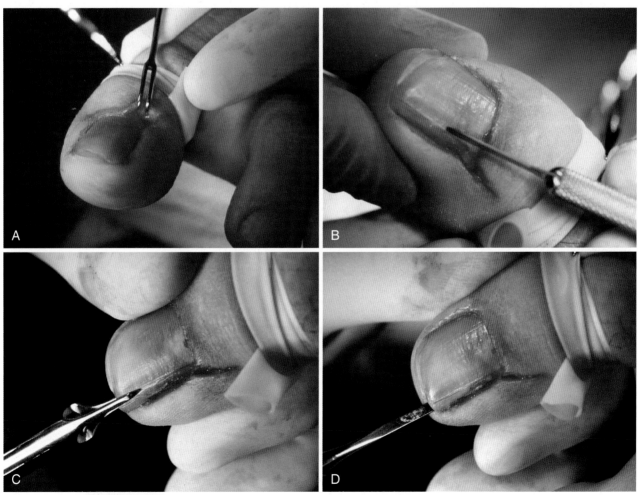

FIGURE 8.26 Winograd technique. **A,** Eponychium is incised. **B,** Nail plate is scored. **C,** Nail splitter is used to divide nail. **D,** Small elevator lifts plate atraumatically from underlying matrix.

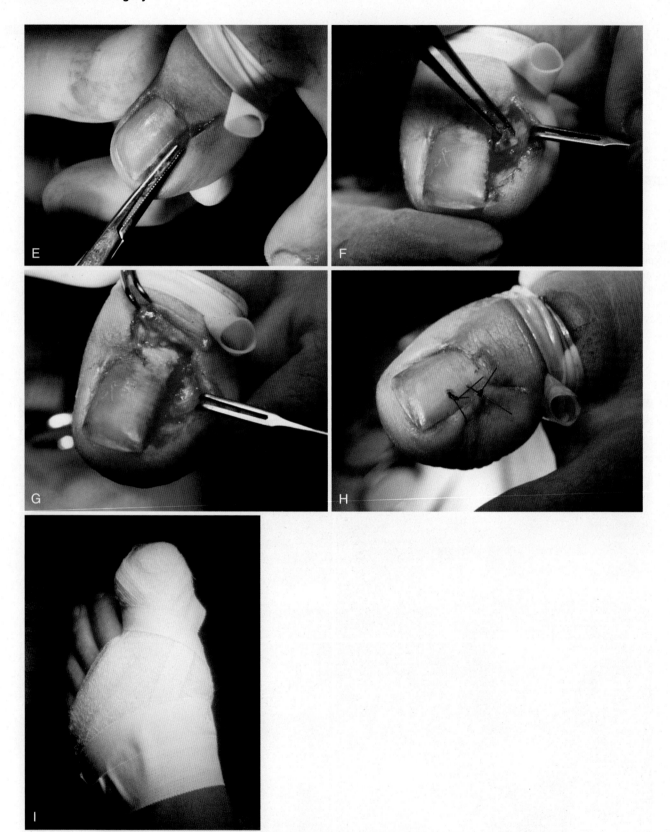

E, Entire portion of plate, which has been removed from body of nail, is removed using straight hemostat. **F,** Pearly colored matrix is exposed. Matrix curves on undersurfaces of paronychium and eponychium. This must be thoroughly removed. **G,** Germinal matrix folding on eponychium and paronychium must be removed by sharp dissection from around nail horns. Nail plate and matrix have been removed completely. **H,** Closing wound is optional, but convalescence is shortened. **I,** Dressing remains in place for 24 to 48 hours. **SEE TECHNIQUE 8.8.**

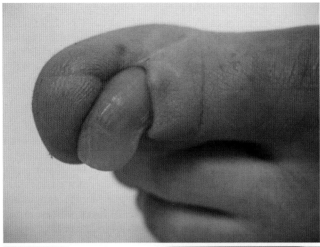

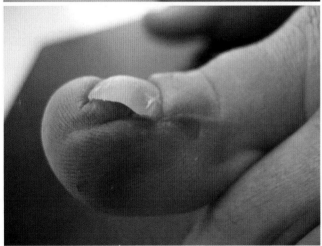

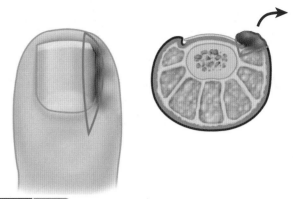

FIGURE 8.29 Wedge resection of nail, nail bed, and nail fold to include nail matrix.

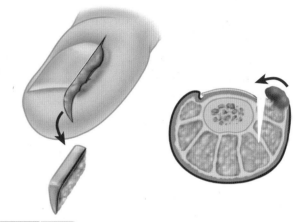

FIGURE 8.30 Watson-Cheyne technique of wedge resection. **SEE TECHNIQUE 8.10.**

FIGURE 8.27 Postoperative appearance of the toenail of 16-year-old girl after wedge excision and nail avulsion. (From Haneke E: Nail surgery, *Clin Dermatol* 31:516–525, 2013.)

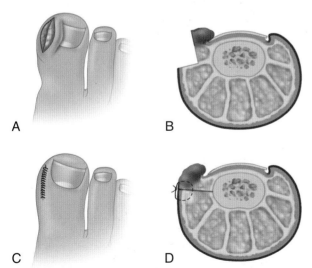

FIGURE 8.28 Soft-tissue wedge resection for ingrown toenail. **A,** Triangular section is removed from lateral aspect of nail groove. **B,** Cross-section after removal. **C,** Nail lip and groove are pulled down after nail margins are sutured. **D,** Cross-section after suturing. (From De Orio JK, Coughlin MJ: Toenail abnormalities. In Coughlin MJ, Mann RA, Saltzman CL, editors: *Surgery of the foot and ankle*, ed 8, Philadelphia, 2007, Elsevier.) **SEE TECHNIQUE 8.9.**

- Approximate the margins of the resulting defect, everting the nail fold and reducing its convexity (Fig. 8.28C and D). The width of the ellipse and, consequently, the extent of the eversion depend on the size of the nail fold.
- Remove the sutures at 10 to 15 days after surgery.

PARTIAL NAIL FOLD AND NAIL MATRIX REMOVAL

The rationale for partial nail fold removal in addition to matrix removal is to eliminate all parts of the pathologic condition that are causing the symptoms yet leave the normal nail and soft tissue intact. The procedure involves wedge resection of the nail, nail bed, and nail fold (Fig. 8.29). The chief complication of wedge resection has been recurrence of nail spicules. These spicules reoccur from inadequate resection of the germinal matrix. Practitioners must recognize that the apex of the wedge, which is the area most crucial to the narrowest area of resection, the wedge apex, is located at the most crucial tissue requiring removal—the matrix (Fig. 8.30). The portion of the nail plate and lateral nail fold removed with the wedge is adequate. We have had no experience with the procedure but believe it to be based on sound reasoning. If the patient understands that part or all of the nail may regrow and be mildly deformed, the procedure is an acceptable treatment.

TECHNIQUE 8.10

(WATSON-CHEYNE AND BURGHARD; O'DONOGHUE; MOGENSEN)

- Remove the lateral fourth of the nail plate by lifting it from its bed with a small, flat dissector that reaches the most proximal end of the nail root. Using straight scissors, remove this portion of the nail.
- With a knife, make a linear incision parallel to the lateral nail fold, extending from 1 cm proximal to the lunula to the hyponychium. Carry this incision to bone.
- Begin the second incision 2 to 3 mm lateral to the inner edge of the lateral nail fold and curve it obliquely at a 45-degree angle to the initial incision to reach the most lateral margin of the germinal matrix. Exposure and removal of this corner of the germinal matrix is important. The whitish hue of the germinal matrix usually contrasts with the reddish color of the sterile matrix, helping delineate the lateral border of the entire nail bed.
- Remove the periosteum with the matrix and expose the fat and subcutaneous tissue in the proximal corner to ensure removal of the germinal matrix.
- When the wedge of nail plate, matrix, and nail fold is removed, cover the wound with a nonadherent dressing followed by a sterile compression wrap.

POSTOPERATIVE CARE The foot is elevated for 48 hours after surgery. The dressing is removed, and warm soaks for 10 to 15 minutes several times a day are begun. The patient should not wear a closed toe shoe, even if the toe box is wide, for 10 to 14 days. The patient should be informed before surgery that it may be 3 to 4 weeks before a shoe can be worn comfortably for 8 hours a day.

LONG-TERM FOLLOW-UP

Long-term follow-up data on these two procedures are difficult to find. One report of partial nail avulsion and elliptical lateral nail fold excision had a recurrence rate of 16.6%.

Another study of nail fold excision without nail plate excision had no recurrences in 23 patients. We have had no experience with the nail-fold procedures without concomitant nail plate or matrix removal. The procedures would seem to be indicated more with incurvated nails (Fig. 8.31), however, in which the nail plate is usually narrow, and further reduction in size by nail plate procedures might not be cosmetically pleasing.

A more extensive lateral nail-fold procedure for severe stage III disease with extensive granulation tissue was described by Vandenbos and Bowers. This more aggressive procedure has been especially popular in the pediatric population. Wide debulking of the involved nail fold is done, leaving an open wound that heals by secondary intention (Figs. 8.32 and 8.33). They reported no recurrences in 124 patients with 212 surgical sites. More recently, other authors reported similar recurrence rates (0%) but with a complication rate close to 20%. Complications include bleeding, severe pain, and infection.

COMPLETE NAIL PLATE AND GERMINAL MATRIX REMOVAL

The procedure for nail plate and germinal matrix removal was originally described by Quenu in 1887 and popularized by Wilson in 1944. The essentials of this procedure are

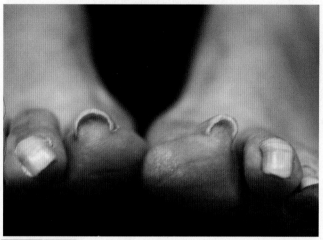

FIGURE 8.31 Incurvatum of nail.

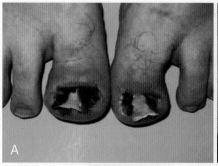 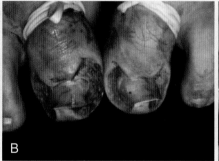 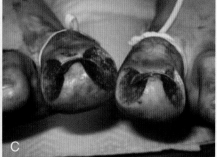

A B C

FIGURE 8.32 Ingrown toenails corrected with soft-tissue nail-fold excision. **A,** Preoperative appearance with extensive medial and lateral nail-fold granulation tissue. **B** and **C,** After nail-fold excision. (From Chapeskie H, Kovac JR: Case Series: Soft-tissue nail-fold excision: a definitive treatment for ingrown toenails, *Can J Surg* 53:282–286, 2010.)

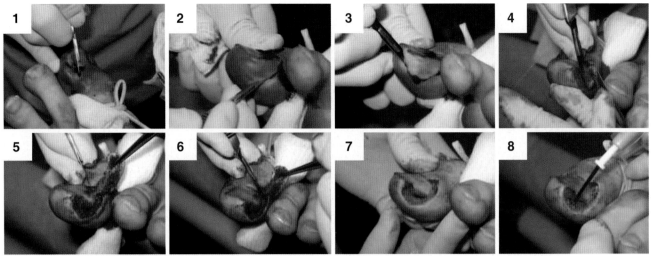

FIGURE 8.33 Nail-fold excision. *1*, Toe is anesthetized, and tourniquet is applied. *2*, Incision 5 to 10 mm long is made proximally from base of nail and 3 to 5 mm from lateral border of nail encompassing proximal nail fold; care is taken to leave nail matrix intact. *3* and *4*, Lateral nail fold is excised with lateral elliptical sweep that proceeds distally to encompass all involved granulation tissue and adjacent soft tissues. *5* and *6*, All skin and subcutaneous tissues at edge of nail are removed. *7*, After excision of soft-tissue nail folds; note intact nail and preservation of nail matrix. *8*, Electrocautery is used to obtain hemostasis, and wound is left open to heal by secondary intension. (From Chapeskie H, Kovac JR: Case Series: Soft-tissue nail-fold excision: a definitive treatment for ingrown toenails, *Can J Surg* 53:282–286, 2010.)

removal of the entire nail plate and germinal matrix while not disturbing the sterile matrix distal to the lunula (Fig. 8.34). The sterile matrix does not form true nail but continues to form flaky cornifications that might be cosmetically displeasing (Fig. 8.35). This procedure is rarely used but can be employed in middle-aged or elderly patients with multiple occurrences of nail problems from a variety of causes (incurvatum, onychogryposis, onychomycosis). Younger patients (usually male) with less concern for cosmesis who have had multiple operations for ingrown toenail are also good candidates for this procedure. It is often a good alternative to the terminal Syme procedure.

TECHNIQUE 8.11

(QUENU; FOWLER; ZADIK)
- Remove the nail plate initially in the same manner as previously described (Fig. 8.21).
- Raise the eponychium as a full-thickness flap by extending oblique incisions from both corners of the proximal nail fold approximately 1 cm proximally (Fig. 8.36A).
- Excise the inner 1 or 2 mm of nail fold on both sides of the nail.
- Excise the germinal matrix (Fig. 8.36B). Begin this incision 1 to 2 mm distal to the lunula or, if the lunula is indistinct, begin the incision one third the distance from the cuticle to the distal nail edge and make it transverse across the sterile matrix.
- Retracting the lateral nail fold, remove each edge of the matrix from the distal phalanx by sharp dissection, being careful not to leave any germinal matrix in the recesses of the lateral grooves. The matrix follows the lateral curvature of the phalanx almost to the midlateral line, and this must be kept in mind during the lateral dissection to remove the matrix.
- With the distal edge and both lateral margins of the germinal matrix detached from the phalanx, the proximal edge and corners can be seen better. Retract the proximal nail fold proximally and complete the removal of the matrix by sharp dissection (Fig. 8.36C).
- The extensor hallucis longus insertion centrally, and fat and subcutaneous tissue at the corners, must be exposed before adequate excision of the germinal matrix is possible. In addition, the periosteum on the dorsal and lateral borders of the distal phalanx should be removed by sharp dissection when the germinal matrix is excised.
- Return the eponychial flap to its previous location (Fig. 8.36D and E). Usually, it does not reach the remaining nail bed, but the gap is small and quickly closes with wound contraction; use of sutures is optional.

POSTOPERATIVE CARE A nonadherent dressing and gently rolled gauze wrap are placed over the wound, and the foot is elevated for 48 hours, at which time the dressing is changed. Warm soaks are started, and an open toe shoe is worn with a light dressing over the phalanx. If the procedure is performed in the presence of gross infection, healing may be delayed but should be complete by 6 to 8 weeks. The patient must be informed before surgery that the new "nail" over the sterile matrix will not look like or grow like the previous normal nail (Fig. 8.36E).

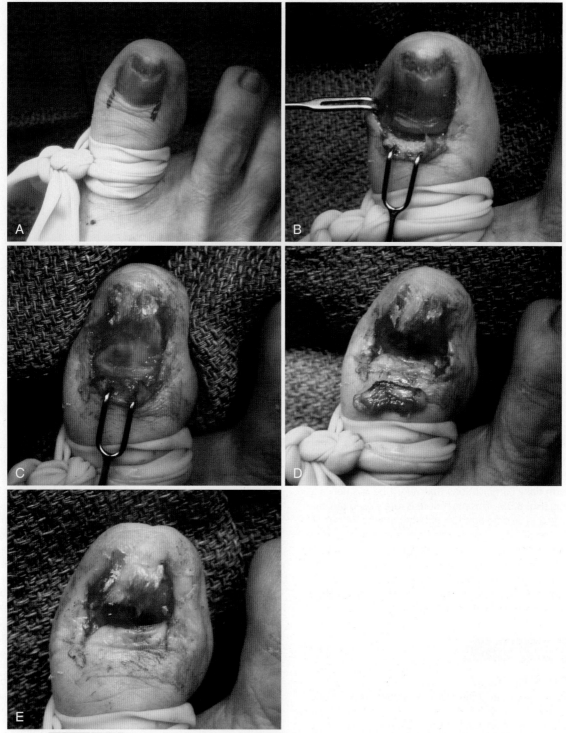

FIGURE 8.34 Chronic, symptomatic stage III ingrown toenail treated with total germinal matrix excision (Quenu). **A,** Skin incisions. **B,** Total nail plate is removed. **C,** Germinal matrix protruding from beneath eponychium can be differentiated from dormant matrix, which is abnormal. **D,** All germinal matrix must be removed. **E,** Eponychium is replaced adjacent to dormant matrix, which remains. In this instance, it has been damaged by the mycotic process.

TERMINAL SYME PROCEDURE

The terminal Syme (Thompson-Terwilliger) procedure involves amputating the distal half of the distal phalanx, including the nail plate, matrix, nail folds, and underlying bone on which these structures rest. The procedure is

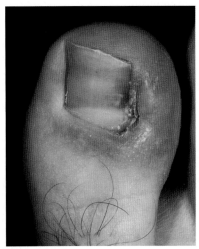

FIGURE 8.35   After germinal matrix nail removal, flaky cornifications may continue to form.

recommended for adults who have had recurrent bouts of infected ingrown toenails that are unrelieved by less extensive procedures. It can also be used for various bone or soft-tissue tumors around the nail and distal phalanx.

Complications of the terminal Syme procedure include osteomyelitis of the distal phalanx, epidermal inclusion cysts along the suture line, and troublesome nail spicules. In our experience, however, this is a dependable procedure, producing an excellent functional and acceptable cosmetic result in most patients (Fig. 8.37). Although the tip of the toe is initially bulbous and unattractive, the final appearance is rarely offensive to the patient. Meticulous technique and attention to detail are mandatory to avoid nail horns. In the presence of an abscess, drainage should be instituted first, and the local wound condition should be improved before performing the procedure. This step should not delay the procedure for more than 2 weeks but usually less.

TECHNIQUE 8.12

- Use sharp dissection throughout the procedure except during the use of a bone cutter or saw to transect the distal phalanx 1 to 2 mm distal to the extensor and flexor hallucis longus insertions. The skin incision is illustrated in Figure 8.38A and B.

Thompson and Terwilliger recommended that a skin margin of 4mm be removed with the entire nail bed and

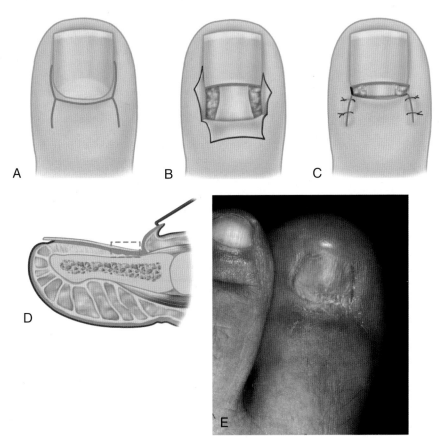

FIGURE 8.36   Nail plate and germinal matrix removal by Quenu technique (Fowler; Zadik). **A,** Skin incision. **B,** Eponychium is raised, and germinal matrix is exposed. **C,** Germinal matrix is removed. **D,** Sagittal section of germinal matrix. **E,** Five years after Quenu technique. **SEE TECHNIQUE 8.11.**

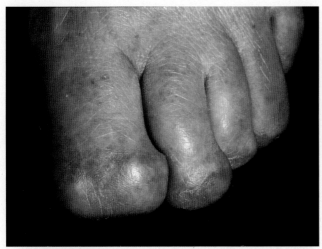

FIGURE 8.37 Result after terminal Syme procedure.

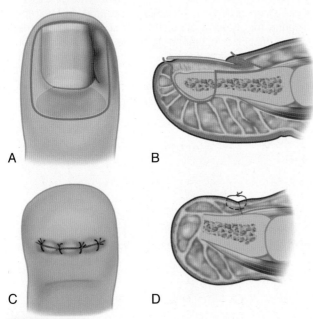

FIGURE 8.38 Terminal Syme procedure. **A** and **B,** Skin incision. **C** and **D,** Removal of distal half of phalanx and closure. **SEE TECHNIQUE 8.12.**

transected part of the phalanx. The proximal margin of skin overlying the germinal matrix may extend more than 4mm proximal to the cuticle, and it is recommended that the skin margin proximally measure 6 to 7 mm because the plantar flap would be long enough to reach the skin dorsally, and the extrinsic tendon insertions lie proximal to this point. In addition, a 2- to 3-mm skin margin distal to the hyponychium would suffice. The goal is to remove the matrix, nail, and bone in one piece and reduce the chance of troublesome nail recurrence.

- Make the incision straight to bone proximally, but on the sides; do not bevel the blade toward the center until plantar to the lateral flares of the phalanx.
- Using a clamp, firmly grasp the phalanx and, with skin hooks retracting the plantar flap, continue sharp

dissection along the plantar surface of the phalanx in a distal-to-proximal direction.
- Transect the phalanx and release any soft tissue remaining to complete the amputation (Fig. 8.38C and D). This method of dissection is similar to removing the heel pad from the calcaneus in a Syme amputation, which is how it got the name *terminal Syme procedure.*
- Smooth any irregularity of the remaining phalanx with a rongeur.
- Maintain strict hemostasis, and close the wound with nonabsorbable sutures without trimming the "dog ears".

The use of a tourniquet was not encouraged by Thompson and Terwilliger; however, a tourniquet allows more precise dissection. It reduces the chance of injury to proper plantar digital nerves at the proximal part of the dissection and aids in identifying small vessels that can be cauterized, reducing the chance of hematoma after surgery.

POSTOPERATIVE CARE The foot is elevated for 48 hours. The dressing is changed, and walking in a wooden-soled or firm-soled shoe with no toe box is allowed. The sutures are removed at 14 to 16 days, and a wide toe box shoe can usually be worn within the next week.

REFERENCES

Aldrich SL, Hong CH, Groves L, et al.: Acral lesions in tuberous sclerosis complex: insights into pathogenesis, *J Am Acad Dermatol* 3:244, 2010.

Altinyazar HC, Dermirel CB, Koca R, Hosnuter M: Digital block with and without epinephrine during chemical matricectomy with phenol, *Dermatol Surg* 36:1568, 2010.

André MS, Caucanas M, André J, et al.: Treatment of ingrowing toenails with phenol 88% or trichloroacetic acid 100%: a comparative, prospective, randomized, double-blind study, *Dermatol Surg* 44:645, 2018.

Baran R, Berker DAR, Holzber M, et al.: *Baran and dawber's diseases of the nails and their management,* ed 4, Hoboken NJ, 2012, Wiley-Blackwell.

Barreiros H, Matos D, Boulao J, et al.: Using 80% trichloroacetic acid in the treatment of ingrown toenails, *An Bras Dermatol* 88:889, 2013.

Bristow IR, de Berker DAR, Acland KM, et al.: Clinical guidelines for the recognition of melanoma of the foot and nail unit, *J Foot Ankle Res* 3:25, 2010.

Chapeskie H, Kovac JR: Case series: Soft-tissue nail-fold excision: a definitive treatment for ingrown toenails, *Can J Surg* 53:282, 2010.

Córdoba-Fernández A, Rayo-Rosado R, Juárez-Jiménez JM: The use of autologous platelet gel in toenail surgery: a within-patient clinical trial, *J Foot Ankle Surg* 49:385, 2010.

Córdoba-Fernández A, Ruiz-Garrido G, Canca-Cabrera A: Algorithm for the management of antibiotic prophylaxis in onychocryptosis surgery, *Foot (Edinb)* 20:140, 2010.

DaCambra MP, Gupta SK, Ferri-de-Barros F: Subungual exostosis of the toes: a systematic review, *Clin Orthop Relat Res* 472:1251, 2014.

Eekhof JA, Van Wijk B, van der Wouden JC: Interventions for ingrowing toenails, *Cochrane Database Syst Rev* 18(4):CD001541, 2012.

Goldberg LH: Chemical matricectomy of nails, *Dermatol Surg* 36:1572, 2010.

Grover C, Khurana A, Bhattacharya SN, et al.: Controlled trial comparing the efficacy of 88% phenol versus 10% sodium hydroxide for chemical matricectomy in the management of ingrown toenail, *Indian J Dermatol Venereol Leprol* 81:472, 2015.

Gupta AK, Versteeg SG: A critical review of improvement rates for laser therapy used to treat toenail onychomycosis, *J Eur Acad Dermatol Venereol* 31(7):1111, 2017.

Gupta 2 AK1, Versteeg SG2, Shear NH3: Confirmatory testing prior to initiating onychomycosis therapy is cost-effective, *J Cutan Med Surg* 22:129, 2018.

Haneke E: Nail surgery, *Clin Dermatol* 31:516, 2013.

Hassel JC, Hassel AJ, Löser C: Phenol chemical matricectomy is less painful, with shorter recovery times but higher recurrence rates, than surgical matricectomy: a patient's view, *Dermatol Surg* 36:1294, 2010.

Imai A, Takayama K, Satoh T, et al.: Ingrown nails and pachyonychia of the great toes impair lower limb functions: improvement of limb dysfunction by medical foot care, *Int J Dermatol* 50:215, 2011.

Koren A1, Salameh F, Sprecher E, et al.: Laser-assisted photodynamic therapy or laser-assisted amorolfine lacquer delivery for treatment of toenail onychomycosis: an open-label comparative study, *Acta Derm Venereol* 98:467, 2018.

Kose O, Celiktas M, Kisin B, et al.: Is there a relationship between forefoot alignment and ingrown toenail? A case-control study, *Foot Ankle Spec* 4:14, 2011.

Kose O, Guler F, Gurcan S, et al.: Cosmetic results of wedge resection of nail matrix (Winograd technique) in the treatment of ingrown toenail, *Foot Ankle Spec* 5:241, 2012.

Kreijkamp-Kaspers S, Hawke KL, van Driel ML: Oral medications to treat toenail fungal infection, *JAMA* 319:397, 2018.

Kücuktas M, Kutluhay Z, Yardimci G, et al.: Comparison of effectiveness of electrocautery and cryotherapy in partial matrixectomy after partial nail extraction in the treatment of ingrown nails, *Dermatol Surg* 39:274, 2013.

Lipner SR1, Scher RK2: Onychomycosis: treatment and prevention of recurrence, *J Am Acad Dermatol* 80:853, 2019.

Livingston MH, Coriolano K, Jones SA: Nonrandomized assessment of ingrown toenails treated with excision of skinfold rather than toenail (NAILTEST): an observational study of the Vandenbos procedure, *J Pediatr Surg* 52:832, 2017.

Matsumoto K, Hashimoto I, Nakanishi H, et al.: Resin splint as a new conservative treatment for ingrown toenails, *J Med Invest* 57:321, 2010.

Mitchell S, Jackson C, Wilson-Storey D: Surgical treatment of ingrown toenails in children: what is best practice? *Ann R Coll Surg Engl*, 93:99, 2011.

Park DH, Singh D: The management of ingrowing toenails, *BMJ* 344:e2089, 2012.

Perez CJ, Maul XA, Catalina Heusser M, Zavala A: Operative technique with rapid recovery for ingrown toenails with granulation tissue formation in childhood, *Dermatol Surg* 39(3 Pt 1):393, 2013.

Pérez-Rey J, Mediavilla-Saldana L, Martinez-Nova A: Exploring postoperative outcomes for ingrown toenails. NaOH vs wedge resection techniques, *Dermatol Surg* 40:281, 2014.

Peyvandi H, Robarti RM, Yegane RA, et al.: Comparison of two surgical methods (Winograd and sleeve method) in the treatment of ingrown toenail, *Dermatol Surg* 37:331, 2011.

Polo C, Borda D, Poggio D, et al.: Glomus tumor of the hallux. Review of the literature and report of two cases, *Foot Ankle Surg* 18:89, 2012.

Romero-Pérez D, Betlloch-Mas, Encabo-Durán B: Onychocryptosis: a long-term retrospective and comparative follow-up study of surgical and phenol chemical matricectomy in 520 procedures, *Int J Dermatol* 56:221, 2017.

Sarifakioglu E, Sarifakioglu N: Crescent excision of the nail fold with partial nail avulsion does work with ingrown toenails, *Eur J Dermatol* 20:822, 2010.

Vaccari S, Dika E, Balestri R, et al.: Partial excision of matrix and phenolic ablation for the treatment of ingrowing toenail: a 36-month follow-up of 197 treated patients, *Dermatol Surg* 36:1288, 2010.

Weber GC1, Firouzi P1, Baran AM, et al.: Treatment of onychomycosis using a 1064-nm diode laser with or without topical antifungal therapy: a single-center, retrospective analysis in 56 patients, *Eur J Med Res* 23:53, 2018.

Yabe T, Takahashi M: A minimally invasive surgical approach for ingrown toenails: partial germinal matrix excision using operative microscope, *J Plast Reconstr Aesthet Surg* 63:170, 2010.

Zaraa I, Dorbani I, Hawilo A, et al.: Segmental phenolization for the treatment of ingrown toenails: technique report, followup of 146 patients, and review of the literature, *Dermatol Online J* 19:18560, 2013.

Zhu X, Shi H, Zhang L, Gu Y: Lateral fold and partial nail bed excision for the treatment of recurrent ingrown toenails, *Int J Clin Exp Med* 5:257, 2012.

The complete list of references is available online at Expert Consult.com.

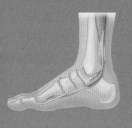

CHAPTER 9

FRACTURES AND DISLOCATIONS OF THE FOOT

Clayton C. Bettin

FRACTURES OF THE CALCANEUS

INTRAARTICULAR FRACTURES

Studies in fracture patterns, soft-tissue management, and outcomes of calcaneal fractures have led to debate about the optimal management of calcaneal fractures. Prospective randomized studies have shown equivocal outcomes with operative and nonoperative treatment. However, recent trends in the literature suggest that restoration of physiologic parameters of length, height, and alignment of the calcaneus may lead to better long-term results. Initial studies using extensile approaches showed higher rates of wound complications with operative treatment; however, recent studies have shown lower complication rates with sinus tarsi and other minimally invasive techniques. Regardless of the treatment, calcaneal fractures are associated with numerous complications and guarded outcomes with significant long-term quality-of-life issues. Outcomes in patients with calcaneal fractures have been shown to be relatively poor, with functional outcome levels similar to patients who underwent organ transplants or sustained myocardial infarctions. Patients with calcaneal fractures should be informed of the potential life-changing nature of this injury and of the prolonged recovery time that is required. Sanders et al. confirmed that the learning curve for operative treatment of this fracture is steep. With substantial literature supporting closed methods of treatment, a thorough knowledge of the anatomy and clearly defined goals are necessary for a successful outcome. Calcaneal fractures present complex challenges for both the orthopaedic surgeon and patient.

■ MECHANISM

Intraarticular fractures account for approximately 75% of calcaneal fractures and historically have been associated with poor functional outcomes. These fractures generally are caused by an axial load mechanism, such as a fall or a motor vehicle accident, and may be associated with other axial load injuries, such as lumbar, pelvic, and tibial plateau fractures. Cadaver studies, anatomic dissections, and the use of CT have allowed a detailed description of the mechanism of injury and the resulting fracture patterns (Fig. 9.1). The contact point of the calcaneus is situated lateral to the weight-bearing axis of the lower extremity. As an axial load force is applied to the posterior facet of the calcaneus through the talus, shear forces are directed through the posterior facet toward the medial wall of the calcaneus (Fig. 9.2). The ensuing fracture (primary fracture line) is almost always present and extends from the proximal-medial aspect of the calcaneal tuberosity, through the anterolateral wall, usually near the crucial angle of Gissane. The most variable aspect of this fracture line is its position through the posterior facet of the calcaneus; it can be in the medial third near the sustentaculum tali, the central third, or the lateral third near the lateral wall.

As the axial force continues, two things happen: (1) the medial spike attached to the sustentaculum is pushed farther toward the medial heel skin, and (2) various secondary fracture lines occur in the region of the posterior facet. Often an anterior fracture extends toward the anterior process and may exit into the calcaneocuboid joint. The additional fractures of the posterior facet can be divided into two types, as described

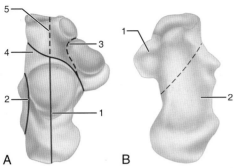

FIGURE 9.1 Dorsal and plantar views illustrating common fracture lines in intraarticular fractures of calcaneus. **A,** Dorsal view: *1,* sagittal fracture through posterior facet; *2,* lateral wall fracture; *3,* fracture line separating remainder of calcaneus from sustentaculum fragment; *4,* transverse fracture through sinus tarsi; *5,* fracture extending into calcaneocuboid joint. **B,** Plantar view: *1,* medial wall fracture in which tuberosity fragment shifts distally and laterally with medial overlap; *2,* tuberosity fragment has variable fracture line or lines.

by Essex-Lopresti (Fig. 9.3). If the fracture line producing the posterior facet fragment exits behind the posterior facet and anterior to the attachment of the Achilles tendon, the injury is called a *joint depression type* (Fig. 9.3C). If it exits distal to the Achilles tendon insertion, it is called a *tongue type* (Fig. 9.3D).

As the talus pushes the posterior facet and the underlying thalamic fragment into the body of the calcaneus, it also pushes out the lateral wall, closing the space for the peroneal tendons and occasionally impinging on the fibula. As the force is removed, recoil of the talus occurs, leaving a depressed thalamic fragment, and the medial spike is retracted into the soft tissues. For this reason, medially open fractures of the calcaneus require deep dissection to expose and irrigate the medial spike thoroughly.

■ RADIOGRAPHIC EVALUATION

Radiographic evaluation of the fracture should include five views. A lateral radiograph is used to assess height loss (loss of Böhler's angle) (Fig. 9.4) and rotation of the posterior facet. The axial (or Harris) view is made to assess varus position of the tuberosity and width of the heel. Anteroposterior and oblique views of the foot are made to assess the anterior process and calcaneocuboid involvement. A single Brodén view, obtained by internally rotating the leg 40 degrees with the ankle in neutral, and then angling the beam 10 to 15 degrees cephalad, is made to evaluate congruency of the posterior facet

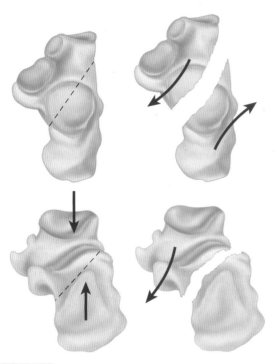

FIGURE 9.2 Primary fracture line occurs as result of shear force.

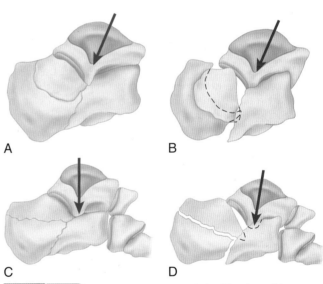

FIGURE 9.3 **A** to **D,** Essex-Lopresti classification of fractures of calcaneus (see text).

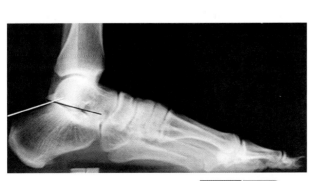

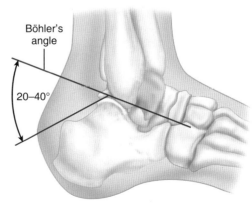

FIGURE 9.4 Böhler's angle (see text).

(Fig. 9.5). CT scans should be obtained for full injury evaluation and surgical planning. The scans should be ordered in multiple planes: the semicoronal plane, oriented perpendicular to the normal position of the posterior facet of the calcaneus (Fig. 9.6), the axial plane, oriented parallel to the sole of the foot, and the sagittal plane oriented perpendicular to the sole of the foot. Three-dimensional reconstructions have also been shown to be useful in evaluation and operative planning of calcaneal fractures. The CT scan should be carefully evaluated for additional fractures in the foot, as well as peroneal tendon dislocations and flexor hallucis longus (FHL) position (best evaluated with soft-tissue windows in the axial plane).

■ CLASSIFICATION

With increasing use of CT, more complex classification systems have been developed for these fractures, which have been shown to have prognostic value in the treatment of these injuries. Although the Essex-Lopresti system has been used for many years and is useful in describing the location of the secondary fracture line, it does not describe the overall energy absorbed by the posterior facet, shown by comminution or displaced fragments (see Fig. 9.3). Classification systems by Crosby and Fitzgibbons and Sanders have become more widely accepted in evaluation of these fractures (Fig. 9.7). Both classifications are based on CT scans and describe comminution and displacement of the posterior facet. The advantage of the Sanders classification is its precision regarding the location and number of fracture lines through the posterior facet. The Sanders system uses a coronal scan through the widest portion of the posterior facet, with Roman numerals I-IV representing the number of fragments. The fragments are then classified further with letters A-C denoting the location of the fracture lines from lateral to medial. Both systems lack descriptions of other important aspects of these fractures, however, including heel height and width, varus-valgus alignment, and calcaneocuboid involvement.

Although CT scans have become valuable in the evaluation and classification of these fractures, correlation with plain radiographs and three-dimensional reformats are helpful because traditional CT cuts may underestimate sagittal-plane rotation of the depressed fragment.

■ TREATMENT

Closed treatment of intraarticular calcaneal fractures includes closed manipulation and casting, compression dressing and early mobilization, traction-fixation, manipulation as recommended by Böhler, and pin fixation as recommended by Essex-Lopresti. Manual reduction methods have been successful in some studies but are rarely used today in place of minimally invasive surgical techniques along with a manipulation.

▌ DECISION-MAKING IN CALCANEAL FRACTURES

Goals common to all types of treatment of calcaneal fractures are as follows: (1) restoration of congruency of the posterior facet of the subtalar joint, (2) restoration of the height of the calcaneus (Böhler's angle), (3) reduction of the width of the calcaneus, (4) decompression of the subfibular space available for the peroneal tendons, (5) realignment of the tuberosity into a valgus position, and (6) reduction of the calcaneocuboid joint if fractured. Factors to be considered in formulating a treatment plan include the following.

Age of the Patient. Most injuries occur in patients younger than the physiologic age of 50 to 55 years. Consideration for operative intervention to restore calcaneal height, alignment, and articular reduction in young patients should be strongly considered. Good results can be obtained with operative treatment of older patients with calcaneal fractures with appropriate patient selection, but nonoperative treatment is advised in patients with severe osteopenia, those with limited ambulatory abilities, and those with significant medical comorbidities.

Health Status. An insensate limb caused by either trauma (sciatic or tibial nerve disruption) or disease (diabetes or other neuropathy) is a strong relative contraindication to open treatment. Patients with limited ambulation because of other medical conditions likewise should be treated conservatively. Tobacco use has been shown to increase complication rates with operative intervention; however, some surgeons consider this only a contraindication to an extensile lateral approach and favor less invasive techniques in this setting.

Fracture Pattern. Sanders types III and IV fractures sustained a significantly higher amount of energy than lesser types, and Park et al. showed that a Sanders type IV is the best

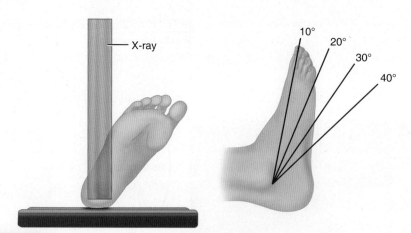

FIGURE 9.5 Brodén view. Three internal rotation views taken in 45 degrees of internal rotation with 10 to 40 degrees of radiographic tube angulation. External rotation view is taken at 45 degrees of external rotation and 30 degrees of radiographic tube angulation.

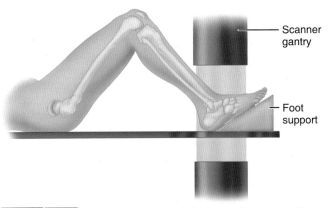

Scanner gantry

Foot support

FIGURE 9.6 Patient positioning for coronal CT of hindfoot.

predictor of compartment syndrome after a fracture of the calcaneus. Concurrent pathologies such as soft-tissue injuries and calcaneocuboid joint involvement are common, while the articular surface, calcaneal bone morphology, and shape are more disrupted than in lesser types. It would follow that higher Sanders types III and IV injuries have poorer outcomes than Sanders types I and II injuries with both operative and nonoperative interventions. Sanders type I or nondisplaced fractures should be treated by a closed method. Type II and type III fractures can be treated with open reduction in consideration with other patient characteristics. Type IV fractures can be treated conservatively or operatively. Long-term studies have shown that type IV injuries are more likely to go on to subtalar arthrodesis in the future. In type IV fractures, consideration should be given to minimally invasive techniques to

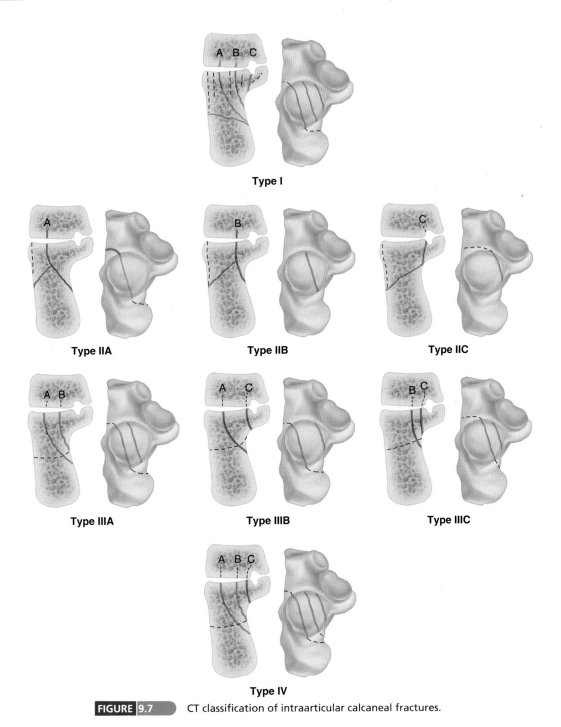

FIGURE 9.7 CT classification of intraarticular calcaneal fractures.

restore the calcaneal architecture for later subtalar arthrodesis or primary subtalar arthrodesis in experienced hands.

❚ SOFT-TISSUE INJURY (OPEN CALCANEAL FRACTURES)

Basic open-fracture care principles apply to calcaneal fractures. Most open injuries are caused by penetration of the sustentacular spike through the plantar medial aspect of the heel. These fractures must be treated aggressively with debridement and irrigation with strong consideration of external or limited internal fixation. There is a significant rate of deep infection in patients with open calcaneal fractures, as high as 39%, occasionally necessitating amputation.

Because of the increased complication rates seen with open calcaneal fractures, a treatment algorithm has been developed to minimize wound problems and subsequent infection. All injuries should undergo the usual care for open fractures, including antibiotics and urgent irrigation and debridement, with subsequent serial irrigation and debridements until the wound is clean. According to this protocol, all patients with lateral wounds should have open reduction through the open wound and percutaneous fixation. Open calcaneal fractures with a medial wound should have the same treatment if the wound is larger than 4 cm, cannot be closed, or is not stable after 7 to 10 days. Otherwise, open calcaneal fractures with medial wounds that are less than 4 cm with closeable, stable wounds can be treated with standard open reduction and internal fixation (ORIF) as done for closed fractures once the soft-tissue swelling subsides. This approach can decrease infection and improve outcomes. Mehta et al. reported a 7% deep infection rate using a similar approach with initial percutaneous provisional fixation and delay of definitive fixation through an extensile lateral approach for an average of 18 days (range, 10 to 28 days) for patients with open types II and IIIA medial wounds.

Open Reduction Techniques. For open reduction techniques, patients either are operated on within the first 12 to 24 hours or, more commonly, surgery is delayed 10 to 14 days to allow soft-tissue swelling to resolve enough for the skin to wrinkle. Minimally invasive techniques are more appropriate options closer to the time of injury. Percutaneous techniques can be used as soon as the patient is medically stable, while the window for sinus tarsi approaches to fixation is within the first 10 to 14 days. After this period, restoration of the calcaneal architecture can be more difficult without extensile approaches. If the soft tissues are not suitable for fixation, a bulky Jones dressing is applied, and the foot is elevated and iced. The foot is checked before surgery to ensure that no fracture blebs are present and that swelling has started to resolve. After 3 weeks, open reduction becomes more difficult, but it is possible up to 4 to 5 weeks.

The extensile lateral technique has traditionally been the gold-standard approach among foot and ankle surgeons and traumatologists. Advantages include wide exposure of the calcaneus, allowing easier access to facet fragments, ability to decompress the lateral wall, exposure of the calcaneocuboid joint, and sufficient area laterally for plate fixation. Disadvantages include injury to the blood supply of the lateral flap and difficulty with assessment of reduction of the medial wall. More soft-tissue dissection is required, and a higher incidence of wound problems occur with this exposure. Attention to fundamentals is required for success with this approach, including careful soft-tissue handling, mobilization, and anatomic restoration of the posterior facet; adequate mobilization and reduction of the tuberosity fragment through the primary fracture line; and stabilization with plates and/or screws.

Multiple orthopaedic manufacturers produce plates specifically for use with extensile lateral techniques. Plates with locking options are popular for this fracture, although it is important to note that cortical screws will allow compression of the plate to the bone and narrowing of the widened heel. A disadvantage of a plate is its increased thickness and the possibility of a subsequent painful implant that requires removal or may block fixation for a later subtalar arthrodesis.

If a large defect remains after elevation of the posterior facet, some surgeons recommend the use of autogenous iliac crest bone graft, allograft, or bone substitutes; however, if internal fixation is secure and the fracture is stable, the defect may be accepted. No significant difference has been found in the maintenance of reduction or subsequent settling of the fracture between fixation with or without bone graft, and good results have been reported with ORIF without the use of bone graft. In a cadaver study, specimens with calcium phosphate bone cement injected into the osseous defect had decreased deformation to cyclical loading when compared with specimens with bone graft. The use of bone graft substitutes may allow patients to bear weight earlier, without loss of reduction and with similar outcomes to those in patients treated with bone graft.

OPEN REDUCTION OF CALCANEAL FRACTURE

TECHNIQUE 9.1

(BENIRSCHKE AND SANGEORZAN)

- Administer preoperative antibiotics and apply a tourniquet.
- Place the patient in a true lateral position on a beanbag or with bolsters and use the lateral approach.
- Carry the incision directly down to the periosteum of the lateral wall with no blunt soft-tissue dissection in the midportion of the wound. The sural nerve may cross the incision at its proximal and its distal end, so soft-tissue dissection should be done in these areas to avoid cutting the nerve (Fig. 9.8A).
- Gently retract the flap while performing subperiosteal dissection along the lateral wall. It is essential to follow the contours of the blown-out lateral wall and not stray into the soft tissues to avoid damage to the peroneal tendons. These tendons should be contained in the flap. Elevate the entire flap in one piece and hold it out of the way with a Kirschner wire placed longitudinally into the fibula, one from lateral to medial in the talus, and one into the cuboid. Bend these wires back to retract the flap, which does not need to be touched again for the remainder of the procedure (Fig. 9.8B).
- Expose the entire lateral wall of the calcaneus distally to the calcaneocuboid joint.
- Carry the dissection above and below the peroneal tendons at the level of the calcaneocuboid joint if necessary.

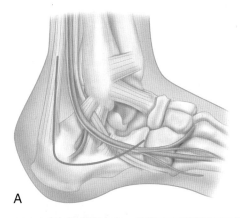

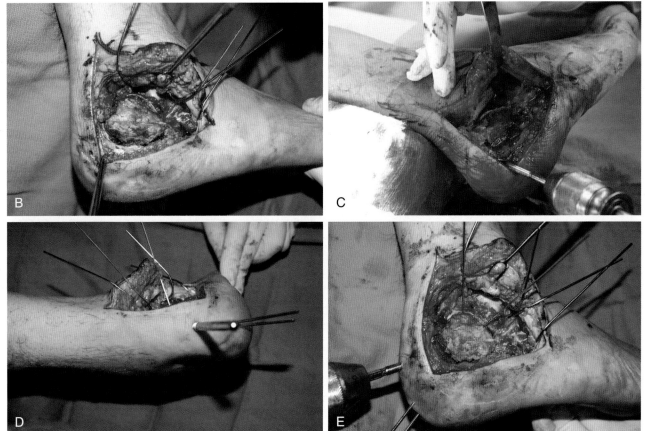

FIGURE 9.8   Open reduction of calcaneal fracture (see text). **A,** Incision. **B,** Retraction of full-thickness flap with Kirschner wires. **C,** Large pin used to manipulate tuberosity fragment. **D,** Provisional fixation from heel into sustentacular fragment. **E,** Reduction and provisional fixation of posterior facet. **SEE TECHNIQUE 9.1.**

This extensile lateral approach exposes the lateral wall of the calcaneocuboid joint and posterior facet. Reduction of the tuber-sustentacular fragment is done indirectly.

- When the exposure is completed, remove the lateral wall and place it in a secure place on the back table for later replacement because this fragment blocks direct observation of the posterior facet. Do not reduce the posterior facet immediately because room for the piece must first be created.
- When a fracture line separates the anterior process from the sustentacular fragment, reduce this part first to allow better exposure of the relationship between the me-

dial part containing the sustentacular fragment and the lateral part with the posterior facet and tuberosity (Fig. 9.8C).

- Reduce the tuberosity to the sustentacular fragment with manipulation of a large threaded Steinmann pin placed into the tuberosity fragment from either lateral to medial or directed posteriorly to correct the varus and loss of height and length; perform a provisional fixation using axially directed Kirschner wires introduced from the heel into the sustentacular fragment (Fig. 9.8D). A large cannulated screw can be placed to continue to hold the tuberosity out of varus.

- With the bone now out to length from these two reduction maneuvers, turn attention to the depression of the posterior facet, reducing it to the intact medial piece and holding it with provisional fixation (Fig. 9.8E).
- Obtain intraoperative radiographs to assess overall reduction.
- A large defect often remains in the substance of the calcaneus beneath the reduced posterior facet. If good stability of the fracture and secure internal fixation are obtained, this defect can be accepted or bone graft or bone cement can be used to fill the void.
- Reduce the lateral wall along the outer edge of the posterior facet and perform fixation, which should take advantage of the known anatomy. The thickened bone in the thalamic portion, which supports the posterior facet, provides the most reliable fixation in most instances.
- Insert small cortical lag screws (2.4 or 2.7 mm) into the sustentacular fragment to maintain the reduction of the posterior facet. A cadaver study showed that the widest safe zone for the starting point of the lag screw is 15 mm below the joint line of the posterior facet, dropping the hand 20 degrees from the perpendicular to the axis of the leg, and aiming from 6 degrees anteriorly at the most anterior starting point to 36 degrees anteriorly from the most posterior starting point to get the sustentaculum without violating the joint.
- Apply a lateral plate that extends from the anterior process of the calcaneus into the most posterior aspect of the tuberosity (Fig. 9.9A and B). The plate helps to maintain a neutral alignment of the calcaneus. When contouring the plate, be careful not to fix the heel in varus. Obtain an intraoperative axial view to confirm neutral alignment before application of the plate. When possible, direct screws from the plate into the sustentacular fragment for maximal fixation. Place the most anterior screw into the subchondral bone supporting the calcaneocuboid articular surface. Place the most posterior screw into the thickened bone at the posterior aspect of the calcaneus.
- Close the flap over a deep drain if desired. It is useful to throw all of the subcutaneous absorbable sutures first and then tie to allow better access and wound edge approximation. A modified Donati-Allgower technique is used for skin closure. Apply a short leg splint.

See also Video 9.1.

POSTOPERATIVE CARE Closed suction drainage is used for 24 to 48 hours if needed. Strict icing and elevation protocols should be maintained to minimize swelling and pain. At the second postoperative week, active range of motion of the ankle and subtalar joint is instituted if the flap shows uncomplicated healing and the wound is sealed. Patients learn to draw the alphabet with the hallux of their injured limb or make progressively larger circles with their feet. Protection is provided by the use of a removable posterior splint or fracture boot. Weight bearing is instituted at 10 to 12 weeks, extensive physical therapy is started, and implants can be removed if the injury is symptomatic at 1 year.

SUBTALAR ARTHRODESIS
TECHNIQUE 9.2

- Carry out ORIF of the calcaneus as described in Technique 9.1 (Fig. 9.10).
- Major bone voids in the posterior side of the calcaneus may require tricortical iliac crest bone graft to restore the normal orientation and height of the calcaneus.
- After internal fixation, use a burr to remove the cartilage and subchondral bone from the posterior facet of the calcaneus and posterior facet of the talus.
- Use extensive autogenous iliac crest bone graft to fill the defect.
- Denude the lateral aspect of the talus to obtain an intraarticular and an extraarticular arthrodesis.
- Fix the arthrodesis with two fully threaded, 6.5-mm cancellous screws (Fig. 9.10).

POSTOPERATIVE CARE The drain, if used, is removed on the first postoperative day, and the sutures are removed at 2 to 3 weeks. A short leg cast or fracture boot is worn until evidence of union is apparent, generally between 10 and 12 weeks. A prefabricated walking brace is applied, and the patient is gradually allowed to return to full activities.

The sinus tarsi approach has become more widely used and can avoid some of the wound complications associated with the extensile lateral approach. There is wide variation in the literature as to what size incision is used in a sinus tarsi approach, ranging from 1 to 2 cm, centered on the posterior facet (Fig. 9.11) for exposure from the posterior fibula to the anterior process of the calcaneus as described by Kocher. Advantages of this approach include direct visualization of the posterior facet (which may be difficult with the extensile lateral approach), lower wound complications, and use of the same incision that would be used for an arthrodesis in the future. Disadvantages of this approach are that lateral wall decompression can be more difficult and reduction of the tuberosity fragment is indirect. In most cases, the lateral approach provides enough exposure for fracture fixation, although this can be combined with a medial approach. The medial approach allows direct reduction of the sustentacular fragment, which may not be "constant" in 42% of patients, according to one study. The medial approach requires careful exposure and mobilization of the medial neurovascular bundle. A variety of sinus tarsi–specific plates have been developed; however, Pitts et al. showed no significant difference in outcomes with plate versus screw-only fixation constructs.

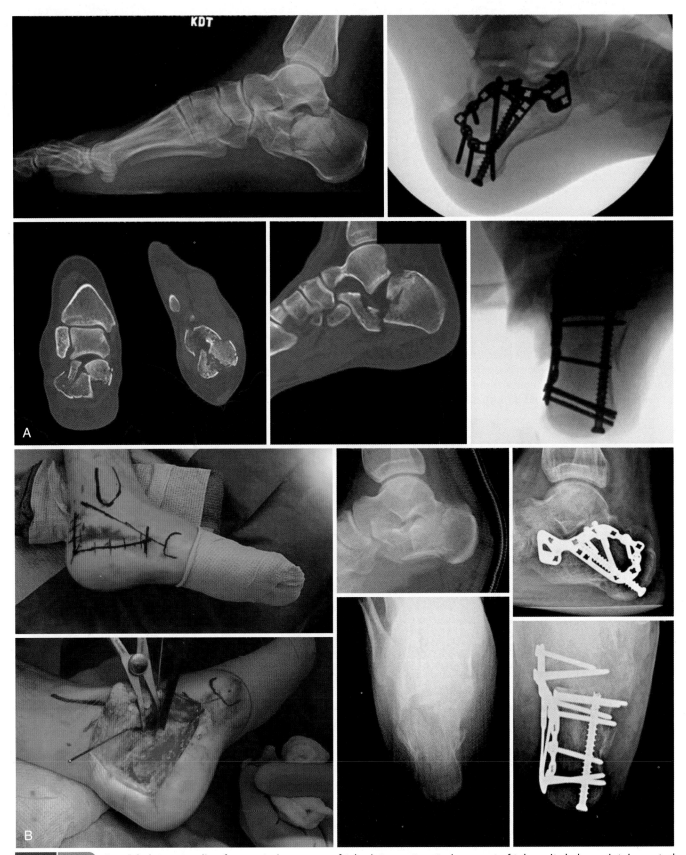

FIGURE 9.9 Lateral plate extending from anterior process of talus into most posterior aspect of tuberosity helps maintain neutral alignment of calcaneus. **SEE TECHNIQUE 9.1.**

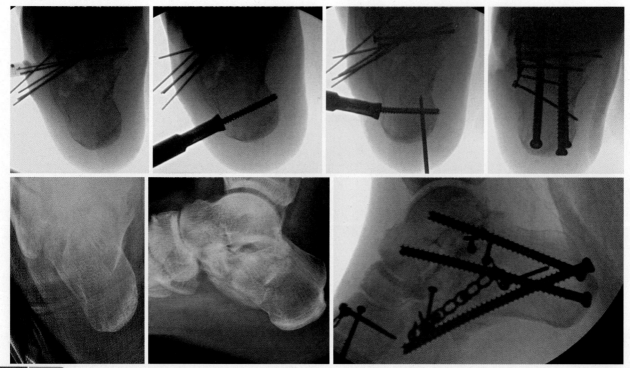

FIGURE 9.10 Subtalar arthrodesis for treatment of calcaneal fracture. Intraoperative correction of varus deformity with joystick along with fixation and double arthrodesis for comminuted calcaneal fracture. Fully threaded screws are used to maintain height of calcaneus. **SEE TECHNIQUES 9.2 AND 9.3.**

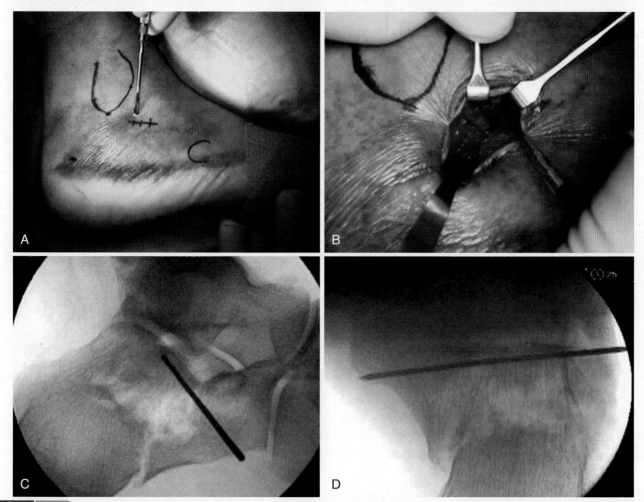

FIGURE 9.11 Percutaneous reduction and fixation of calcaneal fracture (see text). **A** and **B,** Posterior facet is reduced through small stab incision. **C** to **F,** Provisional fixation with Kirschner wires. **G** and **H,** Definitive fixation with cannulated screws. **I,** Skin incision after reduction and fixation. (From Banerjee R, Nickisch F, Easley ME, DiGiovanni CW: Foot injuries. In Browner BD, et al, editors: *Skeletal trauma,* Philadelphia, 2009, Saunders.) **SEE TECHNIQUES 9.3 AND 9.5.**

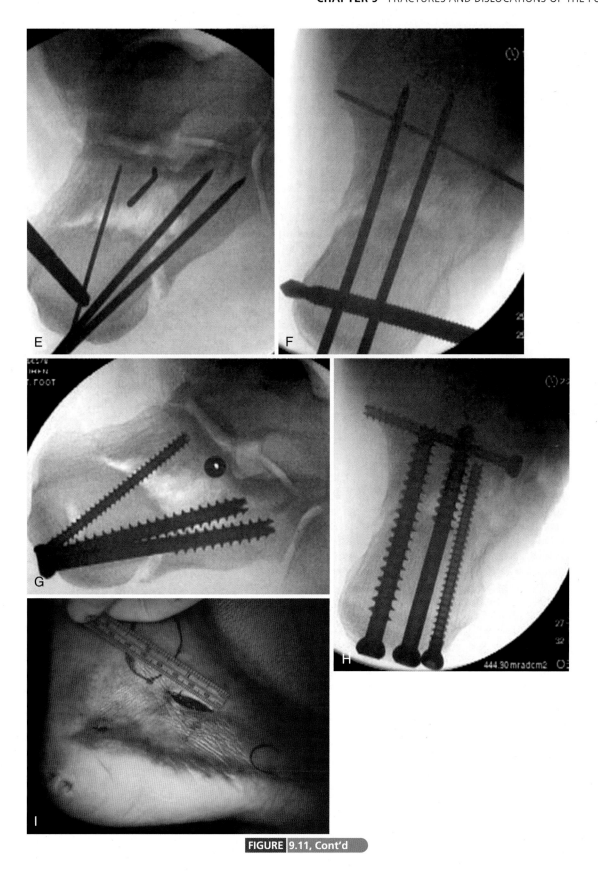

OPEN REDUCTION OF CALCANEAL FRACTURE: SINUS TARSI APPROACH WITH OR WITHOUT MEDIAL APPROACH

TECHNIQUE 9.3

- Two incisions, one medial and one lateral, can be used, although usually the lateral incision provides enough exposure to reduce the major fragments (Fig. 9.12A to C).
- Place the patient in the lateral position on a beanbag or bolsters. If the supine position is chosen, place a large bump beneath the ipsilateral buttock. Apply a tourniquet. Place the patient in a mildly inclined Trendelenburg position and rest the foot on towels or sheets, which at varying times in the procedure allow the foot to hang freely without support when the towels are moved proximal to the ankle joint.
- Make the *lateral incision* along a line from the tip of the fibula toward the base of the fourth metatarsal centered on the posterior facet and as long as needed to allow visualization of the joint reduction.
- Identify the sural nerve in the posterior portion of the incision; it usually lies in a small amount of fat just anterior to the small saphenous vein and overlying the combined sheath of the peroneal tendons. Dissect it distally. Try to preserve both main branches, but if exposure of the lateral aspect of the sinus tarsi and calcaneocuboid joint is incomplete, the medial branch, which usually joins with the lateralmost branch of the superficial peroneal nerve, can be sacrificed without causing significant numbness at the fourth web.
- When the sural nerve and small saphenous vein are retracted, open the inferior peroneal retinaculum on its anterior border where it meets the stem of the inferior extensor retinaculum to expose the anterolateral ridge of the anterior third of the calcaneus, which is the most lateral border of the sinus tarsi.
- Reflect the origin of the extensor digitorum brevis distally to expose the calcaneocuboid joint. Elevate the extensor digitorum brevis only as much as necessary to expose the calcaneocuboid joint.
- Expose the lateral wall of the calcaneus by sharp dissection or with a thin osteotome or periosteal elevator. A small Hohmann retractor can be placed under the peroneal tendons to retract them posteriorly. This is the "door" to the anterior two thirds of the lateral surface of the calcaneus. Stay in this plane with the foot held in valgus and equinus. The lateral wall is thin and frequently comminuted. Distally, the fracture may enter the calcaneocuboid joint.
- Take care to remain lateral to the lateral wall. With lateral wall blowout, it is easy to enter medially to the lateral wall, which will prevent proper placement of a lateral plate.
- A large threaded Steinmann pin can be placed into the posterior tuberosity for traction and manipulation of the large tuberosity fragment (see Fig. 9.10).

- Remove any further hematoma and inspect the posterior facet. If inspection is difficult, place a lamina spreader into the depths of the sinus tarsi, pressing up on the neck of the talus and down on the anterior portion of the calcaneus to give a better view of the posterior facet. This is a pivotal point in the procedure, at which time it should be possible to form a good mental image of the fractures through the posterior facet (usually sagittal) and transversely across the junction of the posterior facet articular surface and the proximal border of the sinus tarsi. This latter fracture frequently communicates medially with the oblique fracture that splits off the large anteromedial sustentacular fragment.
- Insert a Cobb elevator into the primary fracture line to mobilize the fragments, and use the Steinmann pin to manipulate the tuberosity plantarly and posteriorly to regain height and length, and with a valgus moment to correct any varus. Insert provisional fixation with a guidewire for a 5.5-mm or 6.5-mm cannulated screw from the tuberosity into the sustentaculum.
- If a satisfactory medial wall reduction cannot be obtained with manipulation of the tuberosity with the Steinmann pin, a medial approach should be considered.
- For the *medial incision,* tilt the operating table laterally, flex the knee, and abduct the hip. Dorsiflex the foot to 90 degrees at the ankle joint.
- Palpate the most prominent portion of the subcutaneous edge of the tarsal navicular and 1 cm anterior to this begin an incision straight posteriorly that crosses the sustentaculum tali. If the sustentaculum cannot be palpated because of swelling, have the incision cross a point 2 cm distal to the subcutaneous tip of the medial malleolus. Continue the incision posteriorly to 1.5 to 2.0 cm anterior to the Achilles tendon.
- Identify the anterior (distal) and posterior (proximal) borders of the flexor retinaculum (laciniate ligament) that runs from the medial malleolus obliquely plantarward and posteriorly to the posterosuperior border of the calcaneus. The superficial fascia of the leg and foot is continuous with the flexor retinaculum, and this also must be opened the entire length of the incision.
- Dissect the retinaculum anteriorly 1 cm and plantarward to the upper border of the abductor hallucis.
- Identify the neurovascular bundle at the posterior or proximal edge of the flexor retinaculum. Bluntly delineate the posterior aspect of the bundle, ensuring that the lateral plantar artery, vein, and nerve are included in the dissection.
- Pass a Penrose drain around the bundle and gently retract it anteriorly for further exposure of the posterior border of the bundle. Dissect this until it is lost beneath the abductor hallucis.
- Retract the posterior tibial neurovascular bundle anteriorly (usually one or more medial calcaneal branches must be retracted posteriorly) and expose the medial surface of the calcaneus by lifting the abductor hallucis and flexor accessory muscles off the calcaneus with a periosteal elevator.
- Palpate the sustentaculum tali of the calcaneus and clear all soft tissues from the medial surface of the calcaneus

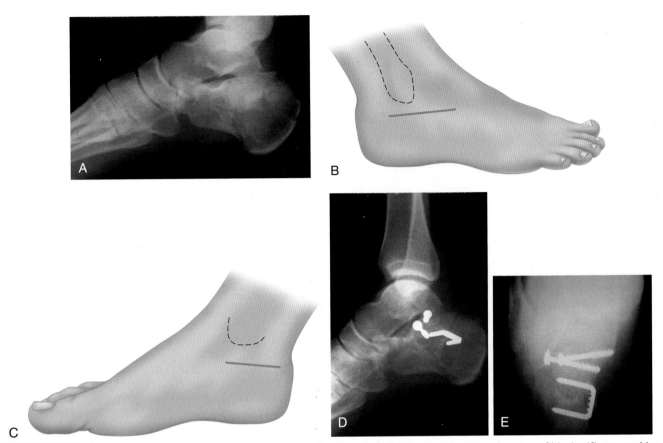

FIGURE 9.12 **A,** Preoperative radiograph. Medial and lateral incisions were chosen in this patient because of his significant smoking history. **B,** Lateral incision. **C,** Medial incision. **D** and **E,** Postoperative radiographs. **SEE TECHNIQUE 9.3.**

from the sustentaculum to the medial ridge of the calcaneal tuberosity.

- The fracture lines delineating the anteromedial and tuberosity fragments should come into view.
- Pass an instrument or finger over the tuberosity fragment and communicate with the lateral wound. Using an instrument or finger, pull down on the tuberosity fragment, disimpacting and dorsiflexing it while holding the ankle in equinus.
- Return to the medial wall of the calcaneus and inspect the fracture lines again. The tuberosity fragment is displaced laterally and distally and must be pulled posteriorly, translated medially, and taken out of varus with help of the Steinmann pin.
- Make a final evaluation of the fracture patterns and plan the fixation.
- While holding the medial wall reduced manually, direct one or two pins from the posterolateral aspect of the posterior tuberosity just lateral to the Achilles tendon and direct the pins upward and medially to engage the sustentacular fragment.
- Through the lateral incision, gently tap a 5- to 6-mm osteotome deep to the depressed posterior facet fragment and, holding the foot in varus for better exposure, lift the posterior facet into its proper position and pin it to the sustentacular fragment with two 0.062-inch Kirschner

wires. Place these wires just below the articular surface in subchondral bone for good purchase. Pass the wires to the medial side, directed distally about 10 to 20 degrees, and locate them by palpation.

- Ensure that a second sagittal fracture through the posterior facet medial to the first fracture is not overlooked because, if present, both depressed fragments need elevation and fixation. Reducing the posterior facet can leave a gap in the cancellous bone beneath the facet; bone grafting of the defect is optional.
- Reduce the anteromedial and tuberosity fragments and the posterior facet; the tuber-joint angle should be within normal limits.
- Place lateral to medial screws (2.4 mm or 2.7 mm) from the posterior facet into the sustentaculum in subchondral bone.
- A small two-hole plate can be used medially if needed, but this is difficult if the temporary fixation pins have been placed too close together or are in the way of optimal plate placement; keep this in mind when placing the wires (Fig. 9.13).
- Place an additional cannulated screw from the tuberosity under the posterior facet screws acting as a kickstand. A third screw can be placed in the lateral calcaneus from the tuberosity into the anterior process to maintain length.

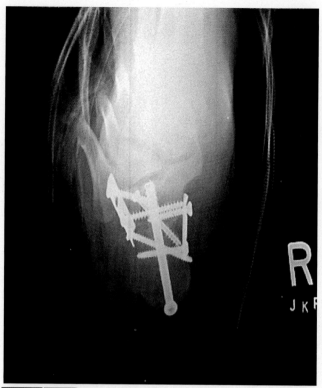

FIGURE 9.13   Fixation of calcaneal fracture with medial and lateral plates. **SEE TECHNIQUE 9.3.**

- A variety of plates designed for the sinus tarsi approach can be used, if desired, and screws inserted subcutaneously (Fig. 9.14). Use of a small 1/3 tubular plate also is an option (Fig. 9.15). Fractures can also be fixed with a screws-only approach (see Fig. 9.11).
- Take axial and lateral radiographs, lavage the wounds, remove the tourniquet, and close the wounds.
- Wrap large, bulky gauze dressings from the toes to the tibial tuberosity and apply a short leg cast.

POSTOPERATIVE CARE The extremity is elevated and iced postoperatively. At 3 weeks, the sutures are removed, and gentle range of motion is initiated. Non–weight bearing is continued until 8 to 12 weeks postoperatively, depending on bone quality and strength of fixation.

Tongue Fracture of the Calcaneus. Although the previously described technique works for joint depression and tongue-type fractures, occasionally a tongue-type fracture does not involve additional fracture lines, widening of the lateral wall, or significant displacement at the primary fracture line. The tongue fracture in this case can be treated by the axial pin fixation described by Gissane, and popularized by Essex-Lopresti, who achieved satisfactory results. Tornetta reported successful outcomes with this technique in 41 patients.

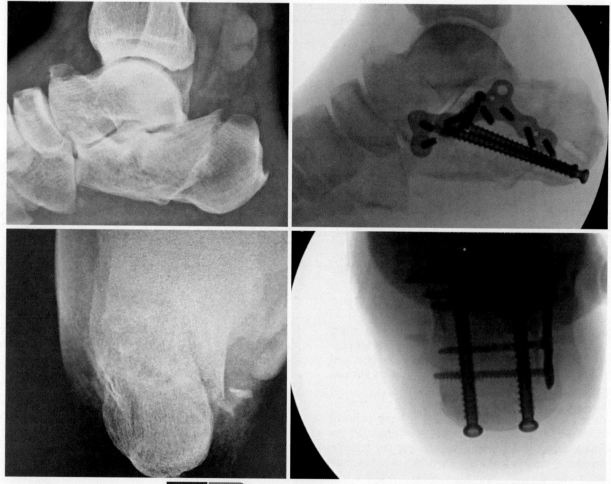

FIGURE 9.14   Lateral plate fixation of calcaneal fracture. **SEE TECHNIQUE 9.3.**

A subset of patients with calcaneal fractures is prone to skin breakdown over the fracture fragment posteriorly. These tend to be patients who did not sustain the injury from a fall, who smoked, who had greater fracture displacement (although it can happen even with minimal displacement), and who were evaluated after a delay. If the threatened soft tissue is recognized early and prompt intervention is instituted, wound problems can be avoided. Otherwise, these patients may require soft-tissue coverage and may eventually require amputation. Similar soft-tissue problems can occur after tuberosity avulsion fractures unless prompt reduction is performed (see Figs. 9.31 and 9.32).

AXIAL FIXATION OF CALCANEAL FRACTURE

TECHNIQUE 9.4

(ESSEX-LOPRESTI)

- With the patient prone, make a small incision over the displaced tuberosity of the calcaneus just lateral to the attachment to the Achilles tendon.
- Introduce a heavy Steinmann pin or Gissane spike into the tongue fragment in a longitudinal direction, angling slightly to the lateral side. Use radiographic or image intensifier control during the insertion of the pin and manipulation of the fracture (Fig. 9.16A).
- With the knee flexed, reduce the fracture by lifting upward on the pin until the knee clears the table; hold the forefoot at the level of the midtarsal joints with the opposite hand and avoid creating a cavus deformity by hyperflexing the forefoot. By this maneuver, the tongue fragment is elevated from its depressed position in the body of the calcaneus.
- Reduce the spreading of the calcaneus by applying pressure on each side of the bone with the heels of the clasped hands. Clear the inferior aspect of the lateral malleolus from contact with any bulging bone fragments that may encroach on the peroneal tendons and produce chronic tenosynovitis.
- Gently rock the calcaneus to settle the smaller fragments into position.
- Make final radiographs to confirm the position (Fig. 9.16B).

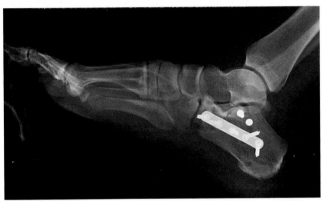

FIGURE 9.15 Use of small 1/3 tubular plate also is option. **SEE TECHNIQUE 8.3.**

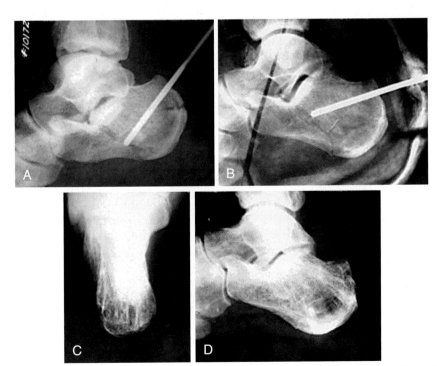

FIGURE 9.16 Essex-Lopresti reduction of fracture of calcaneus by manipulation and pin fixation. **A,** Correct position of pin. **B,** Postoperative radiograph through cast. **C** and **D,** Result after 1 year. Patient returned to work as deckhand on barge. **SEE TECHNIQUE 9.4.**

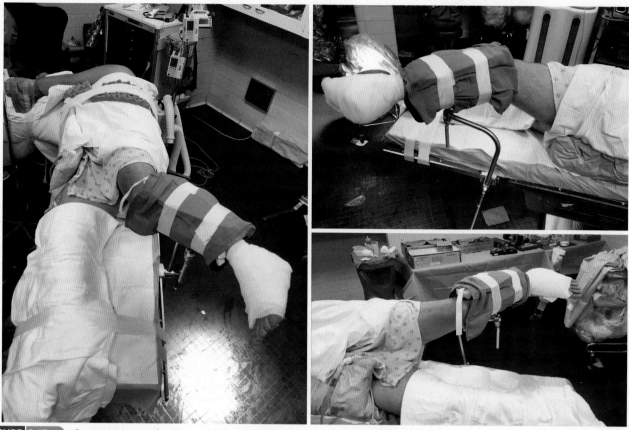

FIGURE 9.17 Percutaneous reduction and fixation of calcaneal fracture. Keeping the leg holder as proximal as possible allows access to ankle.

- Advance the pin or spike across the fracture into the anterior fragment of the calcaneus.

POSTOPERATIVE CARE The foot is carefully padded, and a splint is applied, incorporating the protruding portion of the pin or spike. The initial cast and pin usually are removed at 4 to 6 weeks, and a cast is applied from the tibial tuberosity to the toes. If radiographs confirm union and reconstitution of the depressed cancellous bone beneath the elevated articular surface, weight bearing can be started 8 to 10 weeks after reduction (Fig. 9.16C and D).

Percutaneous Techniques. To minimize wound complications, reduction and percutaneous fixation of calcaneal fractures have become more popular. This approach allows restoration of the basic morphology of the calcaneus and improves the articular reduction; however, it relies heavily on fluoroscopy rather than direct visualization of the joint surfaces. Experience with open fixation of calcaneal fractures is advantageous to understanding the anatomy and interpreting fluoroscopy appropriately to gain the appropriate reduction and fixation. It often is very difficult to obtain a perfect articular reduction with this technique in Sanders types III and IV fractures, although the calcaneal length and height may be restored and provide a better foundation for subtalar arthrodesis in the future. Arthroscopic evaluation may be helpful in evaluating the reduction. If this technique is chosen, it is helpful to perform the surgery as soon as feasible after the injury before the frature fragments consolidate, making reduction more difficult.

PERCUTANEOUS REDUCTION AND FIXATION OF CALCANEAL FRACTURE

TECHNIQUE 9.5

(RODEMUND AND MATTIASSICH)
- Place the patient in a lateral position with a thigh tourniquet, the hip extended, knee flexed, and leg resting on a padded well leg holder (Fig. 9.17). Keeping the leg holder as proximal as possible allows access to the ankle for other procedures such as a heel cord lengthening.
- Place C-arm fluoroscopy on the operative side and angle it at 45 degrees to the operating table. This allows the procedure to be performed in the lateral radiographic view. Rolling the C-arm back allows a Broden view, while swinging through to a traditional lateral C-arm position produces a Harris axial view of the calcaneus (Fig. 9.18).
- Place long 3.0-mm Kirschner wires through the talar neck and calcaneal tuberosity and affix them to dual distractors on both the medial and lateral side of the calcaneus (Fig. 9.19). Take care to be perpendicular to the lateral wall of the tuberosity when inserting the Kirschner wire.
- Generally, there is varus alignment to the fracture, such that the Kirschner wires will form an acute angle and not be parallel initially. With the distractors applied, the wires will become parallel and allow varus alignment to be

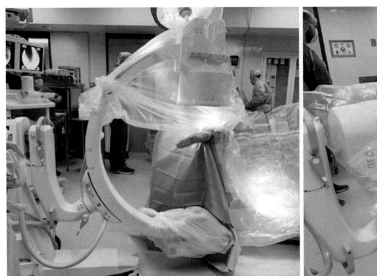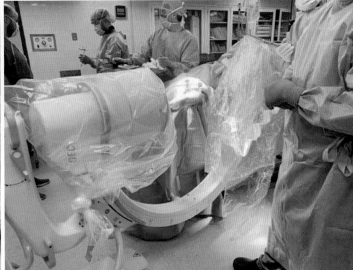

FIGURE 9.18 Rolling C-arm back allows Broden view, while swinging it through to traditional lateral position produces Harris axial view. **SEE TECHNIQUE 9.5.**

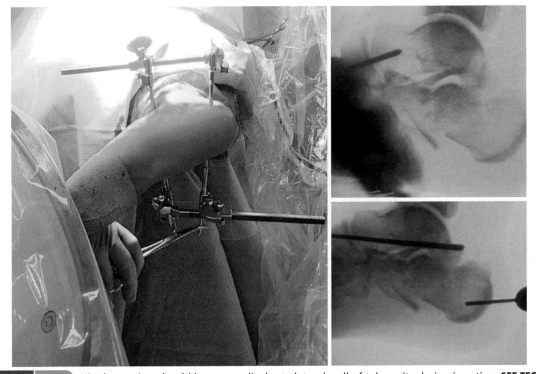

FIGURE 9.19 Kirschner wires should be perpendicular to lateral wall of tuberosity during insertion. **SEE TECHNIQUE 9.5.**

corrected. Continued dual distraction allows restoration of the length and height of the calcaneus (Fig. 9.20).
- A 2.0-mm threaded Kirschner wire can be inserted into the posterior facet and used as a joystick.
- Make a 1-cm incision in the lateral skin so that a Freer elevator or tonsil clamp can be inserted under the posterior facet through the primary fracture line (Fig. 9.21). Under fluoroscopy, the posterior facet fragments can be elevated into appropriate position. Cannulated or solid screws (4.0 mm) can be placed from lateral to medial, anchoring the posterior facet to the sustentaculum tali (Fig. 9.22).

- Insert three larger cannulated screws (5.0, 6.5, or 7.0 mm) from the tuberosity into the sustentaculum, under the posterior facet, and into the anterior process, respectively, based on fracture morphology, to maintain the restored anatomic parameters (Fig. 9.23).

■ COMPLICATIONS AND PREVENTION
▌WOUND NECROSIS, DEHISCENCE, AND INFECTION

Soft-tissue edema and contusion are inherent aspects of calcaneal fractures. Operating through edematous soft tissue,

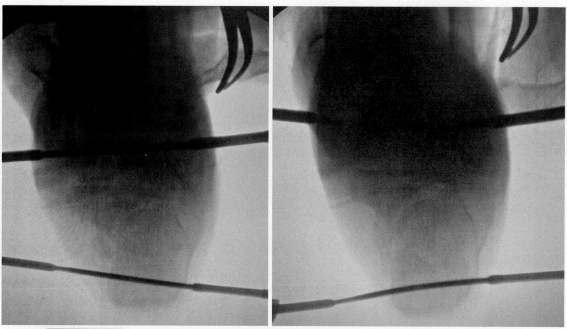

FIGURE 9.20   Continued dual distraction restores length and height of the calcaneus. **SEE TECHNIQUE 9.5.**

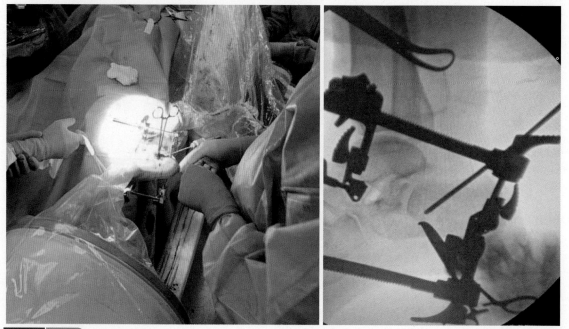

FIGURE 9.21   Freer elevator or tonsil clamp is inserted under posterior facet through primary fracture line. **SEE TECHNIQUE 9.5.**

especially in this area with a tenuous blood supply and no muscle between the skin and bone, entails risk of wound necrosis, dehiscence, and infection. After a standard, extensile, L-shaped approach with two-layer flap closure, wound complications developed in 25% of patients, with 21% requiring surgery for these complications. Other reported rates of marginal wound necrosis vary from 2% to 11%, and soft-tissue infection rates can be as high as 7%. Risk factors for wound complications include diabetes, smoking, open fracture, single layer closure, extended time between injury and surgery, and high body mass index. Although the incidence of mild wound problems is high, serious complications can be minimized in several ways:

1. Wound problems, particularly with fractures of the calcaneus, occur more frequently in active smokers. Patients should be advised not to smoke in the perioperative period and should be informed of the consequences of doing so before surgery is planned.
2. Carefully retracting the soft tissues and maintaining a full-thickness flap with the extensile approach are crucial.
3. A drain under the lateral flap may be considered to prevent hematoma formation postoperatively.
4. A two-layer closure should be performed, closing the wound from both ends to the middle. Throwing all of

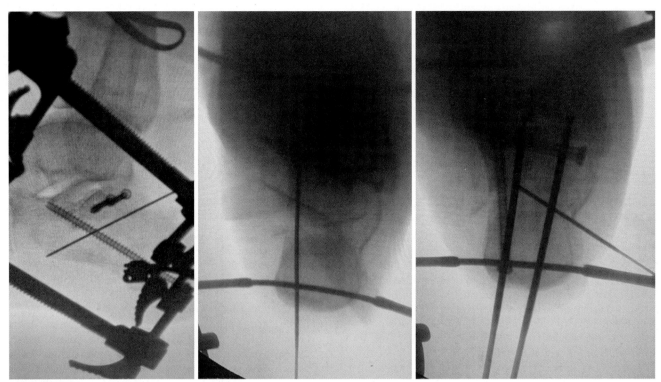

FIGURE 9.22 After elevation of posterior facet fragments into appropriate position, cannulated or solid screws are placed from lateral to medial to anchor posterior facet to sustentaculum tali. **SEE TECHNIQUE 9.5.**

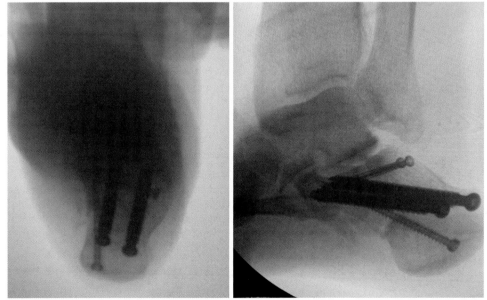

FIGURE 9.23 Three larger cannulated screws are inserted from tuberosity into sustentaculum, under posterior facet, and into anterior process **SEE TECHNIQUE 9.5.**

the sutures first and then tying allows less handing of the soft tissues.

5. Sutures should be left in place for 2 to 3 weeks until the wound is healed, and motion exercises should be avoided during that time to lessen shear forces under the flap.

LOSS OF REDUCTION OF MAJOR FRAGMENTS

Loss of reduction of major fragments can occur if weight bearing is initiated too early. Patients should be kept non–weight bearing for a minimum of 6 to 8 weeks to minimize this complication.

MALREDUCTION

Accurately restoring the proper valgus alignment of the tuberosity fragment is essential. Patients tolerate varus malrotation poorly. Intraoperative Harris radiographs should be obtained to minimize this complication.

SURAL NERVE AND PERONEAL TENDON INJURIES

Sural nerve and peroneal tendon injuries may occur. The sural nerve should be protected at the proximal and distal extremes of the wound in an extensile approach. The sural nerve was shown to be directly under the sinus tarsi surgical incision in 70% of cases reported by Li et al. and should be identified and protected. Peroneal tendons are particularly vulnerable, especially if dislocated, because the extensile flap is elevated over a protruding lateral wall. Limited periosteal elevation and careful retraction should prevent this complication. Peroneal tendons also can subluxate or dislocate out of the fibular groove from the force of the injury. In one study, this occurred in 28% of patients with calcaneal fractures but was addressed in only about 10% of the patients who were treated operatively. Peroneal subluxation or dislocation may lead to later symptoms if missed.

■ RESULTS

Significant controversy remains over the results of nonoperative versus operative treatment. Lack of standardization of results has made it difficult to compare studies that have evaluated outcomes. Numerous studies support the principle that if nonoperative treatment is chosen, early mobilization improves long-term results. Although long-term studies have shown up to 76% good results with early mobilization of displaced intraarticular fractures, other, more recent studies have been considerably more pessimistic about closed treatment.

The results after operative treatment also vary, but most authors judge results by the quality of reduction of the posterior facet. Essex-Lopresti stated that 80% of patients younger than age 50 years who had "successful reduction" had satisfactory results. Most modern studies that directly compare operative and nonoperative treatment conclude that functional outcomes are similar for both groups, but that complication rates are significantly higher in patients treated operatively. One study suggested, however, that there may be a trend for better outcomes in operatively treated patients in longer-term (8- to 10-year) follow-up, and another study showed that early complications do not affect long-term outcomes. These and other studies focusing on operative treatment show that patients with worse functional outcomes include those with a greater severity of injury, those with workers' compensation claims, those involved in heavy labor, and those with bilateral injuries. It is important to note that many studies comparing operative to nonoperative treatment have relied on the extensile lateral approach, whereas more limited techniques of surgical intervention have not been directly compared to nonoperative treatment in a large randomized trial.

Although the debate over open or closed treatment of calcaneal fractures may continue for some time, most authors agree that the inability to surgically obtain an anatomic reduction of the posterior facet is probably associated with a worse outcome than closed treatment. Overall, although there is moderate evidence that there is not a significant difference in pain and functional outcome between operatively treated and nonoperatively treated patients, operative treatment may improve subtalar motion and allow patients to wear regular shoes and return to work. Overall economic impact may be less in operatively treated fractures, especially when costs related to time off from work are included.

Other studies of ORIF through an extensile lateral approach show 73% to 75% good or excellent results, with subjective results clearly better at 10-year than 3-year follow-up. In a study with 10- to 20-year follow-up, 29% of patients required an arthrodesis procedure, with a higher percentage for patients with Sanders type III fractures than those with type II fractures. Patients did reasonably well if they did not develop posttraumatic arthritis, with 77%

scoring within the normal range on the 36-Item Short Form Health Survey (SF-36). A steep learning curve exists for operative treatment of calcaneal fractures, with significantly greater percentages of good and excellent results reported with greater surgeon experience. Ahn et al. suggested that an initial learning period of 20 cases is needed to improve reduction parameters. It is difficult to obtain good results with Sanders type IV fractures. In a small prospective randomized study in which patients with Sanders type IV fractures were treated with either ORIF or ORIF with primary arthrodesis, outcomes were similar for both groups, but patients with ORIF and primary arthrodesis had a shorter healing time.

Operative fixation through a limited lateral approach can produce outcomes similar to those of the extensile lateral approach, with good or excellent results in 59% to 84% of patients, a high accuracy of reduction, and a wound complication rate of 0% to 15%. In multiple retrospective reviews comparing outcomes of calcaneal fractures treated with an extensile lateral approach with those treated with a limited lateral approach, functional and radiographic outcomes were similar; however, those treated with the limited lateral approach had a lower incidence of wound complications and secondary surgeries. With a combined medial and lateral approach, 77% good or excellent results have been achieved. Marsh described 182 calcaneal fractures treated with percutaneous techniques and at final follow-up reported that 54.5% of patients had a residual pain level of 3 or lower.

Percutaneous fixation, with and without the use of arthroscopy, external fixation, and/or dual C-arms, has been reported to lead to reasonable functional outcomes, with 74% to 100% of patients returning to work and a 0% to 15% infection rate. Results were similar when compared with a historical control of patients who had standard ORIF, but patients with percutaneous reductions went back to work earlier and had better range of motion of the subtalar joint. When calcium sulfate cement grafting was added to percutaneous fixation, patients could bear weight earlier and had better range of motion and better outcome scores than those with open reduction without a difference in the quality of reduction.

Most authors reported that regardless of the type of treatment, symptoms should improve for at least 2 years and possibly 6 years. Although anatomic reduction of the posterior facet is correlated with better functional outcomes, eventually enough pain develops in some patients to warrant further treatment.

■ LATE COMPLICATIONS

Regardless of treatment method, chronic pain develops in some patients, limiting their capacity to work and enjoy life. Late problems leading to a painful outcome include posttraumatic arthrosis of the subtalar joint, lateral subfibular impingement with or without problems of the peroneal tendons, anterior ankle impingement from loss of the normal plantarflexed position of the talus, tibial or sural nerve complications, fat pad atrophy, and chronic regional pain syndrome. Classification of calcaneal malunions includes type I, lateral wall exostosis without subtalar arthrosis (Fig. 9.24A); type II, lateral wall exostosis with subtalar arthrosis (Fig. 9.24B); and type III, lateral wall exostosis, subtalar arthrosis, and varus malunion of the calcaneus (Fig. 9.24C).

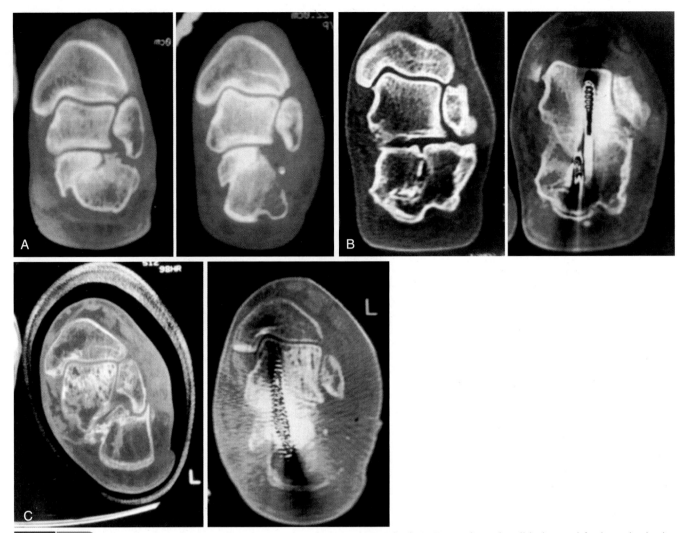

FIGURE 9.24 Classification of calcaneal malunions (Stephens and Saunders). **A,** Type I, lateral wall bulge and far lateral subtalar arthrosis. **B,** Type II, significant subtalar arthrosis. **C,** Type III, varus angulation and subtalar arthrosis. (From Stephens HM, Sanders R: Calcaneal malunions: results of a prognostic computed tomography classification system, *Foot Ankle Int* 17:395, 1996.)

▌CALCANEAL FRACTURE MALUNION

Patients with chronic lateral subtalar pain should be evaluated for two problems: posttraumatic arthrofibrosis or arthrosis and lateral calcaneofibular impingement, the latter of which rarely occurs in isolation. A combination of CT and selective subtalar injection of a local anesthetic can be helpful in determining the cause of the pain. Some patients have a congruous subtalar joint but have impingement or displacement of the peroneal tendons by the extruded lateral calcaneal wall, a type I malunion. This excess bone can be removed through a curved lateral incision along with deepening of the fibular groove for the peroneal tendons (Fig. 9.25). Removing this bone allows the peroneal tendons to assume a more normal position inferior to the fibula and narrows the heel, which assists with shoe fitting and lessens irritation from the lateral shoe counter; this was helpful in 79% of patients in one report. In another report, patients who had this procedure in isolation did not do well if they had concomitant subtalar arthrosis. More commonly, this procedure is done in conjunction with subtalar arthrodesis because many patients have both subtalar arthrosis and lateral impingement.

LATERAL DECOMPRESSION OF A MALUNITED CALCANEAL FRACTURE

TECHNIQUE 9.6

(BRALY, BISHOP, AND TULLOS)

- The procedure can be done with the patient in the lateral position or supine. If supine, place a roll under the ipsilateral hip for greater exposure of the lateral aspect of the foot and ankle. Apply and inflate a pneumatic thigh tourniquet.
- Make a curved incision just plantar to the course of the peroneal tendons, extending from the posterior aspect of the lateral malleolus to the region of the calcaneocuboid joint (Fig. 9.26A). If previous subtalar fusion or open reduction has been performed, attempt to use the existing incision.
- Identify and release the sural nerve from surrounding scar tissue to more normal anatomy proximally and distally (Fig. 9.26B).

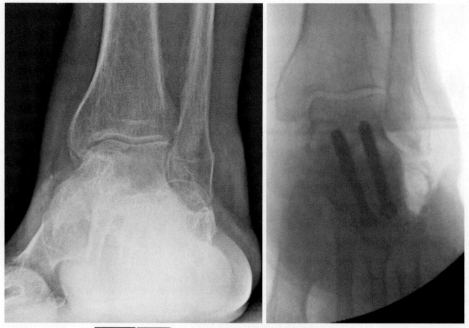

FIGURE 9.25   Lateral wall decompression.

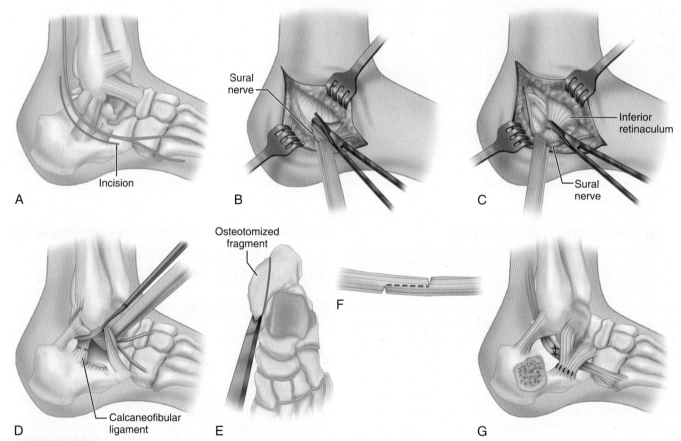

FIGURE 9.26   Technique for malunion of calcaneal fracture (Braly, Bishop, and Tullos). **A,** Incision just plantar to course of peroneal tendons. **B,** Sural nerve decompression. **C,** Inferior retinaculum incised, and peroneal tenolysis performed. **D,** Calcaneofibular ligament is cut to expose lateral calcaneus. **E,** Lateral calcaneal osteotomy. **F,** Z-lengthening of peroneal tendons for anterior dislocation. **G,** Repair or reconstruction of inferior retinaculum with lengthened peroneal tendons relocated.   (Redrawn from Braly WG, Bishop JO, Tullos HS: Lateral decompression for malunited os calcis fractures, *Foot Ankle* 6:90, 1985.) **SEE TECHNIQUE 9.6.**

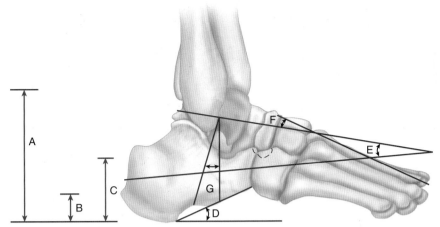

FIGURE 9.27 Radiographic measurements. *A,* Talocalcaneal height. *B,* Cuboid-to-floor distance. *C,* Navicular-to-floor distance. *D,* Calcaneal pitch angle. *E,* Talocalcaneal angle. *F,* First talometatarsal angle. *G,* Talar declination angle. (From Buch BD, Myerson MS, Miller SD: Primary subtalar arthrodesis for the treatment of comminuted calcaneal fractures, *Foot Ankle* 17:61, 1996.)

- Excise any neuromas present and dissect the nerve back to areas where the potential for external irritation over bony prominences during shoe wear is minimized.
- Incise the peroneal tendon sheath, if intact, taking care not to divide completely the superior retinaculum proximally.
- Perform a tenolysis (Fig. 9.26C).
- With the peroneal tendons and sural nerve retracted, incise the calcaneofibular ligament (Fig. 9.26D).
- Incise longitudinally the floor of the peroneal tendon sheath and the periosteum over the lateral calcaneus.
- With subperiosteal dissection, expose the prominent lateral bony mass of the calcaneus and excise it (Fig. 9.26E). Do not attempt to reconstruct the calcaneofibular ligament.
- The amount of bone removed from the calcaneus depends on the degree of lateral impingement of the peroneal tendons and sural nerve evident intraoperatively and on preoperative radiographs. Attempt to narrow the heel, at least laterally, to a more normal width, avoiding violating the subtalar and calcaneocuboid joints during bony resection. Smooth all rough edges with a rongeur and a rasp.
- Repair the reflected overlying periosteum or tendon sheath over the bed of the ostectomy.
- If any raw cancellous bone is left exposed, apply bone wax for hemostasis.
- Close the wounds in routine fashion and apply a soft, compressive dressing.
- If the peroneal tendons are dislocated, Braly et al. recommended Z-lengthening of both tendons before locating them behind the lateral malleolus (Fig. 9.26F); we do not routinely lengthen these tendons. The fibular groove can be deepened in cases of chronic peroneal dislocation.
- Repair the retinaculum or reconstruct it using an osteoperiosteal strip from the lateral malleolus, as described by Zoellner and Clancy (Fig. 9.26G), after the ostectomy.

POSTOPERATIVE CARE Early motion and progressive weight bearing as tolerated are encouraged 2 to 3 days after surgery. If peroneal work was performed, immobilization may be continued until the wound is healed before progressing range of motion and protected weight bearing.

SUBTALAR ARTHRODESIS

With the realization that symptoms should improve for at least 2 years, and as long as a patient is progressing in activity level and work capability, arthrodesis may be avoided, although the psychosocial complications of prolonged disability are profound. If a patient fails to progress with conservative treatment (e.g., bracing, antiinflammatory medications), arthrodesis should be considered. It has been shown that the longer the interval between the injury and the salvage procedure, the longer the interval until the patient returns to full activity or work.

In patients who are candidates for subtalar arthrodesis, bilateral standing radiographs should be scrutinized carefully. The talar angle of declination should be evaluated because it measures excursion of the tibiotalar joint in extension (Fig. 9.27). For patients with a depressed talar angle of declination, Carr et al. modified a procedure originally described by Gallie, the subtalar distraction bone block arthrodesis (Fig. 9.28).

Although the procedure is technically demanding, resulting postoperative appearance of the foot and improved ankle dorsiflexion may be impressive. A number of studies have demonstrated the usefulness of subtalar distraction bone block arthrodesis for the late complications of calcaneal fractures. Failures occurred in patients with transverse tarsal joint arthritis, malunions, and nerve problems. Functional outcomes were better in patients who had a late subtalar arthrodesis after ORIF than in those who were initially treated nonoperatively.

If calcaneal height is normal or minimally depressed and there are no anterior ankle joint impingement symptoms, we prefer in situ subtalar arthrodesis. Lateral wall decompression can be added if widening of the calcaneus is causing subfibular impingement, and use of this local graft for distraction has been shown to have outcomes similar to iliac crest bone grafting. This procedure can be helpful for patients with subtalar arthrosis after calcaneal fractures. No correlation has been identified between final outcome and talar angle declination, talar height, or calcaneal width. Peroneal tendon and subfibular impingement, ankle tenderness, sural nerve injury, and patient smoking all were statistically associated with lower scores.

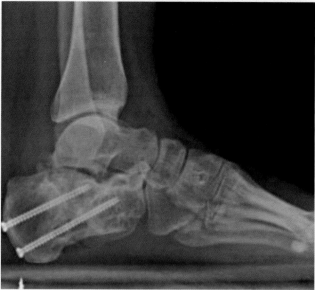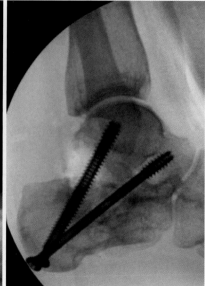

FIGURE 9.28 Talar height restored.

SUBTALAR DISTRACTION BONE BLOCK ARTHRODESIS

TECHNIQUE 9.7

(CARR ET AL.)

- Position the patient prone. Prepare and drape the posterior iliac crest and leg.
- Under tourniquet control, use a longitudinal posterolateral Gallie type of approach to the subtalar joint. Use a vertical incision because, after increasing the height with a bone block, a transverse incision will be more difficult to close. Identify and protect the sural nerve in the proximal incision. Alternatively, it can be excised and buried in surrounding muscle.
- Subperiosteally expose the lateral calcaneal wall and excise to a more normal width with a wide sharp osteotome. This step should ensure peroneal and fibular decompression.
- Identify the subtalar joint.
- A femoral distractor, Kirschner wire distractor, or external fixator with half-pins in the medial subcutaneous tibia and medial calcaneus may need to be applied for exposure. The medial application helps to correct hindfoot varus.
- Apply distraction and denude the subtalar joint to subchondral bone. Use a laminar spreader to aid in subtalar joint exposure. Direct attention to any heel varus or valgus at this point and, if necessary, correct by manipulation. Obtain intraoperative radiographs to ensure correction of the lateral talocalcaneal angle (normally 25 to 45 degrees). A percutaneously placed Kirschner wire distractor can be used to hold the distraction and allow easier instrumentation (Fig. 9.29).
- Measure the subtalar joint gap and harvest an appropriately sized tricortical posterior iliac crest graft. A block 2.5 cm in height may be required for severe deformities. Two separate pieces may be required to fill the gap complete-

ly and help prevent late collapse into varus or valgus. In some cases, the excised lateral wall can serve as sufficient graft material for the measured gap.
- Release the distraction forces.
- Insert a partially threaded cannulated screw (6.5 or 7.0 mm) from the tuberosity into the talar neck to increase talar declination, followed by a fully threaded screw laterally through the graft and into the talar body. A supplemental screw can be placed from the anterior process into the talar head.
- Obtain final radiographs (lateral and axial views) to confirm correct positioning.
- Close the wound in layers with interrupted nylon on the skin.

POSTOPERATIVE CARE The patient is kept in a short leg cast or splint for 6 to 8 weeks followed by weight bearing in a fracture boot for an additional 4 to 6 weeks.

EXTRAARTICULAR FRACTURES

Calcaneal fractures can be extraarticular (not involving the subtalar joint) or intraarticular (involving the subtalar joint). Extraarticular fractures include fractures of the calcaneal tuberosity, the sustentaculum tali, and the anterior process of the calcaneus.

■ FRACTURES OF THE CALCANEAL TUBEROSITY

Avulsion fractures of the calcaneal tuberosity are rare and are thought to be insufficiency fractures through osteoporotic bone and in patients with diabetes. A classification scheme has been proposed, with three types (Fig. 9.30): type I is a sleeve fracture in which a small piece of cortical bone is avulsed; type II is a beak fracture with an oblique fracture line that exits close but posterior to the posterior facet; and type III is an infrabursal fracture that is an avulsion off the middle third of the posterior aspect of the tuberosity. Type II fractures may require prompt reduction and fixation because the fracture fragment may cause soft-tissue compromise (Figs. 9.31 and 9.32). Fixation often is

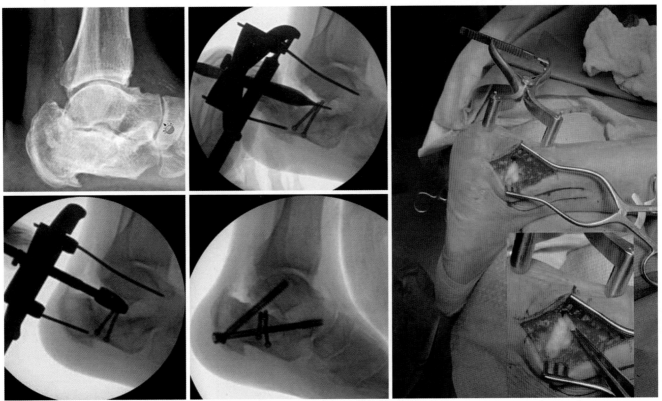

FIGURE 9.29 Subtalar interposition. Inset photo shows the allograft wedge used, with forceps holding a sponge of morphogenic protein (BMP-2). **SEE TECHNIQUE 9.7.**

carried out with screws and plates (Fig. 9.33). Loss of reduction can occur because of the strong pull of the Achilles tendon; suturing the tendon to bone using suture anchors or bone tunnels to augment screw fixation can provide greater fixation strength. In addition, lengthening of the gastrocnemius-soleus muscle (Strayer procedure) in patients with gastrocnemius tightness can help to reduce the deforming force. Because of dissatisfaction with the maintenance of reduction with screws and plates, a lateral tension band technique also has been used (Fig. 9.34). At our institution, avulsions with small to moderate pieces of bone are treated with excision of the bone fragment, smoothing of the dorsal calcaneal surface, and a secondary repair of the Achilles tendon to the remaining calcaneus with suture anchors, often accompanied by a gastrocnemius recession.

■ FRACTURES OF THE SUSTENTACULUM TALI

Isolated fractures of the sustentaculum tali are rare and often are missed on initial radiographs (Fig. 9.35). Although this is considered to be an extraarticular fracture, it can often involve the joint. These fractures often are associated with ipsilateral foot and ankle fractures, and direct ORIF, although a medial approach, yields good results. If not treated operatively, migration of the fragment from nonunion of this fracture can cause tarsal tunnel syndrome.

■ FRACTURES OF THE ANTERIOR PROCESS OF THE CALCANEUS

Fracture of the anterior process of the calcaneus occurs with an inversion injury where the bifurcate ligament causes an avulsion of a bony fragment (Fig. 9.36). It may be seen in the setting of other injuries to the Chopart joint, so close attention should

be paid to the talonavicular joint as well when this injury is found. Delayed diagnosis is common, and the fracture often is found after continued symptoms from what was assumed to be a simple ankle sprain. A type 1 fracture is a nondisplaced fracture, type 2 is a displaced avulsion fracture, and type 3 is a larger fragment involving the calcaneocuboid joint. Most fractures can be treated with cast immobilization; larger displaced fractures can be treated with ORIF. If a symptomatic nonunion occurs, excision of the fracture fragment can be helpful unless delayed excision has allowed arthrosis to occur at the calcaneocuboid joint.

FRACTURES OF THE TALUS

The role of the talus in lower extremity function, the complexity of the anatomy, and the variability of fracture patterns often complicate treatment of talar fractures and often frustrate orthopaedists. To gain full confidence in the treatment of these injuries, one must have thorough knowledge of the osseous and vascular anatomy, have experience with modern methods of fixation, and be prepared to deal with the complications that often occur with talar injuries.

ANATOMY

The vascular anatomy of the talus has been extensively studied (Fig. 9.37). The three major arteries of the leg contribute to a rich, extraosseous, anastomotic plexus, supplying blood to the head, neck, and body of the talus. The head and neck regions are richly supplied by the superior neck vessels, branching off the dorsalis pedis artery and the artery of the sinus tarsi. Osteonecrosis of these areas is extremely rare.

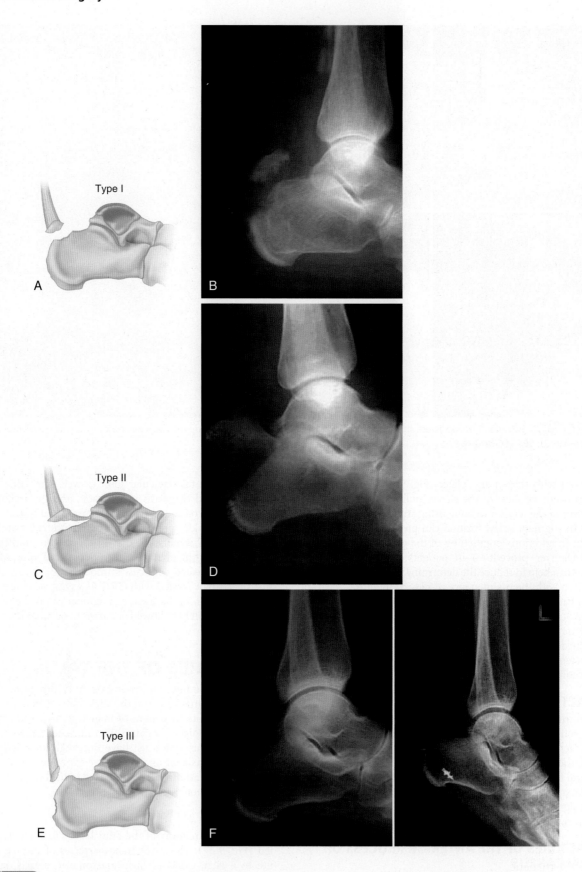

FIGURE 9.30 Classification of calcaneal tuberosity fractures. **A** and **B,** Type I, sleeve fracture. **C** and **D,** Type II, beak fracture. **E** and **F,** Type III, infrabursal fracture.

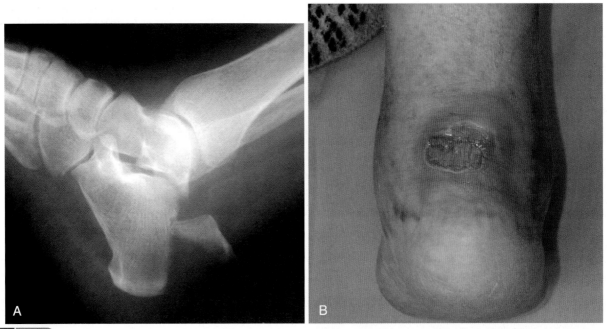

FIGURE 9.31 **A,** Calcaneal avulsion with large fragment. **B,** Open wound on posterior heel that developed when fracture was not treated expediently.

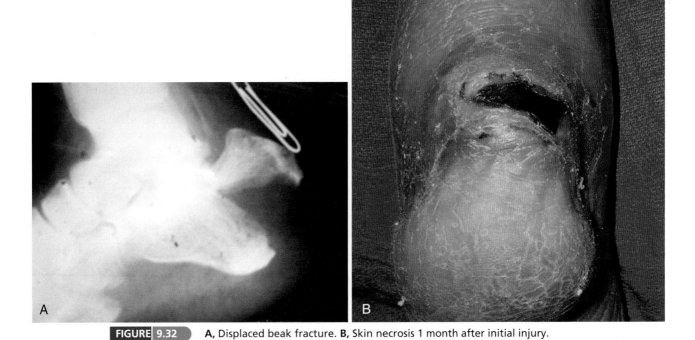

FIGURE 9.32 **A,** Displaced beak fracture. **B,** Skin necrosis 1 month after initial injury.

The tarsal canal is formed by the sulcus on the inferior surface of the talus and the superior sulcus of the calcaneus and contains the artery of the tarsal canal and the talocalcaneal intraosseous ligament. The tarsal canal runs from posteromedial to anterolateral, where it opens into the tarsal sinus. The talar body is vulnerable because of its blood supply. Related primarily to the degree of displacement of the body, the osteonecrosis rates can be 100%. The vascular supply to the talar body can be summarized as follows (Fig. 9.38).

The artery of the tarsal canal, which branches off the posterior tibial artery approximately 1 cm proximal to the division into medial and lateral plantar arteries, is the most consistent major supplier of blood to the body of the talus. In the tarsal canal, it sends four to six direct vessels into the body of the talus.

The deltoid artery, which branches off the artery of the tarsal canal and directly supplies blood to the medial one fourth to one half of the talar body, is the second major blood supply to the talar body. Through intraosseous anastomoses, it has the potential to supply blood to a much greater area.

The artery of the sinus tarsi, which is more variable in its size and origin, supplies the lateral one eighth to one fourth of the talar body. It is formed by branches of the perforating peroneal artery, the dorsalis pedis (or anterior tibial) artery, or anastomoses between the two. The artery of the sinus tarsi forms an anastomosis with the artery of the tarsal canal and has the potential to supply blood to more of the talus.

The posterior tubercle of the talus is supplied by direct branches from the posterior tibial artery (most common) or the peroneal artery. Although quite small, because of intraosseous anastomoses, this region also has the potential to supply blood to more of the body.

A described direct branch to the medial talar neck comes from the posterior tibial artery as demonstrated in a gadolinium-enhanced MRI cadaver study. This artery is at risk during the anteromedial approach for a talar neck fracture but appears to be preserved if a medial malleolar osteotomy is performed

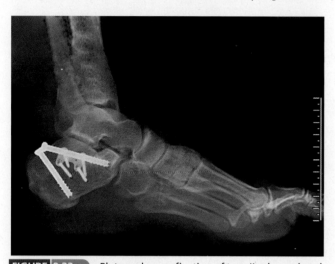

FIGURE 9.33 Plate and screw fixation of type II calcaneal avulsion fracture.

for exposure. Also in this study, the anterolateral approach to the talar neck did not appear to disrupt any major blood supply. The contribution of the blood supply to the talus was 16.9% for the peroneal artery, 36.2% for the anterior tibial artery, and 47.0% for the posterior tibial artery, with the anterior tibial artery being the main blood supply to the anteromedial quadrant of the talus and the posterior tibial artery being the main blood supply to the other three quadrants.

TALAR HEAD FRACTURES

Fractures of the head of the talus have been reported to constitute 5% to 10% of talar injuries. Two mechanisms of injury have been suggested in the literature: axially directed loading and compression of the talar head and a dorsal compression fracture of the anterior tibial plafond. A high index of suspicion should be maintained for posttraumatic tenderness in the anterior ankle region because recognition of this fracture can be difficult. Plain radiographs may define the fracture clearly, but CT often is necessary for definitive diagnosis and evaluation of displacement. The head of the talus with loss of support of the talonavicular joint may be associated with clinical instability of the triple joint complex. Injuries to the calcaneocuboid and subtalar joints are common with this injury.

■ TREATMENT

Displaced fractures of the head of the talus often are a shear type of injury or an impacted injury and should be treated with ORIF. Care should be taken not to strip any remaining vascular supply of the head. For impacted fractures, the articular fragment should be elevated, with bone grafting behind the fragment to minimize collapse. Internal fixation should be used if the fragments are large enough. Shear fractures, although usually medial, often can be adequately exposed through a dorsal incision. Anderson described a two-incision technique that we have used with success as well. Fixation can be placed directly or percutaneously from the medial side as needed (Fig. 9.39). Stable fixation of the talar head is accomplished with partially threaded cancellous lag screws, headless compression screws, or bioabsorbable pins. Care must be

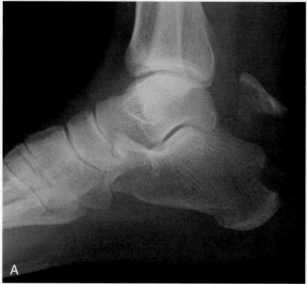
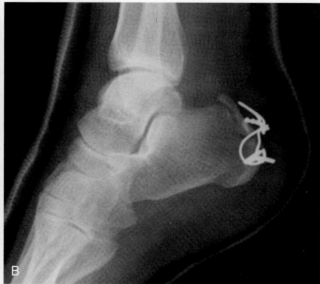

FIGURE 9.34 **A,** Proximally displaced avulsion fracture of calcaneus. **B,** Lateral tension band fixation. (From Nagura I, Fjuioka H, Kurosaka M, et al: Modified tension band wiring fixation for avulsion fractures of the calcaneus in osteoporotic bone: a review of three patients, *J Foot Ankle Surg* 51:330, 2012.)

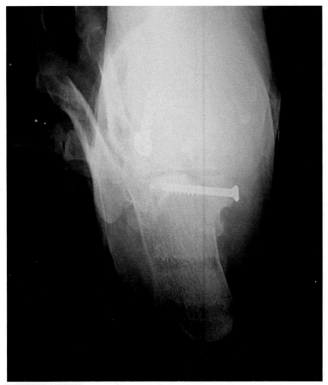

FIGURE 9.35 Internal fixation of sustentaculum fracture with single screw.

taken to be sure that the talonavicular joint is reduced; if the joint is unstable, it may be necessary to place a Kirschner wire across the joint to hold it reduced. Fracture-dislocation of the talar head with shortening of the medial column may require use of an intraoperative external fixator to gain length and reduce the fracture. The external fixator can remain in place or a spanning plate can be applied from the talus onto the cuneiforms to maintain length.

Early motion can be started at approximately 2 weeks after surgery if secure fixation has been obtained, with delay in weight bearing of a minimum of 6 weeks. If fixation is marginal, a short leg cast is used for 6 weeks with no weight bearing. The reported rate of osteonecrosis of this segment of the head is 10%, and if degenerative arthrosis occurs, talonavicular arthrodesis may be indicated. Arthrodesis of the talonavicular joint is reserved for severe fractures because it significantly reduces triple joint complex motion. If isolated talonavicular arthrodesis is necessary, shortening the medial column of the foot must be avoided. An inlay tricortical graft described by Adelaar can be used to avoid medial column shortening of the foot and placement of the hindfoot into varus.

TALAR NECK FRACTURES

Many controversies surround the treatment of talar neck fractures, which reflect the difficulty of assessment, surgical approaches, fixation methods, and frequency of postoperative complications. In 1919, Anderson, having observed 18 patients with talar injuries in the Royal Flying Corps, coined the term *aviator's astragalus*. In 1952, Coltart reviewed 25,000 fractures sustained during World War II. He found 228 talar fractures, 106 of which were classified as talar neck fractures. He reported osteonecrosis rates of 35% with subtalar dislocation and 95% with ankle and subtalar dislocation.

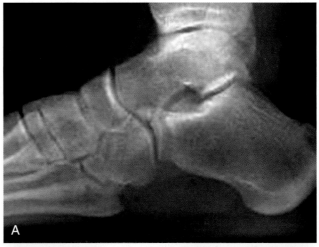

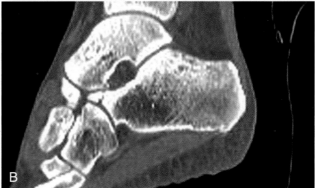

FIGURE 9.36 Fracture of anterior process of calcaneus. **A,** Lateral radiograph. **B,** CT scan.

Since Coltart's report, the incidence of osteonecrosis after talar neck injuries has been widely disputed. Although the actual percentage of osteonecrosis varies among investigators, increasing levels of displacement and dislocation progressively disrupt more vasculature and increase the incidence of this complication.

In 1970, Hawkins published a landmark paper on the results of 57 talar neck fractures in 55 patients. His classification of talar neck fractures, the most widely used today, is simple, provides guidelines for treatment, and is prognostic for development of osteonecrosis and the likelihood of successful outcome. In nondisplaced vertical fractures of the neck (group I fractures), osteonecrosis did not occur and all fractures united. All displaced fractures with subluxation or dislocation of the subtalar joint (group II fractures) united, although osteonecrosis subsequently developed in 42%. In fractures with dislocation of the subtalar and the ankle joints (group III fractures), nonunion occurred in 11% and osteonecrosis developed in 91%. An increasing percentage of fair and poor results (75%) was noted in group III fractures compared with group II fractures. The presence of osteonecrosis also correlated with fair or poor results (88%).

Canale and Kelly at this clinic clinically and radiographically reviewed 71 fractures of the neck of the talus in 70 patients with an average follow-up of 12.7 years. Using the Hawkins classification (Fig. 9.40), there were 15 type I fractures, 30 type II fractures, and 23 type III fractures. An additional type of fracture was described, in which not only the body of the talus was extruded from the ankle mortise but

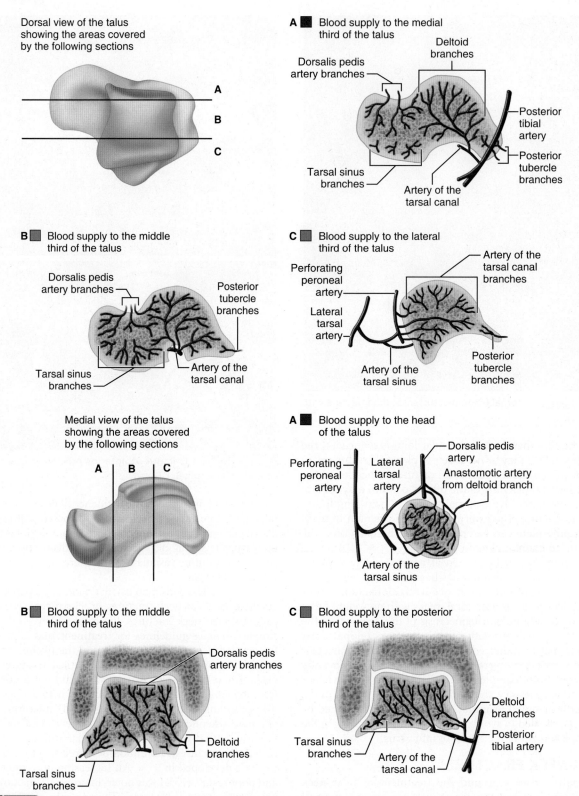

Dorsal view of the talus showing the areas covered by the following sections

A
B
C

A Blood supply to the medial third of the talus

Deltoid branches
Dorsalis pedis artery branches
Posterior tibial artery
Posterior tubercle branches
Tarsal sinus branches
Artery of the tarsal canal

B Blood supply to the middle third of the talus

Dorsalis pedis artery branches
Posterior tubercle branches
Tarsal sinus branches
Artery of the tarsal canal

C Blood supply to the lateral third of the talus

Perforating peroneal artery
Lateral tarsal artery
Artery of the tarsal canal branches
Artery of the tarsal sinus
Posterior tubercle branches

Medial view of the talus showing the areas covered by the following sections

A B C

A Blood supply to the head of the talus

Perforating peroneal artery
Lateral tarsal artery
Dorsalis pedis artery
Anastomotic artery from deltoid branch
Artery of the tarsal sinus

B Blood supply to the middle third of the talus

Dorsalis pedis artery branches
Deltoid branches
Tarsal sinus branches

C Blood supply to the posterior third of the talus

Deltoid branches
Posterior tibial artery
Tarsal sinus branches
Artery of the tarsal canal

FIGURE 9.37 Blood supply to talus in sagittal and coronal sections (see text). (Redrawn from Mulfinger GL, Trueta J: The blood supply of the talus, *J Bone Joint Surg* 52B:160, 1970.)

also the head of the talus was subluxed or dislocated from the navicular articulation. They called this a type IV fracture, and there were three. In two of 13 nondisplaced fractures, osteonecrosis developed, but both had excellent results. The one poor result in a type I fracture was caused by severe degenerative changes in the ankle joint secondary to an unrecognized fracture through the dome of the talus. It is important to tell patients, even patients with type I fractures, that subsequent arthritis and a poor result can occur after a nondisplaced fracture. Of the 30 type II fractures, osteonecrosis developed in

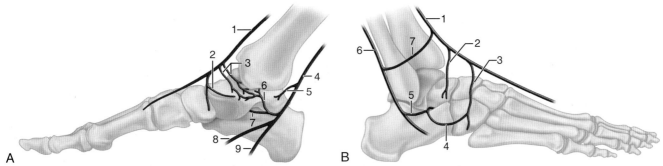

FIGURE 9.38 **A,** Schematic drawing of medial ankle and foot showing extraosseous arterial supply to talus: *1,* anterior tibial artery; *2,* medial recurrent tarsal artery; *3,* medial talar artery; *4,* posterior tibial artery; *5,* posterior tubercle artery; *6,* deltoid branches; *7,* artery of tarsal canal; *8,* medial plantar artery; *9,* lateral plantar artery. **B,** Schematic drawing of lateral ankle and foot with extraosseous arterial supply to talus: *1,* anterior tibial artery; *2,* lateral talar artery; *3,* lateral tarsal artery; *4,* posterior recurrent branch of lateral tarsal; *5,* artery of tarsal sinus; *6,* perforating peroneal; *7,* anterior lateral malleolar artery.

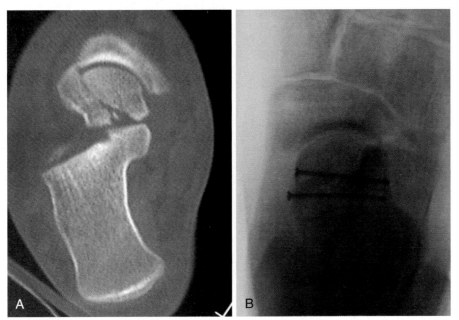

FIGURE 9.39 **A,** CT scan of talar head fracture with medial dislocation of navicular. **B,** Postoperative radiograph showing screw placement. (From Early JS: Talus fracture management, *Foot Ankle Clin North Am* 13:635, 2008.)

50% and 47% had an unsatisfactory result. Of 23 patients with type III fractures, 52% had an unsatisfactory result, with satisfactory results directly related to anatomic reduction of the fracture and the subtalar dislocation.

Vallier et al. further subdivided type II fractures into those with and without subtalar dislocation, type IIA and IIB, respectively. Their data showed that the incidence of osteonecrosis increased with fracture type; it never occurred in a type IIA but did in 25% of type IIB. They demonstrated that the amount of initial displacement correlated more to rates of osteonecrosis than did operative timing.

In early studies, prompt ORIF was advocated for good results. More recent studies suggest that, although prompt reduction is important to relieve tension on the soft tissues, definitive internal fixation can be delayed until soft-tissue swelling has subsided. In a military study in which internal fixation was delayed due to transport times out of theater, fixation was performed an average of 12.9 days after injury.

There was no correlation between the time to fixation and the development of osteonecrosis or posttraumatic arthritis. Other studies have confirmed these findings.

In clinical outcome studies, the rate of osteonecrosis ranged from 20% to 49%, with higher rates in patients with comminuted or open fractures and higher Hawkins classifications. Not all patients with osteonecrosis are symptomatic, especially if collapse does not occur. The rate of posttraumatic arthritis varied from 36% to 94% and again was more common in patients with comminuted and open fractures. Approximately 17% to 44% of patients require secondary surgery, usually for posttraumatic arthritis or malalignment.

■ TREATMENT

Any fracture that involves a joint is a difficult problem, and this is especially true of a weight-bearing joint. Much of the surface of the talus is covered by articular cartilage. For

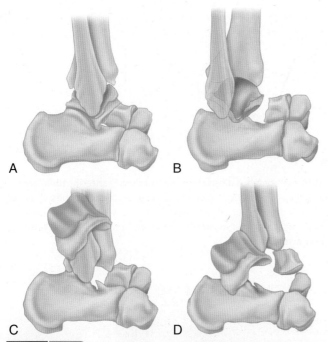

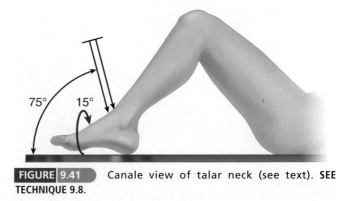

FIGURE 9.41   Canale view of talar neck (see text). **SEE TECHNIQUE 9.8.**

FIGURE 9.40   **A,** Type I talar neck fracture. **B,** Type II. **C,** Type III. **D,** Type IV. (From Canale ST, Kelly FB Jr: Fractures of the neck of the talus: long-term evaluation of 71 cases, *J Bone Joint Surg* 60A:143, 1978.)

this reason, almost any fracture of the talus involves a joint surface. More weight per unit of area is borne by the superior surface of the talus than by any other bone. In fractures of the talus, accurate reduction is essential to reestablish the position of its articular surfaces. Residual irregularity of the joint surfaces can produce arthritic changes with resumption of motion and weight bearing. Impacted fractures of the head, usually associated with compression fractures of the navicular, are difficult to correct surgically and should be considered for non-operative management. Due to the irregularity in the talonavicular joint, arthritis and pain can persist and arthrodesis eventually may be necessary for relief.

Care must be taken to search for local and remote associated fractures. A medial malleolar fracture commonly is associated with a displaced talar neck fracture. Lateral processes of the talar fractures frequently are associated with peroneal tendon dislocations. As with any axial loading injury, the lumbar spine should be evaluated thoroughly.

Radiographic evaluation of talar neck injuries should include anteroposterior, lateral, and oblique views of the ankle, a Canale view, and an anteroposterior view of the foot. Contralateral imaging preoperatively is useful to guide restoration of normal anatomic parameters. Intraoperatively, the view described by Canale, in which the foot is internally rotated 15 degrees and the x-ray beam angled 75 degrees from horizontal, is especially helpful because it profiles the talar neck (Fig. 9.41). This can help prevent malunion and varus.

Although the development of osteonecrosis of the talus may or may not ultimately affect the outcome, most authors agree that varus malunion even of a few degrees is almost uniformly associated with a poor outcome. Because the talar neck is commonly comminuted medially, care must be taken to restore the anatomic alignment of the neck.

TYPE I FRACTURES

Type I fractures, by definition, are nondisplaced. A talar neck fracture must be thoroughly evaluated before labeling it as a type I. Many fractures that appear nondisplaced on radiographs, if examined closely by CT scans, display subtle displacement. All talar fractures should be evaluated with a CT scan to guide treatment. If the subtalar joint is free of displacement and fragments, the fracture should be immobilized in a below-knee cast for 8 to 12 weeks, with weight bearing delayed until trabeculation across the fracture is seen. Close follow-up is imperative to assess for any interval displacement.

TYPES II, III, AND IV FRACTURES

Although there are reports of closed reduction and percutaneous pinning of these fractures, as a rule, displaced fractures of the neck of the talus should be treated with early ORIF because it is difficult to obtain an anatomic reduction by closed means. In the past, a posterolateral approach had been advocated and was supported by a biomechanical study showing that the greatest strength of fixation was achieved with screws placed from a posterior to anterior direction, as opposed to the usual method of fixation, which involved anterior to posterior screws, one medial and one lateral. The current literature, however, supports the use of dual anterior approaches. The anteromedial approach offers good fracture exposure and is easily extended for medial malleolar osteotomy. Often the medial neck is the location of the comminution of the fracture, however, and fracture alignment and reduction can be difficult to assess. Through the anterolateral approach the key to reduction of the neck often can be found, in addition to allowing screw fixation (Fig. 9.42) or the use of mini-fragment plates (Fig. 9.43).

Type III and type IV fractures constitute an orthopaedic emergency for two reasons. First, pressure from the dislocated body on the skin and neurovascular structures can lead to skin slough, neurovascular insult, or both. Second, in theory, the only remaining blood supply to the talus, the deltoid branch, may be rotated and occluded, correctable only through emergency reduction of the talar body. If a reduction of the dislocation can be obtained through closed means, surgical fixation may proceed electively when appropriate resources are available and soft tissues are suitable. An irreducible dislocation should be treated emergently along with operative repair of the fractures. A medial malleolar osteotomy may be needed for exposure of complex talar fractures, especially in types III and IV body fractures where reduction through standard incisions is more difficult (Fig. 9.44).

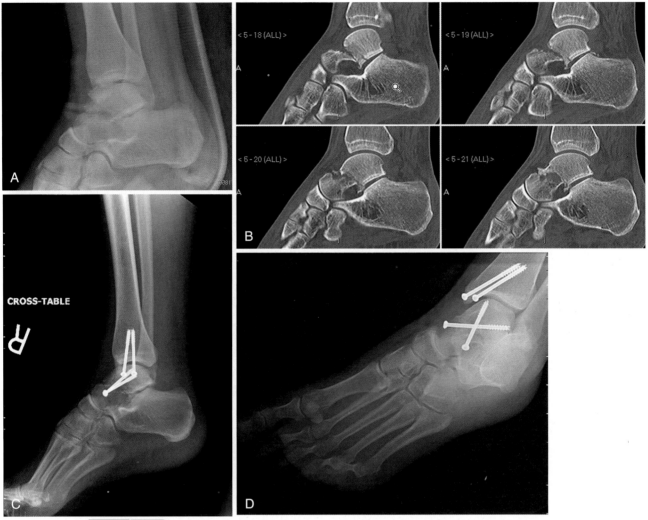

CROSS-TABLE

R

FIGURE 9.42   **A** and **B,** Talar neck fracture. **C** and **D,** Fixation with cannulated screws. **SEE TECHNIQUE 9.8.**

OPEN REDUCTION OF THE TALAR NECK

TECHNIQUE 9.8

- Expose the head and neck of the talus through an incision beginning proximal and just anterior to the medial malleolus, curving distalward and plantarward toward the sole of the foot, and ending on the medial side of the body of the navicular, using the interval between the anterior and posterior tibial tendons (Fig. 9.45A). Avoid incising the posterior tibial tendon and neurovascular structures inferior to the medial malleolus to prevent disruption of the remaining medial blood supply to the talus.
- If the body of the talus is extruded from the ankle mortise, osteotomy of the medial malleolus may make exposure and reduction easier.
- Expose the fracture and the anteromedial aspect of the neck and body of the talus. Preserve intact as much soft tissue as possible around the head and neck of the talus. For the anterolateral approach, expose the lateral neck

through a 5-cm incision over the sinus tarsi, extending toward the base of the fourth metatarsal (Fig. 9.45B). Protect the dorsal intermediate cutaneous nerve in this region.
- After incising the inferior extensor retinaculum, reflect the extensor digitorum brevis plantarly to expose the fracture.
- Two small threaded Kirschner wires can be inserted into the talar head fragment medially and laterally to act as joysticks to assist with fracture reduction. After inserting the wires, distract the fracture and remove any bone debris with irrigation.
- Try to locate interdigitating fracture lines medially or laterally for a guide to reduction, even if a gap remains in the opposite cortex. Although each fracture is different, medial comminution is more common, whereas the key to reduction often will be found laterally. When the reduction is obtained, hold it temporarily with longitudinal Kirschner wires placed along the axis of the talus. Comparing the intraoperative Canale view to the preoperatively obtained contralateral image is useful to prevent varus alignment (see Fig. 9.41).
- Depending on the available space for fixation, a 4.0-mm, 4.5-mm, or 6.5-mm partial or fully threaded cannulated screw can be used (see Fig. 9.42). In each case, care must be taken to countersink the screw head to provide a flat

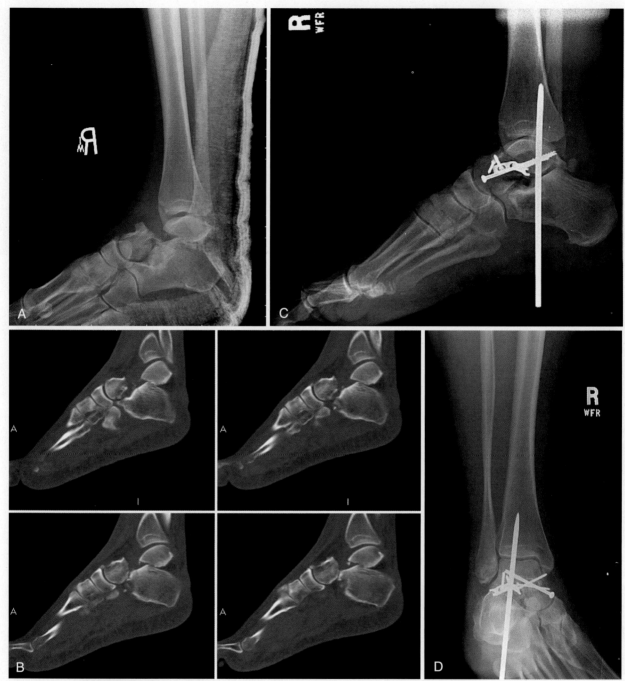

FIGURE | **9.43**   **A** and **B,** Talar neck fracture. **C** and **D,** Fixation with mini-fragment plate and screws. **SEE TECHNIQUE 9.8.**

area for seating of the screw head. If spanning an area of comminution, fully threaded screws should be used to avoid collapse, especially medially. Alternatively, minifragment plates and screws can be placed laterally, especially if there is excessive comminution or limited space for fixation in the head fragment (see Fig. 9.43). We generally prefer a medial position screw along with a lateral mini-fragment plate to maintain length and prevent varus collapse.

- For placement of posterior-to-anterior screws, use the Henry approach from the lateral side of the Achilles tendon and develop the interval between the flexor hallucis longus and the peroneal tendons (Fig. 9.45).

- Place the guidewire above the lateral projection of the posterior process and direct it toward the lateral talar head. Fluoroscopic guidance is essential to avoid the subtalar joint.

- If the cortex is fragile, as in an elderly patient, or if the fracture is more distal, firm fixation may not be secured by placing a screw obliquely. In such patients, drill two Steinmann pins, 3/32-inch or larger, passing proximally from the navicular into the head of the talus, through the fracture site, and deep into the body of the talus. This usually affords good fixation. Transfixing the talonavicular joint in the fracture in this manner is preferable to

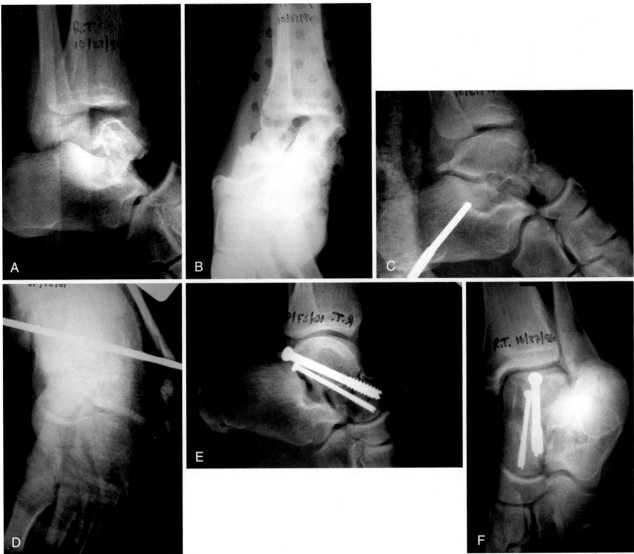

FIGURE 9.44 Type IV talar fracture. **A** and **B,** Injury radiographs showing dislocation of talar body and talar head from talonavicular joint. **C** and **D,** After closed reduction and percutaneous Hoffman pin through tuberosity of calcaneus for leverage. **E** and **F,** Lateral and Canale anteroposterior views after open reduction and internal fixation.

attempting to countersink screws below the surface of the articular cartilage of the head of the talus.

- If the medial malleolus was osteotomized to improve exposure, reduce it and fix it with two malleolar screws.

POSTOPERATIVE CARE The foot is held in a neutral position in a cast, and the ankle is immobilized in a cast from below the knee to the toes, well molded into the arch of the foot. After 6 to 8 weeks, depending on radiographic signs of early union, a walking boot is applied and weight bearing is permitted; however, some patients may have to wait 12 weeks before weight bearing can start.

■ MALUNION OF THE TALAR NECK

Malunion or nonunion of the talar neck is a disabling complication. Zwipp and Rammelt developed a classification system for

these complications and proposed treatment for each type of talar malunion (Table 9.1). To avoid arthrodesis, corrective osteotomy and/or revision of the malunion/nonunion can be done for types I, II, and III if the articular cartilage remains in good condition. This often involves recreating the original fracture, bone grafting to fill the space after realignment of the malunion or debridement of the nonunion, and stable internal fixation. Medial malleolar osteotomy may be needed to obtain adequate exposure and to avoid damage to the medial blood supply to the talus. Studies have shown that good results can be obtained with 90% to 100% patient satisfaction rates and no osteonecrosis, although patients may require further surgery including arthrodesis.

■ OSTEONECROSIS OF THE TALAR BODY AFTER TALAR NECK FRACTURE

In the treatment of fractures and fracture-dislocations of the neck of the talus, satisfactory primary treatment must be emphasized, but early recognition and management of

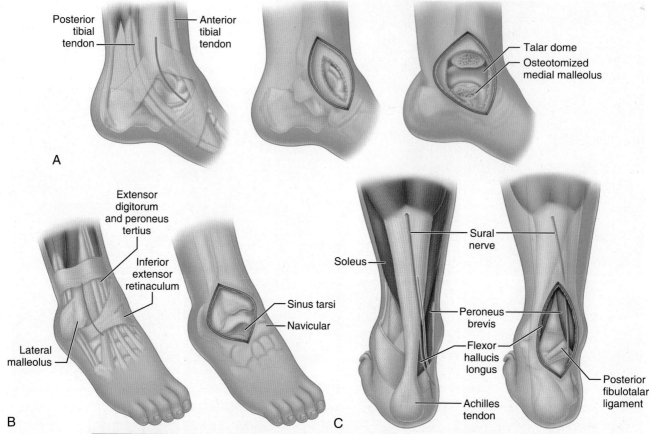

FIGURE 9.45 **A,** Anteromedial approach to ankle. Exposure can be extended from limited capsulotomy in interval between anterior and posterior tibial tendons to wide exposure with malleolar osteotomy. **B,** Anterolateral approach to talus. **C,** Posterolateral approach to talus. (From Mayo KA: Fractures of the talus: Principles of management and techniques of treatment, *Tech Orthop* 2:42, 1987.) **SEE TECHNIQUE 9.8.**

TABLE 9.1

Classification and Treatment Algorithm for Talar Malunions

		TREATMENT OPTIONS	
TYPE	FEATURES	ACTIVE, RELIABLE PATIENTS WITH NO SYMPTOMATIC ARTHRITIS	NONCOMPLIANT PATIENT WITH COMORBIDITIES, ARTHRITIS
I	Malunion with joint displacement	Osteotomy, secondary reconstruction, and internal fixation with joint preservation	Corrective fusion of the affected joint(s)
II	Nonunion with displacement		
III	Type I or II with partial osteonecrosis		
IV	Type I or II with complete osteonecrosis	Neurectomy, (vascularized) bone graft, corrective fusion	
V	Type I or II with septic osteonecrosis	Radial debridement(s), bone grafting, corrective fusion	

Modified from Zwipp H, Rammelt S: Secondary reconstruction for malunions and nonunions of the talar body, *Foot Ankle Clin* 21:95, 2016.

osteonecrosis that may follow also must be considered. It can reasonably be predicted that with fractures of the neck of the talus, a small percentage of nondisplaced fractures and a large percentage of fractures with complete dislocation of the body will be complicated by osteonecrosis. Between 6 and 8 weeks after injury, a thin line of subchondral atrophy along the dome of the talus (Hawkins sign) seen on an anteroposterior radiograph indicates the presence of vascularity and excludes the diagnosis of osteonecrosis (Fig. 9.46). If the Hawkins sign is not present, however, osteonecrosis may or may not occur;

the sign is sensitive but not specific. With osteonecrosis, the bone becomes dense and sclerotic as seen on radiographs, but this may not be evident for several months (Fig. 9.47). MRI can be used to further evaluate for osteonecrosis but should not be obtained for 2 or 3 months postoperatively to allow postoperative edema to resolve.

Bone grafts across the fracture site in the neck of the talus, primary or early subtalar fusion, and ankle fusion generally have been unsuccessful in speeding the revascularization of the body of the talus. Prolonged non–weight bearing in hopes

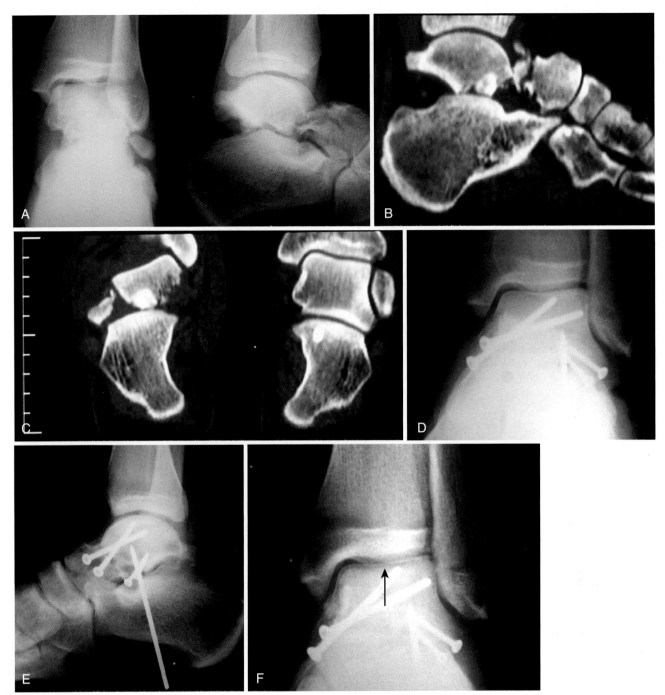

FIGURE 9.46 **A,** Displaced type II talar fracture. **B** and **C,** CT scans show comminution of medial aspect of talar neck and additional fracture of lateral process. **D** and **E,** After open reduction through anteromedial and lateral Ollier approaches, fixation of talar neck with non-lag fragment screw and lateral process with mini-fragment screws. **F,** Positive Hawkins sign at 6 weeks. (From Rammelt S, Zwipp H: Talar neck and body fractures, *Injury* 40:120, 2009.)

of preventing collapse of the dome of the talus has not been sufficiently predictable. In many cases, the talus collapses even though weight bearing is not permitted. In one study, talar revascularization occurred in 44% of those with osteonecrosis, and in another, 59% of patients with osteonecrosis were asymptomatic. When pain develops after osteonecrosis, excision alone of the necrotic body of the talus has not proved useful. Core decompression has shown mixed results. Nunley reported good outcomes with vascularized pedicle

grafts harvested from the cuboid using the proximal lateral tarsal artery as a pedicle. Arthrodesis is most often used to treat this condition, either ankle or subtalar joint, depending on which joint is more involved. Occasionally, tibiotalocalcaneal fusion or tibiocalcaneal fusion after excision of the talus is necessary. The Blair type of ankle fusion with a sliding graft from the anterior aspect of the tibia into the viable neck of the talus with excision of the necrotic body can also be useful (Fig. 9.48).

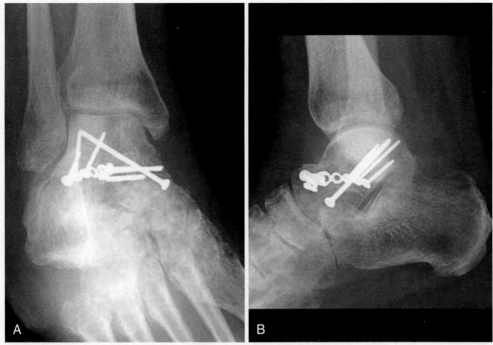

FIGURE 9.47   Anteroposterior **(A)** and lateral **(B)** radiographs of displaced talar neck fracture show bony sclerosis of lateral aspect of talar body, indicative of osteonecrosis, 3 months after injury. (From DiGiovanni CW, Patel A, Calfee R, Nickisch F: Osteonecrosis in the foot, *J Am Acad Orthop Surg* 15:208, 2007.)

In addition to the usual approaches for arthrodesis, we have obtained arthrodesis of this region using an onlay graft technique through a posterior approach as described by Johnson. This procedure allows the placement of much more bone graft than arthrodesis done through other approaches and gives a satisfactory arthrodesis rate, maintaining the length of the limb and the contours of the malleoli (Fig. 9.49).

ONLAY GRAFT TECHNIQUE THROUGH A POSTERIOR APPROACH

TECHNIQUE 9.9

(JOHNSON)
- Using tourniquet control with the patient in the prone position, make a midline incision protecting the sural nerve.
- Enter the Achilles tendon sheath and carefully protect it. Divide the Achilles tendon in the coronal plane to allow better exposure of the posterior ankle and subtalar joints.
- After the deep compartment is entered, develop the interval between the flexor hallucis longus medially and the peroneus longus and brevis laterally.
- Elevate the periosteum from the posterior aspect of the tibia and the dorsal aspect of the tuberosity of the calcaneus. A femoral distractor should be used to assist in the distraction of the ankle and subtalar joints.

- Debride the cartilage from the surfaces of the ankle and subtalar joint with a curet and rongeur.
- Use a 1/2-inch osteotome to create a trough, incorporating the posterior aspect of the tibia, the posterior half of the talar body, the superior portion of the calcaneal tuberosity, and the posterior facet of the calcaneus. This creates one long trough for the onlay graft.
- Harvest cancellous and cortical strips of bone from the posterior superior iliac crest.
- At this point, use the technique for the introduction of an intramedullary arthrodesis nail.
- After stabilization of the arthrodesis in a neutral position with the intramedullary nail, apply the bone graft through the entire posterior aspect of the tibia, talus, and calcaneus.
- Place a drain in the deep wound if desired and repair the Achilles tendon with multiple interrupted 0 braided, absorbable sutures.

POSTOPERATIVE CARE A splint is applied. At 2 to 3 weeks sutures are removed if the wound has healed, and the extremity is placed in a short leg, non–weight-bearing cast. Weight bearing is delayed until there is evidence of union at 10 to 12 weeks. A prefabricated walking boot is applied, and the patient is gradually able to bear weight and transfer to a shoe that has been modified with a full-length steel shank and rocker sole.

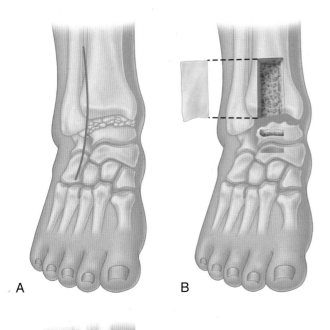

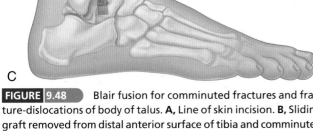

FIGURE 9.48 Blair fusion for comminuted fractures and fracture-dislocations of body of talus. **A,** Line of skin incision. **B,** Sliding graft removed from distal anterior surface of tibia and comminuted fragments excised. **C,** Graft embedded in slot in neck of talus. (From Blair HC: Comminuted fracture and fracture-dislocations of the body of the astragalus: operative treatment, *Am J Surg* 59:37, 1943.)
SEE TECHNIQUE 9.11.

TALAR BODY FRACTURES

It is important to distinguish talar body fractures from talar neck fractures. Although the incidence of osteonecrosis is similar between talar neck and talar body fractures without displacement or displacement without dislocation, a higher incidence of posttraumatic subtalar osteoarthrosis has been noted after talar body fractures. Nondisplaced talar body fractures have a reported incidence of osteonecrosis of 25%; however, with displacement, the rate of osteonecrosis is 50%. Injuries are considered to be talar body fractures if the inferior fracture line is proximal to the lateral process of the talus and as talar neck fractures if the inferior fracture line is distal to the lateral process of the talus.

Sneppen et al. classified talar body fractures into five major types based on anatomic location: type I, osteochondral or transchondral; type II, coronal-sagittal, horizontal, noncomminuted, shear; type III, posterior tubercle; type IV, lateral process; and type V, crush. The noncomminuted, shear fractures may be in the coronal, sagittal, or transverse plane. More recent classification systems include the AO classification (Fig. 9.50) in which fractures are grouped according to increasing severity, with increasing treatment difficulty and worse prognosis. Diagnosis should be made with a plain radiograph, although CT may be indicated for complete evaluation of the fracture pattern and displacement. Displaced fractures should be treated with ORIF. Frequently, these injuries require medial malleolar osteotomy for exposure to obtain an adequate reduction. Use of bioabsorbable pins or headless compression screws may be helpful in fixation. A review of the surgical treatment of talar body fractures confirmed the morbidity of these injuries. An 88% incidence of osteonecrosis or posttraumatic arthritis was noted on radiographs, and worse results occurred with comminuted and open fractures. This study found that all patients who had open fractures and osteonecrosis experienced collapse of the talar body. Another study found only 53% good or excellent results, with worse outcomes in crush injuries, open fractures, and those associated with a talar neck fracture.

The approach to surgical correction of these fractures depends on the fracture pattern. A medial malleolar osteotomy may be needed to expose the fracture (Fig. 9.51). Because the surfaces for fixation in the talar body almost always contain articular cartilage, fixation usually consists of countersunk screws, headless compression screws, or bioabsorbable pins making sure that the implants are not prominent within the joint (Fig. 9.52).

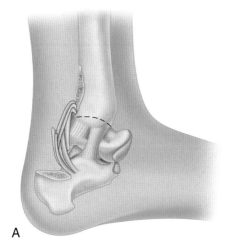

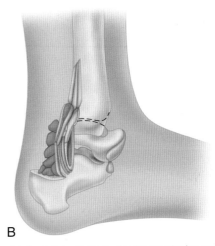

FIGURE 9.49 **A,** Posterior extraarticular arthrodesis of ankle and subtalar joints. **B,** Posterior intraarticular arthrodesis of ankle and subtalar joints.

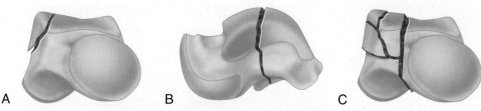

FIGURE 9.50   AO classification of talar body fractures indicates progressive severity, more difficult treatment, and worse prognosis.

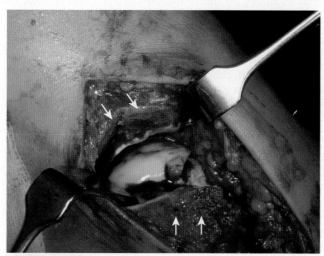

FIGURE 9.51   Chevron osteotomy of medial malleolus provides exposure of talar body fracture. Note predrilled holes *(arrows)* for fixation with small-fragment screws. (From Rammelt S, Zwipp H: Talar neck and body fractures, *Injury* 40:120, 2009.)

Comminuted fractures of the body of the talus with gross displacement are difficult to treat. The long-term result is almost always uniformly bad. Accurate replacement of the fragments often is impossible. In adults, the results of talectomy usually are poor because of pain on weight bearing, instability, and lack of endurance. The results of tibiocalcaneal arthrodesis combined with talectomy are superior to the results of talectomy alone because the foot is stable and enough compensatory movement usually develops in the midtarsal joints to enable the patient to walk with a fairly elastic gait and limp (Fig. 9.53). Timing of surgery is dictated by the condition of the soft tissues and the availability of appropriate resources. Multiple studies have shown that, provided there are no joint dislocations or threatened soft tissues, timing to surgery does not correlate to long-term outcomes.

TIBIOCALCANEAL ARTHRODESIS

TECHNIQUE 9.10

- Expose the operative field through an anterolateral incision.
- Remove the fragments of the body of the talus.
- In comminuted fractures of the talus several months old, or when the junction of the body and neck is intact, divide the

talus with an osteotome into as many pieces as necessary for easy removal. Drive an osteotome through the proximal part of the navicular to remove the proximal articular cartilage and subchondral bone together with the head and neck of the talus.

- Excise the articular surfaces of the tibia and calcaneus. Roughen the medial surface of the lateral malleolus.
- Strip the soft-tissue attachments around both malleoli enough to allow posterior displacement of the foot until the navicular comes in contact with the tibia. It may be necessary to resect a part of both malleoli because the soft tissues collapse like an accordion and resist efforts to appose the calcaneus properly to the tibia.
- Denude the tibia at the point of contact with the navicular.
- If infection is not a concern, a femoral head allograft can be placed into the defect after appropriate contouring of the graft and tibia and calcaneus for proper fit.
- While the foot is held at a right angle to the leg or in 5 degrees of dorsiflexion, insert two Steinmann pins transversely through the calcaneus and tibia, as described for arthrodesis of the ankle, and apply arthrodesis plates, an intramedullary nail, or an external fixation device to maintain firm contact between the two bones. Fix the navicular to the tibia with a screw if desired.
- Denude bone chips obtained during the operation and pack them around the junction of the calcaneus, the navicular, and the tibia.

POSTOPERATIVE CARE The patient is kept non–weight bearing for 6 to 8 weeks and then may bear weight in a cast for another 6 to 8 weeks. The limb is protected for the next several months by a short leg double-upright brace with a locked ankle.

Because of the decrease in height and the rigidity of the ankle joint after calcaneotibial fusion, Blair suggested an alternative procedure: the comminuted fragments of the body of the talus are removed, and a sliding graft from the anterior surface of the tibia is inserted into the remnant of the head and neck of the talus in an attempt to obtain fusion across this area (Fig. 9.54). Blair reported these advantages: the position of the foot is unchanged, backward displacement is unnecessary, the extremity is not shortened, the relationships of the foot and ankle remain near normal, and the weight-bearing thrust is placed on more or less normal, undisturbed joint tissue. After this operation, there is still slight flexion and extension of the foot on the leg, the two subtalar facets, and the talonavicular joint, allowing a rocking motion.

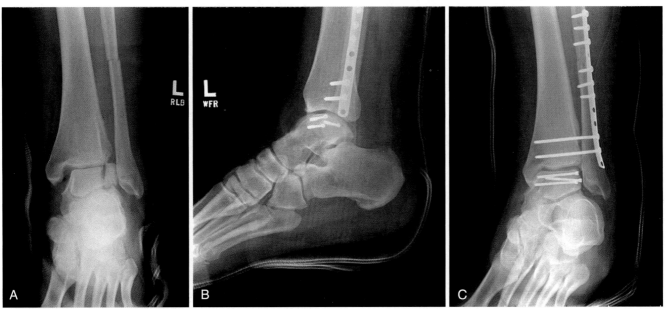

FIGURE 9.52   **A,** Talar body fracture with associated fibular fracture. **B** and **C,** Fixation of talar body with headless compression screws and of fibula with plate and screws.

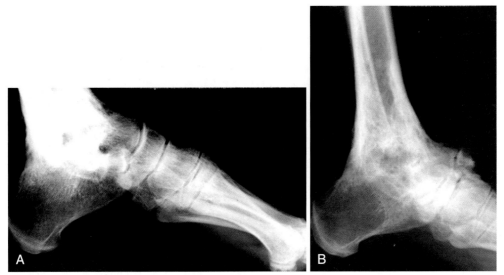

FIGURE 9.53   **A,** Four years after tibiocalcaneal fusion by compression arthrodesis and autogenous iliac bone grafting. **B,** Sixteen years after fusion, degenerative changes at midtarsal joints are present but patient is active with mild symptoms.

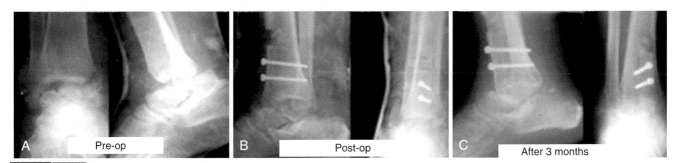

FIGURE 9.54   Results of Blair fusion. **A,** Type III fracture-dislocation of talus. **B,** Immediately after Blair fusion. **C,** Fusion at 3 months. (From Shrivastava MP, Shah RK, Singh RP: Treatment of fracture dislocation of talus by primary tibiotalar arthrodesis [Blair fusion], *Injury* 36:823, 2005.)

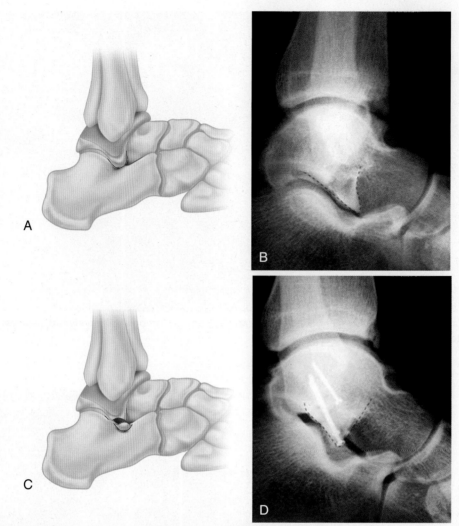

TIBIOTALAR ARTHRODESIS

TECHNIQUE 9.11

(BLAIR)

- Expose the ankle through an anterolateral incision. Remove the fragments of the fractured body of the talus but leave the head and neck fragments undisturbed (see Fig. 9.48). Remove a sliding graft 2.5 cm wide × 5.0 cm long from the anterior aspect of the distal tibia and remove the cartilaginous tip from its end. Introduce the graft into a previously prepared hole about 1.8 cm deep in the neck of the talus.
- With the foot plantarflexed 10 degrees, fix the proximal end of the graft to the tibia with a screw.
- Pack cancellous chips around the distal end of the graft.

POSTOPERATIVE CARE A cast is applied from the groin to the toes with the knee in extension and is worn for 4 to 6 weeks. A short leg cast is applied, and protected walking is allowed depending on the appearance of healing on radiographs. Cast immobilization usually is required for 12 to 16 weeks.

FRACTURES OF THE LATERAL OR POSTERIOR PROCESS OF THE TALUS

Fractures of the talus may involve the lateral or posterior process of the body. Lateral process fractures probably are more common.

■ LATERAL PROCESS FRACTURES

Lateral process fractures have been specifically associated with ankle injuries incurred while snowboarding and often are initially missed in up to 50% of patients. Von Knoch et al. described the V sign as a radiographic indication of lateral process fracture: if the normal V contour of the process is disrupted, the sign is positive (Fig. 9.55). The mechanism of injury is axial loading, dorsiflexion, external rotation, and eversion. A lateral subtalar dislocation may shear off the lateral process of the talus (Fig. 9.56). The lateral

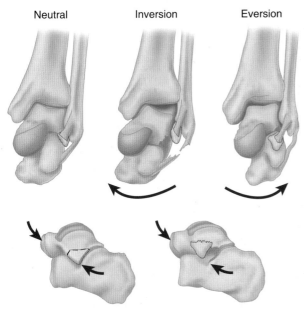

Neutral   Inversion   Eversion

Possible mechanisms of injury in fractures of posterior facet of talus. Probable mechanism is compression. Fragment is sheared off posterior facet by corresponding area of calcaneus as foot is forced into dorsiflexion and slight external rotation. (Redrawn from Dimon JH: Isolated displaced fracture of the posterior facet of the talus, *J Bone Joint Surg* 43A:275, 1961.)

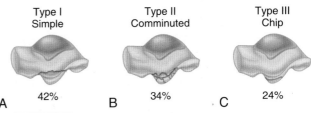

Type I
Simple
42%

Type II
Comminuted
34%

Type III
Chip
24%

A   B   C

FIGURE 9.57 Hawkins classification of fractures of lateral process of talus (see text).

- Protect the communicating branch of the sural nerve and dorsal intermediate cutaneous branch, which sometimes crosses the space.
- Retract the peroneus brevis tendon plantarly and reflect a portion of the extensor brevis origin dorsally, providing exposure to the lateral subtalar joint.
- Reduce the fracture and fix it with standard AO screws, countersinking the heads. Alternatively, use full countersinking screws (Herbert [Acumed, Hillboro, OR], Acutrak [Zimmer, Warsaw, IN]) (Fig. 9.58).
- Apply a bulky compression dressing and a short leg nonwalking cast.

POSTOPERATIVE CARE The compression dressing and short leg nonwalking cast are worn for 3 weeks, and then a walking cast is applied and worn for 3 additional weeks.

process is the site of attachment of three ligaments: the lateral talofibular ligament, the anterior talofibular ligament, and the posterior talofibular ligament. Removing an ununited lateral process fragment can disrupt these attachments but does not cause any ankle or subtalar instability. In the classification of these fractures by Hawkins (Fig. 9.57), type I is a large fragment that involves the talofibular articulation and the subtalar joint, type II is a comminuted fracture that involves these two articulations, and type III is a nonarticular avulsion type of fracture.

Type I lateral process fractures can be treated in a non–weight-bearing cast for 6 weeks, unless they are displaced or involve a significant portion of the talar side of the posterior facet, in which case they should be treated by ORIF. In a review of 109 lateral process fractures, 88% of operatively treated patients had mild or no symptoms, whereas 38% of nonoperatively treated patients had moderate or severe symptoms. Type II fractures may benefit from debridement if the fragments are displaced, which is most often the case. Type III fractures usually are treated nonoperatively. In all types, if a symptomatic nonunion occurs, debridement of the fracture can be done. Using this approach, good outcomes can be obtained, with most patients going back to sporting activities.

OPEN REDUCTION AND INTERNAL FIXATION OF FRACTURES OF THE LATERAL PROCESS OF THE TALUS

TECHNIQUE 9.12

- Approach the lateral process of the talus through a sinus tarsi incision, beginning at the tip of the fibula and extending toward the fourth metatarsal base.

■ POSTERIOR PROCESS FRACTURES

The posterior process of the talus has two tubercles, lateral and medial, with the flexor hallucis longus running between the two. There may be an os trigonum posterior to the lateral tubercle. Posterior process fractures often are difficult to diagnose. Significant attention has been given to posteromedial process fractures, which can result in significant long-term disability if not recognized. These fractures often are associated with subtalar dislocations but can occur with lesser injuries. If a patient has sustained an ankle injury and has not improved after 6 to 8 weeks of conventional treatment, the posterior or lateral talar process may be fractured. CT and bone scans may identify posterior process fractures. A lateral radiograph of the opposite foot for comparison also is helpful. A trial of nonoperative treatment is indicated, but persistence of symptoms and localized tenderness at the posterior process of the talus are indications for excision of the fragment (Fig. 9.59).

In a report on avulsion fractures of the medial tubercle of the posterior process of the talus, patients did well with immobilization and limited weight bearing when the fracture was diagnosed acutely. Fractures that were missed initially did poorly, but when the fractures were discovered, they did well with operative excision.

Posteromedial talar facet fracture also can be associated with a medial subtalar dislocation and often is missed on initial postreduction evaluation. It can be confused with an os trigonum, demonstrating the fact that patients with medial subtalar dislocations should have additional diagnostic imaging studies, such as coronal CT scan. Prognosis is poor if the fracture is through the medial side of the talar body. A fracture through an incomplete medial facet tarsal coalition, easily seen on CT, can be confused with a medial wall fracture of the body of the talus; however, treatment recommendations

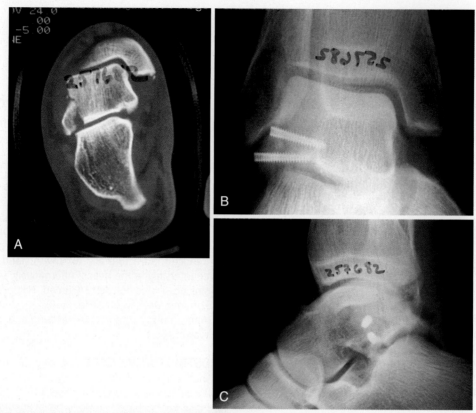

FIGURE 9.58   Displaced lateral process fracture of talus. **A,** Preoperative coronal CT scan showing displacement of lateral process. **B** and **C,** Anteroposterior and lateral views show reduction and stabilization with fully countersinking screws. **SEE TECHNIQUE 9.12.**

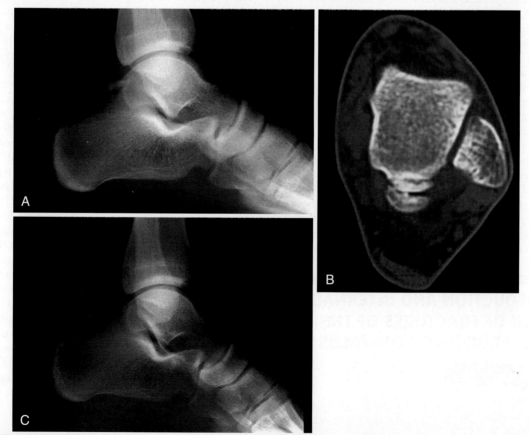

FIGURE 9.59   Posterior process fracture of talus. **A,** Preoperative radiograph. **B,** CT scan showing large posterior process and additional fracture. **C,** Postoperative lateral radiograph after excision. Patient became asymptomatic.

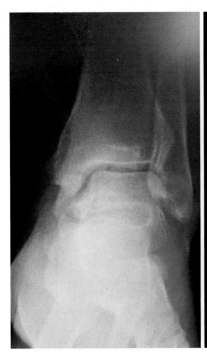 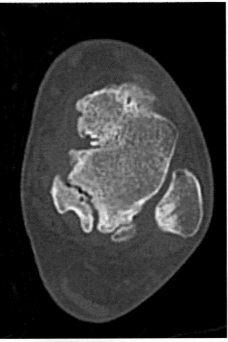 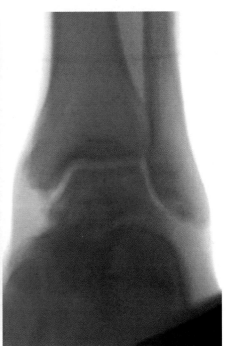

FIGURE 9.60 Posteromedial talus.

are the same. Fractures of the entire posterior process of the talus are rare and may need ORIF because the fragment may involve a large portion of the articular surface. In general, posterior process fractures, if small and/or minimally displaced, can be treated nonoperatively. If the fragment is large enough to involve a significant portion of the articular surface and/or is displaced, surgical fixation through a posterolateral or posteromedial approach (as described by Hsu and Scolaro) can lead to good outcomes. Late excision of symptomatic fractures can be helpful (Fig. 9.60).

TALAR BODY EXTRUSION

Extrusion of the talar body or entire talus typically occurs with high-energy trauma and usually is associated with severely displaced open fractures, severe soft-tissue injury, contamination, and disruption of the talar blood supply (Fig. 9.61A and B). Consensus on the treatment of a completely extruded talar body is lacking. Because the results of talar body excision with or without tibiocalcaneal fusion are most often poor, we believe that maintenance of the limb length and height of the ankle is important enough to warrant replacement of the body. The body should not be replaced in two situations: severe contamination or severe comminution and crushing of the talar body. Open reduction is almost always required, and a fixator or transfixion pins should be used to hold the reduction for 6 to 12 weeks (see Fig. 9.61C and D). In one small series, there was an 83% rate of partial or total osteonecrosis, with two good and four poor results. Although infection rates have been reported to be as high as 50% in some studies, other reports suggest much lower infection rates of 0% to 10%. Total or partial osteonecrosis varies from 11% to 83%. Rates are higher when the extruded talus is fractured: 22% to 37% of patients require subsequent surgery, some requiring multiple procedures. Patients may have persistent disability after this injury, although reasonable results can be obtained.

If the patient presents without a talus, we have had success with initial treatment that consists of irrigation and debridement, placement of antibiotic beads or a spacer, external fixation, and intravenous antibiotics. If the patient remains free of infection, the external fixator can be removed at 2 weeks, with cultures taken of the pin sites and the ankle joint, and the extremity is placed in a splint or cast. If the cultures are negative, a tibiocalcaneal arthrodesis with femoral head allograft can be done (see Fig. 9.61E and F). If the patient does develop an infection, a tibiocalcaneal arthrodesis can be done with external fixation that provides compression on both sides of the fusion, after long-term intravenous antibiotics have been administered. Recent literature suggests that 3D printed anatomic talar replacements may have promise for these difficult clinical scenarios.

SUBTALAR DISLOCATIONS

In dislocation of the subtalar joint, the calcaneus, cuboid, navicular, and all of the forefoot become displaced from the talus. Most often, the foot is dislocated medial to the talus, although lateral, anterior, and posterior dislocations occur (Fig. 9.62).

Medial subtalar dislocations, without marginal fractures of the calcaneus or talus, almost always are reducible by closed means, unless the extensor retinaculum or extensor digitorum brevis becomes interposed and blocks reduction. Open reduction often requires a lateral approach. Lateral subtalar dislocations frequently are irreducible by closed manipulation, and the most common offending structures blocking reduction are the posterior tibial tendon and osteochondral fracture of the talus (Fig. 9.63), which can usually be approached medially. The following treatment algorithm has been outlined: closed dislocations that are reducible should be treated with a non–weight-bearing cast for 6 weeks; open dislocations, dislocations that require operative reduction,

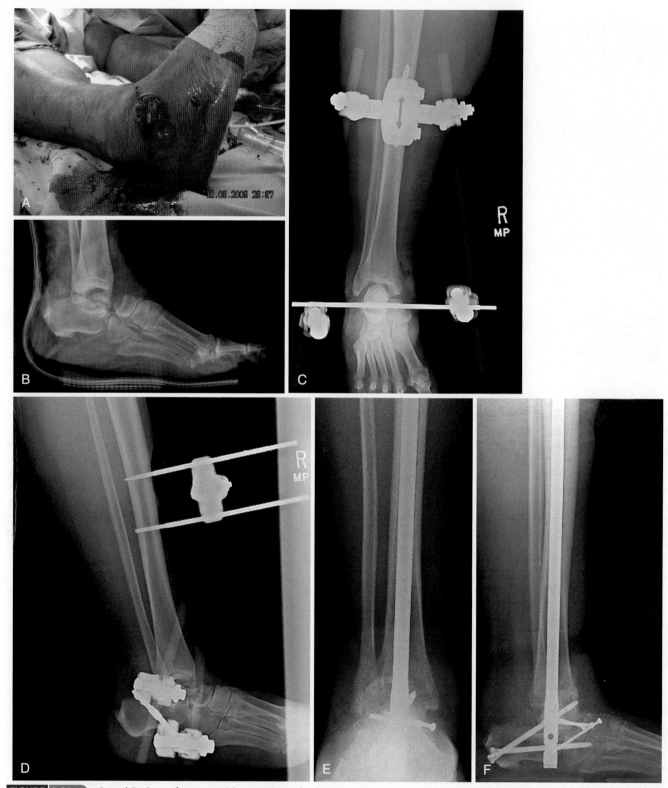

FIGURE 9.61 **A** and **B,** Open fracture with extrusion of talus. **C** and **D,** Fixator applied to hold reduction. **E** and **F,** Tibiocalcaneal arthrodesis with intramedullary nail and femoral head allograft.

and dislocations with severe soft-tissue swelling may require an external fixator or pinning for instability for 6 weeks. For both groups, full weight bearing and rehabilitation should start at 6 weeks, although one study suggests that mobilization at 2 weeks for uncomplicated medial dislocation can lead to successful recovery.

The importance of obtaining a CT scan after reduction of the subtalar dislocation has been emphasized, because patients who have a subtalar dislocation often have additional abnormalities identified on CT scans that are initially missed on plain radiographs. We routinely use CT for further evaluation of these injuries and often find fractures that require

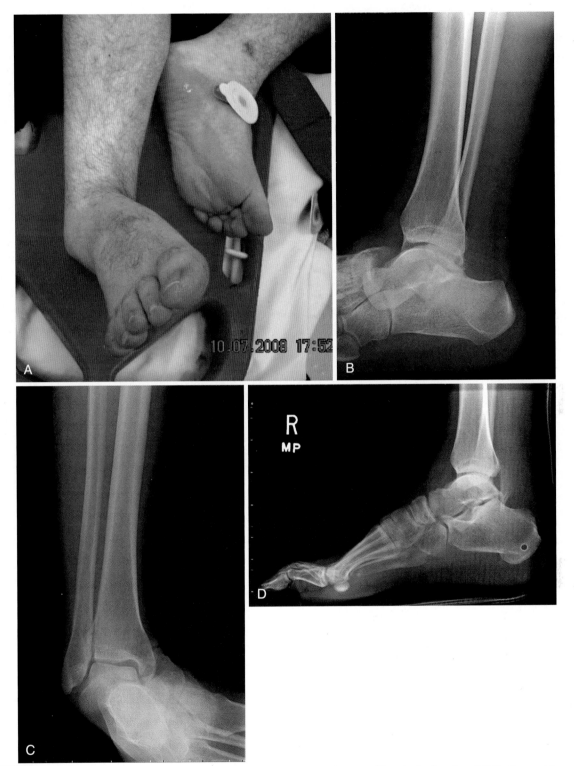

FIGURE 9.62 Medial subtalar dislocation. **A,** Posture of foot. Note prominence of head of talus. **B** and **C,** Radiographic appearance of dislocation. **D,** After reduction of dislocation, no fracture is apparent on lateral radiograph.

treatment because of intraarticular displacement or fragments blocking congruent reduction of the subtalar joint (see Fig. 9.62). If a congruent reduction is obtained and verified on CT, and there are no intraarticular fragments or displaced bone fragments requiring repair, we routinely treat subtalar dislocations nonoperatively.

Lateral dislocations tend to have a poorer prognosis than medial dislocations because there usually is more soft-tissue damage and associated fractures, although in some reports, outcomes are similar for medial and lateral injuries. For both injuries, there is a high incidence of arthritis and associated stiffness of the subtalar joint. Patients with open fractures

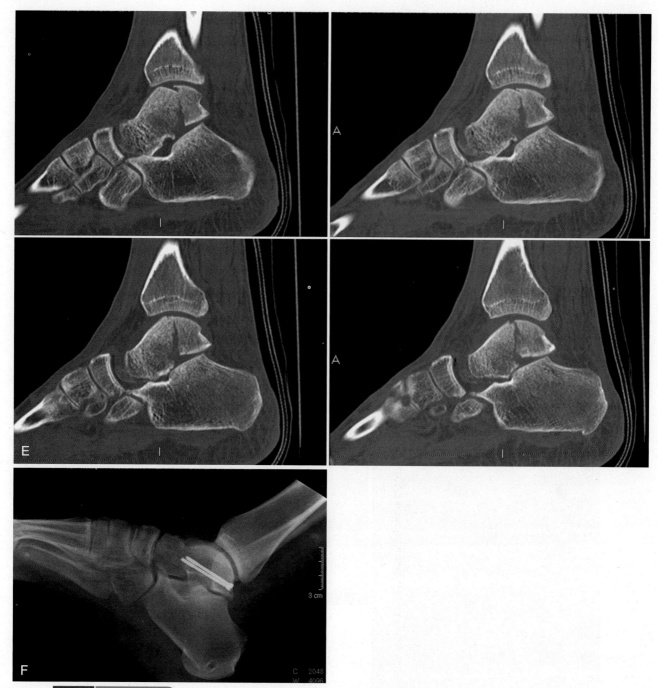

FIGURE 9.62, Cont'd   **E,** CT scans, however, show talar fracture. **F,** After reduction and fixation of fracture.

and associated fractures generally do worse than those with isolated closed dislocations. In a study of 23 isolated subtalar dislocations with no associated fracture, 21 patients had good results and two had satisfactory results. In a long-term review of severe open subtalar dislocations, results were considerably worse than in closed injuries. Associated injuries included tibial nerve injuries, posterior tibial tendon ruptures, and articular fractures. Osteonecrosis occurred in the body of the talus in one third of the patients. Approximately half of the patients eventually had some form of arthrodesis procedure.

OPEN REDUCTION OF SUBTALAR DISLOCATION

TECHNIQUE 9.13

- Make a longitudinal anterolateral incision from just proximal to the ankle joint to the cuboid. Carefully protect

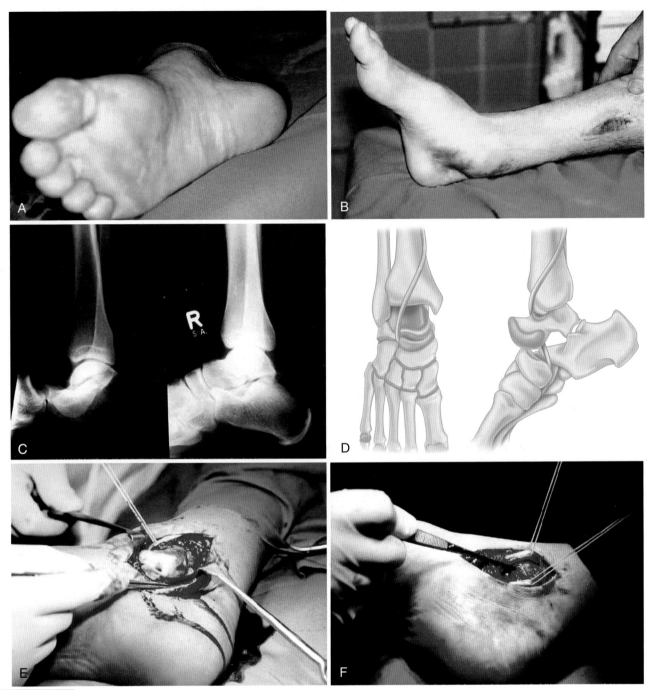

FIGURE 9.63 **A** and **B,** Lateral subtalar dislocation. **C,** Radiographs before and after reduction. **D,** Posterior tibial tendon can be an obstacle to reduction. **E,** Posterior tibial tendon is marked with rubber band. **F,** After removal of tendon and reduction of fracture. (From Wagner R, Blattert TR, Weckbach A: Talar dislocations, *Injury* 35:S-B36, 2004.) **SEE TECHNIQUE 9.13.**

the medial and lateral dorsal cutaneous branches of the superficial peroneal nerve.
- Retract the extensor digitorum longus and extensor hallucis longus tendons medially and the peroneus tertius tendon laterally and expose the talus and midtarsal joints.
- Incise the capsule over the head and neck of the talus and extend the incision into the midtarsus.
- Insert a bone skid or periosteal elevator into the subtalar joint and by leverage and traction reduce the dislocation of the subtalar and the talonavicular joints. When

the dislocation is medial, have an assistant simultaneously abduct and evert the foot; when it is lateral, have the assistant adduct and invert the foot. In a lateral dislocation, the posterior tibial tendon frequently blocks reduction and must be lifted out of the talonavicular joint before reduction is possible (see Fig. 9.63). Also, by extending the medial wound seen in lateral subtalar dislocations and lifting the dorsal neurovascular bundle and offending tendons, the dorsal capsule of the talonavicular joint can be incised. With this structure loosened, the navicular can be levered

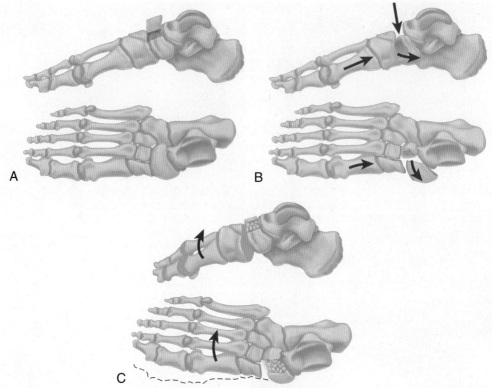

FIGURE 9.64   **A,** Type I fracture. Dorsal fragment usually consists of less than 50% of body of tarsal navicular. Anteroposterior radiographs show only subtle double cortical shadow at joint line. **B,** Type II fracture. Talonavicular joint is most often subluxated dorsally and medially with adduction of forepart of foot. **C,** Type III fracture. Comminuted fracture of body of navicular is associated with disruption of cuneiform-navicular joint, lateral deviation of forepart of foot, and injuries to cuboid or anterior process of calcaneus.   (From Sangeorzan BJ, Benirschke SK, Mosca V, et al: Displaced intraarticular fractures of the tarsal navicular, *J Bone Joint Surg* 71A:1504, 1989.)

around the head of the talus with a periosteal elevator. This may require a separate anterolateral incision.

- If necessary, hold the reduction with an external fixator or longitudinally placed Steinmann pins across the calcaneocuboid and talonavicular joints for 4 to 6 weeks.

POSTOPERATIVE CARE A splint is applied from the base of the toes to the tibial tuberosity over a bulky compression dressing. At 6 weeks, cast immobilization is discontinued; a lace-up foot and ankle leather corset is applied; active inversion, eversion, dorsiflexion, and plantarflexion of the foot and ankle are encouraged; and weight bearing is allowed. The corset is worn for 1 month to control edema, and weight bearing to tolerance with crutches is allowed. Full weight bearing should be comfortable by 6 to 8 weeks after injury. Patients must be advised, however, that the foot and ankle may swell and that the midfoot and hindfoot may feel stiff for several months.

MIDFOOT FRACTURES AND DISLOCATIONS

NAVICULAR/CUBOID/CUNEIFORM FRACTURES

It is rare for these fractures to be nondisplaced, in which case nonoperative treatment with a cast and protected weight bearing may be considered. Displaced fractures of the body of the navicular should be treated with ORIF; the goals are to maintain length of the medial column and to restore articular congruity. Sangeorzan et al. classified navicular body fractures into three types and recommended treatment based on fracture type (Fig. 9.64). In type I fractures, in which the fracture plane is transverse, a satisfactory reduction usually was obtainable. In type II and type III fractures, reduction was more difficult. In each case, an approach was made over the anteromedial hindfoot in the interval between the anterior and posterior tibial tendons. The periosteum of the navicular was not elevated, and the joints were inspected and cleared of debris before fixation. Fixation usually was obtained with smooth Kirschner wires and small fragment AO screws when the size of the fragment permitted (Fig. 9.65). Good results were obtained in only 67% of patients. In a recent study using mini-fragment plates for fixation, there were no nonunions or loss of reduction; one patient developed osteonecrosis of the navicular (Fig. 9.66). Another study showed 61% good results, with 31% of patients needing secondary surgery and 43% of patients with continuing pain.

If collapse of the navicular occurs with medial column shortening, bone grafting (including vascularized pedicle bone grafting), temporary fixation to the talus or cuneiforms, or application of a small external fixator is used for additional fixation. Two incisions, one medial and one dorsolateral,

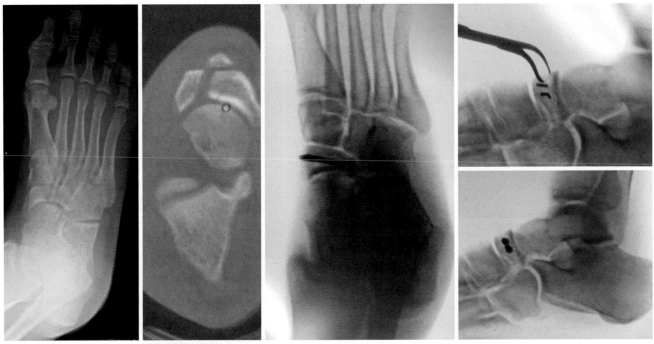

FIGURE 9.65 Open reduction and internal fixation of navicular.

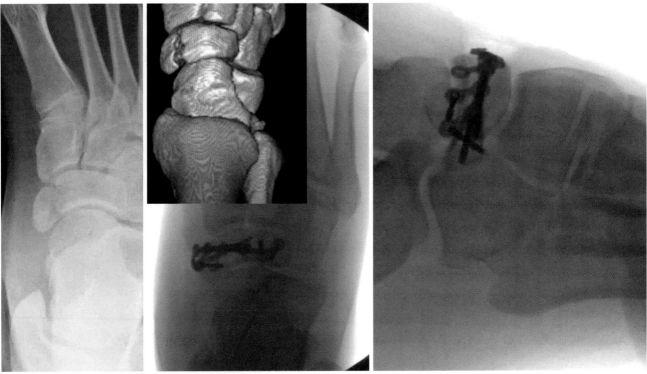

FIGURE 9.66 Plate fixation of navicular fracture.

may be necessary to fully expose the navicular, and plate fixation may be needed because comminution may preclude the use of screws. If an external fixator is used to maintain medial column length (Fig. 9.67), it can be removed at 6 weeks to start range of motion, but the patient is kept non–weight bearing for 12 weeks. Temporary bridge plating from the talar neck to the stable portion of the foot can maintain length in cases of severe comminution but requires a second surgery for removal of implants (Fig. 9.68). Alternatively,

bridge plating from the navicular to the medial and middle cuneiforms can be used, which does not interfere with talonavicular motion (Fig. 9.69). A prolonged recovery and persistent symptoms should be anticipated and the patient counseled accordingly.

Navicular stress fractures are frequent causes of arch pain in athletes. Because many of these fractures are not clearly identified on routine radiographs, a high index of suspicion is necessary for accurate diagnosis. The midfoot

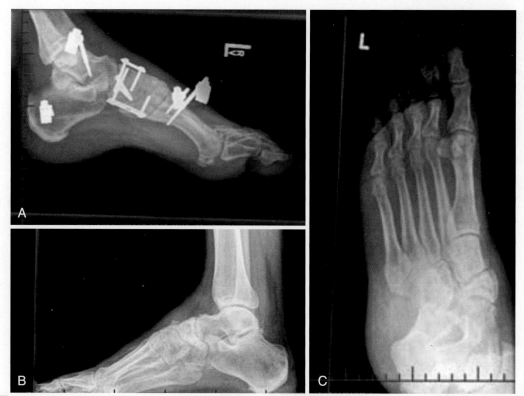

FIGURE 9.67 **A,** Temporary use of external fixator to maintain medial column length in severely comminuted navicular fracture. **B** and **C,** At 2-year follow-up, after implant removal medial column is maintained despite navicular collapse secondary to original injury. (From Apostle KL, Younger ASE: Technique tip: open reduction internal fixation of comminuted fracture of the navicular with bridge plating to the medial and middle columns, *Foot Ankle Int* 29:739, 2008.)

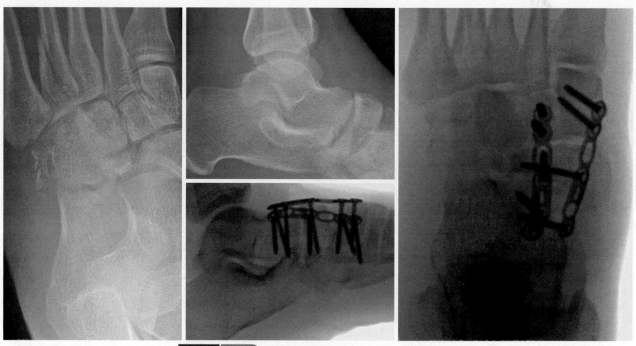

FIGURE 9.68 Bridge plating for navicular fracture.

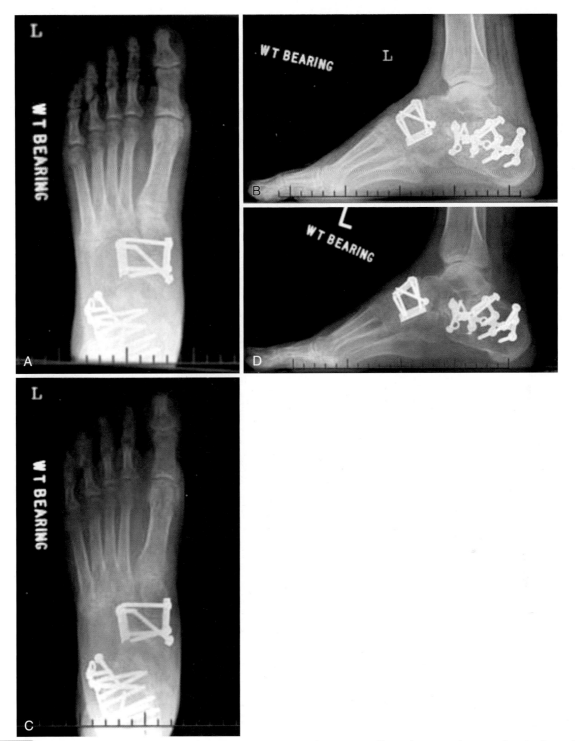

FIGURE 9.69 **A** and **B,** Fixation of navicular fracture with bridging plates to cuneiforms but not talus; associated calcaneal fracture also fixed with mini-fragment plates and screws. **C** and **D,** At latest follow-up fracture had healed and implant removal was planned. (From Apostle KL, Younger ASE: Technique tip: open reduction internal fixation of comminuted fracture of the navicular with bridge plating to the medial and middle columns, *Foot Ankle Int* 29:739, 2008.)

may be tender over the navicular, and the foot may be irritable with eversion and inversion stress. Radiographs may be normal initially, but a bone scan frequently is positive (Fig. 9.70A), and CT (see Fig. 9.70B) or MRI may confirm the diagnosis. The fractures usually are located in the sagittal plane, involving the central third of the navicular bone where there is a relatively avascular zone, although a newer study shows that this avascular zone is not common, suggesting that other factors play a role in the etiology of these stress fractures. The trend has been toward surgical intervention for this condition; however, in a meta-analysis, 6 to 8 weeks of non–weight-bearing cast immobilization was

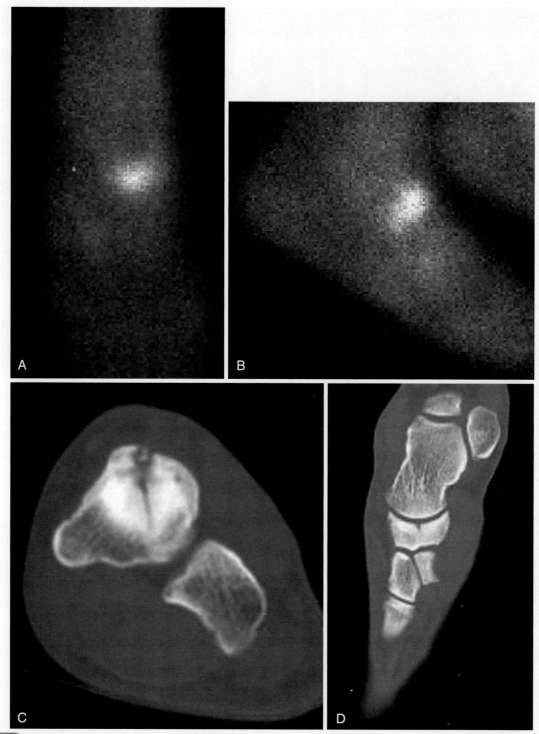

FIGURE 9.70 Although radiographs may be normal initially, navicular stress fracture may be evident on bone scan (**A** and **B**) and CT scan (**C** and **D**).

found to be optimal. There is a trend for better outcomes with non–weight-bearing treatment than with surgery, and allowing the patient to bear weight clearly is inferior to both non–weight bearing and surgical treatment. Although some studies suggest earlier return to activities with surgical treatment, others have found more long-term pain with surgical than with conservative treatment. If surgical treatment is done, a percutaneous technique can be used for nondisplaced fractures and an open technique

for displaced fractures or if bone grafting is required for nonunions.

Cuboid and cuneiform fractures are rare as isolated injuries and often are missed on initial presentation. Suspicion should be heightened for these injuries if the patient presents with ecchymosis in the plantar arch, a sign that was originally described for Lisfranc injuries but can be applied here also. These bones frequently are injured as part of a wider injury pattern involving the Lisfranc (most common) or Chopart joint.

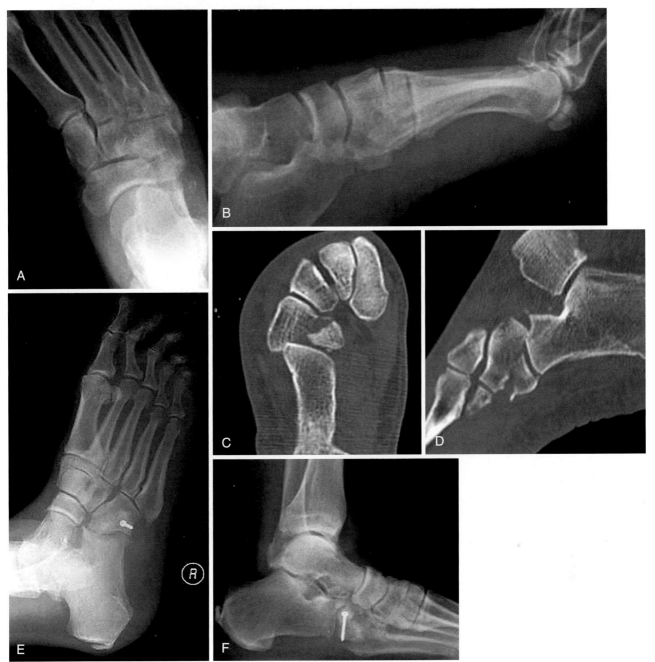

FIGURE 9.71   **A** and **B,** Cuboid fracture was not apparent on radiographs, but because of ecchymosis in area, CT scans (**C** and **D**) were obtained, which showed fracture. **E** and **F,** After open reduction and internal fixation.

Cuboid fractures can be classified into avulsion or compression types. Small avulsions may occur with inversion-type ankle sprains and generally respond to conservative treatment. Compression, or "nutcracker," fractures of the cuboid are associated with Lisfranc and midtarsal disruptions. Most are minimally displaced and can be treated in a non–weight-bearing cast for 4 weeks followed by weight-bearing casts for 4 weeks. A well-molded arch support often is used afterward. For severe displacement with shortening of the lateral column, consideration should be given to ORIF (Fig. 9.71). External fixation may be necessary to restore lateral column length before grafting and fixation (Fig. 9.72). Operative treatment can lead to good results, with minimal long-term pain and disability.

Isolated cuneiform fractures are rare with only a few case reports in the literature. Return to activities can be obtained with nonoperative treatment of nondisplaced fractures and operative treatment of displaced fractures (Fig. 9.73). If the fracture is comminuted, temporary bridge plating or external fixation may be needed to maintain medial column length.

In a review of 155 patients with midfoot fractures and dislocations, there was a relative incidence of isolated midfoot fractures of 35.5%; Lisfranc fracture-dislocations, 31%; Chopart-Lisfranc fracture-dislocations, 16.8%; and pure Chopart fracture-dislocations, 16%. The incidence of this injury at our institution has been markedly higher, especially since the introduction and routine use of airbags in motor vehicles. Patients who may not previously have survived injuries now sustain severe blunt force trauma to the feet, often resulting in dislocations of the Chopart and Lisfranc joints in addition to other injuries. In this study and a similar study from the same

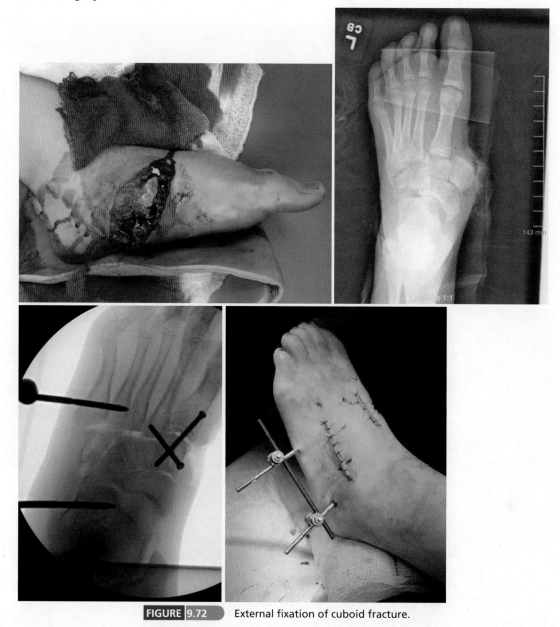

FIGURE 9.72   External fixation of cuboid fracture.

authors, there seemed to be significant improvement in the scores in patients who were treated with early operative intervention and anatomic or near-anatomic alignment and reduction of the joints. The lowest scoring results occurred in patients who had combined Chopart and Lisfranc fracture-dislocations. These injuries often are missed on initial presentation. Most often, the exposure of the Chopart joint is a combination of that described for subtalar dislocation with an anterolateral incision, as described for the Lisfranc fracture-dislocation and dorsomedial incision. Patients should be counseled about the potential for long-term functional impairment because in one study most patients were not able to return to their preinjury levels of activity after 2 years.

FRACTURE-DISLOCATIONS OF THE TARSOMETATARSAL ARTICULATION (LISFRANC JOINT)

Injuries of the tarsometatarsal articulation encompass a wide spectrum, ranging from mild sprains or subtle subluxations to widely displaced debilitating injuries. This part of the foot at the apex of the arch can be difficult to heal because a significant amount of stress passes through this area with weight bearing. The anatomy is unique in this area, with transverse stability provided by the wedge-shaped metatarsal bases and their corresponding cuneiform-cuboid articulations, with the second metatarsal recessed between the medial and lateral cuneiforms as the keystone. These joints have little longitudinal stability, provided only by strong ligamentous support. There are multiple intermetatarsal ligaments at the metatarsal bases except between the first and second metatarsals. Stability in this area is provided by the Lisfranc ligament, which runs from the medial cuneiform to the second metatarsal. The medial column consists of the first metatarsal, medial cuneiform, and navicular facet; the middle column refers to the second and third metatarsals with their corresponding cuneiforms and navicular articulations; and the lateral column refers to the fourth and fifth metatarsals and their cuboid articulations.

■ CLASSIFICATION

Classification of this injury is useful for communication between orthopaedists, and for determining the plane of

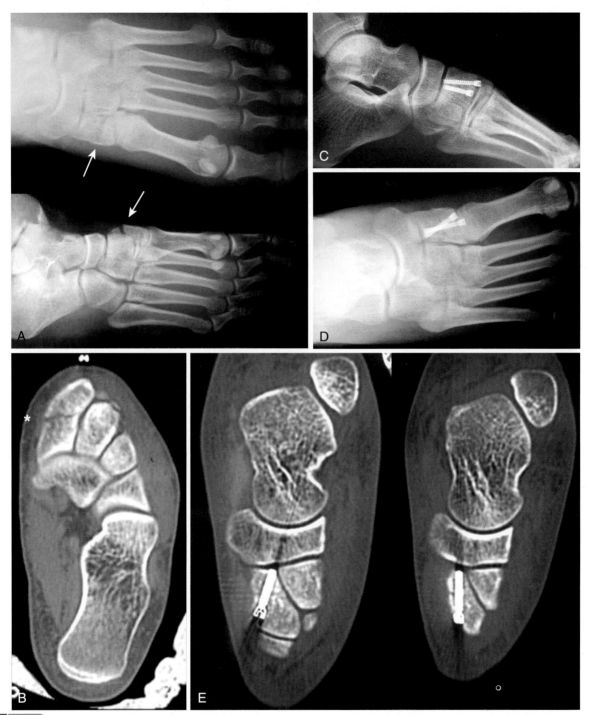

FIGURE 9.73 Appearance of fracture of medial cuneiform on anteroposterior and oblique radiographs **(A)** *(arrows)* and CT scan **(B)** *(asterisk).* Postoperative radiographs **(C and D)** and CT scan **(E).** (From Guler F, Baz AB, Turan A, et al: Isolated medial cuneiform fractures: report of two cases and review of the literature, *Foot Ankle Spec* 4:306, 2011.)

displacement and magnitude of soft-tissue injury. The classification is not prognostic for the result, however. Myerson's modification of the original classification of Quénu and Küss and Hardcastle et al. is presented because it incorporates more proximal injuries to the medial column of the foot (Fig. 9.74). Subtle injuries through the intercuneiform region and the naviculocuneiform joint probably are more common than previously thought.

Type A injuries: Displacement of all five metatarsals with or without fracture of the base of the second metatarsal. The usual displacement is lateral or dorsolateral, and the metatarsals move as a unit. These injuries are referred to as *homolateral.*

Type B injuries: One or more articulations remain intact. Type B1 injuries are medially displaced, sometimes involving the intercuneiform or naviculocuneiform joint. Type B2

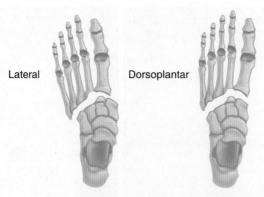

Lateral   Dorsoplantar

Type A: Total incongruity

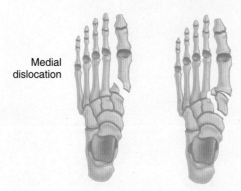

Medial
dislocation

Type B1: Partial incongruity

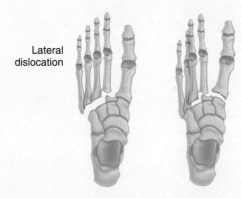

Lateral
dislocation

Type B2: Partial incongruity

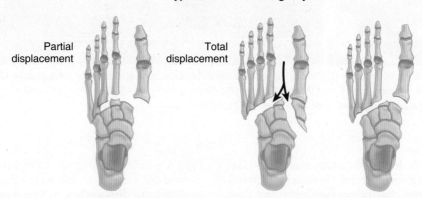

Partial
displacement   Total
displacement

Type C1: Divergent   **Type C2: Divergent**

FIGURE 9.74 **Classification of tarsometatarsal fracture-dislocations.** (From Myerson M, Fisher R, Burgess A, et al: Dislocations of the tarsometatarsal joints: end results correlated with pathology and treatment, *Foot Ankle* 6:225, 1986.)

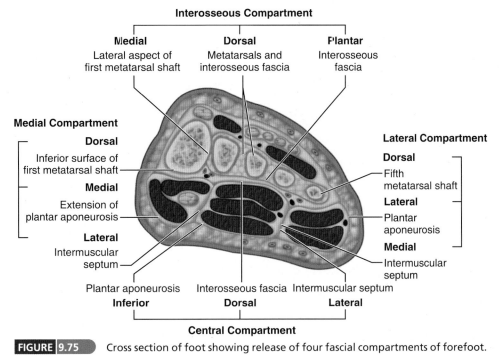

FIGURE 9.75 Cross section of foot showing release of four fascial compartments of forefoot.

injuries are laterally displaced and may involve the first metatarsal-cuneiform joint.

Type C injuries: Divergent injuries that can be partial (C1) or complete (C2). These generally are high-energy injuries, associated with significant swelling, and are prone to complications, especially compartment syndrome.

■ EVALUATION AND TREATMENT

Any injury resulting in midfoot tenderness and swelling merits a careful physical and radiographic examination. Grossly displaced fracture-dislocations are obvious on examination, and closed reduction should be performed urgently to minimize soft-tissue compromise. Care should be taken with subtle injuries to palpate each articulation for tenderness and swelling, especially the medial cuneiform–first metatarsal joint, which often appears nondisplaced on radiographs. Careful observation of the plantar aspect of the foot may reveal ecchymosis, indicating a significant injury. The inability to bear weight on the foot is another sign of potential instability.

Radiographs *must* be obtained with the patient bearing weight. If the radiograph reveals no displacement and the patient cannot bear weight, a short leg cast or fracture boot should be used for 2 weeks, and the radiographs should be repeated with weight bearing, including a standing radiograph of both feet on the same cassette, which allows for comparison and can highlight subtle injuries. Evaluation should be directed to the following areas:

1. The medial shaft of the second metatarsal should be aligned with the medial aspect of the middle cuneiform on the anteroposterior view.
2. The medial shaft of the fourth metatarsal should be aligned with the medial aspect of the cuboid on the oblique view.
3. The first metatarsal–cuneiform articulation should have no incongruency.

4. A "fleck sign" should be sought in the medial cuneiform–second metatarsal space. This represents an avulsion of the Lisfranc ligament.
5. Loss of the arch and/or loss of alignment between the plantar aspect of the fifth metatarsal and medial cuneiform on the lateral view.
6. The naviculocuneiform articulation should be evaluated for subluxation.
7. A compression fracture of the cuboid should be sought.

CT can identify subtle subluxations and occult fractures, and MRI of the Lisfranc ligament can be obtained in the acute setting and if the level of injury cannot be determined by plain radiographs. Weight-bearing CT scans, where available, are very useful in detection of subtle instability.

Compartment syndrome, although rare and usually seen only with higher-energy fracture-dislocations, can cause severe, difficult-to-treat clawing of the toes and chronic pain. We routinely obtain compartmental pressures in patients who have severe swelling, but individual compartments can be difficult to assess (Fig. 9.75), and clinical suspicion alone is enough to warrant decompression. We prefer a long medial incision to decompress the abductor hallucis and deep compartments of the foot, including the calcaneal compartment. In addition, two incisions—one between the second and third metatarsals and one between the fourth and fifth metatarsals—are used for the dorsal intrinsic compartments.

The key to successful outcome in Lisfranc injuries is anatomic alignment of the involved joints. Closed, nondisplaced (<2 mm) injuries can be treated with a non–weight-bearing cast for 6 weeks followed by use of a weight-bearing cast for an additional 4 to 6 weeks. Repeat radiographs should be obtained to ensure that no displacement is occurring in the cast. Displaced fractures should be treated operatively (Fig. 9.76). Closed reduction, using finger traps, countertraction, and/or percutaneous bone clamps, can be successful if displacement is not severe, although open reduction is generally

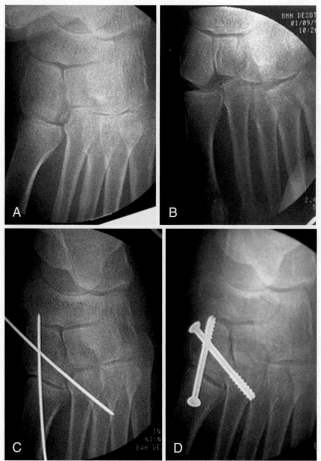

FIGURE 9.76 Subtle Lisfranc instability. **A,** Intraoperative fluoroscopic radiograph showing fleck sign at medial cuneiform–second metatarsal articulation. Patient was taken to operating room because standing radiographs in office showed subtle subluxation, swelling, and tenderness and pointed to more serious instability. **B,** Intraoperative stress radiographs showing subluxation of first through third tarsometatarsal articulations. **C,** Provisional stabilization with guidewires inserted under fluoroscopic control. **D,** Final fixation with cannulated screws.

preferred and can lead to better outcomes. Fixation should be used to maintain the reduction. Kirschner wires can be used, especially for the lateral two joints, but may result in loss of reduction if used in the medial and middle columns; 4-mm cannulated or 4-mm standard, partially threaded cancellous screws provide excellent fixation and can be inserted under image control. Using cannulated screws makes removal easier by employing a guide pin to find the screw head and ultimately to seat the screwdriver. If the reduction is inadequate or significant comminution is present, open reduction should be performed, especially in partial (type B) or divergent (type C) patterns.

Dorsal and/or medial plating also can be used for fixation, which avoids damage to articular surfaces. Studies show that the strength of fixation is similar to that of transarticular screws in cadaver models and that clinically anatomic reduction can be obtained with good clinical outcomes. Fixation with tensioned suture devices also has been described, but there is some controversy in the literature as to whether the biomechanical strength is equal to that of screw fixation, and

there is limited information on clinical outcomes. For high-energy injuries in which soft-tissue compromise is significant, consideration should be given to temporary external fixation after closed reduction until the soft tissues allow for definitive fixation. In one study using this staged treatment, the external fixator was on for an average of 21 days (range, 7 to 144 days) before ORIF or arthrodesis could be performed. For open high-energy injuries, fixation with a Kirschner wire may be the only option, since delayed fixation may interfere with early soft-tissue coverage. However, this may lead to loss of anatomic reduction.

Although the prognosis for this injury is guarded, the literature confirms that the ability to obtain and maintain an anatomic reduction of a fracture-dislocation is associated with improved outcome over nonanatomic reduction. In one study, nonanatomic reduction was associated with the presence of posttraumatic arthrosis in 60%. In patients with anatomic reduction, posttraumatic arthrosis occurred in only 16%. Mora et al. showed that one in three patients might continue to experience pain at the injury site but most were able to return to sports and physical activity. There was a trend toward poorer outcomes for patients with purely ligamentous injuries. Patients with higher-energy injuries, ipsilateral injuries, and type C2 injuries also seemed to fare worse. Primary arthrodesis has been recommended for this injury. A prospective randomized study showed better outcomes for patients who had primary arthrodesis for purely ligamentous Lisfranc injuries than those who had ORIF. Several prospective, randomized studies and meta-analyses of ligamentous and bony Lisfranc injuries found similar outcomes for both open reduction and primary arthrodesis groups, although patients with ORIF required more secondary surgeries, including routine hardware removal. Cochran et al. showed, in a young military population, an earlier return to full military activity, better fitness test scores after 1 year, and lower implant removal rates after primary arthrodesis compared to ORIF. Buda et al. showed isolated plate fixation, smoking, and nonanatomic alignment increased the rate of nonunion in patients undergoing arthrodesis, while autograft decreased this risk.

Low-energy tarsometatarsal injuries such as those incurred by athletes can be difficult to detect. Physical examination findings include pain with pronation and abduction of the forefoot while the hindfoot is stabilized, pain with compression of the midfoot, pain with manipulation of the first metatarsal in the sagittal plane while holding the second metatarsal still, and pain with squeezing of the first and second intermetatarsal space. These subtle injuries are classified as follows: stage I—patients can bear weight but are unable to play sports, and there is little or no displacement seen on weight-bearing radiographs; stage II—similar physical findings to stage I, but radiographs show 2 to 5 mm of diastasis between the first and second metatarsals but no loss of arch height; or stage III—more displacement and collapse of the arch. Stage I injuries can be treated nonoperatively with immobilization and 2 to 6 weeks of non–weight bearing. Stages II and III injuries should be treated operatively. Percutaneous reduction with bone clamps can be attempted. If adequate reduction is obtained, cannulated screws can be placed percutaneously. Open reduction, when necessary, is similar to that for traumatic injuries. Screw fixation is the standard, but dorsal plates can be applied to avoid damage to articular cartilage with transarticular

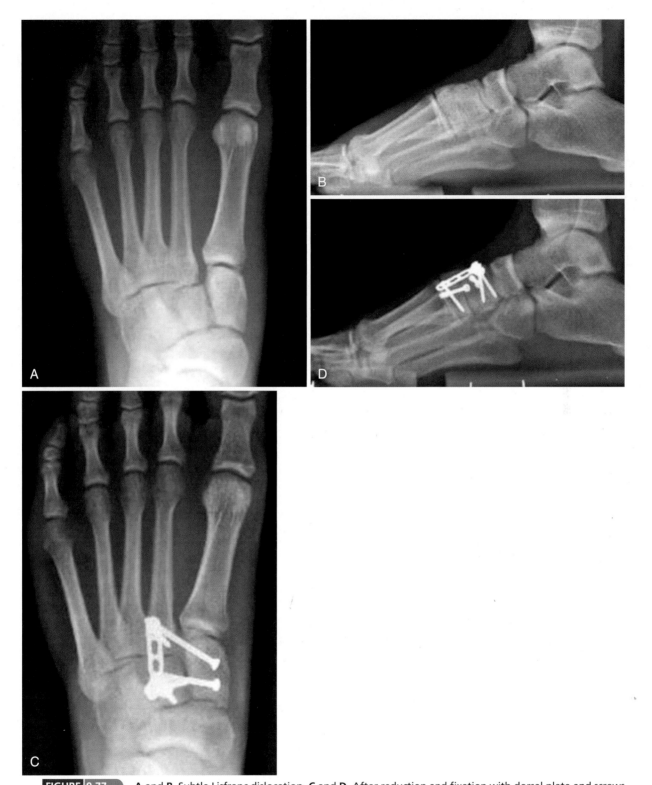

FIGURE 9.77 **A** and **B,** Subtle Lisfranc dislocation. **C** and **D,** After reduction and fixation with dorsal plate and screws.

screws (Fig. 9.77). Alternatively, tensioned suture devices have been used for fixation. Porter et al. showed up to a 50% occurrence of proximal intercuneiform ligament tearing in low-energy Lisfranc athletic injuries, so this joint should be closely inspected during surgery. Postoperative treatment is similar to that for traumatic injuries, although one study has suggested that weight bearing can be started at 3 weeks

after these low-energy injuries. Athletes should not return to cutting activities until at least 6 months after treatment and should be protected with a full-length rigid carbon plate in the shoe.

Degenerative posttraumatic arthrosis can be managed successfully with tarsometatarsal and intermetatarsal arthrodesis as necessary for stabilization of the arthritic joints and reduction of posttraumatic flatfoot deformity. After midfoot arthrodesis, there is significant improvement in the American Orthopaedic Foot and Ankle Society (AOFAS) score for the midfoot and there is a 93% patient satisfaction rate. Arthrodesis of the fourth and fifth tarsometatarsal joints leads to poorer outcomes.

OPEN REDUCTION AND INTERNAL FIXATION OF TARSOMETATARSAL (LISFRANC) FRACTURES

TECHNIQUE 9.14

- With the patient under a regional or general anesthetic, make a dorsal incision lateral to the extensor hallucis longus tendon over the interval between the base of the first and second metatarsals, slightly more lateral if access to the third tarsometatarsal joint is necessary. At the distal extent of the incision, preserve the most medial branch of the dorsal medial cutaneous nerve.
- A second incision may be needed more laterally if open reduction of the fourth and fifth tarsometatarsal joints is necessary (Fig. 9.78A).
- Locate and incise the inferior extensor retinaculum.
- Isolate the dorsalis pedis artery and deep peroneal nerve and use a vessel loop for retraction of these structures medially or laterally to allow inspection of different areas of the Lisfranc joint (Fig. 9.78B).
- Remove any debris from the Lisfranc region between the base of the second metatarsal and the medial cuneiform to allow the space to be reduced. Reduce the first tarsometatarsal joint and hold it with guidewires for cannulated screws. Place a screw from the dorsal aspect of the first metatarsal into the medial cuneiform (Fig. 9.78C). A second screw can be placed from proximal to distal across the first tarsometatarsal joint. A spanning plate also can be used in place of transarticular screws.
- Under fluoroscopic guidance, pass a guidewire from the medial cuneiform into the base of the second metatarsal while holding the reduction with a towel clip. Place the appropriate 4.0-mm cannulated screw over the guidewire (Fig. 9.78D).
- The second and third metatarsal–cuneiform joints can be reduced and fixed similarly with one screw across the joint or a spanning plate. Occasionally, bony comminution may preclude screw fixation. In this case, fixation can be accomplished with dorsal plates (Fig. 9.79).
- If an intercuneiform screw is needed, insert it under fluoroscopic guidance from the medial side of the medial cuneiform into the middle cuneiform.
- Reduce lateral metatarsocuboid disruptions either closed or open through a parallel incision centered dorsolaterally over the articulations, with fixation with Kirschner wires (Fig. 9.80).
- Close the dorsal skin with interrupted nylon sutures.

POSTOPERATIVE CARE A bulky dressing and posterior splint are applied postoperatively. These are converted to a short leg, non–weight-bearing cast at 7 to 10 days postoperatively. Weightbearing may be allowed at 6 to 8 weeks, and laterally placed Kirschner wires are removed at 6 to 8 weeks. Medial screws are removed at 4 to 5 months.

ARTHRODESIS OF LISFRANC INJURIES

- Position the patient supine with a bump under the ipsilateral hip and a thigh tourniquet. Placing a ramp of blankets or a foam positioner along with the knee flexed over a radiolucent triangle on its side allows imaging of the foot in AP and lateral positions with minimal movement of the fluoroscopy unit and eliminates obstruction from the contralateral foot.
- Make a dorsal incision in line with the first web space and identify and protect neurovascular structures. An incision over the medial aspect of the fourth tarsometatarsal joint may also be needed for treatment of third to fifth tarsometatarsal joint injuries.
- Inspect the midfoot joints for stability and cartilaginous injury. Pay specific attention to the first intercuneiform and naviculocuneiform joints where instability indicates a longitudinal Lisfranc injury.
- Denude cartilaginous surfaces from involved joints in the medial column and midfoot with curets and osteotomes, followed by penetration of the subchondral bone with a water-cooled drill bit. Mobility is important in the fourth and fifth metatarsal–cuboid articulation, and, although posttraumatic arthrosis may occur in this region, arthrodesis of these two joints should be avoided.
- Autograft can be harvested from the proximal tibia or calcaneus and inserted into the joints planned for fusion.
- Restore anatomic alignment beginning with the medial column. If the intercuneiform joint is disrupted, restore it and pin it provisionally with a Kirschner wire. Align the first tarsometatarsal joint anatomically, generally with an adduction and internal rotation maneuver, and pin it with a Kirschner wire. Inspect radiographs to assess that Mill's line (a line drawn tangentially along the navicular and medial cuneiform that should intersect the first metatarsal) is restored. Use a Weber clamp or pointed tenaculum to reduce the Lisfranc interval, followed by reduction and provisional pinning of the second to fifth tarsometatarsal joints.
- After provisional fixation with Kirschner wires, obtain multiple fluoroscopic views to assess anatomic reduction of the involved joints.
- Permanent fixation can now be placed either with crossing solid or cannulated cortical screws, spanning plates, or nitinol compression staples (Figs. 9.81 and 9.82).
- Close the wounds, apply sterile dressings, and place the foot into a short leg splint.

POSTOPERATIVE CARE Sutures are removed when the wounds are healed, typically at 2 to 3 weeks. Immobilization is continued in a cast until 6 weeks postoperatively when weight bearing is advanced in a fracture boot. A steel-shank shoe or full-length graphite insert can be used in the shoe to transition out of the boot into normal footwear.

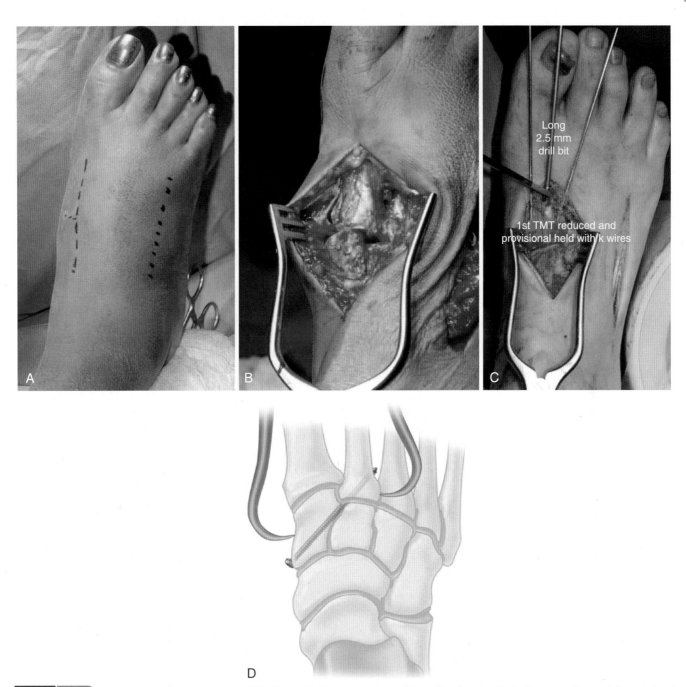

FIGURE 9.78 Open reduction and internal fixation of Lisfranc fracture-dislocation (see text). **A,** Dorsomedial and dorsolateral incisions. **B,** Isolation and retraction of dorsalis pedis artery and deep peroneal nerve. **C,** Reduction and provisional fixation of first tarsometatarsal joint. **D,** Final fixation. (From Sands AK: Open reduction and internal fixation of Lisfranc/tarsometatarsal injuries. In Pfeffer G, Easley M, Frey C, et al, editors: *Operative techniques: foot and ankle surgery,* Philadelphia, 2009, Saunders.) **SEE TECHNIQUE 9.14.**

There is much controversy with regard to the role of primary arthrodesis versus internal fixation for these injuries. Most authors agree that it is the anatomic reduction, whether followed by internal fixation or arthrodesis, that is most important. Consideration for arthrodesis should be given to delayed encounters, comminuted joint surfaces, and poor medical hosts where multiple surgeries should be avoided.

METATARSALS
FRACTURE OF THE PROXIMAL PORTION OF THE FIFTH METATARSAL

A great deal of attention has been directed toward the treatment of fractures of the proximal portion of the fifth metatarsal because of the potentially poor healing in this bone secondary to a watershed area of the blood supply. Three fracture zones have been described (Fig. 9.83).

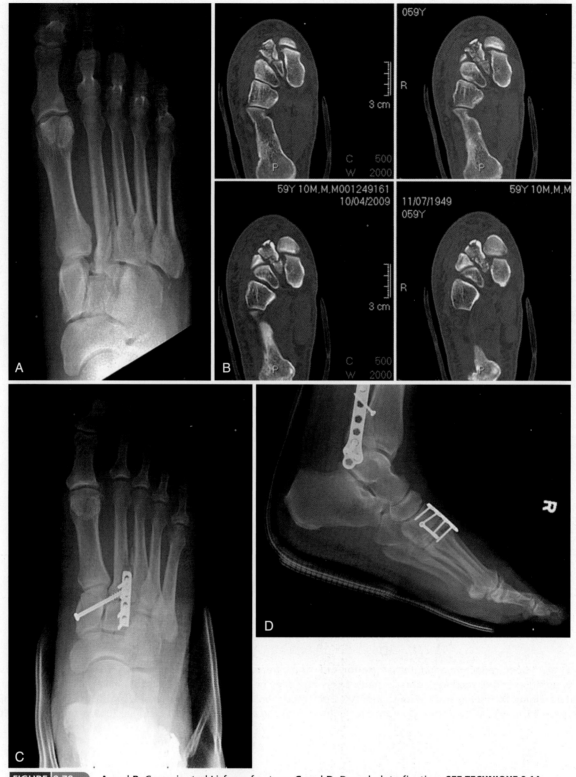

FIGURE 9.79   **A** and **B,** Comminuted Lisfranc fracture. **C** and **D,** Dorsal plate fixation. **SEE TECHNIQUE 9.14.**

Zone I is the most proximal zone and includes the metatarsocuboid articulation, but it is proximal to the fourth and fifth metatarsal articulation. Fractures in this area are avulsion types of injuries, usually secondary to an inversion injury to the foot. Zone II extends from zone I to the metaphyseal/diaphyseal junction and includes the fourth

and fifth metatarsal articulation. This is the area of the true Jones fracture. The mechanism of injury is usually that of a strong abduction force to the forefoot, causing a bending moment at the metaphyseal-diaphyseal junction. Zone III is the proximal 1.5 cm of the diaphysis and is the area where stress fractures usually occur. The Torg

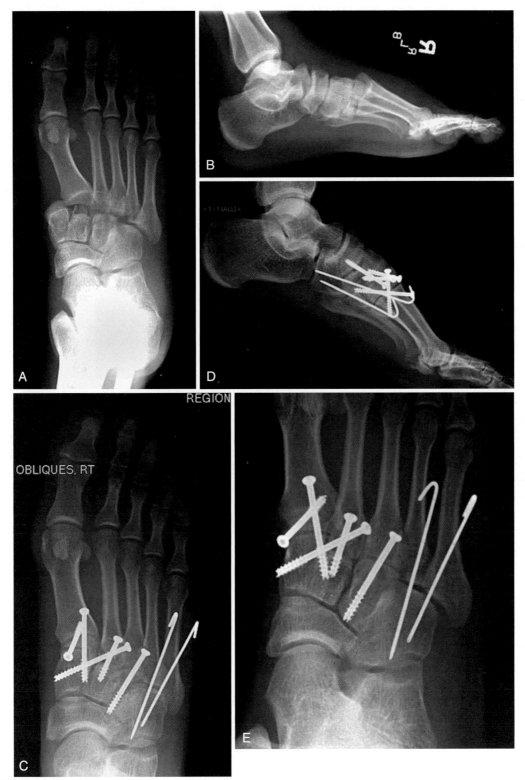

FIGURE 9.80 **A** and **B,** Homolateral Lisfranc dislocation. **C** to **E,** After reduction and fixation. **SEE TECHNIQUE 9.14.**

classification of stress fractures in zone III includes type I, which is an acute fracture; type II, which is a delayed union with some periosteal reaction, widening of the fracture site, and some intramedullary sclerosis; and type III, which is a nonunion with intramedullary sclerosis and blunted fracture edges. One study suggested that no distinction needs to be made between zone II and zone III

fractures because treatment and outcomes are the same in the two groups.

Fractures in zone I generally are treated satisfactorily in a postoperative shoe, walking boot, or short leg walking cast, depending on the level of symptoms of the patient. Although nonunions of these fractures may occur, they rarely are painful and can be treated with excision

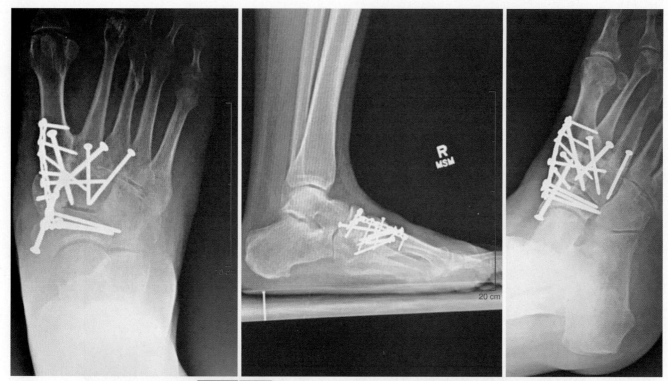

FIGURE 9.81   Arthrodesis with plates and screws. **SEE TECHNIQUE 9.14.**

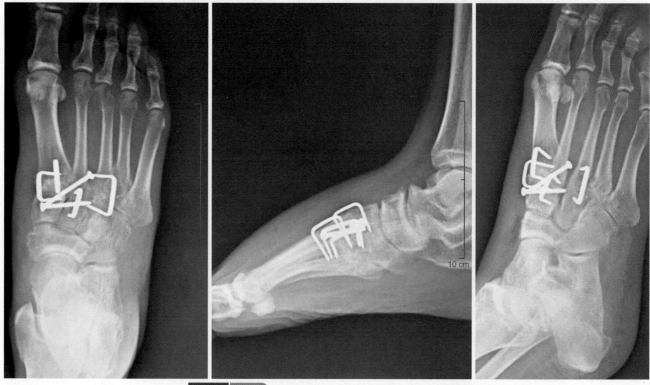

FIGURE 9.82   Arthrodesis with nitinol staples. **SEE TECHNIQUE 9.82.**

of the fragment. In a study of this fracture of the proximal fifth metatarsal, the fracture healed in all 60 patients at an average of 44 days, with no fracture taking longer than 65 days to heal. Patients were randomly assigned to a soft Jones type of dressing or a short leg cast. Patients treated with a compressive soft dressing and allowed to bear weight in a cast boot required a significantly shorter recuperation time and had a better modified foot score than patients treated with cast immobilization. Patients on average missed 22 days of work, and it took 6 months or more for most patients to return to preinjury levels of activities. Another study confirms the shorter recuperation time for patients treated with a walking boot instead of a walking cast.

For zone I fractures with gross displacement or articular involvement in young active patients, open reduction and fixation can be considered. A variety of methods of fixation are described, including plating, screw fixation (Fig. 9.84), and a tension-band technique (Fig. 9.85). In our experience, plates

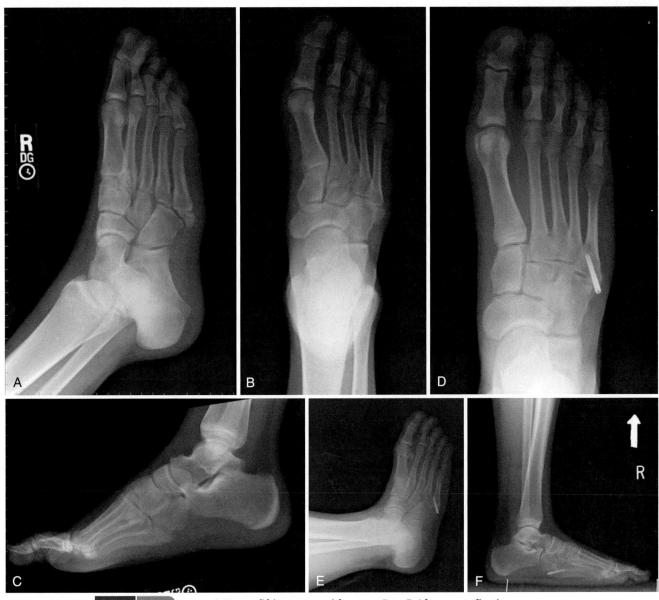

FIGURE 9.83 Fractures of the fifth metatarsal.

- ☐ Tuberosity avulsion fracture
- ☐ Jones fracture
- ☐ Diaphyseal stress fracture

in this area are generally not well tolerated and often require removal.

Treatment of Jones fractures and Torg type I diaphyseal fractures depends on the type of fracture and the activity demands of the patient. An initial non–weight bearing, short leg cast is worn for 6 to 8 weeks followed by a weight-bearing cast until union has been achieved, with a reported healing rate of 75%. In competitive athletes, consideration should be given to early ORIF to decrease disability time. Even with non–weight-bearing immobilization for 6 to 8 weeks, Jones fractures have a reported nonunion rate of 7% to 28%. The use of electrical and pulsed ultrasound bone stimulation for these fractures may improve healing of the fracture; however, they cannot take the place of internal fixation in a high-performance athlete.

In zone III, fractures with clinical or radiographic evidence of chronic injury manifested by partial or complete canal obliteration and sclerosis, non–weight-bearing casting

FIGURE 9.84 **A** to **C,** Zone I fifth metatarsal fracture. **D** to **F,** After screw fixation.

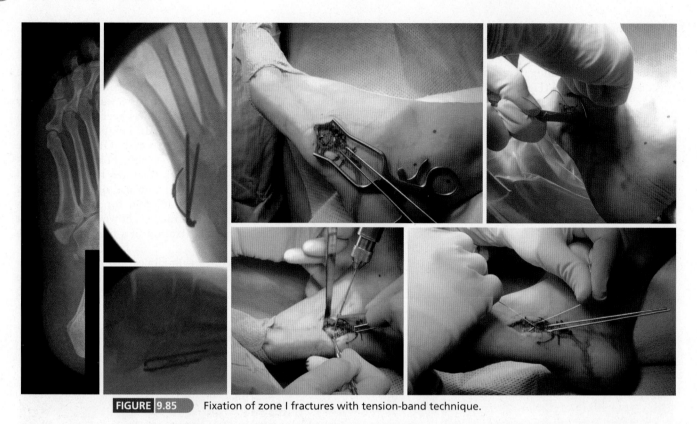

FIGURE 9.85　Fixation of zone I fractures with tension-band technique.

may yield satisfactory results. Generally, the period of immobilization and non–weight bearing is approximately 8 weeks. Refracture is common in this category. It is important to assess for biomechanical or biological reasons why this fracture developed, such as cavovarus foot posture or hypovitaminosis D. A study of 51 elite athletes showed that long, narrow, and straight fifth metatarsals with an adducted forefoot were most at risk for fifth metatarsal fractures. O'Malley et al. showed in 10 professional NBA players that a unique foot type seemed to be associated with higher rates of fifth metatarsal fractures: metatarsus adductus and a curved fifth metatarsal with a prominent base.

Surgery should be considered for zone II and III fractures that are not healing clinically at 8 to 12 weeks and for acute fractures in competitive athletes and others whose occupational demands do not allow prolonged non–weight bearing immobilization. ORIF for zone I fractures rarely is necessary and generally is reserved for displaced intraarticular fractures in highly competitive individuals.

For zones II and III fractures that require surgical intervention, two operative treatments have proved successful: (1) fixation with an intramedullary screw and (2) corticocancellous inlay bone grafting with clearing of the medullary canal of all sclerotic bone. We and most authors currently use an intramedullary screw technique, but we present both methods, each of which has a satisfactory success rate. We have had success using a variety of screw types, including variable pitched compression screws, 5.5-mm and larger cannulated screws, and noncannulated screws with low-profile heads. We believe that

there are many options for screw fixation of the fifth metatarsal, depending on the surgeon's preference and the size of the canal on the preoperative template; however, using a screw smaller than 4.5 mm is not recommended. The largest diameter screw to fill the canal should be used to minimize the risk of refracture. DeSandis et al. showed that, due to the elliptical cross section and distal metaphyseal flare of the fifth metatarsal, the AP radiograph is best to determine the diameter of the screw, whereas the lateral radiograph is best for assessing screw length. In comparing nonoperative and operative treatment of Jones fractures, one study found that up to one fourth of patients treated nonoperatively required later surgical intervention. Another study had a 44% failure rate in patients treated with a cast; patients treated operatively had a quicker time to union and earlier return to sports. Failure rates for refracture or symptomatic nonunion after operative fixation range from 0% to 40%, although in most studies the failure rate is less than 5%, and almost all athletes return to sports. Care should be taken regarding return to full activity because full return to activity before full radiographic union was predictive of failure in operatively treated patients. Intramedullary screw fixation can be used for fractures with fracture site sclerosis or medullary canal obliteration seen on radiographs; however, these patients have a higher complication rate and lower satisfaction than patients without these radiographic changes. Consideration should be given to adding cancellous graft or bone marrow aspirate to the fracture site, especially when treating a nonunion or refracture.

INTERNAL FIXATION WITH AN INTRAMEDULLARY SCREW

As Donley et al. showed, the sural nerve, in particular the dorsolateral branch, lies very close to the insertion point of the screw. Sufficient exposure must be obtained to identify and protect this cutaneous nerve branch.

TECHNIQUE 9.15

(KAVANAUGH, BROWER, AND MANN)

- Position the patient supine with a large bump under the ipsilateral hip and apply a thigh tourniquet. The foot should be resting in an oblique position such that, without moving the fluoroscopy unit, a lateral radiograph can be obtained by elevating and internally rotating the leg, while an AP radiograph is obtained by flexing the knee and externally rotating the leg.
- Use a guidewire to mark the intended screw trajectory with a skin marker to aid as a reference when placing the intramedullary wire.
- Incise the skin proximal to the base of the fifth metatarsal and observe and protect the two branches of the sural nerve (one dorsal and one straight lateral) that are vulnerable. If the peroneus brevis obscures the portal for the drill, raise a portion of it from the bone.
- Use a guidewire to find the medullary canal. This can be difficult, and the wire must lie almost parallel to the hindfoot. Starting slightly dorsal and medial ("high and inside") to what appears to be the center of the bone also helps. Watson et al. showed that adducting the forefoot or osteoplasty of the cuboid may be required to access the center of the base of the fifth metatarsal.
- Drive the wire into the medullary canal and confirm its location by anteroposterior and lateral radiographs (Fig. 9.86C). Take care to slowly advance the wire in the correct position with multiple fluoroscopic views. It is much easier to slowly advance the wire in the correct path rather than trying to redirect a wire with multiple holes in the bone.
- Advance the wire past the fracture and then overdrill it with a cannulated drill.
- Intramedullary taps can be used to measure for the largest screw diameter that can be placed.
- Estimate the length of the screw from the intraoperative radiographs and place the screw over the guidewire, making sure that the head of the screw is buried and that the screw threads are distal to the fracture site (Fig. 9.86D).
- Verify screw placement with radiographs and close the wound (Fig. 9.86E).
- Exposing a nonunion and applying a small cancellous bone graft may or may not enhance union; if cortical thickening and sclerosis are present, we usually do so.

POSTOPERATIVE CARE A well-padded, short leg, nonwalking cast, extending to the toes, is applied. Weight bearing in a cast may be started 2 weeks postoperatively. Return to competitive sports is discouraged until the fracture has healed clinically and radiographically, which usually takes 10 to 12 weeks.

■ INLAY BONE GRAFT

A consistent finding in the presence of nonunion of this fracture is obliteration of the medullary canal by dense, sclerotic bone along the margins of the fracture. Torg et al. suggested that the tendency of this fracture toward nonunion or delayed union or refracture after healing is the result of the formation at the fracture of this poorly organized, sclerotic bone, which impairs healing and the strength of the union. They described a technique to reestablish the continuity of the medullary canal by removing the sclerotic bone and to facilitate healing of the fracture by inserting an inlay bone graft taken from the proximal or distal tibia.

DISTAL FIFTH METATARSAL FRACTURE

Spiral fractures of the distal fifth metatarsal are common and occur frequently in dancers and professional athletes. The mechanism of injury has been reported to be rotational, with rolling over on the outer border of the foot while standing on the ball of the foot with the ankle fully plantarflexed (demi pointe position). A study of dancers with this injury treated both operatively and nonoperatively found that, even in displaced fractures, cast immobilization or symptomatic treatment with bandaging and full weight bearing had no long-term consequences. They reported one delayed union and one refracture, both of which subsequently healed. All of the ballet dancers returned to professional performance without limitations, and no patient reported pain with performance at follow-up. Good functional outcomes also can be obtained with nonoperative treatment of these fractures in nondancers. Aynardi et al. showed only two painful nonunions that required later open treatment with bone grafting and fixation in 142 acute fractures managed nonoperatively.

STRESS FRACTURES OF THE METATARSALS

A variety of factors lead to the development of stress fractures of the metatarsals. They occur most commonly in women, especially during the early years of menopause in the phase of rapid bone resorption. Postmenopausal women often are counseled to begin weight-bearing exercises to diminish loss of bone mass. Stress fractures also have been noted to occur in athletes, especially ballet dancers and athletes engaged in cutting and jumping sports; amenorrheic female athletes are of particular concern. Military recruits in their first few weeks of training also are vulnerable to so-called march fractures. Individuals with diabetes and sensory and motor neuropathy, rheumatoid arthritis, Charcot-Marie-Tooth disease, or stroke may be at risk as well.

Patients often note the gradual onset of pain directly over the second metatarsal neck region 2 to 4 weeks after beginning a running or aerobics program. Swelling over the area usually is noted. The diagnosis is suspected on history and physical examination. Initial radiographs made within 2 weeks after the onset of symptoms may be negative, and bone scan or MRI may assist in the diagnosis in questionable cases. Generally, repeat radiographs at 4 to 6 weeks after injury reveal periosteal new bone formation. Differential diagnoses include entrapment neuritis of the superficial peroneal nerve, radiating pain from a more proximal tarsometatarsal joint arthrosis, and idiopathic or overuse synovitis of the adjacent metatarsophalangeal joint.

A subset of fractures that can be especially difficult to manage are stress fractures of the proximal second

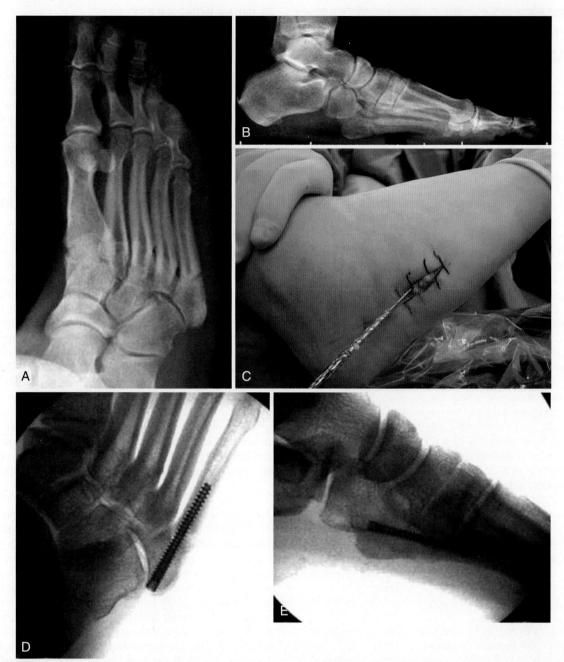

FIGURE 9.86 **A** and **B,** Fifth metatarsal fracture. **C,** Percutaneous screw insertion. **D** and **E,** After fixation. **SEE TECHNIQUE 9.15.**

metatarsal. In a study of ballet dancers with a stress fracture at the base of the second metatarsal, conservative management with relative rest and boot or cast immobilization resulted in resolution of symptoms. Another study had a 50% nonunion rate in nondancers treated nonoperatively who were successfully treated with surgical fixation. It is important to inform the patient that a stress fracture at the second metatarsal occasionally may result in a slight dorsiflexion malunion and transfer of weight to the third metatarsal, which is at risk for the development of a stress fracture. Surgical intervention rarely is required for stress fractures; however, open reduction and plating may be required if there is a nonunion or if significant bony healing has occurred in a malunion (Fig. 9.87A and B).

OPEN REDUCTION AND PLATING OF LESSER METATARSAL STRESS FRACTURE

TECHNIQUE 9.16

- After regional or general anesthesia, place an ankle tourniquet.
- Make a longitudinal incision over the fractured metatarsal. Identify and protect the dorsal medial (superficial

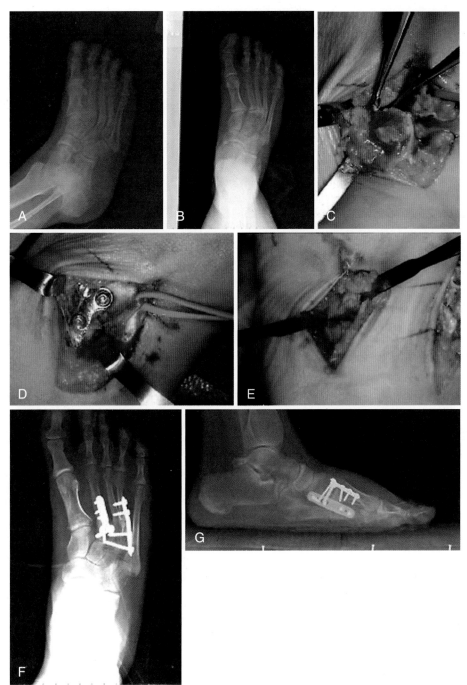

FIGURE 9.87 **A** and **B,** Preoperative oblique and anteroposterior radiographs of lesser metatarsals. **C,** Curettage and preparation of second metatarsal. Note vessel loop around dorsalis pedis and deep peroneal nerve. **D,** Plating of second metatarsal. **E,** Exposure of fourth metatarsal. **F** and **G,** Postoperative anteroposterior and lateral radiographs. (From Murphy GA: Operative treatment of stress fractures of the metatarsals, *Op Tech Sports Med* 14:239, 2006.) **SEE TECHNIQUE 9.16.**

peroneal), dorsal intermediate (superficial peroneal), and dorsal lateral (sural) nerves. For fractures at the base of the second metatarsal, avoid injury to the deep peroneal nerve and dorsalis pedis artery, which lie just medial to the metatarsal.

■ Gently elevate the periosteum and expose the fracture. Use a small curet to remove fibrous tissue if present. Prepare and "freshen" the fracture with a small drill bit (Fig. 9.87C).

■ If bone graft is to be used, pack it into the fracture at this point. Bone graft (3 to 5 cm²) can be obtained from the calcaneus or the distal tibia.

■ Use a small fragment plate for fixation (Fig. 9.87D). When selecting an implant system, choose a low-profile design. Locking plates generally are not required. Although contouring of the plate is unnecessary for the second and third metatarsals, some contouring may be required for fractures

of the fourth or fifth metatarsals, especially if metatarsus adductus is present (Fig. 9.87E). Four cortices of purchase on each side of the metatarsal are ideal (Fig. 9.87F and G).
■ Close the periosteum over the plate and bone if possible. Close the skin with a few subcutaneous 3-0 or 4-0 nylon sutures.

POSTOPERATIVE CARE A well-padded cast or splint is applied over a sterile dressing and sutures are removed at 10 to 14 days. Weight bearing is allowed depending on perceived fracture stability. Pulsing electromagnetic field or ultrasound may be used for high-risk fractures, such as fractures in the base of the fourth or fifth metatarsal and fractures in patients who smoke or have systemic illnesses.

■ COMPLICATIONS

The most frequent complication of open reduction and plating is painful, prominent implants. Generally, this should not be removed earlier than 1 year after surgery, and the mechanical issues that contributed to the fracture in the first place should be treated. Nonunion despite adequate fixation may occur, and if it does, care should be taken to treat all reasons for the nonunion (smoking, poor nutrition [especially vitamin D deficiency], improper footwear, and improper orthotic management).

ACUTE FRACTURES OF THE METATARSALS

Relatively few articles in the literature have addressed fractures of the metatarsals. Because the first metatarsal supports one third of the weight-bearing forces across the forefoot, operative treatment should be considered if there is significant displacement. Because of the potential prominence of implants placed dorsally, medial fixation may be considered. Minimally displaced lesser metatarsal fractures are usually treated nonoperatively and may do better with an elasticized bandage than a short leg weight-bearing cast. Although these fractures generally do well with nonoperative treatment, outcome scores are negatively correlated with increased body mass index and are lower in females, patients with diabetes, and those with fractures with more than 2 mm of displacement. For high-energy fractures of the central metatarsals, treated operatively and nonoperatively, only 32% of patients obtain a good result regardless of the type of treatment. Factors cited as contributing to the poor outcome include sagittal plane displacement, open fracture, and severe soft-tissue injury. It has been our experience that mild lateral plane displacement may be tolerated; however, sagittal plane displacement of a metatarsal head either in extension or plantarflexion or excessive shortening of a metatarsal leads to metatarsalgia and chronic forefoot pain. For this reason, closed reduction and percutaneous pinning from a dorsal approach is recommended. Occasionally, the displacement is severe enough to require ORIF (Fig. 9.88). Care must be taken to realign the metatarsal in the sagittal plane, and this assessment is done primarily while palpating the levels of the metatarsal heads to ensure they are in the same plane. Bryant et al. showed good outcomes with plate fixation of 75 metatarsal fractures with no implant removals.

PHALANGEAL DISLOCATIONS
INTERPHALANGEAL JOINT OF THE HALLUX

Dislocation of the interphalangeal joint of the hallux usually is caused by hyperextension, with the distal phalanx positioned dorsal to the proximal phalanx. Tearing of the plantar skin at the interphalangeal joint flexion crease is common, rendering this an open injury. Most of these dislocations can be reduced closed. If the dislocation is irreducible, two obstacles to reduction may be present: a sesamoid bone or the plantar plate of the interphalangeal joint may be interposed. The FHL also can be displaced into the joint but generally is not the primary deterrent to reduction. Finally, at least one collateral ligament (usually the medial) may be torn.

Two types of interphalangeal dislocations of the hallux have been identified. In the first, the plantar plate, ruptured from one or both of its phalangeal attachments (usually proximally), is trapped within the joint; the interphalangeal joint space is widened (Fig. 9.89), and the deformity is minimal, even deceiving. In the second, more common, type, the distal phalanx lies dorsal to the proximal phalanx, locking the joint in hyperextension. The deformity is obvious. The sesamoid bone within the plantar plate prevents reduction (Fig. 9.90).

Closed reduction under digital block should be attempted. The dislocation can be reduced easily if one or more collateral ligaments are torn and there is no interposition of a sesamoid or plantar plate. Longitudinal traction is applied first in the axial plane of the deformity, followed by flexion when the distal phalanx is level with the articular surface of the proximal phalanx. If the radiograph after reduction shows widening of the joint space, the plantar plate still may be interposed and open reduction is indicated.

Although it has been our experience that interphalangeal joint dislocations of the lesser toes are reducible by closed methods and do well with buddy taping to the adjacent toe for 3 weeks, one study reported that nearly all dislocated lesser toe interphalangeal joints in their study required an open reduction. Approximately 30% of dislocated lesser toe metatarsophalangeal joints required open reduction because they were not reducible by closed means. Lesser toe interphalangeal joints that were reduced were virtually asymptomatic at follow-up; however, residual dislocations at the metatarsophalangeal joints were persistently painful. In most of their patients, the plantar plate prevented closed treatment by being incarcerated within the joint. These injuries can be reduced through a dorsal midline incision. Open reduction is performed for irreducible dislocations or if joint space widening is obvious on radiographs after closed reduction, even if the toe rests in the proper position clinically (Fig. 9.91).

OPEN REDUCTION OF DISLOCATION OF THE INTERPHALANGEAL JOINTS OF THE HALLUX

TECHNIQUE 9.17

■ Make a dorsal inverted L-shaped incision with the transverse limb at the joint and the longitudinal limb dorsomedial. Preserve the extensor hallucis longus insertion into the distal phalanx.
■ On one side of the extensor hallucis longus, identify the plantar plate (identification is easier if the sesamoid is within it) and make a 3- to 4-mm longitudinal incision in it. Reduce the joint with traction.

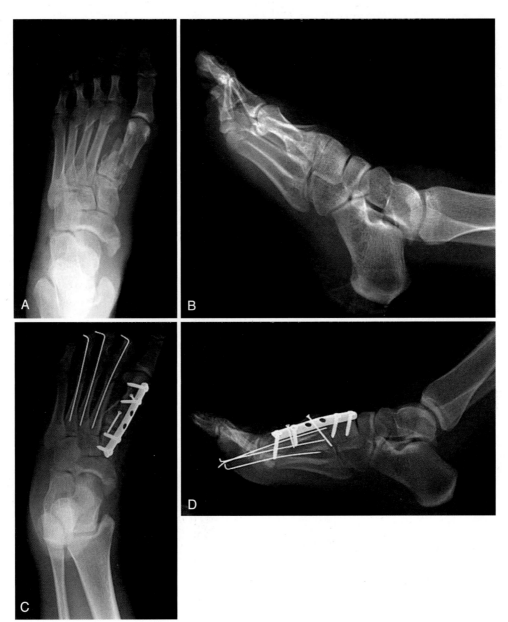

FIGURE 9.88   **A** and **B,** Displaced first metatarsal fracture and fractures of the second to fourth metatarsals. **C** and **D,** After plate and screw fixation of first metatarsal and Steinmann pin fixation of lesser metatarsals.

- If reduction cannot be accomplished, use a probe or small Freer elevator to displace the sesamoid and plantar plate distally while placing traction on the great toe.
- If the joint is stable, no transarticular pin is needed. If the reduction is unstable, hold the joint reduced and drill one or two 0.062-inch Kirschner wires longitudinally distal to proximal to rest in subchondral bone at the base of the proximal phalanx.
- Cut the wires off 2 mm outside the skin and apply a well-padded short leg cast extending past the toes.

POSTOPERATIVE CARE   The patient is instructed to rest and elevate the extremity for 3 days and then to begin partial weight bearing with crutches. At 3 weeks, the wires are removed and weight-bearing to tolerance is allowed in a postoperative wooden-soled shoe. Active and active-assisted range of motion of the interphalangeal joint is begun at that time. At 6 weeks, wearing of a shoe with a wide toe box is allowed.

Marginal wound necrosis and prolonged swelling of the toe are common; however, with rest, elevation, reduction of edema, and time, these are not alarming problems. Some permanent limitation of interphalangeal joint motion is common after this injury. Initial radiographs should be reviewed carefully because other injuries to the forefoot are common.

FIRST METATARSOPHALANGEAL JOINT DISLOCATION

Dislocation of the first metatarsophalangeal joint is rare. The mechanism of injury is hyperextension of the great toe,

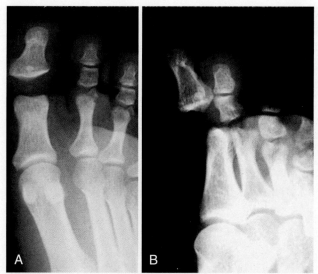

FIGURE 9.89   **A,** Anteroposterior radiograph shows marked widening of interphalangeal joint. **B,** Lateral view shows wide joint space; distal phalanx is not hyperextended. (From Miki T, Yamamuro T, Kitai T: An irreducible dislocation of the great toe: report of two cases and review of the literature, *Clin Orthop Relat Res* 230:200, 1988.)

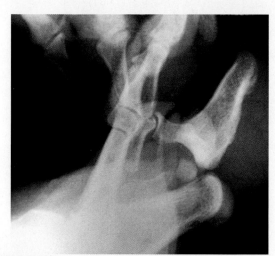

FIGURE 9.90   Anteroposterior radiograph shows overlapping of proximal phalangeal head and distal phalangeal base. (From Miki T, Yamamuro T, Kitai T: An irreducible dislocation of the great toe: report of two cases and review of the literature, *Clin Orthop Relat Res* 230:200, 1988.)

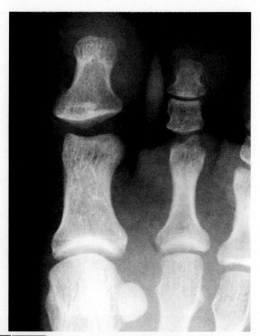

FIGURE 9.91   Interphalangeal joint space remains wider than normal after closed reduction; this is indication for open reduction. (From Miki T, Yamamuro T, Kitai T: An irreducible dislocation of the great toe: report of two cases and review of the literature, *Clin Orthop Relat Res* 230:200, 1988.)

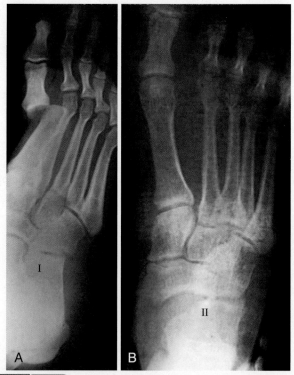

FIGURE 9.92   Dorsomedial dislocation of first metatarsophalangeal joint. **A,** Dislocation could not be reduced by closed means. **B,** After open reduction, joint was stable.

causing displacement of the proximal phalanx onto the dorsum of the first metatarsal head and neck (Fig. 9.92). The head of the first metatarsal becomes trapped between the flexor hallucis brevis and abductor hallucis tendons medially and the lateral head of the flexor hallucis brevis and adductor tendons laterally. Dorsally, the metatarsal head is held by the plantar plate and the deep transverse metatarsal ligament. On the plantar surface, the plantar aponeurosis prevents further reduction. The FHL tendon usually lies lateral to the metatarsal head. Type I dislocations are those in which the intersesamoid ligament is intact but displaced dorsally over the metatarsal neck, making this irreducible by closed means; in type IIA injuries, the intersesamoid ligament is ruptured, causing widening of the sesamoids; in type IIB injuries, the

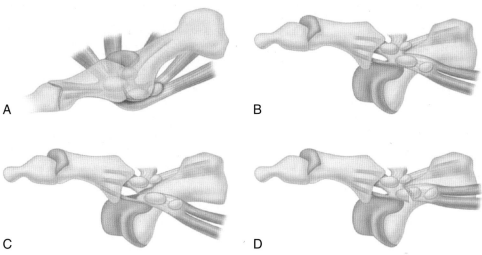

FIGURE 9.93 **A,** Normal anatomy of first metatarsophalangeal joint. **B,** Type I dislocation. **C,** Type IIA dislocation. **D,** Type IIB dislocation.

intersesamoid ligament is intact but there is a sesamoid fracture, usually of the tibial sesamoid, and the distal fragment is pulled distally (Fig. 9.93).

In a report of 11 complex dislocations of the metatarsophalangeal joints, tarsometatarsal joint injuries frequently were present, and more than half of the injuries were open dislocations that required open debridement and relocation. One closed injury required open reduction, but the remaining five were reduced by closed methods. One recurrent dislocation was noted in a patient who went back to jogging too soon. All patients except one complained of decreased metatarsophalangeal joint motion, however, not to the extent of significantly reducing endurance to work or exercise. Many patients had plantar sensitivities; four required the use of a full-time orthosis.

According to Jahss, closed reduction usually is impossible in dorsal dislocations of the great toe in which the intersesamoid ligament is not disrupted. If this ligament is torn with wide separation of the tibial and fibular sesamoids, or if one of the sesamoids is fractured transversely, the dislocation frequently can be reduced closed. We recommend a midline medial approach.

OPEN REDUCTION OF FIRST METATARSOPHALANGEAL JOINT DISLOCATION USING A MIDLINE MEDIAL APPROACH

TECHNIQUE 9.18

- Make a medial longitudinal incision on the great toe about 5 cm long centered over the first metatarsophalangeal joint. Use sharp dissection through the skin only to avoid injuring any displaced cutaneous nerves.
- Elevate the dorsal flap in the same manner as in hallux valgus repair and assess the magnitude of injury to the collateral ligaments, the plantar plate with the enclosed sesamoids, and the dorsal capsule.
- Use a small Freer or periosteal elevator while hyperextending the great toe and applying traction and guide the base of the proximal phalanx over the metatarsal head and into the reduced position.
- Repair the collateral ligament (usually the medial collateral) and dorsal capsule with absorbable sutures.
- Assess the stability of the metatarsophalangeal joint by gentle flexion and extension and by flexing and extending the ankle to produce a pull on the long flexor tendons.
- If the reduction appears unstable, drill a small Kirschner wire across the joint to maintain reduction. It should be removed 3 weeks after surgery.
- Remove the tourniquet, secure hemostasis, and close the skin with nonabsorbable, interrupted sutures.

POSTOPERATIVE CARE Apply a short leg cast that extends distal to the toes over a bulky forefoot dressing that has been applied to hold the toe congruously on the metatarsal head and in 10 to 15 degrees of extension. Partial weight bearing with crutches is allowed during the first 3 weeks, after which time the cast is removed and full weight bearing is allowed while wearing a shoe with a wide toe box. Active and active-assisted range of motion of the first metatarsophalangeal joint is begun, and a toe spacer in the first web space is used for another 3 weeks. Permanent reduction in range of motion of the first metatarsophalangeal joint can be expected, but functional motion should be regained after several months.

FIRST METATARSOPHALANGEAL JOINT SPRAIN

If the hyperextension force at the first metatarsophalangeal joint is not enough to cause a dislocation, it may result in a sprain of that joint, also known as turf toe. It often is an athletic injury and occurs with an axial load to a dorsiflexed forefoot (Fig. 9.94). Turf toe is classified as grade 1—minimal stretch, plantar/medial tenderness, no ecchymosis, and

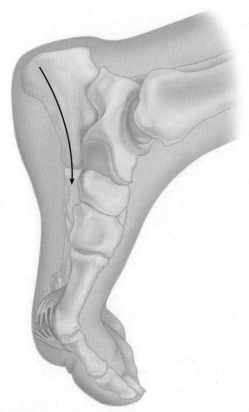

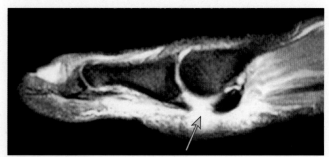

FIGURE 9.95   Sagittal fast-spin-echo MRI of elite athlete with clinically suspected turf toe demonstrates disruption of plantar plate *(arrow)* and full-thickness cartilage loss over first metatarsal head. (From McCormick JJ, Anderson RB: The great toe: failed turf toe, chronic turf toe, and complicated sesamoid injuries, *Foot Ankle Clin* 14:135, 2009.)

Follow-up after turf toe injuries has shown that 50% of patients continue to experience some pain and stiffness. In a study of 19 patients, 9 of whom were treated operatively, all but 2 returned to full athletic activities.

FIGURE 9.94   Turf toe injury occurs with an axial load to dorsiflexed forefoot.

minimal restriction of range of motion of the joint; grade 2—partial tear of the plantar plate, with swelling and ecchymosis and restriction of range of motion, and patient walks with a limp; or grade 3—complete tear of the plantar plate that may be associated with a sesamoid fracture or diastasis of a bipartite sesamoid, and patient is unable to bear weight. Radiographs may show an avulsion fracture of the proximal phalanx, an impacted fracture of the metatarsal, or a sesamoid fracture. There also may be proximal migration of the sesamoids, which is easier to detect when compared with radiographs of the uninjured foot. Examination of the joint under fluoroscopy may demonstrate lack of migration of the sesamoids when the joint is dorsiflexed, suggestive of plantar plate rupture, especially when compared with the contralateral side. A cadaver study suggests that when measuring the distance from the distal margin of the sesamoids to the most proximal margin of the proximal phalanx on a lateral dorsiflexion stress view, a 3-mm difference when compared with the contralateral foot may be indicative of injury to three of the four ligaments of the plantar plate complex. MRI may demonstrate rupture of the plantar plate (Fig. 9.95). Grade 1 and 2 injuries usually are treated nonoperatively, with initial rest, followed by mobilization of the joint and protection with a full-length rigid carbon plate. If the patient's symptoms persist, further workup should be done to exclude other conditions, such as an osteochondral lesion of the metatarsal head, loose body, sesamoid fracture, or plantar plate rupture. Grade 3 injuries are initially treated with cast or boot immobilization and rarely may require operative treatment to repair the plantar plate.

PLANTAR PLATE REPAIR (ANDERSON)

TECHNIQUE 9.19

- Make medial and plantar-lateral incisions for full access to the plantar plate (Fig. 9.96A).
- On the medial side, identify and protect the plantar-medial nerve (Fig. 9.96B), while deeper dissection exposes the plantar plate rupture.
- With the plantar-lateral incision, take care to avoid injury to the common plantar digital nerve and the branch to the great toe.
- Expose the defect in the plantar plate.
- Through both incisions, pass sutures to repair the capsule and then tie them with the toe in 15 degrees of plantarflexion (Fig. 9.97A to C). If there is not enough tissue present on the proximal phalanx for a direct repair, suture anchors or bone tunnels may be needed.
- If there is a sesamoid fracture or diastasis of a bipartite sesamoid, partial or complete sesamoidectomy may be needed. Repair the soft-tissue defect, and if the defect is too large for direct repair, transfer of the abductor hallucis can be done.

POSTOPERATIVE CARE The toe is immobilized in 5 to 10 degrees of plantarflexion, and the patient is non–weight bearing. Careful joint mobilization, avoiding excessive dorsiflexion, can be started at 1 week in a reliable patient. Weight bearing can be initiated at 4 weeks in a boot, with further careful joint mobilization. Approximately 1 month later, the patient can be weaned from the boot into a shoe with a full-length rigid carbon plate. Full recovery may take 6 to 12 months.

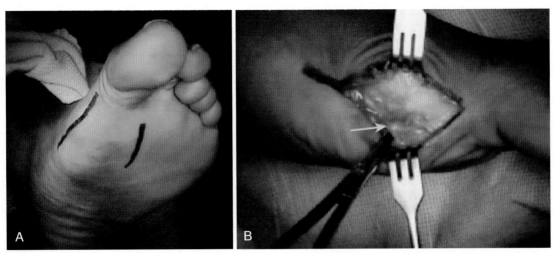

FIGURE 9.96 Open repair of turf toe injury. **A**, Placement of incisions. **B**, Medial exposure with arrow identifying the plantar-medial digital nerve. (From McCormick JJ, Anderson RB: The great toe: failed turf toe, chronic turf toe, and complicated sesamoid injuries, *Foot Ankle Clin N Am* 14:135, 2009.) **SEE TECHNIQUE 9.19.**

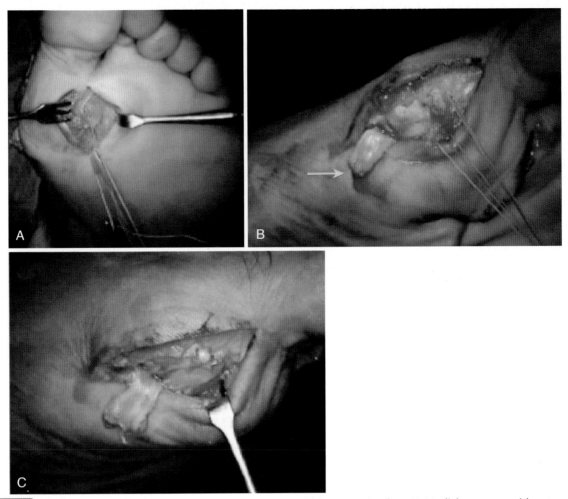

FIGURE 9.97 Open repair of turf toe injury. **A**, Lateral exposure with sutures in place. **B**, Medial exposure with sutures in place. Arrow points to the abductor hallucis tendon, which was avulsed in this patient. **C**, Medial view with sutures tied (three knots are visible). (From McCormick JJ, Anderson RB: The great toe: failed turf toe, chronic turf toe, and complicated sesamoid injuries, *Foot Ankle Clin N Am* 14:135, 2009.) **SEE TECHNIQUE 9.19.**

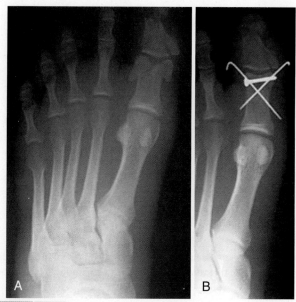

FIGURE 9.98   Phalangeal fracture. Preoperative **(A)** and post-operative **(B)** radiographs.

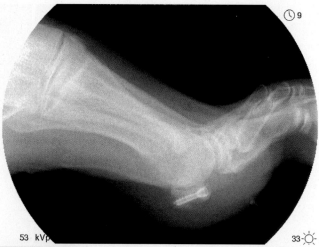

FIGURE 9.99   Mini-fragment screw fixation of sesamoid fracture (see text). (From Pagenstret GI, Valderrabano V, Hintermann B: Internal fixation of the sesamoid bone of the hallux. In Pfeffer G, Easley M, Frey C, et al, editors: *Operative techniques: foot and ankle surgery,* Philadelphia, 2009, Saunders.)

PHALANGEAL FRACTURES

Surgical treatment of phalangeal fractures of the toes is rarely required because most phalangeal fractures can be treated successfully by conservative measures. Occasionally, an intraarticular fracture severely displaced into the interphalangeal or metatarsophalangeal joint of the great toe may require ORIF to prevent deformity and arthritic changes. The fracture and the joint are exposed, the fracture is reduced anatomically, and, with a power drill, small 0.045-inch Kirschner wires are inserted for internal fixation (Fig. 9.98). These pins are bent and left outside the skin and generally removed 3 to 4 weeks after surgery when the fracture has stabilized. Alternatively, mini-fragment screws may be used for fixation. No cast is required, and protected weight bearing can begin as soon as soft-tissue healing permits.

SESAMOID FRACTURES

Fractures of the hallucal sesamoids most often are seen in an acute setting with dislocations of the metatarsophalangeal joint after high-energy injuries. Chronic stress fractures of the sesamoids, most commonly seen in long-distance runners and ballet dancers, can be difficult to diagnose and differentiate from other conditions affecting the hallucal sesamoids. The medial or tibial sesamoid is the more commonly injured sesamoid because it generally is larger than the fibular sesamoid and is seated more directly beneath the metatarsal head. The sesamoids are reported to be multipartite in 5% to 30% of asymptomatic individuals. Although the bipartite sesamoid can be bilateral, a singular sesamoid in the contralateral foot does not absolutely confirm the presence of fracture and can represent symptomatic synchondrosis of the bipartite sesamoid in an injured foot. Fractures and the bipartite condition occur more frequently in the tibial sesamoid.

Two features might distinguish a fracture from a bipartite sesamoid. Fractured sesamoid bones tend to be roughly divided into equally sized sections; bipartite sesamoids tend to have one larger fragment and one smaller fragment. Bipartite sesamoids tend to have smooth, rounded edges; fractured sesamoids tend to have irregular, jagged edges. Simple separation of a synchondrosis of a bipartite sesamoid may have symptoms similar to

a fractured sesamoid. If the fracture is not widely displaced, the differential diagnosis of a fractured sesamoid includes a painful bipartite sesamoid, osteochondritis dissecans, and osteonecrosis of the sesamoid.

The mechanism of injury to the sesamoids can be either direct, which generally involves an axial loading force on the sesamoid and produces a comminuted multifragmented bone, or indirect, in which the first metatarsophalangeal joint is hyperextended violently, as can be seen most commonly in football and soccer players. Physical examination usually shows tenderness and swelling in the region of the sesamoid. Limited extension of the great toe and pain with passive extension of the great toe usually are present. The patient may have a shortened stance phase of gait and usually descends stairs with the injured foot leading. Radiographic evaluation should include standard anteroposterior and lateral views along with other specialized views. The forefoot should be in slight pronation while obtaining a lateral radiograph to profile the sesamoids. The medial oblique sesamoid view is helpful in evaluating the tibial sesamoid, and the lateral oblique view is helpful in evaluating the fibular sesamoid. In addition, the axial sesamoid view can be helpful in showing sclerosis and joint space narrowing associated with osteochondritis of the sesamoid. MRI or CT scans can be of assistance. Radionuclide bone scanning can be used in confirming the diagnosis; however, caution is recommended in interpreting increased bone scan activity because a significant percentage (26% to 29%) of asymptomatic individuals had some increased activity and because the difference between one foot and the other was significant.

TREATMENT

Widely displaced tibial or fibular sesamoid fractures generally are associated with either dislocation or traumatic subluxation with spontaneous reduction of the metatarsophalangeal joint. Disruption of the flexor brevis musculotendinous unit with wide displacement of the sesamoid is not tolerated well by patients. If the sesamoid fragments are of roughly equal size and the displacement is significant (>5 mm), open reduction with internal fixation using the approach described subsequently is necessary. Internal fixation generally involves mini-fragment screws (Fig. 9.99) or use of an 18-gauge wire looped around the proximal and distal poles and placed in a figure-of-eight over the sesamoid. Bone grafting from the calcaneus or the supramalleolar area of the distal tibia may be helpful in achieving union.

Minimally displaced or nondisplaced fractures of the sesamoid and stress fractures can be treated initially with cast immobilization, incorporating a toe plate for 3 to 4 weeks. Repeat casting for another 3 to 4 weeks may be necessary if symptoms have not resolved. After this, the toe is protected by placing a full-length rigid carbon plate and an orthotic with a dancer's pad in an athletic shoe. Patients who do not respond to this treatment are candidates for operative treatment of the sesamoid. The following options are available for surgical treatment: (1) complete excision of the sesamoid, (2) partial excision of a painful bipartite sesamoid or nonunion of a sesamoid fracture, and (3) cancellous bone grafting to promote union. Although traditionally we have excised the involved sesamoid after failure of conservative treatment, the tibial sesamoid has a significant function in increasing the lever arm and action of the flexor hallucis brevis muscle and in protecting the FHL tendon.

We have been gaining experience with excising the smaller fragment of a painful bipartite sesamoid or trying to preserve most of the sesamoid with a nonunion. If a partial sesamoid excision is done, the patient should be informed preoperatively that the remaining sesamoid fragment may need to be excised as well. Repairing the flexor hallucis brevis mechanism is crucial regardless of which treatment method is chosen. In one report, all patients returned to sports after excision of the proximal pole of the sesamoid. Indications for complete sesamoidectomy are comminuted fractures with no large fragments and the loss of articulating cartilage, either on the articular side of the sesamoid or on the overlying surface of the metatarsal head.

In a review of sesamoidectomies in athletically active patients, athletes were able to return to sports at a mean time of 7.5 weeks and the remainder of "active" patients returned to activity at 12 weeks. Complications included hallux varus in one and postoperative scarring with neuroma-like symptoms in two patients after fibular sesamoidectomy. Hallux valgus deformity developed late in one patient after tibial sesamoidectomy. In another report on tibial sesamoidectomies, 90% of patients returned to preoperative activity levels, and there were no cases of hallux varus or valgus, which was attributed to careful soft-tissue repair. In a more recent report, 22 of 24 patients returned to activities after sesamoidectomy; 1 patient developed hallux valgus.

SESAMOIDECTOMY

TECHNIQUE 9.20

- Make a medial longitudinal incision centered just plantar to midline and incise the capsule longitudinally in line with the skin.
- Evaluate the intraarticular portion of the tibial sesamoid for the quality of the cartilage and mobility of the fragments.
- Examine the plantar surface of the metatarsal head for cartilage damage.

- Approach the sesamoid through an extracapsular approach. Protect the proper medial plantar nerve to the hallux, which emerges plantarly at the musculotendinous junction of the abductor hallucis muscle.
- Retract this nerve plantarly.
- Make an incision over the sesamoid and perform either a complete sesamoidectomy or a partial sesamoidectomy.
- Repair the flexor brevis defect using 2-0 nonabsorbable polyethylene suture. If a portion of the sesamoid is left, use suture or a mini-suture anchor to secure the flexor hallucis brevis tendon to the cancellous surface of the remaining sesamoid fragment.
- Repair the capsule with 2-0 absorbable sutures and close the skin with nylon.

POSTOPERATIVE CARE A short leg cast with a toe plate is applied over a bulky dressing. Weight bearing is delayed for 2 to 3 weeks, followed by weight bearing in a walking brace. Range-of-motion exercises are performed at 2 to 3 weeks, and the resumption of light jogging is allowed at 8 weeks.

Anderson and McBryde reported their experience with autogenous bone grafting for nonunions of the hallux sesamoid in 21 patients. They reported successful bony union in all but two patients, and most patients obtained pain relief and returned to their preinjury level of activity. These authors advocated bone grafting as opposed to sesamoid excision in select patients.

BONE GRAFTING OF SESAMOID NONUNION

TECHNIQUE 9.21

(ANDERSON AND MCBRYDE)
- Make a 5-cm longitudinal skin incision along the medial plantar aspect of the first ray centered in the metatarsophalangeal joint. Identify the capsule and abductor hallucis tendon and subsequently divide them in line with the skin incision, entering the joint dorsal to the tibial hallucal sesamoid.
- Use retraction to expose the articular surface of each sesamoid.
- Excision is justified when severe cartilaginous destruction is present.
- If the surface is intact, as is usually the case, proceed with bone grafting through an extraarticular approach.
- Through the same skin incision, dissect plantar to the abductor hallucis tendon for extraarticular exposure of the tibial sesamoid. Avoid injury to the plantar digital nerve.
- After sharp periosteal elevation, identify the nonunion within the midportion of the sesamoid. Gross motion at the nonunion site may be seen.
- Avoiding disruption of the articular surface, curet fibrous and necrotic tissue with a small dental curet.

- Pack the defect with autogenous bone graft, harvested locally through a cortical window in the medial eminence of the first metatarsal head. As a result of the tendinous expansion that surrounds the sesamoid, the proximal and distal fragments remain in close apposition.
- Approximate the periosteal layers and close the wound with an absorbable suture.

POSTOPERATIVE CARE The patient is placed immediately into a short leg plaster splint, rendering the entire hallux immobile. The patient remains non–weight bearing for 3 to 4 weeks, at which time a short leg walking cast is applied, again immobilizing the hallux. The cast is removed at 8 weeks. A soft medial longitudinal arch support is prescribed and used in conjunction with a firm-soled shoe. Active exercises are initiated, followed by gentle passive range of motion if symptoms permit.

OSTEOCHONDRITIS OF THE SESAMOID

Osteochondritis of the sesamoid is characterized by a deformed sesamoid with irregular areas of increased bone density modeling a fragmentation. This may be apparent on an axial radiograph or a CT scan of the sesamoid. Although the exact cause is unknown, trauma probably is the most frequent cause. As in all sesamoid disorders, nonsurgical treatment consisting of a well under the sesamoid or a dancer's pad and full-length rigid carbon plate should be used before sesamoidectomy is recommended.

OTHER CONDITIONS OF THE SESAMOID

Other conditions associated with sesamoids include sesamoiditis, which is a poorly understood and fairly vague diagnosis. Surgical treatment should be delayed until all conservative measures have been exhausted. Arthritis, intractable plantar keratoses, and nerve impingement also may affect the sesamoid.

REFERENCES

CALCANEUS

Agren PH, Wretenberg P, Sayed-Noor AS: Operative versus nonoperative treatment of displaced intra-articular calcaneal fractures: a prospective, randomized, controlled multicenter trial, *J Bone Joint Surg* 95A:1351, 2013.

Ahn J, Kim TY, Kim TW, et al.: Learning curve for open reduction and internal fixation of displaced intra-articular calcaneal fracture by extensile lateral approach using the cumulative summation control chart, *Foot Ankle Int* 40:1052, 2019.

Aly T: Management of valgus extra-articular calcaneus fracture malunions with a lateral opening wedge osteotomy, *J Foot Ankle Surg* 50:703, 2011.

Banerjee R, Chao J, Sadeghi C, et al.: Fractures of the calcaneal tuberosity treated with suture fixation through bone tunnels, *J Orthop Trauma* 25:685, 2011.

Beltran MJ, Collinge CA: Outcomes of high-grade open calcaneus fratures managed with open reduction via the medial wound and percutaneous wire fixation, *J Orthop Trauma* 26:662, 2012.

Berberian W, Sood A, Karanfilian B, et al.: Displacement of the sustentacular fragment in intra-articular calcaneal fractures, *J Bone Joint Surg* 95A:995, 2013.

Blake MH, Owen JR, Sanford TS, et al.: Biomechanical evaluation of a locking and nonlocking reconstruction plate in an osteoporotic calcaneal fracture model, *Foot Ankle Int* 32:432, 2011.

Brunner A, Müller J, Regazzoni P, Babst R: Open reduction and internal fixation of OTA C2-C4 fractures of the calcaneus with a triple-plate technique, *J Foot Ankle Surg* 51:299, 2012.

Buckley R, Leighton R, Sanders D, et al.: Open reduction and internal fixation compared with ORIF and primary subtalar arthrodesis for treatment of Sanders type IV calcaneal fractures: a randomized multicenter trial, *J Orthop Trauma* 28:577, 2014.

Chen I, Zhang G, Johng J, et al.: Comparison of percutaneous screw fixation and calcium sulfate cement grafting versus open treatment of displaced intra-articular calcaneal fractures, *Foot Ankle Int* 32:979, 2011.

De Groot R, Frima SJ, Schepers T, Roerdink WH: Complications following the extended lateral approach for calcaneal fractures do not influence mid- to longterm outcome, *Injury* 44:1596, 2013.

de Vroome SW, van der Linden FM: Cohort study on the percutaneous treatment of displaced intra-articular fractures of the calcaneus, *Foot Ankle Int* 35:156, 2014.

Dhillon MS, Ball K, Prabhakar S: Controversies in calcaneus fracture management: a systematic review of the literature, *Musculoskelet Surg* 95:171, 2011.

El-Hawary A, Kandil YR, Ahmed M, et al.: Distraction subtalar arthrodesis for calcaneal malunion: comparison of local *versus* iliac bone graft, *Bone Joint J* 101-B:596, 2019.

Epstein N, Chandran S, Chou L: Current concepts review: intra-articular fractures of the calcaneus, *Foot Ankle Int* 33:79, 2012.

Firoozabadi R, Kramer PA, Benirschke SK: Plantar medial wounds associated with calcaneal fractures, *Foot Ankle Int* 34:941, 2013.

Gaskill T, Schweitzer K, Nunley J: Comparison of surgical outcomes of intra-articular calcaneal fractures by age, *J Bone Joint Surg* 92A:2884, 2010.

Gotha HE, Zide JR: Current controversies in management of calcaneus fractures, *Orthop Clin N Am* 48:91, 2017.

Griffin D, Parsons N, Shaw E, et al.: Operative care did not benefit closed, displaced, intra-articular calcaneal fractures, *J Bone Joint Surg Am* 97:341, 2015.

Griffin D, Parsons N, Shaw E, et al.: Operative versus non-operative treatment for closed, displaced, intra-articular fractures of the calcaneus: randomised controlled trial, *BMJ* 349:g4483, 2014.

Hirschmann A, Walter WR, Alaia EF, et al.: Acute fracture of the anterior process of the calcaneus: does it herald a more advanced injury to Chopart joint? *AJR* 210:1123, 2018.

Illert T, Rammelt S, Drewes T, et al.: Stability of locking and non-locking plates in an osteoporotic calcaneal fracture model, *Foot Ankle Int* 32:307, 2011.

Jiménez-Almonte JH, King JD, Luo D, et al.: Classifications in brief: Sanders classification of intraarticular fractures of the calcaneus, *Clin Orthop Relat Res* 477:467, 2019.

Kikuchi C, Charlton TP, Thordarson DB: Limited sinus tarsi approach for intra-articular calcaneus fractures, *Foot Ankle Int* 34:1689, 2013.

Kinner B, Tetz S, Müller F, et al.: Outcome after complex trauma of the foot, *J Trauma* 70:159, 2011.

Kline AJ, Anderson RB, Davis WH, et al.: Minimally invasive technique versus an extensile lateral approach for intra-articular calcaneal fractures, *Foot Ankle Int* 34:773, 2013.

Kwon JY, Diwan A, Susarla S: Effect of surgeon training, fracture, and patient variables on calcaneal fracture management, *Foot Ankle Int* 32:262, 2011.

Li S: Wound and sural nerve complilcations of the sinus tarsi approach for calcaneus fractures, *Foot Ankle Int* 39:1106, 2018.

López-Oliva F, Forriol F, Sánchez-Lorente T, Sanz YA: Treatment of severe fractures of the calcaneus by reconstruction arthrodesis using the Vira system: prospective study of the first 37 caes with over 1 year follow-up, *Injury* 41:804, 2010.

Mehta S, Mirza AJ, Dunbar RP, et al.: A staged treatment plan for the management of type II and type IIIA open calcaneus fractures, *J Orthop Trauma* 24:142, 2010.

Nosewicz T, Knupp M, Barg A, et al.: Mini-open sinus tarsi approach with percutaneous screw fixation of displaced calcaneal fractures: a prospective computed tomography-based study, *Foot Ankle Int* 33:925, 2012.

Park YH, Lee JW, Hong JY, et al.: Predictors of compartment syndrome of the foot after fracture of the calcaneus, *Bone Joint J* 100-B:303, 2018.

Phisitkul P, Sullivan JP, Goetz JE, Marsh JL: Maximizing safety in screw placement for posterior facet fixation in calcaneus fratures: a cadaveric radio-anatomical study, *Foot Ankle Int* 34:1279, 2013.

Pitts CC, Almaguer A, Wilson JT, et al.: Radiographic and postoperative outcomes of plate versus screw constructs and open reduction and internal fixation of calcaneus fractures via the sinus tarsi, *Foot Ankle Int* 40:929, 2019.

Potenza V, Caterini R, Farsetti P, et al.: Primary subtalar arthrodesis for the treatment of comminuted intra-articular calcaneal fractures, *Injury* 41:702, 2010.

Rammelt S, Amlang M, Barthel S, et al.: Percutaneous treatment of less severe intraarticular calcaneal fractures, *Clin Orthop Relat Res* 468:983, 2010.

Roll C, Schirmbeck J, Müller F, et al.: Value of 3D reconstructions of CT scans for calcaneal fracture assessment, *Foot Ankle Int* 37:1211, 2016.

Romeson T, Biert J, Frolke JPM: Treatment of displaced intra-articular calcaneal fractures with closed reduction and percutaneous screw fixation, *J Bone Joint Surg* 93A:920, 2011.

Sanders R, Vaupel ZM, Erdogan M, Downes K: Operative treatment of displaced intraarticular calcaneal fractures: long-term (20-20 years) results in 108 fractures using a prognostic CT classification, *J Orthop Trauma* 28:551, 2014.

Schepers T: The sinus tarsi approach in displaced intra-articular calcaneal fractures: a systematic review, *Int Orthop* 35:697, 2011.

Schepers T, Backes M, Dingemans SA, et al.: Similar anatomical reduction and lower complication rates with the sinus tarsi approach compared with the extended lateral approach in displaced intra-articular calcaneal fractures, *J Orthop Trauma* 31:293, 2017.

Sivakumar BS, Wong P, Dick CG, et al.: Arthroscopic reduction and percutaneous fixation of selected calcaneus fractures: surgical technique and early results, *J Orthop Trauma* 28:569, 2014.

Song JH, Kang C, Hwang DS, et al.: Extended sinus tarsi approach for treatment of displaced intraarticular calcaneal fractures compared to extended lateral approach, *Foot Ankle Int* 40:167, 2019.

SooHoo NF, Garng E, Krenek L, Zingmond DS: Complication rates following operative treatment of calcaneus fractures, *Foot Ankle Surg* 17:233, 2011.

Tantavisut S, Phisitkul P, Westerlind BO, et al.: Percutaneous reduction and screw fixation of displaced intra-articular fractures of the calcaneus, *Foot Ankle Int* 38:367, 2017.

Tomesen T, Biert J, Frölke JP: Treatment of displaced intra-articular calcaneal fractures with closed reduction and percutaneous screw fixtiaon, *J Bone Joint Surg* 93A:920, 2011.

Toussaint RJ, Lin D, Ehrlichman LK, et al.: Peroneal tendon displacement accompanying intra-articular calcaneal fractures, *J Bone Joint Surg* 96A:310, 2014.

van Hoeve S, de Vos J, Verbruggen JPAM, et al.: Gait analysis and functional outcome after calcaneal fracture, *J Bone Joint Surg Am* 97:1879, 2015.

Wiersema B, Brokaw D, Weber T, et al.: Complications associated with open calcaneus fractures, *Foot Ankle Int* 32:1052, 2011.

Woon CY, Chong KW, Yeo W, et al.: Subtalar arthroscopy and fluoroscopy in percutaneous fixation of intra-articular calcaneal fractures: the best of both worlds, *J Trauma* 71:917, 2011.

TALUS

Abdelgaid SM, Ezzat FF: Percutaneous reduction and screw fixation of fracture neck talus, *Foot Ankle Surg* 18:219, 2012.

Anderson MR, Ketz JP, Flemister AS: Operative treatment of talar head fractures: surgical technique, *J Orthop Trauma* 32:e344, 2018.

Bellamy JL, Keeling JJ, Wenke J, Hsu JR: Does a longer delay in fixation of talus fractures cause osteonecrosis? *J Surg Orthop Adv* 20:34, 2011.

Buckwalter JA, Westermann R, Mooers B, et al.: Timing of surgical reduction and stabilization of talus fracture-dislocations, *Am J Orthop (Belle Mead NJ)* 46:E408, 2017.

Chen H, Liu W, Deng L, Song W: The prognostic value of the Hawkins sign and diagnostic value of MRi after talar neck fractures, *Foot Ankle Int* 35:1255, 2014.

Cody EA, Nunley JA: Vascularized pedicle graft for talar osteonecrosis, *Foot Ankle Clin N Am* 24:121, 2019.

Fernandez ML, Wade AM, Dabbah M, Juliano PJ: Talar neck fractures treated with closed reduction and percutaneous screw fixation: a case series, *Am J Orthop (Belle Mead NJ)* 40:72, 2011.

Fournier A, Barba N, Steiger V, et al.: Total talar fracture – long-term results of internal fixation of talar fractures. A multicentric study of 114 cases, *Orthop Traumatol Surg Res* 98(Suppl 4):S48, 2012.

Grear BJ: Review of talus fractures and surgical timing, *Orthop Clin N Am* 47:625, 2016.

Gross CE, Sershon RA, Frank JM, et al.: Treatment of osteonecrosis of the talus, *JBJS Reviews* 4:e2, 2016.

Hsu AR, Scolaro JA: Posteromedial approach for open reduction and internal fixation of talar process fractures, *Foot Ankle Int* 37:446, 2016.

Huang P, Lundgren M, Garapati R: Complete talar extrusion treated with an antibiotic cement spacer and staged femoral head allograft, *J Am Acad Orthop Surg* 26:e324, 2018.

Jungbluth P, Wild M, Hakimi M, et al.: Isolated subtalar dislocation, *J Bone Joint Surg* 92A:890, 2010.

Karampinas PK, Kavroudakis E, Polyzois V, et al.: Open talar dislocations without associated fractures, *Foot Ankle Surg* 20:100, 2014.

Lasanianos NG, Lyras DN, Mouzopoulos G, et al.: Early mobilization after uncomplicated medial subtalar dislocation provides successful functional results, *J Orthop Traumatol* 12:37, 2011.

Maceroli MA, Wong C, Sanders RW, et al.: Treatment of comminuted talar neck fractures with use of minifragment plating, *J Orthop Trauma* 30:572, 2016.

Maher MH, Chauhan A, Altman GT, et al.: The acute management and associated complication of major injuries of the talus, *JBJS Reviews* 5:e2, 2017.

Marsh JL: Percutaneous reduction, screw fixation, and calcium sulfate cement grafting was effective for displaced intra-articular calcaneal fractures, *J Bone Joint Surg Am* 94(10):941, 2012..

Miller AN, Prasarn ML, Dyke JP, et al.: Quantitative assessment of the vascularity of the talus with gadoinium-enhanced magnetic resonance imaging, *J Bone Joint Surg* 93A:1116, 2011.

Ohl X, Haeisvoure A, Hemery X, Dehoux E: Long-term follow-up after surgical treatment of talar fractures, *Int Orthop* 35:93, 2011.

Perera A, Baker JF, Lui DF, Stephens MM: The management and outcome of lateral process fracture of the talus, *Foot Ankle Surg* 16:15, 2010.

Prasarn ML, Miller AN, Dyke JP, et al.: Arterial anatomy of the talus: a cadaver and gadolinium-enhanced MRI study, *Foot Ankle Int* 31:987, 2010.

Rammelt S: Secondary correction of talar fractures: asking for trouble? *Foot Ankle Int* 33:359, 2012.

Rodemund C, Mattiassich G: Minimal invasive Therapie von intraartikulären Fersenbeinfrakturen, Referat Innovationen, www.researchgate.net.

Rodemond C, Krenn R, Kihm C, et al: Minimally infasive surgery for intra-articular calcaneus fractures: a 9-year single-center, retrospective stdy of a standardized technique using a 2-point distractor, *BMC Musculoskel Disord*, Revision under review Jul 2020.

Sultan AA, Mont MA: Core decompression and bone grafting for osteonecrosis of the talus: a critical analysis of the current evidence, *Foot Ankle Clin N Am* 24:107, 2019.

Suter T, Barg A, Knupp M, et al.: Surgical technique: talar neck osteotomy to lengthen the medial column after talar neck fracture, *Clin Orthop Relat Res* 471:1356, 2013.

Vallier HA: Fractures of the talus: state of the art, *J Orthop Truama* 29:385, 2015.

Valliier HA, Reichard SG, Boyd AJ, Moore TA: A new look at the Hawkins classification for talar neck fractures: which features of injury and treatment are predictive of osteonecrosis? *J Bone Joint Surg* 96A:192, 2014.

Vints W, Matricali G, Geusens E, et al.: Long-term outcome after operative management of talus fractures, *Foot Ankle Int* 39:1432, 2018.

Xue Y, Zhang H, Pei F, et al.: Treatment of displaced talar neck fractures using delayed procedures of plate fixtion through dual approaches, *Int Orthop* 38:149, 2014.

CHOPART/MIDFOOT

Ahmed S, Bolt B, McBryde A: Comparison of standard screw fixation versus suture button fixation in Lisfranc ligament injuries, *Foot Ankle Int* 31:892, 2010.

Alcelik I, Fenton C, Hannant G, et al.: A systematic review and meta-analysis of the treatment of acute lisfranc injuries: open reduction and internal fixation versus primary arthrodesis, *Foot Ankle Surg* 2019, [Epub ahead of print].

Benirschke SK, Meinberg EG, Anderson SA, et al.: Fractures and dislocations of the midfoot: lisfranc and Chopart injuries, *Instr Course Lect* 62:79, 2013.

Brin YS, Nyska M, Kish B: Lisfranc injury repair with the TightRope device: a short-term case series, *Foot Ankle Int* 31:624, 2010.

Buda M, Hagemeijer NC, Kink S, et al.: Effect of fixation type and bone graft on tarsometatarsal fusion, *Foot Ankle Int* 39:1394, 2018.

Buda M, Kink S, Stavenuiter R, et al.: Reoperation rate differences between open reduction internal fixation and primary arthrodesis of Lisfranc injuries, *Foot Ankle Int* 39:1089, 2018.

Cochran G, Renninger C, Tompane T, et al.: Primary arthrodesis versus open reduction and internal fixation for low-energy Lisfranc injuries in a young athletic population, *Foot Ankle Int* 38:957, 2017.

Coulibaly MO, Jones CB, Sietsema DL, Schildhauer TA: Results and complications of operative and non-operative navicular fracture treatment, *Injury* 46:1669, 2015.

Evans J, Beingessner DM, Agel J, Beirschke SK: Minifragment plate fixation of high-energy navicular body fractures, *Foot Ankle Int* 32:S485, 2011.

Fishman FG, Adams SB, Easley ME, Nunley 2nd JA: Vascularized pedicle bone grafting for nonunions of the tarsal navicular, *Foot Ankle Int* 33:734, 2012.

Guler F, Baz AB, Turan A, et al.: Isolated medial cuneiform fractures: report of two cases and review of the literature, *Foot Ankle Spec* 4:306, 2011.

Kadow TR, Siska PA, Evans AR, et al.: Staged treatment of high energy midfoot fracture dislocations, *Foot Ankle Int* 35:1287, 2014.

Kalia V, Fishman EK, Carrino JA, Fayad LM: Epidemiology, imaging, and treatment of Lisfranc fracture-dislocations revisited, *Skeletal Radiol* 41:129, 2012.

Kösters C, Bockholt S, Müller C, et al.: Comparing the outcomes between Chopart, Lisfranc and multiple metatarsal shaft fractures, *Arch Orthop Trauma Surg* 134:1397, 2014.

Marsland D, Belkoff SM, Solan MC: Biomechanical analysis of endobuttone versus screw fixation after Lisfranc ligament complex sectioning, *Foot Ankle Surg* 19:267, 2013.

McKeon KE, McCormick JJ, Johnsn JE, Klein SE: Intraosseous and extraosseous arterial anatomy of the adult naviculara, *Foot Ankle Int* 33:859, 2012.

Mora AD, Kao M, Alfred T, et al.: Return to sports and physical activities after open reduction and internal fixation of Lisfranc injuries in recreational athletes, *Foot Ankle Int* 38:801, 2018.

Nithyananth M, Boopalan PR, Titus VT, et al.: Long-term outcome of high-energy open Lisfranc injuries: a retrospective study, *J Trauma* 70:710, 2011.

Pelt CE, Bachus KN, Vance RE, Beals TC: A biomechanical analysis of a tensioned suture device in the fixataion of the ligamentous Lisfranc injury, *Foot Ankle Int* 32:422, 2011.

Porter DA, Barnes AF, Rund A, et al.: Injury pattern in ligamentous Lisfranc injuries in competitive athletes, *Foot Ankle Int* 40:185, 2019.

Purushothaman B, Robinson E, Lakshmanan P, Siddique M: Extra-articular fixation for treatment of Lisfranc injury, *Surg Technol Int* 19:199, 2010.

Reinhardt KR, Oh LS, Schottel P, et al.: Treatment of Lisfranc fracture-dislocations with primary partial arthrodesis, *Foot Ankle Int* 33:50, 2012.

Rosenbaum A, Dellenbaugh S, Dipreta J, Uhl R: Subtle injuries to the Lisfranc joint, *Orthopedics* 34:882, 2011.

Schepers T, Oprel PP, Van Lieshout EM: Influence of approach and implant on reduction accuracy and stability in Lisfrance fracture-dislocation at the tarsometatarsal joint, *Foot Ankle Int* 34:705, 2013.

Stern RE, Assal M: Dorsal multiple plating without routine transarticular screws for fixation of Lisfranc injury, *Orthopedics* 37:815, 2014.

Torg JS, Moyer J, Gaughn JP, Boden BP: Management of tarsal navicular stress fractures: conservative versus surgical treatment: a meta-analysis, *Am J Sports Med* 38:1048, 2010.

van Dorp KB, de Vries MR, van der Elst M: Chopart joint injury: a study of outcome and morbidity, *J Foot Ankle Surg* 49:541, 2010.

van Raaij TM, Duffy PJ, Buckley RE: Displaced isolated cuboid fractures: results of four caes with operative treatment, *Foot Ankle Int* 31:242, 2010.

Wagner E, Ortiz C, Villalón IE, et al.: Early weight-bearing after percutaneous reduction and screw fixation for low-energy Lisfranc injury, *Foot Ankle Int* 34:978, 2013.

Wilson MG, Gomez-Tristan A: Medial plate fixation of Lisfranc injuries, *Tech Foot Ankle Surg* 9:110, 2010.

METATARSALS

Aynardi M, Pedowitz DI, Saffel H, et al.: Outcome of nonoperative management of displaced oblique spiral fractures of the fifth metatarsal shaft, *Foot Ankle Int* 34:1619, 2013.

Bryant T, Beck DM, Daniel JN, et al.: Union rate and rate of hardware removal following plate fixation of metatarsal shaft and neck fractures, *Foot Ankle Int* 39:326, 2018.

Cakir H, Van Vliet-Koppert ST, Van Lieshout EM, et al.: Demographics and outcome of metatarsal fractures, *Arch Orthop Trauma Surg* 131:241, 2011.

DeSandis B, Murphy C, Rosenbaum A, et al.: Multiplanar CT analysis of fifth metatarsal morphology: implications for operative management of zone II fractures, *Foot Ankle Int* 37:528, 2016.

Hunt KJ, Anderson RB: Treatment of Jones fracture nonunions and refractures in the elite athlete: outcomes of intramedullary screw fixation with bone grafting, *Am J Sports Med* 39:1948, 2011.

Karnovsky SC, Rosenbaum AJ, DeSandis B, et al.: Radiographic analysis of National Football League players' fifth metatarsal morphology relationashi9 to proximal fifth metatarsal fracture risk, *Foot Ankle Int* 40:318, 2019.

Kim HN, Park WY: Reduction and fixation of metatarsal neck fractures using closed antegrade intramedullary nailing: technique tip, *Foot Ankle Int* 32:1098, 2011.

Lee KT, Park YU, Young KW, et al.: Surgical results of 5th metatarsal stress fracture using modified tension band wiring, *Knee Surg Sports Traumatol Arthrosc* 19:853, 2011.

Metzl J, Olson K, Davis WH, et al.: A clinical and radiographic comparison of two hardware systems used to treat Jones fracture of the fifth metatarsal, *Foot Ankle Int* 34:956, 2013.

Murawski CD, Kennedy JG: Percutaneous internal fixation of proximal fifth metatarsal Jones fractures (zones II and III) with Charlotte Carolina screw and bone marrow aspirate concentrate: an outcome study in athletes, *Am J Sports Med* 39:1295, 2011.

Nagao M, Saita Y, Kameda S, et al.: Headless compression screw fixation of Jones fractures: an outcomes study in Japanese athletes, *Am J Sports Med* 40:2578, 2012.

O'Malley M, DeSandis B, Allen A, et al.: Operative treatment of fifth metatarsal Jones fractures (zones II and III) in the NBA, *Foot Ankle Int* 37:488, 2016.

Orr JD, Glisson RR, Nunley JA: Jones fracture fixation: a biomechanical comparison of partially threaded screws versus tapered variable pitch screws, *Am J Sports Med* 40:691, 2012.

Polzer H, Polzer S, Mutschler W, Prall WC: Acute fractures to the proximal fifth metatarsal bone: development of classification and treatment recommendations based on the current evidence, *Injury* 43:1626, 2012.

Ritchie JD, Shaver JC, Anderson RB, et al.: Excision of symptomatic nonunions of proximal fifth metatarsal avulsion fractures in elite athletes, *Am J Sports Med* 39:2466, 2011.

Rongstad KM, Tueting J, Rongstad M, et al.: Fourth metatarsal base stress fractures in athletes: a case series, *Foot Ankle Int* 34:962, 2013.

Shadid MK, Punwar S, Boulind C, Bannister G: Aircast walking boot and below-knee walking cast for avlusion fractures of the base of the fifth metatarsal: comparative cohort study, *Foot Ankle Int* 34:75, 2013.

Shindle MK, Endo Y, Warren RF, et al.: Stress fractures about the tibia, foot, and ankle, *J Am Acad Orthop Surg* 20:167, 2012.

Smith TO, Clark A, Hing CB: Interventions for treating proximal fifth metatarsal fractures in adults: a meta-analysis of the current evidence base, *Foot Ankle Surg* 17:300, 2011.

Watson GI, Karovsky SC, Konin G, et al.: Optimal starting point for fifth metatarsal zone II fractures: a cadaveric study, *Foot Ankle Int* 38:802, 2017.

PHALANGES, TURF TOE, SESAMOIDS

Bichara DA, Henn 3rd RF, Theodore GH: Sesamoidectomy for hallux sesamoid fractures, *Foot Ankle Int* 33:704, 2012.

Patel T, Song AJ, Lomasney LM, et al.: Acute fibular sesamoid fracture: one part of the spectrum of sesamoid pathologies, *Orthopedics* 37:650, 2014.

Simons P, Klos K, Loracher C, et al.: Lateral soft-tissue release through a medial incision: anatomic comparison of two techniques, *Foot Ankle Surg* 21:113, 2015.

Van Vliet-Koppert ST, Cakir H, Van Lieshout EM, et al.: Demographics and functional outcome of toe fractures, *J Foot Ankle Surg* 50:307, 2011.

Waldrop 3rd NE, Zirker CA, Wijdicks CA, et al.: Radiographic evaluation of plantar plate injury: as in vitro biomechanical study, *Foot Ankle Int* 34:403, 2013.

Woon CYL: Dislocation of the interphalangeal joint of the great toe: is percutaneous reduction of an incarcerated sesamoid an option? Surgical technique, *J Bone Joint Surg* 93A:109, 2011.

The complete list of references is available online at Expert Consult.com.

SUPPLEMENTAL REFERENCES

CALCANEUS

Abidi NA, Dhawan S, Gruen GS, et al.: Wound-healing risk factors after open reduction and internal fixation of calcaneal fractures, *Foot Ankle Int* 19:856, 1998.

Aitken AP: Fractures of the os calcis—treatment by closed reduction, *Clin Orthop Relat Res* 30:67, 1963.

Aktuglu K, Ayodogan U: The functional outcome of displaced intra-articular calcaneal fractures: a comparison between isolated cases and polytrauma patients, *Foot Ankle Int* 23:314, 2002.

Aldridge 3rd JM, Easley M, Nunley JA: Open calcaneal fractures: results of operative treatment, *J Orthop Trauma* 18:7, 2004.

Amendola A, Lammens P: Subtalar arthodesis using interposition iliac crest bone graft after calcaneal fracture, *Foot Ankle* 17:608, 1996.

Attinger C, Cooper P: Soft-tissue reconstruction for calcaneal fractures or osteomyelitis, *Orthop Clin North Am* 32:135, 2001.

Bajammal S, Tornetta P, Sanders D, Bhandari M: Displaced intra-articular calcaneal fractures, *J Orthop Trauma* 19:360, 2005.

Barla J, Buckley R, McCormack R, et al.: Displaced intraarticular calcaneal fractures: long-term outcome in women, *Foot Ankle Int* 25:853, 2004.

Beavis EC, Rourke K, Court-Brown C: Avulsion fracture of the calcaneal tuberosity: a case report and literature review, *Foot Ankle Int* 29:863, 2008.

Bednarz PA, Beals TC, Manoli A: Subtalar distraction bone block fusion: an assessment of outcome, *Foot Ankle Int* 18:785, 1997.

Benirschke SK, Sangeorzan BJ: Extensive intraarticular fractures of the foot: surgical management of calcaneal fractures, *Clin Orthop Relat Res* 292:128, 1993.

Berry GK, Stevens DG, Kreder HJ, et al.: Open fractures of the calcaneus: a review of treatment and outcome, *J Orthop Trauma* 18:202, 2004.

Bezes H, Massart P, Delvaux D, et al.: The operative treatment of intraarticular calcaneal fractures: indications, technique and results in 257 cases, *Clin Orthop Relat Res* 290:55, 1993.

Bibbo C, Patel DV: The effect of demineralised bone matrix-calcium sulfate with vancomycin on calcaneal fracture healing and infection rates: a prospective study, *Foot Ankle Int* 27:487, 2006.

Böhler L: Diagnosis, pathology, and treatment of fractures of the os calcis, *J Bone Joint Surg* 13:75, 1931.

Braly WG, Bishop JO, Tullos HS: Lateral decompression for malunited os calcis fractures, *Foot Ankle* 6:90, 1985.

Brauer CA, Manns BJ, Ko M, et al.: An economic evaluation of operative compared with nonoperative management of displaced intra-articular calcaneal fractures, *J Bone Joint Surg* 87A:2741, 2005.

Buch BD, Myerson MS, Miller SD: Primary subtalar arthrodesis for the treatment of comminuted calcaneal fractures, *Foot Ankle* 17:61, 1996.

Buckley R, Tough S, McCormack R, et al.: Operative compared with nonoperative treatment of displaced intra-articular calcaneal fractures: a prospective, randomized, controlled multicenter trial, *J Bone Joint Surg* 84A:1733, 2002.

Buckley RE, Meek RN: Comparison of open versus closed reduction of intraarticular calcaneal fractures: a matched cohort in workmen, *J Orthop Trauma* 6:216, 1992.

Burdeaux BD: Reduction of calcaneal fractures by the McReynolds medial approach technique and its experimental basis, *Clin Orthop Relat Res* 177:87, 1983.

Burdeaux Jr BD: Fractures of the calcaneus: open reduction and internal fixation from the medial side a 21-year prospective study, *Foot Ankle Int* 18:685, 1997.

Carr JB: Mechanism and pathoanatomy of the intraarticular calcaneal fracture, *Clin Orthop Relat Res* 290:36, 1993.

Carr JB: Surgical treatment of the intraarticular calcaneus fracture, *Orthop Clin North Am* 25:665, 1994.

Carr JB, Hansen ST, Benirschke SK: Subtalar distraction bone block fusion for late complications of os calcis fractures, *Foot Ankle* 9:81, 1988.

Chan SCF, Alexander IJ: Subtalar arthrodesis with interposition tricortical iliac crest graft for late pain and deformity after calcaneus fracture, *Foot Ankle Int* 18:613, 1997.

Chandler JT, Bonar SK, Anderson RB, et al.: Results of in situ subtalar arthrodesis for late sequelae of calcaneus fractures, *Foot Ankle Int* 20:18, 1999.

Clare MP, Lee 3rd WE, Sanders RW: Intermediate to long-term results of a treatment protocol for calcaneal fracture malunion, *J Bone Joint Surg* 87A:963, 2005.

Coughlin MJ: Calcaneal fractures in the industrial patients, *Foot Ankle Int* 21:896, 2000.

Crosby LA, Fitzgibbons T: Computerized tomography scanning of acute intraarticular fractures of the calcaneus, *J Bone Joint Surg* 72A:852, 1990.

Crosby LA, Fitzgibbons T: Intraarticular calcaneal fractures: results of closed treatment, *Clin Orthop Relat Res* 290:47, 1993.

Crosby LA, Fitzgibbons T: Open reduction and internal fixation of type II intraarticular calcaneus fractures, *Foot Ankle* 17:253, 1996.

Crosby LA, Kamins P: The history of the calcaneal fracture, *Orthop Rev* 20:501, 1991.

Csizy M, Buckley R, Tough S, et al.: Displaced intra-articular calcaneal fractures: variables predicting late subtalar fusion, *J Orthop Trauma* 17:106, 2003.

Day FG: Treatment of fracture of the os calcis, *Can Med Assoc J* 63:373, 1950.

Degan TJ, Morrey BF, Braun DP: Surgical excision for anterior process fractures of the calcaneus, *J Bone Joint Surg* 64A:519, 1982.

Della Rocca GJ, Nork SE, Barei DP, et al.: Fractures of the sustentaculum tali: injury characteristics and surgical technique for reduction, *Foot Ankle Int* 30:1037, 2009.

Deyerle WM: Long-term follow-up of fractures of the os calcis: diagnostic peroneal synoviogram, *Orthop Clin North Am* 4:213, 1973.

Dooley P, Buckley R, Tough S, et al.: Bilateral calcaneal fractures: operative versus nonoperative treatment, *Foot Ankle Int* 25:47, 2004.

Ebraheim NA, Biyani A, Padanilam T, et al.: A pitfall of coronal computed tomographic imaging in evaluation of calcaneal fractures, *Foot Ankle* 17:503, 1996.

Ebraheim NA, Elgafy H, Sabry FF, et al.: Sinus tarsi approach with transarticular fixation for displaced intraarticular fractures of the calcaneus, *Foot Ankle Int* 21:105, 2000.

Ebraheim NA, Sabry FF, Haman S, et al.: Congruity of the subtalar joint in tongue fracture of the calcaneus: an anatomical study, *Foot Ankle Int* 21:665, 2000.

Elsner A, Jubel A, Prokop A, et al.: Augmentation of intraarticular calcaneal fractures with injectable calcium phosphate cement: densitometry, histology, and functional outcome in 18 patients, *J Foot Ankle Surg* 44:390, 2005.

Essex-Lopresti P: Results of reduction in fractures of the calcaneum, *J Bone Joint Surg* 33B:284, 1951.

Essex-Lopresti P: The mechanism, reduction technique, and results in fractures of the os calcis, *Br J Surg* 39:395, 1952.

Flemister Jr AS, Infante AF, Sanders RW, et al.: Subtalar arthrodesis for complications of intra-articular calcaneal fractures, *Foot Ankle Int* 21:392, 2000.

Folk JW, Starr AJ, Early JS: Early wound complications of operative treatment of calcaneus fractures: analysis of 190 fractures, *J Orthop Trauma* 13:369, 1999.

Gallie WE: Subastragalar arthrodesis of the os calcis, *J Bone Joint Surg* 25:731, 1943.

Gardner MJ, Nork SE, Barei DP, et al.: Secondary soft-tissue compromise in tongue-type calcaneus fractures, *J Orthop Trauma* 22:439, 2008.

Gatha M, Pedersen B, Buckely R: Fractures of the sustentaculum tali of the calcaneus: a case report, *Foot Ankle Int* 29:237, 2008.

Geel CW, Flemister Jr AS: Standardized treatment of intra-articular calcaneal fractures using an oblique lateral incision and no bone graft, *J Trauma* 50:1083, 2001.

Gehrmann RM, Rajan S, Patel DV, Bibbo C: Athletes' ankle injuries: diagnosis and management, *Am J Orthop* 34:551, 2005.

Gilmer PW, Herzenberg J, Frank JL, et al.: Computerized tomographic analysis of acute calcaneal fractures, *Foot Ankle* 6:184, 1986.

Gupta A, Bhalambor N, Nihal A, Trepman E: The modified Palmer lateral approach for calcaneal fractures: wound healing and postoperative computed tomographic evaluation of fracture reduction, *Foot Ankle Int* 24:744, 2003.

Hammesfar R, Fleming LL: Calcaneal fractures: a good prognosis, *Foot Ankle* 2:161, 1981.

Harding D, Waddell JP: Open reduction in depressed fractures of the os calcis, *Clin Orthop Relat Res* 199:124, 1985.

Harvey EJ, Grujic L, Early JS, et al.: Morbidity associated with ORIF of intra-articular calcaneus fractures using a lateral approach, *Foot Ankle Int* 22:868, 2001.

Heckman JD: Fractures and dislocations of the foot. In Rockwood CA, Green DP, editors: *Fractures in adults* (vol. 2). Philadelphia, 1984, Lippincott.

Heier KA, Infante AF, Walling AK, Sanders RW: Open fractures of the calcaneus: soft-tissue injury determines outcome, *J Bone Joint Surg* 85A:2276, 2003.

Herscovici Jr D, Widmaier J, Scaduto JM, et al.: Operative treatment of calcaneal fractures in elderly patients, *J Bone Joint Surg* 87A:1260, 2005.

Hess M, Booth B, Laughlin RT: Case report: calcaneal avulsion fractures: complications from delayed treatment, *Am J Emerg Med* 26:254.e1, 2008.

Howard JL, Buckley R, McCormack R, et al.: Complications following management of displaced intra-articular calcaneal fractures: a prospective randomized trial comparing open reduction internal fixation with nonoperative management, *J Orthop Trauma* 17:241, 2003.

Huang PJ, Fu YC, Cheng YM, et al.: Subtalar arthrodesis for late sequelae of calcaneal fractures: fusion in situ versus fusion with sliding corrective osteotomy, *Foot Ankle Int* 20:166, 1999.

Huefner T, Thermann H, Geerling J, et al.: Primary subtalar arthrodesis of calcaneal fractures, *Foot Ankle Int* 22:9, 2001.

Hutchinson III F, Huebner MK: Treatment of os calcis fractures by open reduction and internal fixation, *Foot Ankle* 15:225, 1994.

Ibrahim T, Rowsell M, Rennie W, et al.: Displaced intra-articular calcaneal fractures: 15-year follow-up of a randomised controlled trial of conservative versus operative treatment, *Injury* 38:848, 2007.

Järvholm U, Körner L, Thoren O, et al.: Fractures of the calcaneus: a comparison of open and closed treatment, *Acta Orthop Scand* 55:652, 1984.

Johal HS, Buckley RE, Le IL, Leighton RK: A prospective randomized controlled trial of a bioresorbable calcium phosphate paste (alpha-BSM) in treatment of displaced intra-articular calcaneal fractures, *J Trauma* 67:875, 2009.

Johnson EE: Intraarticuar fractures of the calcaneus: diagnosis and surgical management, *Orthopedics* 13:1091, 1990.

Jung HG, Yoo MJ, Kim MH: Late sequelae of secondary Haglund's deformity after malunion of tongue type calcaneal fracture: report of two cases, *Foot Ankle Int* 23:1014, 2002.

Khazen GE, Wilson AN, Ashfaq S, et al.: Fixation of calcaneal avulsion fractures using screws with and without suture anchors: a biomechanical investigation, *Foot Ankle Int* 28:1183, 2007.

Kingwell S, Buckley R, Willis M: The association between subtalar motion and outcome satisfaction in patients with displaced intraarticular calcaneal fractures, *Foot Ankle Int* 25:666, 2004.

Kitaoka HB, Schaap EJ, Chao EY, et al.: Displaced intraarticular fractures of the calcaneus treated nonoperatively: clinical results and analysis of motion and ground-reaction and temporal forces, *J Bone Joint Surg* 76A:1531, 1994.

Koski A, Kuokkanen H, Tukiainen E: Postoperative wound complications after internal fixation of closed calcaneal fractures: a retrospective analysis of 126 consecutive patients with 148 fractures, *Scand J Surg* 94:243, 2005.

Kundel K, Brutscher M, Bickel R: Calcaneal fractures: operative versus nonoperative treatment, *J Trauma* 41:839, 1996.

Lance EM, Carey Jr EJ, Wade PA: Fractures of the os calcis: treatment by early mobilization, *Clin Orthop Relat Res* 30:76, 1963.

Laughlin RT, Carson JG, Calhoun JH: Displaced intraarticular calcaneus fractures treated with the Galveston plate, *Foot Ankle* 17:71, 1996.

Letournel E: Open treatment of acute calcaneal fractures, *Clin Orthop Relat Res* 290:60, 1993.

Leung KS, Yuen KM, Chan WS: Operative treatment of displaced intraarticular fractures of the calcaneum: medium-term results, *J Bone Joint Surg* 75B:196, 1993.

Levin LS, Nunley JA: The management of soft-tissue problems associated with calcaneal fractures, *Clin Orthop Relat Res* 290:151, 1993.

Lindsay WKN, Dewar FP: Fractures of the os calcis, *Am J Surg* 95:555, 1958.

Longino D, Buckley RE: Bone graft in the operative treatment of displaced intraarticular calcaneal fractures: is it helpful? *J Orthop Trauma* 15:280, 2001.

Loutzenhiser L, Lawrence SJ, Donegan RP: Treatment of select open calcaneus fractures with reduction and internal fixation: an intermediate-term review, *Foot Ankle Int* 29:825, 2008.

Lowery RBW, Calhoun JH: Fractures of the calcaneus, part I: anatomy, injury, mechanism, and classification, *Foot Ankle* 17:230, 1996.

Lowery RBW, Calhoun JH: Fractures of the calcaneus, part II: treatment, *Foot Ankle* 17:360, 1996.

Martinez S, Herzenberg JE, Apple JS: Computed tomography of the hindfoot, *Orthop Clin North Am* 16:481, 1985.

McReynolds IS: Trauma to the os calcis and heel cord. In Jahss M, editor: *Disorders of the foot and ankle*, Philadelphia, 1984, Saunders.

Melcher G, Degonda F, Leutenegger A, et al.: Ten-year follow-up after operative treatment for intraarticular fractures of the calcaneus, *J Trauma* 38:713, 1995.

Miller ME: Surgical management of calcaneus fractures: indications and techniques, *Instr Course Lect* 39:161, 1990.

Monsey RD, Levine BP, Trevino SG, et al.: Operative treatment of acute displaced intraarticular calcaneus fractures, *Foot Ankle* 16:57, 1995.

Myerson M, Quill GE: Late complications of fractures of the calcaneus, *J Bone Joint Surg* 75A:331, 1993.

Myerson MS: Primary subtalar arthrodesis for the treatment of comminuted fractures of the calcaneus, *Orthop Clin North Am* 26:215, 1995.

Myerson MS, Berger BI: Nonunion of a fracture of the sustentaculum tali causing a tarsal tunnel syndrome: a case report, *Foot Ankle Int* 16:740, 1995.

O'Brien J, Buckley R, McCormack R, et al.: Personal gait satisfaction after displaced intraarticular calcaneal fractures: 2-8 year followup, *Foot Ankle Int* 25:657, 2004.

O'Connell F, Mital MA, Rowe CR: Evaluation of modern management of fractures of the os calcis, *Clin Orthop Relat Res* 83:214, 1972.

Omoto H, Nakamura K: Method for manual reduction of displaced intraarticular fracture of the calcaneus: technique, indications, and limitations, *Foot Ankle Int* 24:724, 2003.

Omoto H, Sakurada K, Sugi M, et al.: A new method of manual reduction for intraarticular fracture of the calcaneus, *Clin Orthop Relat Res* 177:104, 1983.

Paley D, Hall H: Intraarticular fractures of the calcaneus: a critical analysis of results and prognostic factors, *J Bone Joint Surg* 75A:342, 1993.

Parkes II JC: Injuries of the hindfoot, *Clin Orthop Relat Res* 122:28, 1977.

Parmar HV, Triffitt PD, Gregg PJ: Intraarticular fractures of the calcaneum treated operatively or conservatively: a prospective study, *J Bone Joint Surg* 75B:932, 1993.

Pennal GF, Yadav MP: Operative treatment of comminuted fractures of the os calcis, *Orthop Clin North Am* 4:197, 1973.

Pozo JL, Kirwan EO, Jackson AM: The long-term results of conservative management of severely displaced fractures of the calcaneus, *J Bone Joint Surg* 66B:386, 1984.

Randle JA, Kreder JH, Stephen D, et al.: Should calcaneal fractures be treated surgically? A meta-analysis, *Clin Orthop Relat Res* 377:217, 2000.

Redfern DJ, Oliveira ML, Campbell JT, Belkoff SM: A biomechanical comparison of locking and nonlocking plates for the fixation of calcaneal fractures, *Foot Ankle Int* 27:196, 2006.

Richter M, Gosling T, Zech S, et al.: A comparison of plates with and without locking screws in a calcaneal fracture model, *Foot Ankle Int* 26:309, 2005.

Robbins MI, Wilson MG, Sella EJ: MR imaging of anteroposterior calcaneal process fractures, *AJR Am J Roentgenol* 172:475, 1999.

Romash MM: Calcaneal fractures: three-dimensional treatment, *Foot Ankle* 8:180, 1988.

Romash MM: Reconstructive osteotomy of the calcaneus with subtalar arthrodesis for malunited calcaneal fractures, *Clin Orthop Relat Res* 290:157, 1993.

Romash MM: Calcaneal osteotomy and arthrodesis for malunited calcaneal fracture. In Johnson KA, editor: *Master techniques in orthopaedic surgery: the foot and ankle*, New York, 1994, Raven.

Sanders R: Intraarticular fractures of the calcaneus: present state of the art, *J Orthop Trauma* 6:252, 1992.

Sanders R, Fortin P, DiPasquale T, et al.: Operative treatment in 120 displaced intraarticular calcaneal fractures: results using a prognostic computed tomography scan classification, *Clin Orthop Relat Res* 290:87, 1993.

Sanders R, Gregory P: Operative treatment of intraarticular fractures of the calcaneus, *Orthop Clin North Am* 26:203, 1995.

Sanders R, Hansen ST, McReynolds IS: Trauma to the calcaneus and its tendon. In Jahss MH, editor: *Disorders of the foot and ankle*, Philadelphia, 1991, Saunders.

Sangeorzan BJ: Salvage procedures for calcaneus fractures, *Instr Course Lect* 46:339, 1997.

Savva N, Saxby TS: In situ arthrodesis with lateral-wall ostectomy for the sequelae of fracture of the os calcis, *J Bone Joint Surg* 89B:919, 2007.

Schepers T, Vogels LM, Schipper IB, Patka P: Percutaneous reduction and fixation of intraarticular calcaneal fractures, *Oper Orthop Traumatol* 20:168, 2008.

Schildhauer TA, Bauer TW, Josten C, et al.: Open reduction and augmentation of internal fixation with an injectable skeletal cement for the treatment of complex calcaneal fractures, *J Orthop Trauma* 14:309, 2000.

Scranton Jr PE: Comparison of open isolated subtalar arthrodesis with autogenous bone graft versus outpatient arthroscopic subtalar arthrodesis using injectable bone morphogenic protein-enhanced graft, *Foot Ankle Int* 20:162, 1999.

Segal D, Marsh JL, Leiter B: Clinical applications of computerized axial tomography (CAT) scanning of calcaneus fractures, *Clin Orthop Relat Res* 199:114, 1985.

Shereff MJ: Radiographic anatomy of the hindfoot, *Clin Orthop Relat Res* 177:16, 1983.

Simpson LA, Schulak DJ, Spiegel PG: Intraarticular fractures of the calcaneus: a review, *Contemp Orthop* 6:19, 1983.

Squires B, Allen PE, Livingstone J, Atkins RM: Fractures of the tuberosity of the calcaneus, *J Bone Joint Surg* 83B:55, 2001.

Stephens HM, Sanders R: Calcaneal malunions: results of a prognostic computed tomography classification system, *Foot Ankle Int* 17:395, 1996.

Stephenson JR: Displaced fractures of the os calcis involving the subtalar joint: the key role of the superomedial fragment, *Foot Ankle* 4:91, 1983.

Stephenson JR: Treatment of displaced intraarticular fractures of the calcaneus using medial and lateral approaches, internal fixation, and early motion, *J Bone Joint Surg* 69A:115, 1987.

Stephenson JR: Surgical treatment of displaced intraarticular fractures of the calcaneus: a combined lateral and medial approach, *Clin Orthop Relat Res* 290:68, 1993.

Stoffel K, Booth G, Rohrl SM, Kuster M: A comparison of conventional versus locking plates in intraarticular calcaneus fractures: a biomechanical study in human cadavers, *Clin Biomech* 22:100, 2007.

Stulik J, Stehlik J, Rysavy M, Sozniak A: Minimally-invasive treatment of intraarticular fractures of the calcaneum, *J Bone Joint Surg* 88B:1634, 2006.

Thompson KR: Treatment of comminuted fractures of the calcaneus by triple arthrodesis, *Orthop Clin North Am* 4:189, 1973.

Thordarson DB, Bollinger M: SRS cancellous bone cement augmentation of calcaneal fracture fixation, *Foot Ankle Int* 26:347, 2005.

Thordarson DB, Greene N, Shepherd L, et al.: Facilitating edema resolution with a foot pump after calcaneus fracture, *J Orthop Trauma* 13:43, 1999.

Thordarson DB, Hedman TP, Yetkinler D, et al.: Superior compressive strength of a calcaneal fracture construct augmented with remodelable cancellous bone cement, *J Bone Joint Surg* 81A:239, 1999.

Thordarson DB, Krieger LE: Operative vs. nonoperative treatment of intraarticular fractures of the calcaneus: a prospective randomized trial, *Foot Ankle* 17:2, 1996.

Thordarson DB, Latteier M: Open reduction and internal fixation of calcaneal fractures with a low profile titanium calcaneal perimeter plate, *Foot Ankle Int* 24:217, 2003.

Thoron SJ, Cheleuitte D, Ptaszek AJ, Early JS: Treatment of open intraarticular calcaneal fractures: evaluation of a treatment protocol based on wound location and size, *Foot Ankle Int* 27:317, 2006.

Tornetta 3rd P: Percutaneous treatment of calcaneal fractures, *Clin Orthop Relat Res* 375:91, 2000.

van Tetering EA, Buckley RE: Functional outcome (SF-36) of patients with displaced calcaneal fractures compared to SF-36 normative data, *Foot Ankle Int* 25:733, 2004.

Walde TA, Sauer B, Degreif J, Walde HJ: Closed reduction and percutaneous Kirschner wire fixation for the treatment of dislocated calcaneal fractures: surgical technique, complications, clinical and radiological results after 2-10 years, *Arch Orthop Trauma Surg* 128:585, 2008.

Zmurko MG, Karges DE: Functional outcome of patients following open reduction internal fixation for bilateral calcaneus fracture, *Foot Ankle Int* 23:917, 2002.

Zoellner G, Clancy Jr W: Recurrent dislocation of the peroneal tendon, *J Bone Joint Surg* 61A:292, 1979.

Zwipp H, Tscherne H, Thermann H, et al.: Osteosynthesis of displaced intraarticular fractures of the calcaneus: results in 123 cases, *Clin Orthop Relat Res* 290:76, 1993.

TALUS

Adelaar RS: Fractures of the talus, *Instr Course Lect* 39:147, 1990.

Adelaar RS: Complex fractures of the talus, *Instr Course Lect* 46:323, 1997.

Anderson HG: *The medical and surgical aspects of aviation*, London, 1919, Henry Frowde Oxford University Press1919.

Baumhauer JF, Alvarez RG: Controversies in treatment talus fractures, *Orthop Clin North Am* 26:335, 1995.

Beals TC, Holmes JR, Manoli II A: *Longitudinal Lisfranc fracture-dislocations*, San Francisco, February 1997, Paper presented at the twenty-seventh annual meeting of the American Orthopaedic Foot and Ankle Society, February 1997.

Bibbo C, Anderson RB, Davis WH: Injury characteristics and the clinical outcome of subtalar dislocations: a clinical and radiographic analysis of 25 cases, *Foot Ankle Int* 24:158, 2003.

Bibbo C, Lin SS, Abidi N, et al.: Missed and associated injuries after subtalar dislocation: the role of CT, *Foot Ankle Int* 22:324, 2001.

Blair HC: Comminuted fracture and fracture-dislocations of the body of the astragalus: operative treatment, *Am J Surg* 59:37, 1943.

Bradshaw C, Khan K, Brukner P: Stress fracture of the body of the talus in athletes demonstrated with computer tomography, *Clin J Sport Med* 6:48, 1996.

Brand JC, Brindle T, Nyland J, et al.: Does pulsed low-intensity ultrasound allow early return to normal activities when treating stress fractures: a review of one tarsal navicular and eight tibial stress fractures, *Iowa Orthop J* 19:26, 1999.

Brennan MJ: Subtalar dislocations, *Instr Course Lect* 39:157, 1990.

Canale ST, Belding RH: Osteochondral lesions of the talus, *J Bone Joint Surg* 62A:97, 1980.

Canale ST, Kelly Jr FB: Fractures of the neck of the talus: long-term evaluation of 71 cases, *J Bone Joint Surg* 60A:143, 1978.

Cantrell MW, Tarquinio TA: Fracture of the lateral process of the talus, *Orthopedics* 23:55, 2000.

Chen YJ, Hsu RW, Shih HN, Huang TJ: Fracture of the entire posterior process of the talus associated with subtalar dislocation: a case report, *Foot Ankle Int* 17:226, 1996.

Coltart WD: Aviator's astragalus, *J Bone Joint Surg* 34B:545, 1952.

Comfort TH, Behrens F, Gaither DW, et al.: Long-term results of displaced talar neck fractures, *Clin Orthop Relat Res* 199:81, 1985.

Dabezies EJ, Shackleton R: Orthopaedic grand rounds: subtalar dislocation, *Orthopedics* 5:348, 1982.

DeLee JC, Curtis R: Subtalar dislocation of the foot, *J Bone Joint Surg* 64A:433, 1982.

De Palma L, Santucci A, Marinelle M: Irreducible isolated subtalar dislocation: a case report, *Foot Ankle Int* 29:523, 2008.

Dhillon MS, Nagi ON: Total dislocations of the navicular: are they ever isolated injuries? *J Bone Joint Surg* 81B:881, 1999.

DiGiovanni CW, Langer PR, Nickisch F, Spenciner D: Proximity of the lateral talar process to the lateral stabilizing ligaments of the ankle and subtalar joint, *Foot Ankle Int* 28:175, 2007.

Dimon JH: Isolated displaced fracture of the posterior facet of the talus, *J Bone Joint Surg* 43A:275, 1961.

Early JS: Talus fracture management, *Foot Ankle Clin* 13:635, 2008.

Ebraheim NA, Patil V, Owens C, Kandimalla Y: Clinical outcome of fractures of the talar body, *Int Orthop* 32:773, 2008.

Ebraheim NA, Padanilam TG, Wong FY: Posteromedial process fractures of the talus, *Foot Ankle* 16:734, 1995.

Ebraheim NA, Sabry FF, Nadim Y: Internal architecture of the talus: implication for talar fracture, *Foot Ankle Int* 20:794, 1999.

Ebraheim NA, Skie MC, Podeszwa DA: Medial subtalar dislocation associated with fracture of the posterior process of the talus: a case report, *Clin Orthop Relat Res* 303:226, 1994.

Ebraheim NA, Skie MC, Podeszwa DA, et al.: Evaluation of process fractures of the talus using computed tomography, *J Orthop Trauma* 8:332, 1994.

Elgafy H, Ebraheim NA, Tile M, et al.: Fractures of the talus: experience of two level 1 trauma centers, *Foot Ankle Int* 21:1023, 2000.

Fitch KD, Blackwell JB, Gilmour WN: Operation for non-union of stress fracture of the tarsal navicular, *J Bone Joint Surg* 71B:105, 1989.

Fleuriau Chateau PB, Brokaw DS, Jelen BA, et al.: Plate fixation of talar neck fractures: preliminary review of a new technique in twenty-three patients, *J Orthop Trauma* 16:213, 2002.

Fortin PT, Balazsy JE: Talus fractures: evaluation and treatment, *J Am Acad Orthop Surg* 9:114, 2001.

Frawley PA, Hart JA, Young DA: Treatment outcome of major fractures of the talus, *Foot Ankle* 16:339, 1995.

Gelberman RH, Mortensen WW: Arterial anatomy of the talus, *Foot Ankle* 4:64, 1983.

Gissane W: A dangerous type of fracture of the foot, *J Bone Joint Surg* 33B:535, 1951.

Giuffrida AY, Lin SS, Abidi N, et al.: Pseudo os trigonum sign: missed posteromedial talar facet fracture, *Foot Ankle Int* 25:372, 2004.

Goldner JL, Poletti SC, Gates HS, Richardson WJ: Severe open subtalar dislocations, *J Bone Joint Surg* 77A:1075, 1995.

Gregory P, DiPasquale T, Herscovici D, et al.: Ipsilateral fractures of the talus and calcaneus, *Foot Ankle* 17:701, 1996.

Grob D, Simpson LA, Weber BG, et al.: Operative treatment of displaced talus fractures, *Clin Orthop Relat Res* 199:88, 1985.

Haliburton RA, Sullivan CR, Kelly PJ, et al.: The extra-osseous and intra-osseous blood supply of the talus, *J Bone Joint Surg* 40A:1115, 1958.

Hawkins LG: Fracture of the lateral process of the talus: a review of thirteen cases, *J Bone Joint Surg* 47A:1170, 1965.

Hawkins LG: Fractures of the neck of the talus, *J Bone Joint Surg* 52A:991, 1970.

Heck BE, Ebraheim NA, Jackson WT: Anatomical considerations of irreducible medial subtalar dislocation, *Foot Ankle Int* 17:103, 1996.

Heckman JD, McLean MR: Fractures of the lateral process of the talus, *Clin Orthop Relat Res* 199:108, 1985.

Higgins TF, Baumgaertner MR: Diagnosis and treatment of fractures of the talus: a comprehensive review of the literature, *Foot Ankle Int* 20:595, 1999.

Inokuchi S, Ogawa K, Usami N: Classification of fractures of the talus: clear differentiation between neck and body fractures, *Foot Ankle Int* 17:748, 1996.

Inokuchi S, Ogawa K, Usami N, et al.: Long-term follow-up of talus fractures, *Orthopedics* 19:477, 1996.

Johnson KA, editor: *Surgery of the foot and ankle*, New York, 1989, Raven.

Johnstone AJ, Maffulli N: Primary fusion of the talonavicular joint after fracture dislocation of the navicular bone, *J Trauma* 45:1100, 1998.

Karasick D, Schweitzer M: The os trigonum syndrome: imaging features, *AJR Am J Roentgenol* 166:125, 1996.

Khan KM, Fuller PJ, Brukner PD, et al.: Outcome of conservative and surgical management of navicular stress fracture in athletes: eighty-six cases proven with computerized tomography, *Am J Sports Med* 20:657, 1992.

Kim DH, Berkowitz MJ, Pressman DN: Avulsion fractures of the medial tubercle of the posterior process of the talus, *Foot Ankle Int* 24:172, 2003.

Kim DH, Hrutkay JM, Samson MM: Fracture of the medial tubercle of the posterior process of the talus: a case report and literature review, *Foot Ankle Int* 17:186, 1996.

Kirkpatrick DP, Hunter RE, Janes PC, et al.: The snowboarder's foot and ankle, San Francisco, February 1997, Paper presented at the twenty-seventh annual meeting of the American Orthopaedic Foot and Ankle Society, February 1997.

Langer P, Nickisch F, Spenciner D, et al.: In vitro evaluation of the effect lateral process talar excision on ankle and subtalar joint stability, *Foot Ankle Int* 28:78, 2007.

Lemaire RG, Bustin W: Screw fixation of fractures of the neck of the talus using a posterior approach, *J Trauma* 20:669, 1980.

Lin PP, Roe S, Kay M, et al.: Placement of screws in the sustentaculum tali, *Clin Orthop Relat Res* 352:194, 1998.

Lindvall E, Haidukewych G, DiPasquale T, et al.: Open reduction and stable fixation of isolated, displaced talar neck and body fractures, *J Bone Joint Surg* 86A:2229, 2004.

Marsh JL, Saltzman CL, Iverson M, Shapiro DS: Major open injuries of the talus, *J Orthop Trauma* 9:3791, 1995.

McCrory P, Bladin C: Fractures of the lateral process of the talus: a clinical review: "snowboarder's ankle, *Clin J Sport Med* 6:124, 1996.

McKeever FM: Fracture of the neck of the astragalus, *Arch Surg* 46:720, 1943.

Miller WE: Operative intervention for fracture of the talus. In Bateman JE, Trott AW, editors: *Foot and ankle*, New York, 1980, Marcel Dekker.

Morris HD, Hand WL, Dunn AS: The modified Blair fusion for fractures of the talus, *J Bone Joint Surg* 53A:1289, 1971.

Mulfinger GL, Trueta J: The blood supply of the talus, *J Bone Joint Surg* 52B:160, 1970.

Nadim Y, Tosic A, Ebraheim N: Open reduction and internal fixation of fracture of the posterior process of the talus: a case report and review of the literature, *Foot Ankle Int* 20:50, 1999.

Naranja Jr RJ, Mohaghan BA, Okereke E, Williams Jr GR: Open medial subtalar dislocation associated with fracture of the posterior process of the talus, *J Orthop Trauma* 10:142, 1996.

Patel R, Van Bergeyk A, Pinney S: Are displaced talar neck fractures surgical emergencies? A survey of orthopaedic trauma experts, *Foot Ankle Int* 26:378, 2005.

Quirk R: Stress fractures of the navicular, *Foot Ankle Int* 19:494, 1998.

Rammelt S, Winkler J, Heineck J, Zwipp H: Anatomical reconstruction of malunited talus fractures: a prospective study of 10 patients followed for 4 years, *Acta Orthop* 76:588, 2005.

Ries M, Healy Jr WA: Total dislocation of the talus: case report with a 13-year follow-up and review of the literature, *Orthop Rev* 17:76, 1988.

Ritsema GH: Total talar dislocation, *J Trauma* 28:692, 1988.

Rockett MS, Brage ME: Navicular body fractures: computerized tomography findings and mechanism of injury, *J Foot Ankle Surg* 36:185, 1997.

Sanders DW, Busam M, Hattwick E, et al.: Functional outcomes following displaced talar neck fractures, *J Orthop Trauma* 18:265, 2004.

Sanders R: Displaced intra-articular fractures of the calcaneus, *J Bone Joint Surg* 83A:1438, 2001.

Sangeorzan BJ, Benirschke SK, Mosca V, et al.: Displaced intraarticular fractures of the tarsal navicular, *J Bone Joint Surg* 71A:1504, 1989.

Smith CS, Nork SE, Sangeorzan BJ: The extruded talus: results of implantation, *J Bone Joint Surg* 88A:2418, 2006.

Sneppen O, Christensen SB, Krogsoe O, et al.: Fracture of the body of the talus, *Acta Orthop Scand* 48:317, 1977.

Swanson TV, Bray TJ, Holmes GB: Fractures of the talar neck, *J Bone Joint Surg* 74A:544, 1992.

Szyszkowitz R, Reschauer R, Seggl W: Eighty-five talus fractures treated by ORIF with five to eight years of follow-up study of 69 patients, *Clin Orthop Relat Res* 199:97, 1985.

Tezval M, Dumont C, Stürmer KM: Prognostic reliability of the Hawkins sign in fractures of the talus, *J Orthop Trauma* 21:538, 2007.

Thomason K, Eyres KS: A technique of fusion for failed total replacement of the ankle: tibio-allograft-calcaneal fusion with al locked retrograde intramedullary nail, *J Bone Joint Surg* 90B:885, 2008.

Thordarson DB, Triffon MJ, Terk MR: Magnetic resonance imaging to detect avascular necrosis after open reduction and internal fixation of talar neck fractures, *Foot Ankle Int* 17:742, 1996.

Torg JS, Pavlov H, Cooley LH, et al.: Stress fractures of the tarsal navicular: a retrospective review of twenty-one cases, *J Bone Joint Surg* 64A:700, 1982.

Trillat A, Bousquet G, Lapeyre B: Displaced fractures of the neck or of the body of the talus: value of screwing by posterior surgical approach, *Rev Chir Orthop Reparatrice Appar Mot* 56:529, 1970.

Trnka HJ, Zetti R, Ritschl P: Fracture of the anterior superior process of the calcaneus: an often misdiagnosed fracture, *Arch Orthop Trauma Surg* 117:300, 1998.

Tucker DJ, Feder JM, Boylan JP: Fractures of the lateral process of the talus: two case reports and a comprehensive literature review, *Foot Ankle Int* 19:641, 1998.

Valderrabano V, Perren T, Ryf C, et al.: Snowboarder's talus fracture: treatment outcome of 20 cases after 3.5 years, *Am J Sports Med* 33:871, 2005.

Vallier HA, Nork SE, Barei DP, et al.: Talar neck fractures: results and outcomes, *J Bone Joint Surg* 86A:1616, 2004.

Vallier HA, Nork SE, Benirschke SK, et al.: Surgical treatment of talar body fractures, *J Bone Joint Surg* 86A:180, 2004.

Viladot A, Lorenzo JC, Salazar J, et al.: The subtalar joint: embryology and morphology, *Foot Ankle* 5:54, 1984.

von Knoch F, Reckord U, von Knoch M, Summer C: Fracture of the lateral process of the talus in snowboarders, *J Bone Joint Surg* 89B:772, 2007.

Wagner R, Blatttert TR, Wickbach A: Talar dislocations, *Injury* 35:SB36, 2004.

Wildenauer E: Die Blutversorgung der Talus, *Z Anat* 115:32, 1950.

Zimmer TJ, Johnson KA: Subtalar dislocations, *Clin Orthop Relat Res* 238:190, 1989.

Ziran BH, Abidi NA, Scheel MJ: Medial malleolar osteotomy for exposure of complex talar body fractures, *J Orthop Trauma* 15:513, 2001.

MIDFOOT

Aitken AP, Poulson D: Dislocations of the tarsometatarsal joint, *J Bone Joint Surg* 45A:246, 1963.

Anderson LD: Injuries of the forefoot, *Clin Orthop Relat Res* 122:118, 1977.

Arntz CT, Hansen Jr ST: Dislocations and fracture dislocations of the tarsometatarsal joints, *Orthop Clin North Am* 18:105, 1987.

Apostle KL, Younger ASE: Technique tip: open reduction internal fixation of comminuted fractures of the navicular with bridge plating to the medial and middle cuneiforms, *Foot Ankle Int* 29:739, 2008.

Baravarian B, Geffen D: Lisfranc tightrope, *Foot Ankle Spec* 2:249, 2009.

Boden BB, Osbahr DC: High-risk stress fractures: evaluation and treatment, *J Am Acad Orthop Surg* 8:344, 2000.

Buzzard BM, Briggs PJ: Surgical management of acute tarsometatarsal fracture dislocation in the adult, *Clin Orthop Relat Res* 353:125, 1998.

Coss S, Manos RE, Buoncristiani A, et al.: Abduction stress and AP weight-bearing radiography of purely ligamentous injury in the tarsometatarsal joint, *Foot Ankle Int* 19:537, 1998.

Curtis MJ, Myerson M, Szura B: Tarsometatarsal joint injuries in the athletes, *Am J Sports Med* 21:497, 1993.

DeLee JC: Fractures and dislocations of the foot. In Mann RA, editor: *Surgery of the foot* (vol. 5). St. Louis, 1986, Mosby.

DePalma L, Santucci A, Sabetta SP, et al.: Anatomy of the Lisfranc joint complex, *Foot Ankle Int* 18:356, 1997.

Fitch KD, Blackwell JB, Gilmour WN: Operation for nonunion of stress fracture of the tarsal navicular, *J Bone Joint Surg* 71B:105, 1989.

Goosens M, De Stoop N: Lisfranc's fracture dislocations: etiology, radiology and results of treatment, *Clin Orthop Relat Res* 176:154, 1983.

Hardcastle PH, Reschauer R, Kutscha-Lissberg E, et al.: Injuries to the tarsometatarsal joint: incidence, classification and treatment, *J Bone Joint Surg* 64B:349, 1982.

Heckman JD: Fractures and dislocations of the foot. In Rockwood Jr CA, Green DP, editors: *Fractures in adults* (vol. 2). Philadelphia, 1984, Lippincott.

Henning JA, Jones CB, Sietsema DL, et al.: Open reduction internal fixation versus primary arthrodesis for Lisfranc injuries: a prospective randomized study, *Foot Ankle Int* 30:913, 2009.

Hesp WL, Van der Werken C, Goris RJA: Lisfranc dislocations: fractures and/or dislocations through the tarsometatarsal joints, *Injury* 15:261, 1983.

Johnson JE, Johnson KA: Dowel arthrodesis for degenerative arthritis of the tarsometatarsal (Lisfranc) joints, *Foot Ankle* 5:243, 1986.

Komenda GA, Myerson MS, Biddinger KR: Results of arthrodesis of the tarsometatarsal joints after traumatic injury, *J Bone Joint Surg* 78A:1665, 1996.

Kuo RS, Tejwani NC, DiGiovanni CW, et al.: Outcome after open reduction and internal fixation of Lisfranc joint injuries, *J Bone Joint Surg* 82A:1609, 2000.

Latterman C, Goldstein JL, Wukich DK, et al.: Practical management of Lisfranc injuries in athletes, *Clin J Sport Med* 17:311, 2007.

Lin SS, Bono CM, Treuting R, Shereff MJ: Limited intertarsal arthrodesis using bone grafting and pin fixation, *Foot Ankle Int* 21:742, 2000.

Lu J, Ebraheim NA, Skie M, et al.: Radiographic and computed tomographic evaluation of Lisfranc dislocation: a cadaver study, *Foot Ankle Int* 18:351, 1997.

Ly TV, Coetzee JC: Treatment of primarily ligamentous Lisfranc joint injuries: primary arthrodesis compared with open reduction and internal fixation. A prospective, randomized study, *J Bone Joint Surg* 88A:514, 2006.

Mann RA, Prieskorn D, Sobel M: Midtarsal and tarsometatarsal arthrodesis for primary degenerative osteoarthrosis or osteoarthrosis after trauma, *J Bone Joint Surg* 78A:1376, 1996.

Monteleone Jr GP: Stress fractures in the athlete, *Orthop Clin North Am* 26:423, 1995.

Mulier T, Reynders P, Sioen W, et al.: The treatment of Lisfranc injuries, *Acta Orthop Belg* 63:82, 1997.

Myerson M: The diagnosis and treatment of injuries to the Lisfranc joint complex, *Orthop Clin North Am* 20:655, 1989.

Myerson MS: The diagnosis and treatment of injury to the tarsometatarsal joint complex, *J Bone Joint Surg* 81B:756, 1999.

Myerson MS, Cerrato RA: Current management of tarsometatarsal injuries in the athlete, *J Bone Joint Surg* 90A:2522, 2008.

Nunley JA, Vertullo CJ: Classification, investigation, and management of midfoot sprains: lisfranc injuries in the athlete, *Am J Sports Med* 30:871, 2002.

Panchbhavi VK, Vallurupalli S, Yang J, Andersen CR: Screw fixation compared with suture-button fixation of isolated Lisfrance ligament injuries, *J Bone Joint Surg* 91A:1143, 2009.

Patterson RH, Petersen D, Cunningham R: Isolated fracture of the medial cuneiform, *J Orthop Trauma* 7:94, 1993.

Petje G, Steinböck G, Landsiedl F: Arthrodesis for traumatic flat foot, *Acta Orthop Scand* 67:359, 1996.

Potter HG, Deland JT, Gusmer PB, et al.: Magnetic resonance imaging of the Lisfranc ligament of the foot, *Foot Ankle Int* 19:438, 1998.

Potter NJ, Brukner PD, Makdissi M, et al.: Navicular stress fractures: outcomes of surgical and conservative management, *Br J Sports Med* 40:692, 2006.

Preidler KW, Brossmann J, Daenen B, et al.: MR imaging of the tarsometatarsal joint: analysis of injuries in 11 patients, *AJR Am J Roentgenol* 167:1217, 1996.

Rajapakse B, Edwards T, Hong T: A single surgeon's experience of treatment of Lisfranc joint injuries, *Injury* 37:914, 2007.

Quénu E, Küss G: Étude sur les luxations du metatarse (luxations métatarsotarsiennes) du diastasis entre le 1er et le 2e metatarsien, *Rev Chir* 39:281, 1909.

Resch S, Stenström A: The treatment of tarsometatarsal injuries, *Foot Ankle* 11:117, 1990.

Richter M, Thermann H, Huefner T, et al.: Chopart joint fracture-dislocation: initial open reduction provides better outcome than closed reduction, *Foot Ankle Int* 25:340, 2004.

Richter M, Wippermann B, Krettek C, et al.: Fractures and fracture dislocations of the midfoot: occurrence, causes, and long-term results, *Foot Ankle Int* 22:392, 2001.

Ross G, Cronin R, Hauzenblaz J, et al.: Plantar ecchymosis sign: a clinical aid to diagnosis of occult Lisfranc tarsometatarsal injuries, *J Orthop Trauma* 10:119, 1996.

Sangeorzan BJ, Swiontkowski MK: Displaced fractures of the cuboid, *J Bone Joint Surg* 72B:376, 1990.

Sangeorzan BJ, Veith RG, Hansen Jr ST: Salvage of Lisfranc's tarsometatarsal joint by arthrodesis, *Foot Ankle* 10:193, 1990.

Saxena A, Fullem B: Navicular stress fractures: a prospective study on athletes, *Foot Ankle Int* 27:917, 2006.

Schenck Jr RC, Heckman JD: Fractures and dislocations of the forefoot: operative and nonoperative treatment, *J Am Acad Orthop Surg* 3:70, 1995.

Schildhauer TA, Nork SE, Sangeorzan BJ: Temporary bridge plating of the medial column in severe midfoot injuries, *J Orthop Trauma* 17:513, 2003.

Shapiro MS, Wascher DC, Finerman GA: Rupture of Lisfranc's ligament in athletes, *Am J Sports Med* 22:687, 1994.

Shereff MJ: Compartment syndromes of the foot, *Instr Course Lect* 39:127, 1990.

Shereff MJ: Fractures of the forefoot, *Instr Course Lect* 39:133, 1990.

Swords MP, Schramski M, Switzer K, Nemec S: Chopart fractures and dislocations, *Foot Ankle Clin* 13:679, 2008.

Taylor SF, Heidenreich D: Isolated medial cuneiform fracture: a special forces soldier with a rare injury, *South Med J* 101:848, 2008.

Teng AL, Pinzur MS, Lomasney L, et al.: Functional outcome following anatomic restoration of tarsal-metatarsal fracture dislocation, *Foot Ankle Int* 23:922, 2002.

Weber M, Locher S: Reconstruction of the cuboid in compression: sort to midterm results in 12 patients, *Foot Ankle Int* 23:1008, 2002.

METATARSALS

Adelaar RS: The treatment of tarsometatarsal fracture-dislocations, *Instr Course Lect* 39:141, 1990.

Alepuz ES, Carsi VV, Alcántara P, et al.: Fractures of the central metatarsal, *Foot Ankle Int* 17:200, 1996.

Boden BP, Osbahr DC: High-risk stress fractures: evaluation and treatment, *J Am Acad Orthop Surg* 6:344, 2000.

Brukner P, Bennell K: Stress fractures in female athletes: diagnosis, management, and rehabilitation, *Sports Med* 6:419, 1997.

Brunet JA: Pathomechanics of complex dislocations of the first metatarsophalangeal joint, *Clin Orthop Relat Res* 332:126, 1996.

Brunet JA, Tubin S: Traumatic dislocation of lesser toes, *Foot Ankle Int* 18:406, 1997.

Brunet JA, Wiley JJ: The late results of tarsometatarsal joint injuries, *J Bone Joint Surg* 69B:437, 1987.

Chuckpaiwong B, Cook C, Nunley JA: Stress fractures of the second metatarsal base occur in nondancers, *Clin Orthop Relat Res* 461:197, 2007.

Chuckpaiwong B, Queen RM, Easley ME, Nunley JA: Distinguishing Jones and proximal diaphyseal fractures of the fifth metatarsal, *Clin Orthop Relat Res* 466:1966, 2008.

Clapper MF, O'Brien TJ, Lyons PM: Fractures of the fifth metatarsal: analysis of a fracture registry, *Clin Orthop Relat Res* 315:238, 1995.

Curtis MJ, Myerson M, Szura B: Tarsometatarsal joint injuries in the athlete, *Am J Sports Med* 21:497, 1993.

Donahue SW, Sharkey NA: Strains in the metatarsals during the stance phase of gait: implications for stress fractures, *J Bone Joint Surg* 9A:1236, 1999.

Donley BG, McCollum MJ, Murphy GA, Richardson EG: Risk of sural nerve injury with intramedullary screw fixation of fifth metatarsal fractures: a cadaver study, *Foot Ankle Int* 20:182, 1999.

Egol K, Walsh M, Rosenblatt K, et al.: Avulsion fractures of the fifth metatarsal base: a prospective outcome study, *Foot Ankle Int* 28:581, 2007.

Faciszewski T, Burks RT, Manaster BJ: Subtle injuries of the Lisfranc joint, *J Bone Joint Surg* 72A:1519, 1990.

Fam AG, Shuckett R, McGillivray DC, et al.: Stress fractures in rheumatoid arthritis, *J Rheumatol* 10:722, 1983.

Frey C, Andersen GD, Feder KS: Plantarflexion injury to the metatarsophalangeal joint ("sand toe"), *Foot Ankle Int* 17:576, 1996.

Glasgow MT, Naranja RJ, Glasgow SG, et al.: Analysis of failed surgical management of fractures of the base of the fifth metatarsal distal to the tuberosity: the Jones fracture, *Foot Ankle Int* 17:449, 1996.

Josefsson PO, Karlsson M, Redlund-Johnell I, et al.: Closed treatment of Jones fracture: good results in 40 cases after 11-26 years, *Acta Orthop Scand* 65:545, 1994.

Josefsson PO, Karlsson M, Redlund-Johnell I, et al.: Jones fracture: surgical versus nonsurgical treatment, *Clin Orthop Relat Res* 299:252, 1994.

Kavanaugh JH, Brower TD, Mann RV: The Jones' fracture revisited, *J Bone Joint Surg* 60A:776, 1978.

Kaye RA: Insufficiency stress fractures of the foot and ankle in postmenopausal women, *Foot Ankle Int* 4:221, 1998.

King RE: Dislocation of the tarsometatarsal joints, *Bull Hosp Jt Dis* 47:190, 1987.

Larson CM, Almekinders LC, Taft TN, Garrett WE: Intramedullary screw fixation of Jones fractures: analysis of failures, *Am J Sports Med* 30:55, 2002.

Maenpaa H, Lehto MU: Belt EA: stress fractures of the ankle and forefoot in patients with inflammatory arthritides, *Foot Ankle Int* 9:833, 2002.

Manoli A: Compartment syndromes of the foot: current concepts, *Foot Ankle* 10:340, 1990.

Mologne TS, Lundeen JM, Clapper MF, O'Brien TJ: Early screw fixation versus casting in the treatment of acute Jones fracture, *Am J Sports Med* 33:970, 2005.

Moshirfar A, Campbell JT, Molloy S, et al.: Fifth metatarsal tuberosity fracture fixation: a biomechanical study, *Foot Ankle Int* 24:630, 2003.

Muscolo L, Migues A, Slullitel G, et al.: Stress fracture nonunion at the base of the second metatarsal in a ballet dancer: a case report, *Am J Sports Med* 6:1535, 2004.

Myerson M: The diagnosis and treatment of injuries to the Lisfranc joint complex, *Orthop Clin North Am* 20:655, 1989.

Myerson M, Fisher R, Burgess A, et al.: Dislocations of the tarsometatarsal joints: end results correlated with pathology and treatment, *Foot Ankle* 6:225, 1986.

O'Malley MJ, Hamilton WG, Munyak J: Fractures of the distal shaft of the fifth metatarsal: "dancer's fracture", *Am J Sports Med* 24:240, 1996.

O'Malley MJ, Hamilton WG, Munyak J, et al.: Stress fractures at the base of the second metatarsal in ballet dancers, *Foot Ankle Int* 17:89, 1996.

Pietropaoli MP, Wnorowski DC, Werner FW, et al.: Intramedullary screw fixation of Jones fractures: a biomechanical study, *Foot Ankle Int* 20:560, 1999.

Porter DA, Duncan M, Meyer SJ: Fifth metatarsal Jones fracture fixation with a 4.5-mm cannulated stainless steel screw in the competitive and recreational athlete: a clinical and radiographic evaluation, *Am J Sports Med* 33:726, 2005.

Prieskorn D, Graves S, Yen M, et al.: Integrity of the first metatarsophalangeal joint: a biomechanical analysis, *Foot Ankle Int* 16:357, 1995.

Quill GE: Fractures of the proximal fifth metatarsal, *Orthop Clin North Am* 26:353, 1995.

Reese K, Litsky A, Kaeding C, et al.: Cannulated screw fixation of Jones fractures: a clinical and biomechanical study, *Am J Sports Med* 32:1736, 2004.

Resch S, Stenström A: The treatment of tarsometatarsal injuries, *Foot Ankle* 11:117, 1990.

Rosenberg GA, Sferra JJ: Treatment strategies for acute fractures and nonunions of the proximal fifth metatarsal, *J Am Acad Orthop Surg* 8:332, 2000.

Sammarco GJ: The Jones fracture, *Instr Course Lect* 42:201, 1993.

Sangeorzan BJ, Veith RG, Hansen ST: Salvage of Lisfranc's tarsometatarsal joint by arthrodesis, *Foot Ankle* 10:193, 1990.

Shah SN, Knoblich GO, Lindsey DP, et al.: Intramedullary screw fixation of proximal fifth metatarsal fractures: a biomechanical study, *Foot Ankle Int* 22:581, 2001.

Torg JS, Balduini FC, Zelko RR, et al.: Fractures of the base of the fifth metatarsal distal to the tuberosity: classification and guidelines for non-surgical and surgical management, *J Bone Joint Surg* 66A:209, 1984.

Trevino SG, Kodros S: Controversies in tarsometatarsal injuries, *Orthop Clin North Am* 26:229, 1995.

Vuori JP, Aro HT: Lisfranc joint injuries: trauma mechanisms and associated injuries, *J Trauma* 35:40, 1993.

Weinfeld SB, Haddad SL, Myerson MS: Metatarsal stress fractures, *Clin Sports Med* 16:319, 1997.

Wiener BD, Linder JF, Giattini JFG: Treatment of fractures of the fifth metatarsal: a prospective study, *Foot Ankle Int* 18:267, 1997.

Wright RW, Fischer DA, Shively RA, et al.: Refracture of proximal fifth metatarsal (Jones) fracture after intramedullary screw fixation in athletes, *Am J Sports Med* 28:732, 2000.

Yue JJ, Marcus RE: The role of internal fixation in the treatment of Jones fractures in diabetics, *Foot Ankle Int* 17:559, 1996.

Zelko RR, Torg JS, Rachun A: Proximal diaphyseal fractures of the fifth metatarsal—treatment of the fractures and their complications in athletes, *Am J Sports Med* 7:95, 1979.

Zenios M, Kim WY, Sampath J, Muddu BN: Functional treatment of acute metatarsal fractures: a prospective randomized comparison of management in a cast versus elasticated support bandage, *Injury* 36:832, 2005.

PHALANGES

Hojyo F, Nagata K, Narahara T, et al.: Two cases of irreducible dislocation of the interphalangeal joint of the great toe with interposition of sesamoid bone, *J Orthop Surg* 34:820, 1983.

Jahss MH: Traumatic dislocations of the first metatarsophalangeal joint, *Foot Ankle* 1:15, 1980.

Jahss MH: Chronic and recurrent dislocations of the fifth toe, *Foot Ankle* 1:275, 1981.

Katayama M, Murakami Y, Takahashi H: Irreducible dorsal dislocation of the toe: report of three cases, *J Bone Joint Surg* 70A:769, 1988.

Kursunoglu S, Resnick D, Goergen T: Traumatic dislocation with sesamoid entrapment in the interphalangeal joint of the great toe, *J Trauma* 27:959, 1987.

Lewis AG, DeLee JC: Type-I complex dislocation of the first metatarsophalangeal joint: open reduction through a dorsal approach, *J Bone Joint Surg* 66A:1120, 1984.

Miki T, Yamamuro T, Kitai T: An irreducible dislocation of the great toe: report of two cases and review of the literature, *Clin Orthop Relat Res* 230:200, 1988.

Nelson TL, Uggen W: Irreducible dorsal dislocation of the interphalangeal joint of the great toe, *Clin Orthop Relat Res* 157:110, 1981.

Salamon PB, Gelberman RH, Huffer JM: Dorsal dislocation of the metatarsophalangeal joint of the great toe: a case report, *J Bone Joint Surg* 56A:1073, 1974.

Sarrafian SK: *Anatomy of the foot and ankle*, Philadelphia, 1983, Lippincott.

Yu EC, Garfin SR: Closed dorsal dislocation of the metatarsophalangeal joint of the great toe, *Clin Orthop Relat Res* 185:237, 1983.

SESAMOIDS

Anderson RB: McBryde AM: autogenous bone grafting of hallux sesamoid nonunions, *Foot Ankle Int* 18:293, 1997.

Aper RL, Saltzman CL, Brown TD: The effect of hallux sesamoid resection on the effective moment of the flexor hallucis brevis, *Foot Ankle* 15:462, 1994.

Aper RL, Saltzman CL, Brown TD: The effect of hallux sesamoid excision on the flexor hallucis longus moment arm, *Clin Orthop Relat Res* 325:209, 1996.

Biedert R, Hintermann B: Stress fractures of the medial great toe sesamoids in athletes, *Foot Ankle Int* 24:137, 2003.

Brown TIS: Avulsion fractures of the fibular sesamoid in association with dorsal dislocation of the metatarsophalangeal joint of the hallux: report of a case and review of the literature, *Clin Orthop Relat Res* 149:229, 1980.

Burman MS, Lapidus PW: The functional disturbances caused by the inconstant bones and sesamoids of the foot, *Arch Surg* 22:936, 1931.

Chisin R, Peyser A, Milgrom C: Bone scintigraphy in the assessment of the hallucal sesamoids, *Foot Ankle Int* 16:291, 1995.

deBritto SR: The first metatarso-sesamoid joint, *Int Orthop* 6:61, 1982.

Fleischli J, Cheleuitte E: Avascular necrosis of the hallucal sesamoids, *J Foot Ankle Surg* 34:358, 1995.

Glass B: Fractured fibular sesamoid: a case report, *J Foot Surg* 19:19, 1980.

Helal B: Surgery of the forefoot, *Br Med J* 1:276, 1977.

Helal B: The great toe sesamoid bones: the lux or lost souls of Ushia, *Clin Orthop Relat Res* 157:82, 1981.

Hussain A: Dislocation of the first metatarsophalangeal joint with fracture of fibular sesamoid, *Clin Orthop Relat Res* 359:209, 1999.

Inge GAL, Ferguson AB: Surgery of the sesamoid bones of the great toe: an anatomical and clinical study with a report of 41 cases, *Arch Surg* 27:466, 1933.

Irwin AS, Maffulli N, Wardlaw D: Traumatic dislocation of the lateral sesamoid of the great toe: nonoperative management, *J Orthop Trauma* 180:2, 1995.

Jahss MH: The sesamoids of the hallux, *Clin Orthop Relat Res* 157:88, 1981.

Kaiman ME, Piccona R: Tibial sesamoidectomy: a review of the literature and retrospective study, *J Foot Surg* 22:286, 1983.

Lee S, James WC, Cohen BE, et al.: Evaluation of hallux alignment and functional outcome after isolated tibial sesamoidectomy, *Foot Ankle Int* 26:803, 2005.

Morris JM: Biomechanics of the foot and ankle, *Clin Orthop Relat Res* 122:10, 1977.

Nuber GW, Anderson PR: Acute osteomyelitis of the metatarsal sesamoid, *Clin Orthop Relat Res* 167:212, 1982.

Richardson EG: Hallucal sesamoid pain: causes and surgical treatment, *J Am Acad Orthop Surg* 7:270, 1999.

Saxena A, Krisdakumtorn T: Return to activity after sesamoidectomy in athletically active individuals, *Foot Ankle Int* 24:415, 2003.

Van Hal ME, Keene JS, Lange TA, et al.: Stress fractures of the great toe sesamoids, *Am J Sports Med* 10:122, 1982.

Weiss JS: Fracture of the medial sesamoid bone of the great toe: controversies in therapy, *Orthopedics* 14:1003, 1991.

Zinman H, Keret D, Reis ND: Fracture of the medial sesamoid bone of the hallux, *J Trauma* 21:581, 1981.

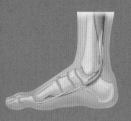

CHAPTER 10

SPORTS INJURIES OF THE ANKLE

David R. Richardson

Participation in sports is associated with foot and ankle injuries; however, one does not need to be an athlete to experience a twisting, impaction, contusive, or repetitive traumatic event. In addition, some conditions are initiated by antecedent trauma; the history of the condition may be nonspecific, and symptoms of injury may have subsided (e.g., chondromalacia or osteochondritis dissecans of the ankle). Other than fractures or dislocations, trauma produces at least three kinds of joint affections: (1) acute severe ligamentous injuries with joint disruptions, (2) ligamentous injuries of lesser magnitude from a single episode or from repetitive "overuse" producing nondisruptive and microscopic abnormalities of the joint, and (3) aggravation of preexisting joint abnormalities. Miscellaneous affections of joints probably not caused by trauma but possibly aggravated by athletic, recreational, or occupational activities are discussed in other chapter.

ACUTE LIGAMENTOUS INJURIES

Sprains constitute 85% of all ankle injuries, and 85% of those involve a lateral inversion mechanism. Ankle injuries account for 14% to 21% of all sports-related injuries; approximately 40% of basketball injuries and 25% of soccer injuries involve the ankle. Volleyball and football also have especially high risks of ankle ligament injury. Compared with men, women have a slightly higher overall incidence of ankle injuries in similar sports activities. Men, however, have a higher incidence of medial ankle and syndesmotic sprains. Greater mean height and weight, increased body mass index, and certain athletic activities (e.g., basketball, cheerleading, rugby) may be risk factors for ankle sprains as well.

Ankle ligamentous injuries, as classified by O'Donoghue, occur as minor ligamentous "stretch" injuries (type I sprain), incomplete ligamentous tears (type II sprain), or complete disruption of the ligament or ligaments (type III sprain). A more practical approach is based on the stability of the ankle as determined by stress testing and the functional level of the patient (Box 10.1). Eversion and abduction of the foot may result in disruption of the deltoid ligament; however, more commonly the inversion stress results in ligamentous disruption on the lateral side of the ankle (usually the anterior talofibular ligament or calcaneofibular ligament). Diagnosis and treatment depend on an understanding of the ligamentous and muscular structures around the ankle.

ANATOMY

Stabilizing the medial side of the ankle anteriorly and posteriorly is the strong, flat, triangular deltoid ligament consisting of five components. The deep portion of the deltoid ligament is probably the most important and provides the greatest restraint against lateral translation. The two components, the anterior and posterior deep tibiotalar ligaments, attach

---

BOX 10.1

Ankle Ligament Injury and Treatment Recommendations

Acute
Stable ankle (clinical and radiographic studies with anesthesia as needed)
  Symptomatic treatment
Unstable ankle (+ anterior drawer or talar tilt clinically and radiographically)
  Low-demand patient
    Functional treatment
  High-demand patient
    Surgical intervention

Chronic
Continued pain or functional instability
  Surgical intervention based on examination and imaging studies

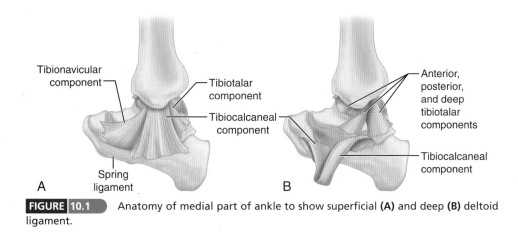

FIGURE 10.1 Anatomy of medial part of ankle to show superficial **(A)** and deep **(B)** deltoid ligament.

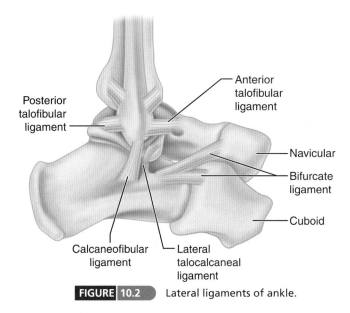

FIGURE 10.2 Lateral ligaments of ankle.

to the undersurface of the medial malleolus and the body of the talus (Fig. 10.1). Both deep components are intraarticular but extrasynovial. The posterior deep tibiotalar ligament is the strongest of the entire deltoid complex. The superficial portion of the deltoid ligament consists of the other three components: the tibionavicular component anteriorly, the tibiocalcaneal component in the middle, and the posterior tibiotalar component posteriorly. Both the superficial and deep components resist valgus tilting of the talus and are secondary restraints against anterior translation of the talus.

Laterally, the three primary ligaments that stabilize the ankle vary in structure (Fig. 10.2). The anterior talofibular ligament is 2.0 to 2.5 mm thick, 15 to 20 mm long, and 6 to 8 mm wide and is attached posteriorly to the anterior border of the lateral malleolus and anteriorly to the neck of the talus, where it blends with the anterolateral joint capsule. It is the weakest and most often injured of the lateral ligaments. It primarily functions to resist anterior translation of the talus when the ankle is in a relatively neutral position. The calcaneofibular ligament is 20 to 25 mm long, 6 to 8 mm wide, and 3 to 4 mm thick and is stronger than the anterior talofibular ligament. It is attached superiorly to the tip of the lateral malleolus, extends deep to the peroneal tendons, and inserts

inferiorly on the lateral surface of the calcaneus (it is the only lateral ligament that is extracapsular). The posterior talofibular ligament is 30 mm long, 5 mm wide, and 5 to 8 mm thick and is the strongest of the lateral ligaments. It is attached anteriorly to the digital fossa of the fibula and posteriorly to the lateral tubercle on the posterior aspect of the talus. The bifurcate ligament does not assist in maintaining stability of the ankle, but injury to this ligament often is misdiagnosed because of its proximity to the lateral ankle ligaments. The bifurcate ligament is attached to the anterior process of the calcaneus. Just distal to the origin, the ligament divides in a Y-shaped manner to insert on both the dorsomedial aspect of the cuboid and the dorsolateral aspect of the navicular.

The relationship of the distal tibiofibular syndesmosis is maintained by four ligaments (Fig. 10.3). The anterior inferior tibiofibular ligament attaches medially to the anterior tibial tubercle, extends inferior and lateral, and inserts on the anterior fibula. Occasionally, a slip of this ligament (Bassett's ligament) inserts distally on the fibula and may cause impingement symptoms at the anterolateral aspect of the talus (see Fig. 10.36). The posteroinferior tibiofibular ligament is the strongest component (the interosseous membrane is not part of the distal tibiofibular syndesmosis) and runs in a similar direction as the anteroinferior tibiofibular ligament. The inferior transverse tibiofibular ligament is deep and inferior to the posteroinferior tibiofibular ligament. On its anterior surface, the inferior transverse tibiofibular ligament forms a labrum that articulates with the posterolateral talus, effectively deepening the tibiotalar joint. The interosseous tibiofibular ligament attaches to the contiguous rough surfaces of the tibia and fibula and is continuous with the interosseous membrane proximally. With dorsiflexion of the ankle, the syndesmosis allows the fibula to translate, rotate, and proximally migrate. This ligamentous complex also allows the fibula to share approximately 16% of the axial load.

DIAGNOSIS

A careful physical examination is essential to avoid misdiagnosis. The following structures must be palpated because they may be associated with a complaint of ankle pain: the anterior talofibular, calcaneofibular, bifurcate, syndesmotic, and deltoid ligaments; the medial and lateral malleoli; the fifth metatarsal base and the insertion of the peroneus tertius onto the dorsal fifth metatarsal base; the anterior process of the calcaneus and lateral process of the talus; and the

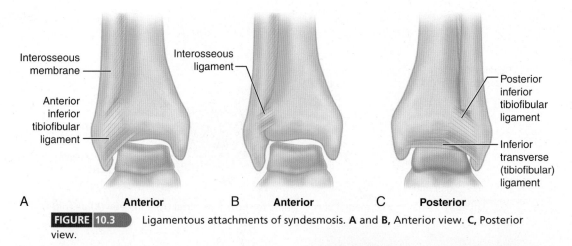

Interosseous
membrane

Interosseous
ligament

Posterior
inferior
tibiofibular
ligament

Anterior
inferior
tibiofibular
ligament

Posterior
inferior
tibiofibular
ligament

Inferior
transverse
(tibiofibular)
ligament

A   **Anterior**   B   **Anterior**   C   **Posterior**

FIGURE 10.3 Ligamentous attachments of syndesmosis. **A** and **B,** Anterior view. **C,** Posterior view.

Achilles, peroneal, posterior tibial, flexor hallucis longus, and flexor digitorum longus tendons. Frey et al. found that physical examination was 100% accurate in the diagnosis of grade III ligament injuries but only 25% accurate in the diagnosis of grade II injuries compared with MRI findings. Clinicians most often underestimate the damage with a grade II ligament tear. Van Dijk et al. suggested that a more accurate diagnosis is possible if physical examination is performed 5 days after injury rather than within 48 hours.

In acute injuries, diagnosis by stressing the ankle for instability is often difficult but may be improved with an appropriate regional block. Injection of local anesthetic into the peroneal sheath and lateral gutter of the ankle before provocative maneuvers of the ankle often improves the examination of the lateral ligaments by decreasing guarding and muscle spasm. Inversion-eversion and anteroposterior stress testing (anterior drawer sign) can be used to evaluate acute and chronic instability and to help determine the extent of the injury, but stress tests must clearly show a significant difference between the abnormal and normal ankles before they can be considered diagnostic.

■ INVERSION AND EVERSION STRESS TESTS

Complete rupture of the deltoid ligament, including the deep portion, is less common. When the deltoid ligament is completely disrupted with rupture of the tibiofibular syndesmosis or fracture of the lateral malleolus, the talus can shift laterally with eversion stress. External rotation stress radiographs allow the accurate diagnosis of deltoid incompetence in patients with supination-eversion (Lauge-Hansen) fibular fractures with a reduced mortise. Direct examination around the medial malleolus for tenderness, swelling, and ecchymosis are poor predictors of instability. Some shift of the talus laterally may occur when the syndesmosis alone has been ruptured. Eversion stress radiographs of normal ankles have been reported to reveal little talar shift or tilt.

If the lateral ligaments are completely disrupted, the talus tilts with inversion stress (Fig. 10.4). Inversion stress is best applied with the ankle plantarflexed. Tilting of the talus 15 degrees may indicate rupture of the anterior talofibular ligament alone, tilting 15 to 30 degrees indicates rupture of the anterior talofibular and calcaneofibular ligaments, and tilting more than 30 degrees may indicate that all three of the lateral ligaments (anterior and posterior talofibular as well as calcaneofibular ligaments) were ruptured. However, there is

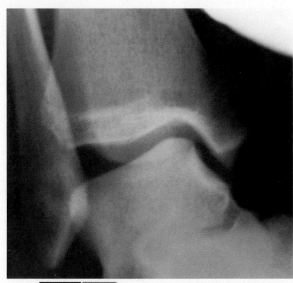

FIGURE 10.4 Positive inversion stress test.

no absolute endpoint to distinguish a positive talar tilt from a negative one. At our institution, we stress both ankles and believe that more than 10 degrees of talar tilt over that of the normal side indicates a significant lateral ligamentous injury. Stress radiographs do not need to be obtained routinely because most unstable ligamentous injuries are treated functionally with good results. "Functional" treatment usually refers to the use of RICE (*r*est, *i*ce, *c*ompression, *e*levation) and a short semirigid brace. This is followed by early range-of-motion exercises and early weight bearing with an emphasis on neuromuscular training.

An os subfibulare (an ossicle adjacent to the fibula inferiorly) may represent an avulsion fracture instead of a normal variant and may or may not be associated with laxity of the anterior talofibular ligament. Recurrent inversion sprains of the ankle and continuous discomfort are indications for stress films to determine any tibiotalar joint laxity and any movement of the os subfibulare.

■ ANTEROPOSTERIOR STRESS TEST (ANTERIOR DRAWER SIGN)

The anterior drawer sign (Fig. 10.5) indicates a tear of the anterior talofibular ligament. Clinically, it is helpful to place the tip of the thumb on the tip of the lateral malleolus while

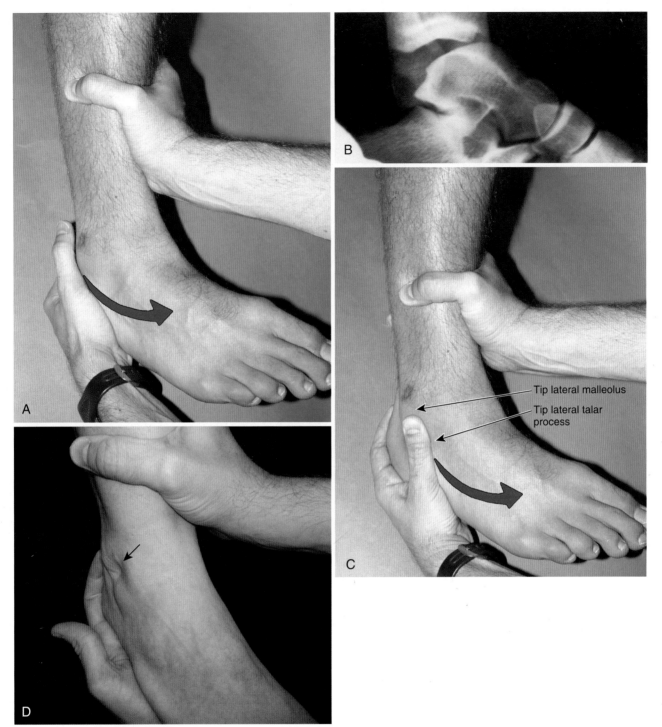

FIGURE 10.5 **A,** Demonstration of anterior drawer sign positioning for radiograph. **B,** Positive anterior drawer test. **C,** Clinical demonstration of anterior draw sign. **D,** Sulcus, or suction, sign *(arrow)* indicating disruption of the anterior talofibular ligament.

palpating the lateral talar process with the base of the thumb. The ankle is held in neutral or slight plantarflexion and is allowed to internally rotate. With gentle stress, one can assess the degree of anterior displacement of the talus relative to the tibia (Fig. 10.5C). A sulcus sign may be present with disruption of the anterior talofibular ligament (Fig. 10.5D). A relatively low-magnitude load is all that is required when evaluating the integrity of the anterior talofibular ligament in an acute ligamentous ankle injury. More important than the number of millimeters of displacement is the clinical impression that the talus is subluxating out of the mortise.

Recently, subtalar sprains have garnered more attention. Although it is difficult to differentiate between a subtalar and ankle sprain, negative stress films in the presence of a clinically serious ankle injury or patient-reported chronic functional instability should arouse suspicion of an underlying subtalar sprain. Most subtalar ligamentous injuries occur in combination with injuries of the lateral ligament of the ankle.

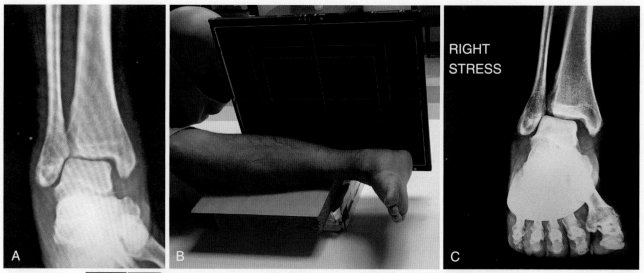

FIGURE 10.6   **A,** Non–weight bearing standard mortise view of ankle. **B,** Limb placed over bolster with distal third of leg off the table, with cassette positioned for a cross table lateral image, allowing external rotation stress of mortise **(C).**

Sectioning of the interosseous talocalcaneal ligament along with the anterior talofibular ligament produces a significant change in subtalar motion compared with injury to the anterior talofibular ligament alone. To determine the appropriate treatment in a symptomatic patient, subtalar stress radiographs (inversion stress Broden view) in addition to routine talar stress radiographs to quantify the relative contributions of each of these joints to inversion laxity may be useful. Several authors, however, have questioned the validity of these tests to diagnose subtalar instability.

■ STRESS VIEW OF THE ANKLE MORTISE AND SYNDESMOSIS

If not pronounced a stress view of the mortise may help in diagnosing syndesmotic injuries (Fig. 10.6A). Gravity and manual external rotation stress views are both effective, although radiographic measurements are influenced by position. We usually opt for the gravity stress view because this causes less discomfort to the patient. To perform the gravity stress view, the patient is placed in a semilateral position with the affected side down. The injured limb is placed over a bolster, with the distal third of the leg "floating" off the table and the cassette positioned for a cross table lateral image (Fig. 10.6B). This allows for external rotation stress of the mortise and diagnosis of the instability (Fig. 10.6C).

■ MAGNETIC RESONANCE IMAGING

More powerful and three-dimensional MRI studies have allowed for greater accuracy in the diagnosis of ankle and hindfoot injuries. Axial MRI with a local gradient provides optimal views of the anterior and posterior talofibular ligaments and the deep layers and tibionavicular component of the deltoid ligament, whereas MRI coronal imaging allows a complete view of the calcaneofibular, posterior talofibular, tibiocalcaneal, and posterior tibiotalar ligaments. In both imaging planes, differentiation of the deep and superficial layers of the medial collateral ligament, as well as between the syndesmotic complex and the lateral collateral ligaments, was possible. Nielson et al. found no correlation between tibiofibular

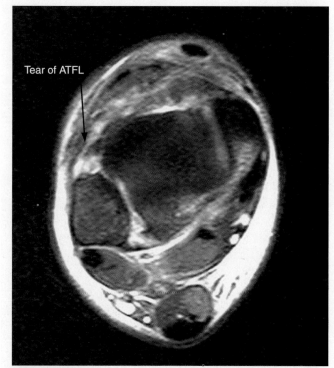

FIGURE 10.7   MRI of patient with syndesmosis injury; note tear of the anterior tibiofibular ligament *(arrow).*

clear space and overlap measurements in patients with syndesmotic injuries seen on MRI (Fig. 10.7). A medial clear space measurement of more than 4 mm correlated with disruption of the deltoid and tibiofibular ligaments (Fig. 10.8).

MRI has been shown to be more specific than sensitive, especially as it relates to the calcaneofibular ligament. Note that bone bruises occur in a significant number of ankle sprains and that multiple bone bruises occur more frequently in patients with multiple ligaments injured. Although bone bruise–like lesions may be seen at an average of 8.4 weeks, they often are present more than 1 year after injury. MRI has

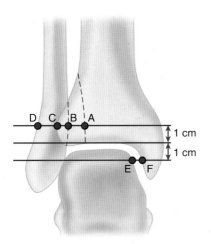

A = Lateral border of posterior tibial malleolus
B = Medial border of fibula
C = Lateral border of anterior tibial prominence
D = Lateral border of fibula
E = Medial border of talus
F = Lateral border of medial malleolus
AB = Tibiofibular clear space
BC = Tibiofibular overlap
EF = Medial clear space

FIGURE 10.8 Radiographic relationships important in evaluating tibiofibular articulation. Line *EF* represents medial clear space; line *AB* represents tibiofibular clear space.

been shown to be effective by several authors in identifying and differentiating lateral ankle ligament injuries; however, many believe that the costs outweigh the benefits. If a peroneal pathologic process is suspected, MRI may be beneficial, but it is not routinely necessary to diagnose lateral ligament injury.

TREATMENT

Most type I and type II sprains or ligamentous injuries can be treated by functional bracing and early rehabilitation. This treatment allows stretched and attenuated ligaments to be in reasonable anatomic alignment and length during the healing process. Although immobilization quickly relieves pain and may be beneficial in reducing the swelling, early mobilization for these injuries produces results that are superior to immobilization. Proprioceptive training after usual care appears beneficial as well. Regardless, most sprains do not need surgical repair. Even patients with complete grade III tears may obtain good results with functional treatment consisting of a short period of protection with taping or bracing that allows early weight bearing, followed by functional range-of-motion exercises and neuromuscular training of the ankle. High-demand patients will benefit from a sport-specific rehabilitation program developed with the collaboration of the physician, trainer, therapist, and coaches. Advantages of this method include quick recovery of functional range of motion and early return to work and physical activity. However, acute surgical intervention may improve long-term results if instability is present clinically and radiographically. Secondary operative reconstruction or delayed repair of the ruptured ligaments can be done years after the injury if necessary, and the results may be comparable with primary repair. Competitive athletes can be treated functionally, although 10% to 20% require later secondary repair. Although functional treatment

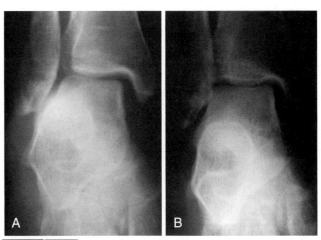

FIGURE 10.9 **A,** Acute tear of deltoid ligament with oblique fracture of fibula and lateral shift of talus in ankle mortise. **B,** After repair of deltoid ligament.

avoids the additional trauma to the tissues and complications inherent in surgical treatment, in high-demand patients with clinical and radiographic instability, acute surgical intervention is a reasonable approach. Indications for surgical treatment are large bony avulsions, unstable osteochondral injuries, severe ligamentous incompetence on the medial or lateral sides of the ankle, and recurrent ankle injuries.

The goal of treatment is to prevent chronic instability of the ankle. A 1-mm lateral shift of the talus in the mortise has been shown to produce a 42% reduction in the area of contact between the tibia and the talus. Because stress per unit area increases as the total contact area decreases, displacement may contribute to a poor result and give support to the contention that joint instability leads to traumatic arthritis. Ankle instability may result from fracture or ligamentous injury or a combination of both, and what may appear at the ankle to be a pure ligamentous injury with talar shift may include a fracture of the proximal fibula (e.g., Maisonneuve fracture).

■ REPAIR OF ACUTE RUPTURE OF THE DELTOID LIGAMENT

In active patients, acute ruptures of the deltoid ligament, shown by abnormal tilt or shift of the talus in the ankle mortise and a palpable defect in the ligament, usually should be repaired. Often, the lateral malleolus is fractured or the distal tibiofibular joint is disrupted (Fig. 10.9). Crim et al., in a review of patients with chronic lateral ankle instability, found that 72% had an injury of the deltoid ligament as seen on MRI; 43% of all patients had injuries to both the deep and superficial components. Isolated partial ruptures of the deltoid ligament have been reported, but isolated complete ruptures are rare. Varus and valgus stress testing may show some widening of the clear space of the medial malleolus and some tilting of the talus in deltoid ligament rupture without fracture, and comparison MRI can determine the extent and location of the deltoid tear. For isolated complete disruption, immobilization in a below-knee, non–weight bearing plaster cast for 4 to 6 weeks, followed by use of a molded shoe orthosis for 4 to 6 months, has been recommended. Surgical exploration for patients with evidence of significant displacement at the time of injury is often warranted. This condition should not be confused with isolated rupture of the posterior tibial tendon, which also causes medial ankle pain in pronation.

Satisfactory functional results have been reported after surgical treatment in patients with complete disruption or incompetency of the deltoid ligament, without deltoid repair as part of the initial operation as long as surgical reduction of the medial joint space and lateral malleolus was accurate and maintained until bone repair was complete. Hsu et al. reviewed 14 cases of direct repair of the deltoid ligament in professional American football athletes after ankle fracture fixation. Each patient underwent a dynamic arthroscopic examination with removal of loose bodies and debridement of osteochondral lesions as indicated followed by fixation of the lateral malleolar fracture. The deltoid ligament was then repaired directly by approximating the tibionavicular and tibial calcaneal portion of the deltoid to its native attachment on the medial malleolus. Each patient followed a standard postoperative rehabilitation protocol. Good results were noted in these high-performance athletes after this treatment regimen. Note that the posterior tibial tendon or the proximal end of the avulsed deltoid ligament may be caught between the medial malleolus and the talus with attempted reduction of the laterally displaced talus (see Fig. 10.9). The technique of repair of acute rupture of the deltoid ligament is described in other chapter.

REPAIR OF ACUTE RUPTURE OF THE LIGAMENTS OF THE DISTAL TIBIOFIBULAR JOINT

When the ligaments binding the distal tibia to the fibula are ruptured, the medial malleolus usually is fractured or the fibula is fractured proximal to the lateral malleolus or both injuries may occur. Occasionally, however, the associated injury is rupture of the deltoid ligament. Syndesmotic sprains reportedly account for approximately 1% of all ankle injuries and 18% of all ankle sprains; however, because diastasis is rare in isolated injuries, this may be underreported. Male sex and higher level of competition are risks factors for syndesmotic ankle sprain during athletics. Diastasis after an isolated syndesmotic injury is rare, and rupture of the ligaments of the distal tibiofibular joint usually can be treated by closed methods. However, if widening of the ankle mortise remains after manipulation, surgery is necessary (Fig. 10.10). In surgically treated syndesmosis injuries, malreduction results in poor functional outcomes. Open reduction of the syndesmosis results in a significantly lower incidence of malreduction compared with closed reduction with percutaneous fixation (Fig. 10.11). In patients treated operatively and with acceptable risks for a larger incision, we advocate open treatment of the syndesmosis. Direct visualization or palpation of the syndesmosis has been shown to be equally effective in achieving syndesmotic reduction, but neither method is perfect. If the ankle mortise was dislocated or significantly subluxed, we recommend routinely opening it medially with sweeping of the medial clear space and repair of the deltoid ligament as necessary.

Several authors have described the sequelae of syndesmosis ankle sprains in military cadets and professional and college football players. They concluded that this is a more serious injury with a longer recovery time than a third-degree lateral ankle sprain. Accurate diagnosis of a syndesmosis sprain can be made by a positive squeeze test (Fig. 10.12), but this should be done only after other injuries to the leg are ruled out by examination and radiographs. According to the study by Teitz and Harrington, compression (squeezing) of the calf caused

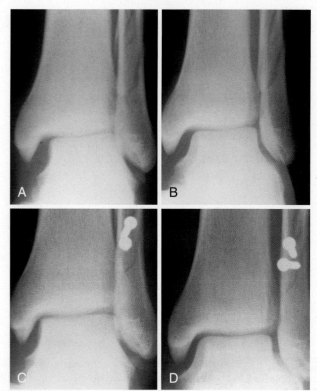

FIGURE 10.10 Tear of deltoid ligament associated with fibular fracture. **A,** Anteroposterior view shows small fragment off medial malleolus and shift of talus within ankle mortise. **B,** Oblique view shows widening of joint space on medial side of ankle. **C** and **D,** Open reduction and internal fixation of fracture of lateral malleolus, with reduction of talus into ankle mortise; deltoid ligament was not repaired.

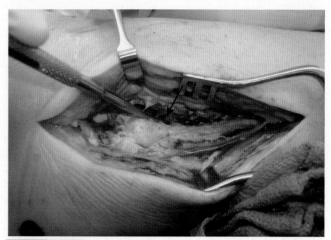

FIGURE 10.11 Disruption of the syndesmotic ligaments is directly visualized.

separation of the distal fibula and tibia. External rotation stress testing (Fig. 10.13) also is helpful in making the diagnosis. At follow-up, many patients in these series had developed ossification of the syndesmosis (Fig. 10.14); however, in the absence of frank synostosis, functional ankle results were excellent or good. Chronic ankle instability did not seem to result from the syndesmosis sprains, but recurrent sprains were common if heterotopic ossification occurred. In some patients, syndesmosis ossification may be symptomatic, thus requiring

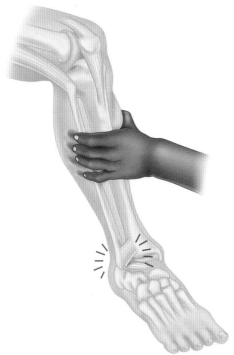

FIGURE 10.12   Squeeze test is performed by compressing fibula to tibia above midpoint of calf. Test is considered positive if proximal compression produces distal pain in interosseous ligaments or supporting structures.

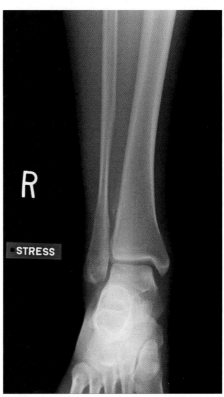

FIGURE 10.14   Chronic syndesmosis disruption with deltoid incompetence and early syndesmotic calcification.

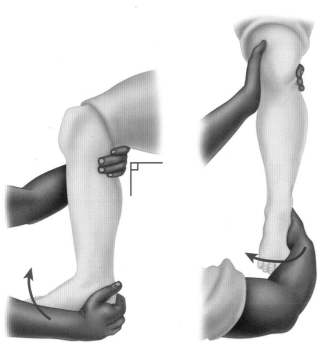

FIGURE 10.13   External rotation testing is performed by applying external rotation stress to involved foot and ankle while knee is held in 90 degrees of flexion and ankle is in neutral position. Positive test produces pain over anterior or posterior tibiofibular ligaments and over interosseous membrane.

surgical excision. Yasui et al. reported good results with anatomic reconstruction of the anteroinferior tibiofibular ligament using an autologous gracilis tendon in six patients with chronic disruption of the syndesmosis after a pronation and external rotation type IV injury. Surgical fusion of the syndesmosis may be required in patients with chronic instability.

Most authors have advocated the use of metal screws or suture buttons for the stabilization of syndesmotic injuries with persistent diastasis. The outcomes with titanium or stainless steel screws, as well as with tricortical or quadricortical fixation, have not been shown to be significantly different. Although 4.5-mm screws have not demonstrated improved biomechanical properties when placed in a tricortical fashion, they have demonstrated improved resistance to shear stress on the distal tibiofibular joint when placed across four cortices. More recent literature indicates that suture button fixation of the syndesmosis may result in improved American Orthopaedic Foot and Ankle Society (AOFAS) scores, lower postoperative complications, and earlier time to full weight bearing. Ideal placement of the fixation device has not been established. We advocate placement of the screw or suture button 3 cm proximal and parallel to the distal tibial articular surface (just proximal to the incisura), angled 20 to 30 degrees anteromedially and starting on the posterolateral aspect of the fibula. In theory suture button fixation (Fig. 10.15) provides secure, but not rigid, fixation of the syndesmosis, allowing for spontaneous reduction of the syndesmosis even if there is mild initial malreduction.

Hardware removal is common for both screw and suture button techniques. A review found that approximately 50% of screws and 10% of suture buttons require removal. When screw removal is planned, it most often is done before full weight bearing, 3 to 4 months after the initial procedure. Screw breakage, button subsidence, and early or late loss of

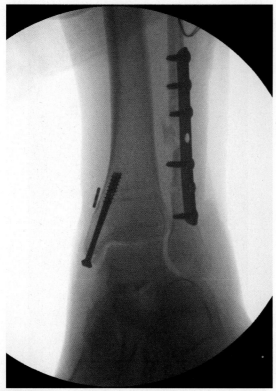

FIGURE 10.15 Fixation of syndesmosis with suture button.

reduction have been reported as some of the most common complications after surgical repair of the syndesmosis. Our institution favors suture button fixation in active individuals, allowing for earlier weight bearing and obviating the need for routine implant removal. Alternatively, the syndesmosis can be directly repaired through fixation of bony avulsion injuries or suture anchor repair. We do not recommend suture button fixation when the fibular fracture is not rigidly fixed (e.g., Maisonneuve fractures). Suture fixation allows for a small amount of motion and may result in the fibula healing slightly shortened.

REPAIR OF ACUTE RUPTURE OF LIGAMENTS OF DISTAL TIBIOFIBULAR JOINT

TECHNIQUE 10.1

- Position the patient supine with a bump under the ipsilateral hip. A more lateral decubitus position with a beanbag may be necessary to visualize the posteroinferior tibiofibular ligament, if desired. External rotation of the hip allows access to the medial structures as needed.
- Place a bolster under the ankle while allowing the heel to "float" off the operating table. This will prevent anterior subluxation of the talus on the tibial plafond.
- Make an incision 5 cm long parallel to the anterior border of the distal fibula, and expose the distal tibiofibular joint.

- Press the fibula into the groove in the tibia (incisura fibularis) to shift the fibula and the talus medially into normal position. With this technique, suturing or reattaching the ligaments is unnecessary.
- Once reduced, maintain the syndesmosis in position with a large clamp under gentle compression (if the mortise is anatomically reduced, a clamp may be unnecessary) and ensure that the fibula does not sublux or rotate. Use intraoperative fluoroscopy to further assess fibular position and reduction of the syndesmosis and ankle mortise.
- Under fluoroscopic visualization, drill an appropriate-sized tunnel for placement of either a screw or a suture button. This can be placed through a fibular plate or directly against the fibula. A plate may decrease the risk of a stress injury or implant subsidence but may increase lateral irritation. Direct the drill in a 25% anteromedial direction beginning on the posterior aspect of the fibula. Drill 3 cm proximal and parallel to the tibial plafond. Combined use of a metal screw and a suture button provides rigid fixation for 10 to 12 weeks and protects against late loss of reduction.
- If the screw is to be removed, placement across four cortices may facilitate retrieval should the screw break (Fig. 10.16).
- Check the position of the implant and the reduction of the talus by radiographs in the operating room to ensure that the talus has been replaced precisely against the medial malleolus; if not, it is likely that some soft structure, such as a tendon or the deltoid ligament, is obstructing reduction (Fig. 10.17) (see discussion of irreducible fracture or fracture-dislocation of the ankle in other chapter).
- For an associated proximal fibular fracture, apply a small, lightweight, semitubular plate to fix the fracture. One of the screws for the plate on a more distal fracture can be used to transfix the distal tibiofibular joint. This AO technique is described in other chapter.

ALTERNATIVE TECHNIQUE FOR DIRECT ANATOMIC REPAIR
- Position the patient as described previously.
- Repair lateral malleolar injury as needed.
- If syndesmotic instability is associated with a bony avulsion, attempt bony fixation because this will provide a stronger repair (Fig. 10.18A-D). If the fragment is too small to allow for bony fixation, excise it and place a suture anchor at the fibular or tibial footprint of the anteroinferior tibiofibular ligament or posteroinferior tibiofibular ligament, as indicated (Fig. 10.19A-C).

POSTOPERATIVE CARE A splint is applied from the base of the toes to the tibial tuberosity. At 2 weeks, the splint is removed, and a cast is applied and worn for an additional 3 weeks. At 5 weeks, a walking boot is placed and the patient is instructed on active, touch-down–weight-bearing range-of-motion exercises. Weight bearing in the boot is begun at 8 to 10 weeks. The boot is worn until the screw (if used) is removed at 14 weeks postoperatively. Weight bearing should be limited until/if hardware is removed because it may become loose or break within the tibiofibular joint.

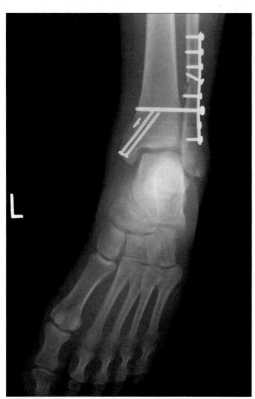

FIGURE 10.16 In young active individual who wishes to have syndesmosis screw removed, we often add suture button fixation to allow earlier removal of metal screw without risk of loss of reduction. Placement of syndesmotic screw across four cortices to allow retrieval from medial aspect of ankle in case of screw breakage. **SEE TECHNIQUE 10.1.**

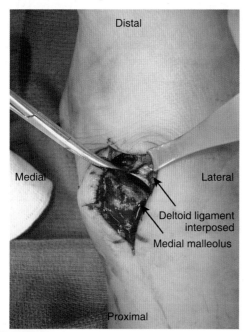

FIGURE 10.17 Deltoid ligament preventing reduction of ankle fracture-dislocation. **SEE TECHNIQUE 10.1.**

■ REPAIR OF ACUTE RUPTURE OF THE LATERAL LIGAMENTS

The anterior talofibular ligament is the most important stabilizing ligament of the ankle; however, isolated rupture of the anterior talofibular ligament can be treated by immobilization. Although 10% to 20% of athletes may have chronic symptoms related to an ankle sprain, the cause of functional instability of the ankle after injury of the ligaments is unknown. After healing of a ruptured anterior talofibular ligament, some patients still have lateral pain and swelling even though they can return to full activity. It has been postulated that the presence of a localized synovitis, painful scar in the ligament, weakness of the peroneal musculature, or even a proprioceptive deficit involving the nerves of the ankle joint may be the cause of residual symptoms. Articular cartilage lesions also may cause pain after healing or stabilization of the joint. Intraarticular chondral lesions larger than one half the thickness of the articular cartilage and more than 5 mm in diameter are associated with postoperative pain, indicating that ligament reconstruction alone may not relieve pain if large intraarticular lesions are present and that the two problems (ligamentous insufficiency and intraarticular lesion) must be evaluated and treated separately.

When at least two of the lateral ligaments, the anterior talofibular and the calcaneofibular, are torn, support exists for surgical repair. Disruption of the calcaneofibular ligament results in de facto alterations to subtalar joint kinematics, although the literature suggests repair is not always required. Several authors have reported better results with acute surgical repair of ruptured lateral ligaments, especially in young athletic patients. One study of 388 patients randomized to functional treatment (taping or elastic bandaging, followed by functional rehabilitation) or operative treatment found that the risk of giving way, recurrent sprains, and residual pain was reduced in the surgically treated group. There was no difference in swelling, subjective outcome, or return to sports. Despite the better results, the authors did not recommend routine primary repair of the lateral ankle ligaments, partly because of the higher costs involved and the risk of complications associated with surgery. In other series of patients, not necessarily athletes, operative repair resulted in a higher incidence of early complications that slightly delayed the patients' return to work, and there was no evidence that operative repair offered improved symptomatic or functional benefit. A comprehensive literature evaluation and meta-analysis concluded that conservative treatment of acute lateral ligament tears results in outcomes similar to those with surgical treatment. The excellent results found after delayed repairs or reconstruction of the lateral ligaments perhaps allow for a more conservative approach to acute injuries. Conservative treatment should consist of functional therapy. Rest, ice, compression, and elevation (RICE) should begin immediately after injury. In most instances, a functional brace should be placed and physical rehabilitation begun as soon as weight bearing is tolerated. Athletes with a significant ligament injury should consider the indefinite use of a functional brace because they are at increased risk of recurrent sprains.

Several authors have reported good results with the Gould modification of the Broström procedure. This modification includes mobilization and reattachment of the lateral portion of the extensor retinaculum to the tip of the fibula after direct capsular reefing or repair of the anterior talofibular and calcaneofibular ligaments as originally described by Broström.

If the lateral ligaments are significantly disrupted, of the patient demonstrates hyperlaxity or weighs more than 240 lb, we often add suture tape augmentation over the primary repair.

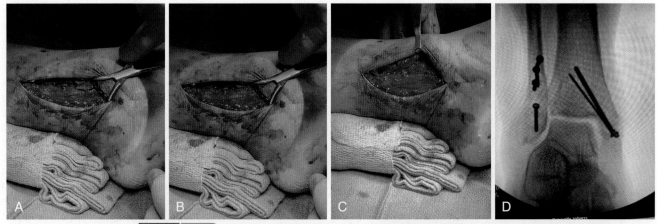

FIGURE 10.18 **A-D,** Repair of syndesmosis with fixation of Wagstaffe fracture.

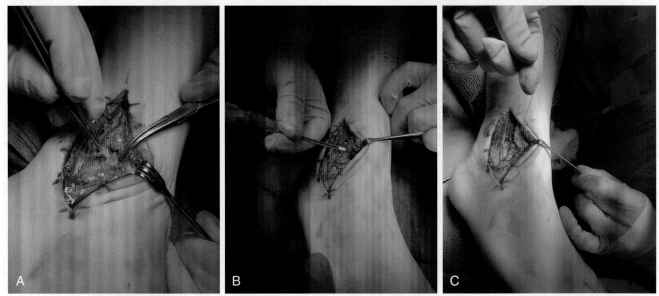

FIGURE 10.19 **A** and **B,** Stabilization of syndesmosis with repair of the anterior talofibular ligament. **C,** Primary anatomic repair.

REPAIR OF ACUTE RUPTURE OF LATERAL LIGAMENTS

TECHNIQUE 10.2

(BROSTRÖM, GOULD)

- Begin a curved incision 5 cm proximal to the distal tip of the fibula and 1.5 cm anterior to its margin and curve it distally and posteriorly to end distal to the fibula half the distance from the tip of the fibula to the tip of the heel (Fig. 10.20).
- Section the aponeurotic tissue overlying the tibiofibular joint and the ankle joint capsule.
- Identify and preserve the branches of the superficial peroneal nerve anteriorly, which often lies near the talar end of the anterior talofibular ligament, and the sural nerve lying over the peroneal tendons. Identify the lateral portion of the extensor retinaculum and mobilize it for attachment to the distal fibula at the end of the procedure. Preserve as many superficial veins as possible.

- If needed, nonabsorbable suture tape secured to the talus and fibula with anchors may be used for augmentation (Fig. 10.20E). The anchor is placed at the proximal aspect of the talar neck directed slightly posteriorly and superiorly (Fig. 10.20F).
- Repair the joint capsule and peroneal sheath, close the wound (Fig. 10.20G), and apply a plaster posterior splint with a U-shaped stirrup with the ankle in a neutral position in the sagittal plane and mildly everted.

POSTOPERATIVE CARE Sitting is allowed with the leg dependent for only a few minutes each half hour for the first few days postoperatively, and when dependency is tolerated well, crutch walking is instituted. After 2 weeks the sutures should be removed and the patient is allowed to touch-down weight bear in a walking boot with crutches and asked to begin gentle active range-of-motion exercises without inversion of the ankle. At 5 weeks the patient should be fully weight bearing with no crutches and range-of-motion exercises and manual resistive exercises to gain eversion strength are begun. Inversion past neutral is not allowed until 8 weeks after surgery.

CHRONIC INSTABILITY AFTER INJURY

Chronic instability of the ankle from an earlier rupture of a ligament should first be treated conservatively if it is symptomatic. Symptoms in women often may be decreased by broadening and lowering the heel of the shoe and in men by applying a lateral wedge to the shoe heel or on an orthotic. In sports activities, high-top athletic shoes or taping of the ankle for chronic instability may be symptomatically beneficial, although they provide only limited protection. A semirigid orthosis has been found to be more effective than taping in providing initial ankle protection and in guarding against reinjury and has a higher satisfaction rate among athletes.

For severe disability and instability, a muscle-strengthening program may be tried for several months, and some patients may improve enough to make a reconstructive operation unnecessary. However, it is also reasonable to proceed with reconstruction of the lateral ligaments because this is still often required and recurrent sprains are associated with a risk of associated injuries to other structures (e.g., osteochondral lesions). With mechanical instability, stress radiographs show 8 to 10 degrees of increased tilt of the talus in the ankle mortise compared with the normal ankle. When this is not the case, other causes for the disability, such as a stress fracture, should be sought (Fig. 10.21). Functional instability may occur as well and is defined as the subjective feeling of ankle instability or recurrent ankle sprain caused by neuromuscular or proprioceptive deficits. Dixon et al. described an excrescent lesion, a symptomatic anterolateral exostosis at the insertion of the anterior talofibular ligament, found by a CT scan in patients with chronic ankle pain after an inversion injury. Physical examination and oblique radiographs were suggestive in most cases. Surgical excision and, in some cases, repair of the anterior talofibular ligament (Broström procedure) usually were required. Arthroscopic examination at the time of ligament reconstruction has been recommended to determine if symptoms are caused by a chondral lesion that requires treatment in addition to the ligament reconstruction. Others have suggested, however, that arthroscopic examination of the ankle joint is unnecessary in the absence of any defined intraarticular pathologic process clinically and after imaging, and extravasation of fluid into the lateral soft tissues makes defining tissue planes more difficult at surgery.

■ LATERAL REPAIR OF CHRONIC INSTABILITY

Satisfactory results have been obtained from the Watson-Jones, Evans, and Elmslie operations (Fig. 10.22). These procedures use the peroneus brevis tendon to reconstruct the anterior talofibular and the calcaneofibular ligaments. The Watson-Jones technique may present two technical difficulties: the tunnel in the neck of the talus may be difficult to drill, and the peroneus brevis tendon may be too short. The Evans technique was designed to overcome these difficulties, but it primarily reconstructs the calcaneofibular ligament, whereas the Watson-Jones technique attempts reconstruction of the calcaneofibular and the anterior talofibular ligaments. Chrisman and Snook showed experimentally that subtalar instability still may be present after the Watson-Jones procedure. They postulated that with this reconstruction the line of pull of the peroneus brevis to the base of the fifth metatarsal is at an oblique angle to the fibers of the original calcaneofibular ligament. For this reason, they modified the Elmslie procedure to enhance lateral ankle and subtalar stability (Fig. 10.23).

Excellent and good results have been reported in 80% to 93% of patients after the Watson-Jones procedure. Fair and poor results generally were attributed to preexisting arthritis in the ankle or subtalar joint, because the ankles were stable after surgery. The Evans procedure has been reported to obtain excellent or good results in 80% to 95% of patients; however, in one series of 42 patients, only 50% had satisfactory long-term results. A comparison of the Watson-Jones and Evans procedures determined that long-term clinical results were similar but that the Evans technique controlled talar tilt better and the Watson-Jones procedure was more effective in reducing anteroposterior instability.

Several modifications of the Evans and Watson-Jones procedures have been described. One such modification involves securing the peroneus brevis in the standard fibular tunnel and using the remaining tendon to cross the subtalar joint posteriorly (Fig. 10.24). The direction of the tendon in relationship to the calcaneus and talus varied depending on the type of instability. Reported results were satisfactory. Kaikkonen et al. and Rosenbaum et al. stated that, although surgical treatment of chronic ankle instability using this modified Evans procedure restored the mechanical stability of the joint, too frequently the function of the ankle did not return to the preinjury level. Persistent clinical problems and functional changes indicated that the disturbed ankle joint kinematics permanently altered foot function and may have contributed to the development of arthrosis. They recommended that the Evans procedure be used only if anatomic reconstruction of the lateral ankle ligaments is not feasible.

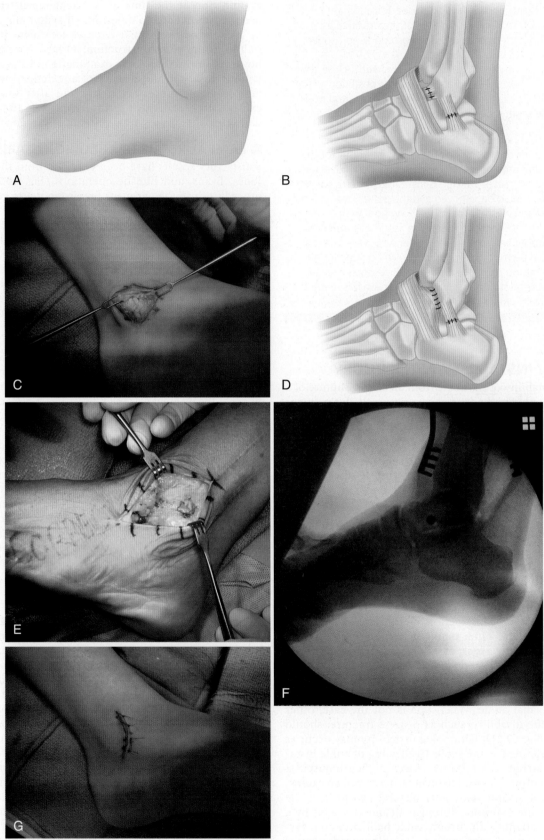

FIGURE 10.20 Modified Broström procedure. **A,** Skin incision. **B** and **C,** Shortening and reattachment of attenuated anterior talofibular and calcaneofibular ligaments. **D,** Suture of extensor retinaculum over repair. **E,** Nonabsorbable suture tape secured to talus and fibula with anchors. **F,** Anchor placed in proximal aspect of talar neck. **G,** Wound closure. **SEE TECHNIQUE 10.2.**

Snook, Chrisman, and Wilson described a modification of the Elmslie procedure in which the anterior talofibular and calcaneofibular ligaments were reconstructed using half of the peroneus brevis tendon. Their long-term results reported in 1985 indicated that 45 of 48 ankles had excellent

or good results. The three fair and poor results were caused by persistent lateral instability. They modified the procedure by (1) drilling a tunnel in the calcaneus that is stronger and easier to make than the original "trapdoor" tunnel; (2) suturing the end of the graft in front of the lateral malleolus, rather than at the base of the fifth metatarsal, providing a stronger repair; and (3) putting the foot and ankle in mild rather than forced eversion while the graft is sutured in place. According to these investigators, these minor changes in technique did not make any difference in the results compared with those obtained in their original study. A cadaver study comparing the Evans, Watson-Jones, and Chrisman-Snook procedures found that, with inversion-eversion loading, all three reconstructions increased ankle stability over the anterior talofibular and calcaneofibular ligament cut state. Only the Chrisman-Snook reconstruction resulted in a significantly more stable ankle joint complex than the ankles with cut anterior talofibular ligaments; however, it resulted in ankles with significantly less motion than intact ankles.

Reconstruction of chronically lax lateral ligaments by shortening procedures has been described. The primary advantages of these procedures are that they attack the basic defect and morbidity is less because part or all of a tendon is not sacrificed. Transection and imbrication of the lateral ligaments results in improved mechanical stability in approximately 80% of patients. Unsatisfactory results may occur in patients with generalized joint hypermobility or long-standing ligamentous laxity, which must be recognized and discussed with patients preoperatively. Unsatisfactory results also are frequent in patients with prior ankle surgery. Better functional results may be obtained with reconstruction of both ligaments than with reconstruction of the anterior talofibular ligament alone, although the literature is inconclusive. Karlsson et al. recommended combined reconstruction if there is any doubt regarding the involvement of both ligaments.

Studies have compared simple anatomic repair with the modified Broström approach and found that most patients with chronic ankle instability were successfully treated with anatomic reconstruction of the lateral ankle ligaments by either procedure, although the surgical exposure was greater, length of operation longer, and complications more frequent with the modified Broström technique.

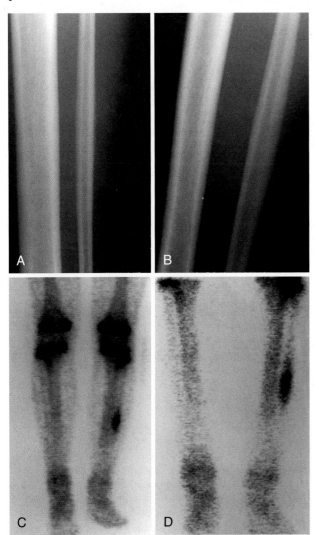

FIGURE 10.21   **A** and **B,** Plain films of fibula in patient with chronic, recurrent pain over distal third of leg and ankle and long history of chronic ankle sprains. **C** and **D,** Bone scans reveal increased uptake in middle third of fibula, indicating stress fracture.

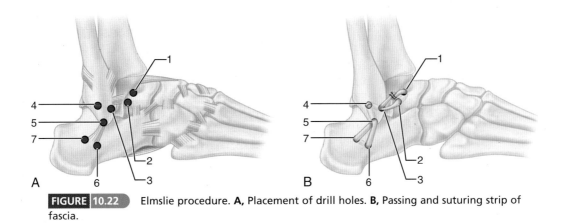

FIGURE 10.22   Elmslie procedure. **A,** Placement of drill holes. **B,** Passing and suturing strip of fascia.

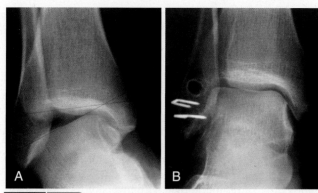

FIGURE 10.23 **A,** Stress radiograph showing lateral tilt of talus caused by chronic lateral instability of ankle joint. **B,** Two years after Chrisman-Snook procedure.

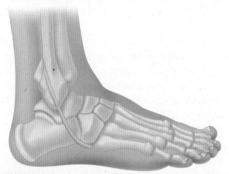

FIGURE 10.24 Larsen technique of transfer of peroneus brevis tendon for chronic lateral ankle instability.

Liu and Baker used cadaver specimens to test stability after the Chrisman-Snook, Watson-Jones, and modified Broström procedures. They found that all three procedures reduced anterior drawer and talar tilt. The modified Broström procedure produced the least amount of anterior talar displacement and talar tilt angle and the greatest mechanical strength. No significant differences were noted between the Watson-Jones and Chrisman-Snook procedures.

Historically, we have had satisfactory results with the Watson-Jones procedure; however, when subtalar instability and ankle instability can be shown and the patient is engaged in strenuous activities, the modified Elmslie procedure (Chrisman-Snook) may be considered. We have obtained good results using the modified Broström procedure in patients with moderate or severe instability (Fig. 10.25). The modified Broström technique is our treatment of choice and produces good results and fewer complications. We reserve tendon augmentation for patients with hypermobility, long-standing ligamentous insufficiency, high body mass index (usually >240 lb), or as a salvage procedure in patients with a failed modified Broström procedure. Tendon augmentation usually is accomplished using a third to half of the peroneus brevis left attached to the base of the fifth metatarsal and placed through a bone tunnel in the distal fibula (Fig. 10.26).

LATERAL REPAIR OF CHRONIC INSTABILITY (WATSON-JONES, MODIFIED)

TECHNIQUE 10.3

- Make a lateral incision over the ankle beginning proximally at the junction of the middle and distal thirds of the fibular shaft, continue it distally along the anterior border of the shaft, curve it gently anteriorly, and end it 5 cm anterior to the tip of the lateral malleolus.
- Open the peroneal sheath as far proximally as possible, sharply separate the peroneus brevis tendon from the muscle, and dissect proximally an extension of the muscle fascia with the tendon to make the transfer long enough.
- Suture the severed end of the muscle to the adjacent peroneus longus tendon.
- Free the peroneus brevis tendon as far distally as the lateral malleolus, but do not disturb the peroneal retinaculum.
- Drill two tunnels through the bone as follows, making them large enough to receive the tendon. Drill the first tunnel in an oblique anteroposterior direction through the lateral malleolus about 2.5 cm proximal to its tip. Drill the second in the longitudinal axis of the leg through the lateral part of the neck of the talus just anterior to the talofibular joint; here it is easier to drill a hole in the superolateral margin of the neck and another in the inferolateral margin so that they join to form the tunnel. Finally, a tunnel is created by drilling distal to the first fibular tunnel.
- Guide the peroneus brevis tendon through the first tunnel from posterior to anterior and through the second from inferior to superior; finally, deliver the remaining tendon into the distal fibular tunnel from anterior to posterior and secure with an anchor or tenodesis screw.

POSTOPERATIVE CARE A cast or splint is applied from the base of the toes to the tibial tuberosity and is worn for 2 weeks. At 2 weeks, a boot is placed to permit touchdown weight bearing and gentle range of motion in dorsiflexion, plantarflexion, and eversion. Inversion is not begun until 7 weeks postoperatively. Full weight bearing is allowed in a boot at 5 weeks, and a laced ankle corset is placed at 7 weeks when a formal functional rehabilitation program is begun.

LATERAL REPAIR OF CHRONIC INSTABILITY (EVANS)

TECHNIQUE 10.4

- Make a lateral incision over the ankle beginning proximally at the junction of the middle and distal thirds of the fibular

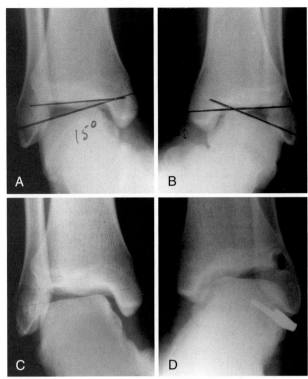

FIGURE 10.25 **A** and **B**, Stress views of right and left ankles with chronic, recurrent sprains. **C** and **D**, Stress views after Broström procedure on right ankle and modified Watson-Jones procedure on left ankle (note fibular drill hole for Watson-Jones procedure).

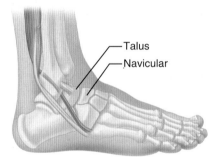

—Talus
—Navicular

FIGURE 10.26 Augmentation of collateral ligaments with peroneus brevis as described by Eyring and Guthrie.

shaft and continue it distally along the posterior border of the fibular shaft, curving it gently anteriorly toward the base of the fifth metatarsal. Find and protect the sural nerve as it crosses anteriorly in the distal aspect of the incision.

■ Incise the peroneal tendon sheath and superior peroneal retinaculum.

■ As far proximately as possible, harvest the anterior half of the peroneus brevis and place a grasping suture. Use this grasping suture to split the tendon distally 4 cm distal to the lateral malleolus (Fig. 10.27A). The hemostat marks the distal extent of the divided tendon. A suture may be placed at this junction to prevent further tearing of the tendon.

■ Drill a tunnel through the fibula large enough to receive the tendon, beginning at the tip of the fibula and emerging posteriorly 3.2 cm proximal to the tip.

■ Guide the tendon through the tunnel from inferior to superior (Fig. 10.27B) and secure it with a tenodesis screw (shown) or suture it under tension to the adjacent soft tissue at both ends of the tunnel.

■ If enough length is present, suture the remaining tendon back to itself distally and/or to fibular periosteum (Fig. 10.27B).

■ Repair the peroneal sheath and superior peroneal retinaculum (Fig. 10.27C).

POSTOPERATIVE CARE A cast or splint is applied from the base of the toes to the tibial tuberosity and is worn for 2 weeks. At 2 weeks, a boot is placed to permit touchdown weight bearing and gentle range of motion in dorsiflexion, plantarflexion, and eversion. Inversion is not begun until 7 weeks postoperatively. Full weight bearing is allowed in a boot at 5 weeks, and a laced ankle corset is placed at 7 weeks when a formal functional rehabilitation program is begun.

LATERAL REPAIR OF CHRONIC INSTABILITY (CHRISMAN-SNOOK)

TECHNIQUE 10.5

■ Make a long, curved incision over the course of the peroneal tendons from their musculotendinous junctions to the base of the fifth metatarsal.

■ Divide the ligament holding the tendons in their groove behind the fibula.

■ Identify the sural nerve and dissect it from above downward, leaving some fatty subcutaneous tissue around it. Free the nerve sufficiently to allow gentle retraction.

■ Retract the peroneus longus tendon, which overlies the peroneus brevis tendon in the groove, and expose the peroneus brevis.

■ Split the peroneus brevis in half longitudinally from its insertion upward to its musculotendinous junction. Leave the anterior and posterior halves of the tendon attached to the base of the fifth metatarsal. Divide the half with the longest tendon component at the musculotendinous junction (Fig. 10.28A and B). Clean most of the muscle tissue away from the cut end proximally.

■ Alternatively, a semitendinosus or gracilis autograft or allograft can be used to avoid harvesting a tendon that contributes to the stability of the lateral ankle.

■ If a free graft is used, it must be first secured in the neck of the talus using a drill to create a bone tunnel large enough to accept the graft. The Arthrex biotenodesis set (Arthrex, Naples, FL) allows precise measurement of the tendon diameter and multiple drill sizes to create the tun-

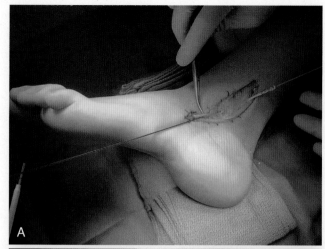

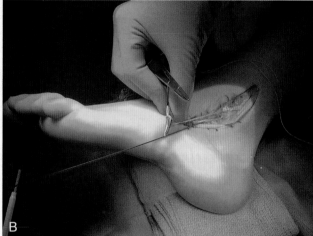

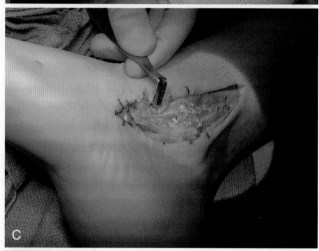

FIGURE 10.27 **A,** Grasping suture used to split tendon distally. **B,** Suture remaining tendon onto itself distally or to fibular periosteum. **C,** Peroneal sheath and superior peroneal retinaculum repaired. **SEE TECHNIQUE 10.4.**

nel. A tenodesis screw or anchor is used for graft fixation in the talus.

- Drill an appropriate-sized tunnel through the fibula in an anteroposterior direction at or just proximal to the level of the tibiotalar joint (see Fig. 10.28A and B).
- Pass a suture through the end of the graft in a grasping fashion, and use a suture passer to thread it through the

tunnel. Thread the graft from anterior to posterior. Make the hole slightly larger than the diameter of the graft.

- After the tendon graft has been pulled through the tunnel (Fig. 10.28C), place the ankle in neutral position and the foot in mild eversion, obtained by gentle manual positioning.
- Pull the graft taut and, using a strong, nonabsorbable suture, secure the graft to the periosteal ligamentous tissues adjacent to the anterior end of the drill hole. Alternatively, use a biotenodesis screw in the bone tunnel to secure the graft. This portion of the tendon graft replaces the anterior talofibular ligament.
- If a stump of the original ligament on the talus remains, suture it firmly to the contiguous tendon graft.
- Return the peroneus longus tendon and the remaining half of the peroneus brevis tendon to the fibular groove, allowing the graft to pass superficial to them to prevent dislocation of the tendons.
- Expose by dissecting distally and posteriorly the lateral border of the calcaneus. Periosteal elevation reveals a constant vertical ridge.
- Drill two holes, 1.5 cm apart and the same size as the hole in the fibula, anterior and posterior to the ridge (Fig. 10.28D), and join them using curved curets.
- Pass the tendon through this tunnel from posterior to anterior (Fig. 10.28D and E) and place sutures at both ends of the tunnel through the graft and adjacent soft tissues. The posterior and inferior direction of the graft from the fibula to the calcaneus duplicates that of the original calcaneofibular ligament.
- If the graft is short, drill a single hole completely through the calcaneus from the lateral to the medial side and then make a stab wound on the medial side of the heel and use the suture to pull the graft tautly into the hole. Tie the suture to a padded button on the medial side of the heel, a tenodesis screw, or an anchor to secure the graft to the calcaneus.
- If the remaining graft is long enough, suture it at the insertion of the peroneus brevis on the fifth metatarsal (Fig. 10.28F), as Chrisman and Snook originally described, or suture it onto itself at the anterior end of the fibula tunnel, as is now recommended, to gain additional support (Fig. 10.28F and G).
- After the graft is sutured in place, close the fascia and ligament over the fibular groove and close the skin in a routine fashion.

POSTOPERATIVE CARE A cast or splint is applied from the base of the toes to the tibial tuberosity and is worn for 2 weeks. At 2 weeks, a boot is placed to permit touchdown weight bearing and gentle range of motion in dorsiflexion, plantarflexion, and eversion. Inversion is not begun until 7 weeks postoperatively. Full weight bearing is allowed in a boot at 5 weeks, and a laced ankle corset is placed at 7 weeks when a formal functional rehabilitation program is begun.

Karlsson et al. compared their results after anatomic reconstruction of the lateral ankle ligaments using early mobilization, range of motion, and air casting with ligaments treated with 6 weeks of immobilization in a plaster cast. They concluded that after the reconstruction the functional and stability results were equally good with early

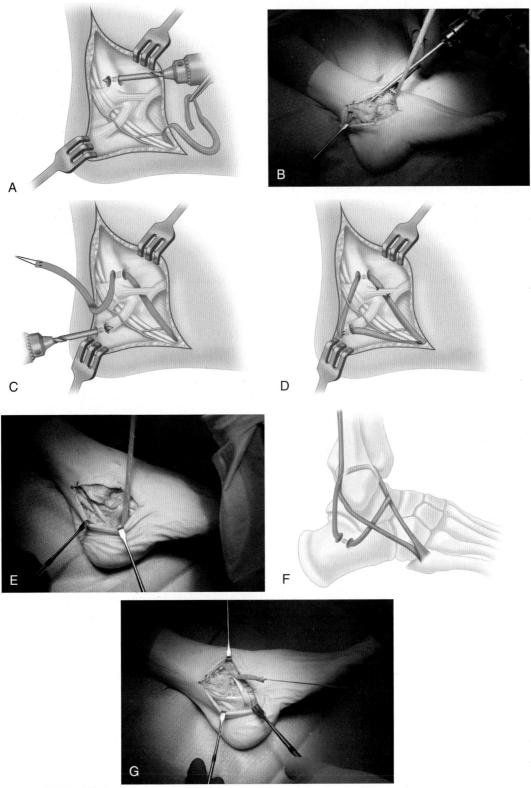

FIGURE 10.28   Modified Elmslie operation (Chrisman-Snook). **A,** Split of peroneus brevis tendon. **B,** Mobilized half of peroneus brevis tendon threaded through anterior talocalcaneal ligament (held by sutures) and through hole in fibula. **C,** Completed reconstruction (see text). **D,** Modification of original operation with end of graft sutured to its anterior portion at anterior end of fibular tunnel. **E to G,** As an alternative, a semitendinosus allograft can be used. **SEE TECHNIQUE 10.5.**

postoperative mobilization and 6-week immobilization. With early mobilization, however, plantarflexion strength was regained earlier than with cast immobilization, without any risk of short-term or medium-term complications, such as increased ankle laxity. They recommended early mobilization after lateral ankle reconstruction.

Split lesions of the peroneal brevis tendon can be associated with chronic ankle instability and should be checked during every surgical procedure for ankle laxity. After ligamentous repair, residual pain can be caused by neglected peroneus brevis "split" tear.

■ MEDIAL REPAIR OF CHRONIC INSTABILITY

Because chronic medial instability often does not cause severe disability that cannot be treated conservatively, and because the reconstructive options have had less success than those laterally, there is little information concerning the best treatment options for this difficult problem. Patients with chronic medial ankle instability may give a history of a pronation-type injury but more often report having had multiple ankle sprains without clearly remembering the mechanism. One cadaver study found that sectioning of the deltoid ligament resulted in a 43% increase in tibiotalar contact area while peak pressures increased 30%. Sectioning of the deltoid ligament alone results in valgus tilt of the talus and therefore chronic incompetence, which may lead to tibiotalar arthrosis. It is important to assess for incompetence of the medial tendons of the ankle, especially the posterior tibial tendon. The combination of posterior tibial insufficiency and deltoid incompetence has been described previously and categorized by Myerson as a stage IV adult-acquired flatfoot. This combination is most commonly seen in the older population. Medial ankle ligament reconstruction is indicated after failed conservative treatment in patients with chronic symptomatic mechanical instability.

We agree with Myerson that primary repair of a chronic deltoid tear, either end-to-end, "vest-over-pants," or advancement to bone, does not usually work. Because of the short fibers of the deep deltoid and the increased tension placed on the medial aspect of the ankle, anatomic primary repair of the chronically deficient deltoid ligament is less satisfactory than repair of the lateral ankle ligament. Several authors have described reconstructive techniques for chronic deltoid instability. Deland described a deltoid ligament reconstruction with a peroneus longus autograft. The peroneus longus was used instead of the peroneus brevis because of its insertion on the medial aspect of the foot and increased length. The peroneus longus is difficult to reach on the plantar aspect of the foot, and we recommend cadaver dissection to become familiar with the anatomy.

PERONEAL TENDON SUBLUXATION AND DISLOCATION

Subluxation and dislocation of the peroneal tendons are discussed in chapter 3.

INTERNAL DERANGEMENTS

As mentioned previously, if stress tests of the ankle are negative, some occult derangement other than ligamentous instability may be causing pain and disability. These conditions include (1) occult hindfoot lesions, (2) sinus tarsi syndrome, (3) osteochondral ridges (impingement overuse syndromes), and (4) osteochondritis dissecans of the talus.

OCCULT LESIONS OF THE TALUS AND CALCANEUS

Tarsal coalition may produce symptoms that mimic chronic ankle sprain. Snyder et al. also noted that adolescents with tarsal coalitions had an increased number of ankle sprains. Peroneal spasm may be noted, and CT scans are helpful in determining the type and location of the tarsal coalition (Fig. 10.29). Techniques for treatment of tarsal coalition are described in chapter 3.

We have seen osteoid osteoma (Fig. 10.30), eosinophilic granuloma (Fig. 10.31A), and simple bone cyst all mimic symptoms of chronic ankle sprain. Finally, fractures of the lateral process of the talus or anterior process of the calcaneus (Fig. 10.32) may mimic chronic ankle sprain. Treatment of these injuries is described in other chapter. Bone scanning as a screening technique may be helpful in determining the location of the fracture (Fig. 10.33A), and CT can disclose the type of fracture (Fig. 10.33B).

SINUS TARSI SYNDROME

In 1958, O'Connor described what he called the "sinus tarsi syndrome," in which pain in the sinus tarsi persists for many months or years after nonoperative treatment of an ankle sprain. Since then, very little has been written about sinus tarsi syndrome, and the condition is poorly defined. Pain in the lateral region of the ankle and sinus tarsi usually is listed as the characteristic physical finding. Some authors have suggested that sinus tarsi syndrome is a subtle variation of subtalar instability, although anatomic studies have shown scarring, fat atrophy, or degenerative changes in the soft-tissue elements of the sinus tarsi. Others have proposed nerve injury that results in loss of proprioceptive function as contributing to the development of the syndrome. Subtalar arthrography has been suggested as a modality for establishing the diagnosis. An absence of microrecesses and an abrupt cutoff of dye at the interosseous ligament correlate with sinus tarsi syndrome; however, this has not been fully substantiated. Ganglions at the anterior aspect of the subtalar joint, retraction of the joint recesses, a smooth and rounded appearance of the capsule, and a frozen subtalar joint also have been described. On normal MRI studies, the absence of the anterior microrecesses of the posterior subtalar joint is a common finding (i.e., 46 of 90 studies), suggesting that this may reflect a lack of iatrogenic joint distention. In addition, MRI studies consistent with fibrosis, chronic synovitis, nonspecific inflammatory changes, and synovial cysts have been noted. Initial and reconstructed MRI arthrograms along and perpendicular to the interosseous talocalcaneal and cervical ligaments are useful for diagnosing tears in patients with sinus tarsi syndrome. Ganglions in the sinus tarsi also have been cited as a potential source of pain.

If injection of an anesthetic agent and cortisone into the sinus tarsi does not provide at least temporary relief, the diagnosis is questionable. Often, this treatment provides permanent resolution of symptoms. If significant pain recurs despite temporary relief after injection, surgery may be indicated. Results after surgery are good, with complete or partial pain relief after excision of the fat pad

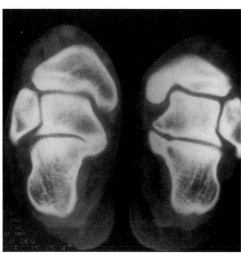

FIGURE 10.29 CT scan shows medial facet tarsal coalition of calcaneus and talus in young patient with frequent ankle sprains.

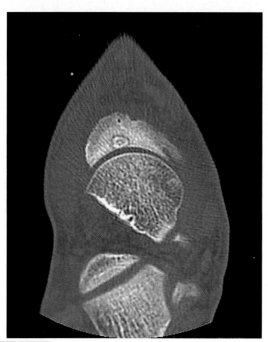

FIGURE 10.30 Osteoid osteoma of navicular. After excision and bone grafting, patient was asymptomatic.

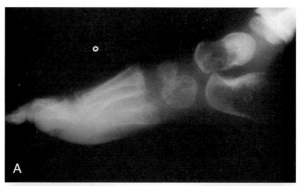

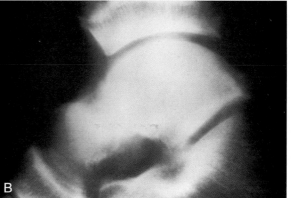

FIGURE 10.31 Talar neoplasms, which may mimic chronic ankle sprain. **A,** Eosinophilic granuloma. **B,** Pigmented villonodular synovitis.

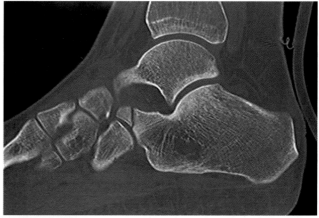

FIGURE 10.32 Fracture of anterior process of calcaneus. After conservative treatment failed, fracture fragment was excised with good results.

and resection of the superficial ligaments, taking care to avoid damage to the talar blood supply. Others advised curettage of the fatty neurovascular tissue of the sinus with preservation of the interosseous ligament unless it is obviously damaged. Yet others preserve the interosseous talocalcaneal and cervical ligaments if possible and resect the fibrofatty tissue and the extensions from the inferior extensor retinaculum.

We have had three patients who might have been considered to have sinus tarsi syndrome because for many months after sprain of the ankle they continued to have pain in the region of the sinus tarsi for which no reason could be found. Eventually each calcaneus developed a discrete osteoblastic lesion that was excised, with subsequent relief.

OSTEOCHONDRAL RIDGES OF THE TALUS AND TIBIA (ANTERIOR AND POSTERIOR IMPINGEMENT SYNDROMES)

In 1957, O'Donoghue called attention to a cause of disability in the ankle that had previously been reported but had received little attention. Osteochondral ridges (exostoses) may form just proximal to the anterior lip of the distal articular surface of the tibia and on the opposing area of the dorsal surface of the neck of the talus. They develop most often in athletes and, according to O'Donoghue, are caused by direct injury during strong dorsiflexion of the foot in which the neck of the talus is thrust against the tibia. Repeated minor

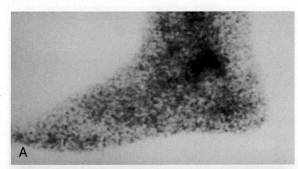

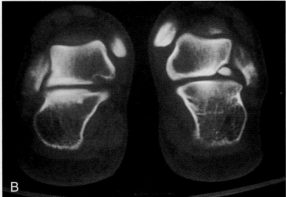

FIGURE 10.33 Avulsion fracture of talus. **A,** Bone scan. **B,** CT scan.

injuries cause the ridges to become larger and make collision between the talus and tibia easier. Such a ridge may develop on the tibia or talus or both.

This condition has been termed an *anterior impingement syndrome* caused by overuse of the dorsiflexors in athletes. When posterior, it is termed *posterior compression syndrome* or *os trigonum syndrome* in athletes who constantly plantar-flex the ankle. The patient complains of an aching in the ankle that is greatly increased by strong dorsiflexion of the foot. Examination usually reveals tenderness in the anterolateral part of the ankle joint and pain in this region when the foot is strongly dorsiflexed or plantarflexed. Radiographs reveal either that the anterior margin of the distal tibia has lost its rounded character and is sharp or that a distinct ridge or bony spur projects anteriorly from this margin (Fig. 10.34). A similar ridge or spur of varying size may or may not be present on the dorsal surface of the neck of the talus. "Tram track" lesions often are present and aid in locating the corresponding impingement lesion. Scranton and McDermott categorized ankle spurs according to their size and degree of involvement of the ankle and showed that treatment and recovery correlated with the grade (Fig. 10.35).

Both these overuse syndromes usually can be treated with antiinflammatory medication, immobilization, and curtailment of the aggravating activity. O'Donoghue recommended excising the ridges or spurs when they cause a definite disability. The ankle is exposed arthroscopically or through an open anterolateral approach.

Successful arthroscopic resection of anterior bone spurs causing anterior impingement syndrome has resulted in significant pain relief; decreased swelling, stiffness, and limping; and increased activity and range of dorsiflexion, although plantarflexion may not improve and numbness of the anterior foot has been described.

Anterior lateral impingement caused by chronic synovitis from overuse syndromes, chronic ankle sprains, and nondisplaced fractures have been noted. Excellent results have been reported after arthroscopic synovectomy. According to Hauger et al., CT arthrography provided evidence of anterolateral soft-tissue impingement and corresponded to that seen at arthroscopy: nodular formation in the lateral groove (discoid meniscal lesions) and irregular appearance of the edges of the lateral groove (abundant fibrous reaction).

A separate distal fascicle of the anterior inferior tibiofibular ligament present in most human ankles may cause talar impingement, abrasion of the articular cartilage, and pain in the anterior aspect of the ankle. Resection of this ligament and any abraded cartilage, either arthroscopically or by arthrotomy, usually alleviates pain caused by the impingement. The amount to be resected can be determined by dorsiflexing the ankle during the operative procedure (Fig. 10.36). Adjacent talar or fibular chondromalacia and inflammatory synovitis also may be present (Fig. 10.37).

BONE SPUR RESECTION AND ANTERIOR IMPINGEMENT SYNDROME

TECHNIQUE 10.6

(OGILVIE-HARRIS)

- With the patient under general anesthesia, apply and inflate a thigh tourniquet.
- Insert a needle just medial to the anterior tibial tendon and distend the ankle joint with 15 to 20 mL of saline.
- Make a small longitudinal incision to allow insertion of a 2.7- or 4.0-mm, 30-degree angle arthroscope through an anteromedial portal just medial to the anterior tibial tendon. Take care to pass the arthroscope across the anterior aspect of the joint and not across the dome of the talus.
- Make a separate anterolateral portal just lateral to the peroneus tertius tendon to allow inflow and outflow of saline. Be aware of the superficial peroneal nerve in this area. Instruments and the arthroscope can be switched to either portal as necessary.
- Fully examine the ankle with the use of a noninvasive ankle distraction device as necessary (Fig. 10.38). Distraction may need to be removed to identify and gain access to large anterior osteophytes, especially on the talus, because distraction may cause the anterior capsule to tighten.
- Use a pressure irrigation system with a 3.5-mm full-radius resector to clear the anterior synovium and define the anterior tibial and superior talar bony spurs.
- Use a 3-mm burr to remove the spurs, resecting them back to the level of normal cartilage.
- Smooth off the tibial surface with a 3.5-mm full-radius resector.
- Carry out a similar procedure on the superior neck of the talus.
- Examine the whole ankle by passing the arthroscope gently over the dome of the talus. This can be accomplished with the use of manual distraction in mid-plantarflexion or with a commercially available noninvasive ankle distraction device.
- Davis described a modification of this technique in which a trough is made with a 3-mm arthroscopic burr approximately 1 mm proximal and parallel to the anterior edge of

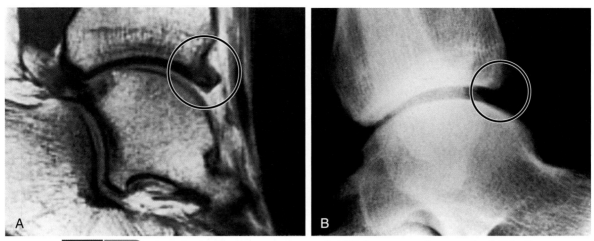

FIGURE 10.34 Anterior impingement syndrome. **A,** MRI shows osteophyte on distal tibia. **B,** Radiograph after excision of osteophyte.

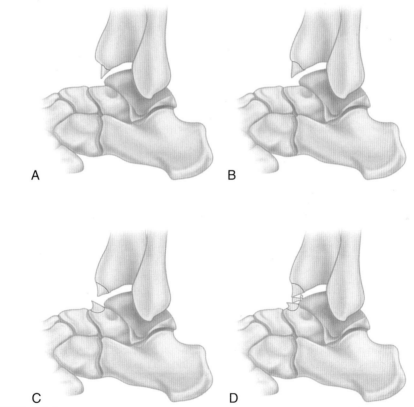

FIGURE 10.35 Scranton and McDermott classification of ankle spurs. **A,** Grade I, synovial impingement. Radiographs show inflammatory reaction with spurs 3 mm. **B,** Grade II, osteochondral reaction exostosis. Radiographs show spurs larger than 3 mm. No talar spur is seen. **C,** Grade III, severe exostosis with or without fragmentation. Secondary spur is noted on dorsum of talus, often with fragmentation of osteophytes. **D,** Grade IV, pantalocrural osteoarthritic destruction. Radiographs suggest degenerative osteoarthritic changes medially, laterally, or posteriorly.

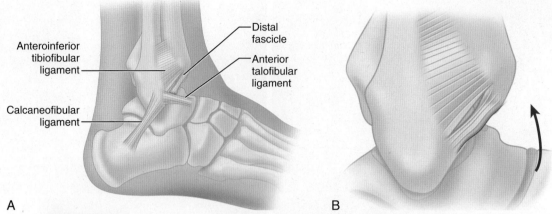

FIGURE 10.36 Lateral aspect of ankle joint. **A,** Distal fascicle of anteroinferior tibiofibular ligament is parallel and distal to anterior tibiofibular ligament proper and is separated from it by fibrofatty septum. **B,** With dorsiflexion of ankle, distal fascicle (Bassett's ligament) may impinge on anterolateral aspect of talus.

the tibia. This trough is taken down to subchondral bone to the level of surrounding normal cartilage. An arthroscopic bone-biter is used to remove the bony spur. This allows for more control of the burr with less potential for inadvertent damage to the articular surface than may occur with the use of an arthroscopic shaver, with which it often is difficult to gain purchase on the intact chondral surface of a spur.

POSTOPERATIVE CARE Ambulation is allowed immediately. A vigorous rehabilitation program is begun at 1 week, including ice packs and active and passive range-of-motion exercises. A tilt board is used for proprioceptive training and to strengthen the anterior and posterior muscles of the calf and foot. At 6 weeks, sports activities can be resumed in a gradual, protected fashion, taking care that the footwear is adequate for its purpose (e.g., properly fitted running shoes).

OSTEOCHONDRAL LESIONS OF THE TALUS (OSTEOCHONDRAL FRACTURE, TRANSCHONDRAL FRACTURE, DOME FRACTURE OF THE TALUS)

In 1959, Berndt and Harty, in an exhaustive review, determined that osteochondritis dissecans of the talus was in reality a "transchondral" (osteochondral) fracture caused by trauma. They classified the "lesion" into four different stages: stage I, a small area of compression of subchondral bone; stage II, a partially detached osteochondral fragment; stage III, a completely detached osteochondral fragment remaining in the crater; and stage IV, a displaced osteochondral fragment (Fig. 10.39).

A number of studies have documented that medial lesions are more common than lateral lesions. In cadaver experiments, the lateral lesion was produced by inversion and strong dorsiflexion, whereas the mechanism of injury in the medial lesion was inversion, plantarflexion, and lateral rotation of the tibia on the talus. In general, medial lesions are more posterior and lateral lesions are more anterior. Morphologically, medial lesions tend to be deeper and cup shaped, whereas lateral lesions are usually shallow and wafer shaped. Medial lesions usually are nondisplaced, and lateral lesions often are displaced.

Suggested causes of osteochondral lesions of the talus have included local osteonecrosis, systemic vasculopathies, acute trauma, chronic microtrauma, endocrine or metabolic factors, degenerative joint disease, joint malalignment, and genetic predisposition. A history of trauma is documented in more than 85% of patients with osteochondral lesions of the talus (98% of lateral lesions and 70% of medial lesions).

Although the incidence of osteochondral lesions of the talus has been reported as approximately 4% of all osteochondral lesions, the true incidence may be higher. Some studies have suggested that osteochondral lesions of the talus may occur in up to 50% of acute ankle sprains and fractures, particularly in association with sports injuries. Nearly half of osteochondral lesions of the talus were reported to be missed on radiographs by emergency department physicians, who usually make a diagnosis of "sprained ankle."

Persistent effusion, delayed synovitis, and locking or giving way of the joint 4 to 5 weeks after ankle injury are indications for radiographic examination. Oblique and plantarflexion views that avoid tibial overlap generally show the osteochondral lesion more clearly than standard plain films. If osteochondral fracture is suspected, a technetium bone scan should be done. If the bone scan is positive, a CT scan helps determine the exact size and location of the lesion and any related cystic lesions. CT scans should be made with 2-mm cuts in the axial and coronal planes to help determine the location of the lesion. CT scans also should be ordered with contrast medium if possible. MRI also is useful in patients who have not responded adequately to conservative management. Advantages of MRI include its ability to identify Berndt and Hardy stage I lesions and provide detail of the articular cartilage. Several useful imaging classifications have been developed. The arthroscopic staging systems described by Pritsch et al. and Cheng et al. are the most definitive, however, because they use direct inspection and probing of the lesion. These classifications are based on inspection of the articular cartilage (Table 10.1).

Treatment of an osteochondral lesion depends on a variety of factors, including the characteristics of the patient

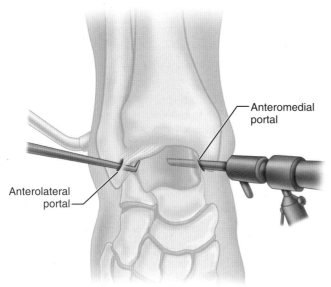

FIGURE 10.37 Anterior soft-tissue impingement is observed through anteromedial portal while probe is inserted through anterolateral portal to palpate area of synovitis and fibrosis in anterolateral gutter.

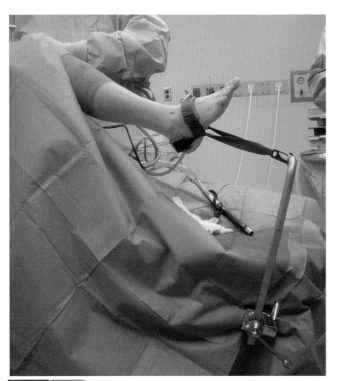

FIGURE 10.38 Noninvasive ankle distraction. **SEE TECHNIQUE 10.6.**

(activity level, general health, age) and the lesion (size, location, associated degenerative changes). Most lesions initially should be treated conservatively with immobilization and physical therapy. Operative treatment is of three general types: debridement of the lesion with stimulation of the underlying subchondral bone (microfracture, drilling, abrasion, curettage), direct repair of the lesion (retrograde drilling and bone grafting, internal fixation), or repair of the lesion with osteochondral autografts or allografts or chondrocyte transplantation. If surgery is considered, preoperative planning can

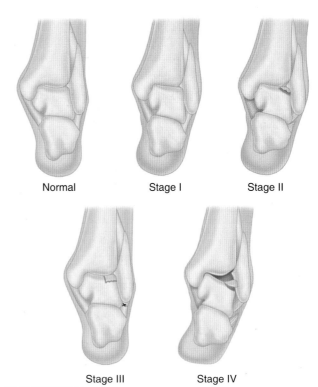

FIGURE 10.39 Four stages of osteochondritis dissecans of talus. Lateral lesions characteristically appear shallow and horizontal and frequently are elevated or detached. Medial lesions are characteristically deeper; and although they may appear to be detached, most frequently they sit in their crater.

be aided by CT; axial and coronal 2-mm cuts determine the location of the lesion (anterior, medial, or posterior) and the necessity of osteotomy of the medial malleolus. If the fragment appears to be floating in the crater, it usually is inverted so that cartilage apposes the crater and cancellous bone apposes the ankle joint. MRI is helpful in localizing a floating lesion (Fig. 10.40) and may help to determine whether a lesion is still attached or loose in the crater.

Several authors have reported that a trial of conservative therapy does not affect the outcome in patients requiring future surgery. In one series of 35 ankles with chronic, cystic talar lesions, only 54% had good or excellent results with nonoperative treatment, and a systematic review of the literature found that only 45% of those treated nonoperatively had successful outcomes. We believe, however, all displaced lesions with symptoms should have the fragment excised and the crater curetted and drilled to prevent the development of arthritis. Completely detached (stage III) lateral lesions, because of their high rate of failure to unite and high incidence of becoming displaced and causing early arthritis, also should be considered for early surgery (Fig. 10.41). In acute stage III and IV lesions, the osteochondral fragment often can be reattached and internally fixed with retrograde Kirschner wires or bioabsorbable screws or pins.

Incomplete medial and lateral lesions (stage II), completely detached but undisplaced (stage III) medial lesions, and lesions occurring in children (Fig. 10.42) may be treated by plaster immobilization or by a patellar tendon–bearing brace. If after 4 to 6 months the lesion is not healing or has progressed, surgical excision and curettage should be performed.

TABLE 10.1

Classification Systems for Osteochondral Lesions of the Talus

PLAIN RADIOGRAPHS	COMPUTED TOMOGRAPHY
BRENDT AND HARTY (1959)	*FERKEL AND SGAGLIONE (1994)*
I: Compressed II: Chip avulsed but attached III: Chip detached but undisplaced IV: Chip detached and displaced	I: Cystic lesion within dome of talus, intact roof on all views IIA: Cystic lesion with communication to talar dome surface IIB: Open articular surface lesion with overlying nondisplaced fragment III: Undisplaced lesion with lucency IV: Displaced fragment

Loomer et al. (1993)

V: Radiolucent cystic lesion seen on CT

MRI				
Anderson (1989)	Dipaola et al. (1991)	Taranow et al. (1999)	Hepple et al. (1999)	Mintz et al. (2003)
1. Bone marrow edema (subchondral trabecular compression; radiographs negative, bone scan positive) 2a. Subchondral cyst 2b. Incomplete separation of fragment 3. Fluid around undetached, undisplaced fragment 4. Displaced fragment	1. Thickening of articular cartilage and low signal changes on intermediate/spin density images 2. Articular cartilage breached with low-signal rim behind fragment indicating fibrous attachment 3. Articular cartilage breached high-signal changes behind fragment indicating synovial fluid between fragment and underlying subchondral bone 4. Loose body	1. Subchondral compression/bone bruise appearing as high signal on T2-weighted images 2. Subchondral cysts that are not seen acutely (arise from stage 1) 3. Partially separated or detached fragments in situ 4. Displaced fragments	1. Articular cartilage damage only 2a. Cartilage injury with underlying fracture and surrounding bony edema 2b. Stage 2a without surrounding bony edema 3. Detached but undisplaced fragment 4. Detached and displaced fragment 5. Subchondral cyst formation	0. Normal 1. Hypointense but morphologically intact cartilage surface 2. Fibrillation or fissures not extending to bone 3. Flap present or bone exposed 4. Loose undisplaced fragment 5. Displaced fragment

ARTHROSCOPY	
Pritsch et al. (1986)	*Cheng et al. (1995)*
1. Intact overlying cartilage 2. Soft overlying cartilage 3. Frayed overlying cartilage	1. Smooth, intact but soft or ballotable 2. Rough surface 3. Fibrillation/fissuring 4. Flap present or bone exposed 5. Loose, undisplaced fragment 6. Displaced fragment

As an alternative to surgical excision in the early stages and for medial lesions and lesions in children that have not healed, percutaneous arthroscopic drilling has been recommended to promote healing. Arthroscopic drilling for the treatment of medial osteochondral lesions of the talus does not require osteotomy of the medial malleolus or postoperative immobilization; the procedure is less invasive than other types of operative treatment for the condition, and it allows early resumption of daily activities and sports. The procedure is reported to be as effective and useful in young patients, especially patients with open physes. A specific indication for the procedure is an early lesion with only mild osteosclerosis of the surrounding talar bone, continuity of the cartilaginous surface, and stability of the osteochondral fragment. Retrograde percutaneous drilling through the sinus tarsi preserves the intact articular cartilage (Figs. 10.43 and 10.44). Because of the difficulty of adequately filling the contours of the lesion, bone grafts have been used in conjunction with retrograde drilling to prevent articular collapse.

More recently, surgical-grade calcium sulfate in a liquid form has been injected into the defect after drilling, and some authors have reported the use of a bone-marrow aspirate harvested from the iliac crest, centrifuged to isolate pluripotent cells, and mixed with the calcium graft to promote more rapid healing.

When surgery is planned, CT with 2-mm cuts in the coronal and axial planes determines whether the lesion is in the anterior third, middle third, or posterior third of the talar dome. This is especially helpful in planning surgery on the medial side, where an osteotomy of the medial malleolus may be necessary (Fig. 10.45). Because the lateral malleolus is posterior to the tibia, lateral lesions, even when they are in the middle or posterior third, usually can be approached anteriorly and removed without an osteotomy. Flick and Gould described an anteromedial approach for posteromedial lesions, "grooving" the anteromedial distal tibial articular surface 6 to 8 mm to expose the lesion without osteotomy of the medial malleolus

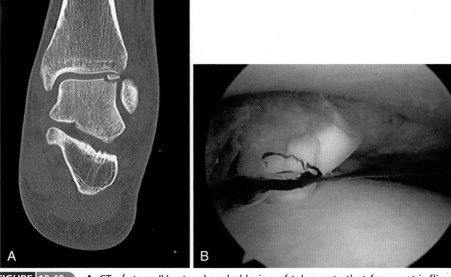

FIGURE 10.40 **A,** CT of stage IV osteochondral lesion of talus; note that fragment is flipped, with articular cartilage adjacent to subchondral bone. **B,** Stage IV osteochondral lesion as seen arthroscopically.

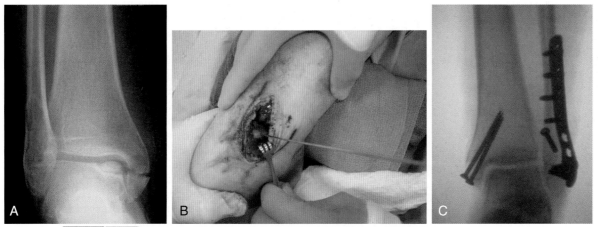

FIGURE 10.41 **A,** Large osteochondral lesion on medial aspect of talus in patient with bimalleolar ankle fracture. **B,** Osteochondral lesion secured with absorbable pin. **C,** Healed ankle fracture and osteochondral lesion several months postoperatively.

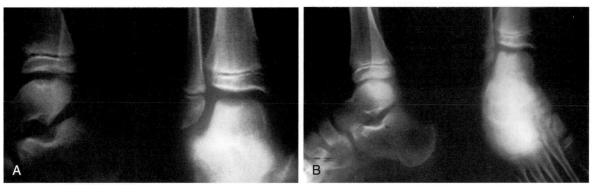

FIGURE 10.42 **A,** Early evidence of osteochondritis dissecans of talus in child with open physes. **B,** After 6 months of conservative treatment, area of osteochondritis is smaller and appears to be consolidating.

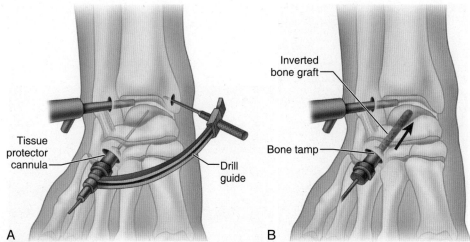

FIGURE 10.43 Arthroscopic drilling and bone grafting for osteochondral lesion of posteromedial talar dome as described by Stone and Guhl. **A,** Through a small incision, a guide pin is placed through sinus tarsi with use of modified ligament guide. **B,** Graft is placed into channel and gently compressed into position with tamp and mallet.

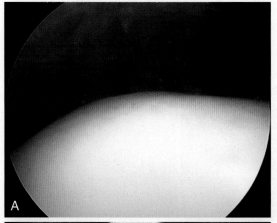

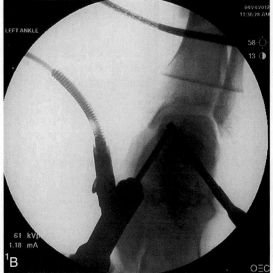

FIGURE 10.44 Retrograde drilling of osteochondral lesion. **A,** After confirming intact articular cartilage, subchondral lesion was drilled in retrograde fashion **(B)** and bone grafted.

(Fig. 10.46A). A gouge is used to make a groove in the tibia 5 to 6 mm wide and 6 to 8 mm long (Fig. 10.46B). At follow-up, no ankle arthritis was noted as a result of the "grooving" of the distal tibia. We have had only limited experience with this procedure. Several authors have reported good results with the use of an inverted-V type of osteotomy or a proximally based chevron medial malleolar osteotomy. If a talar osteochondral lesion occurs with an ankle fracture, it is often relatively easy to gain access and treat (Fig. 10.47).

Thompson and Loomer described a posteromedial arthrotomy through an anteromedial approach to expose posteromedial lesions of the talus and avoid a medial malleolar osteotomy. Bassett et al. described a simple approach to the posteromedial ankle through the posterior portion of the posterior tibial tendon sheath (see Fig. 10.53). This approach allows exposure of the talar dome and the tibial articular surface of the posterior joint and the posterior capsule while protecting the posteromedial tendons, the neurovascular structures, and the deep posterior fibers of the deltoid ligament.

Healing is uneventful for most patients in whom osteotomy of the medial malleolus is used to approach a posteromedial lesion (Fig. 10.48). The malleolar screw often needs to be removed (Fig. 10.49A-C). Patients are immobilized in a cast for 6 weeks and then allowed weight bearing in a walking boot until 12 weeks after surgery. A patellar tendon–bearing brace is sometimes used after surgery to unload the ankle joint and decrease pressure on the defect (Fig. 10.50). The surgical approaches to medial and lateral lesions and the techniques for osteotomy of the medial malleolus are described subsequently. We have limited experience with the combined anteromedial and posteromedial approach of Thompson and Loomer; it is a "large" exposure but may be necessary in some patients.

Large lesions can be replaced and fixed with pinning and grafting similar to the techniques used for osteochondral lesions in the knee, but the fragment must have viable subchondral cancellous bone. Kumai et al. reported treating 27 large lesions (>8 × 8 mm) with cortical bone pegs harvested from the distal tibia. They reported 89% good clinical results at an average 7 years of follow-up. Pinning and grafting are technically difficult, and nonunion may necessitate later removal of the pins and the fragment.

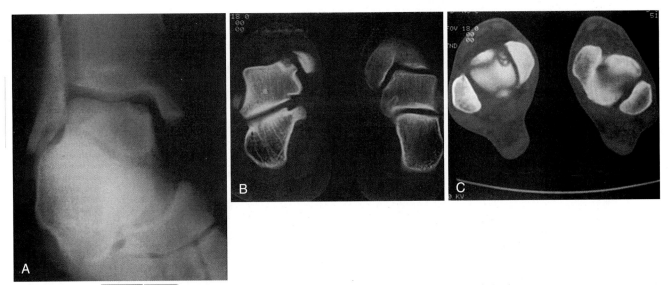

FIGURE 10.45 **A,** Anteroposterior radiograph shows stage III lesion of medial talus. **B,** CT scan reveals extent and depth of lesion. **C,** Scan cut in coronal plane shows location of lesion anteriorly.

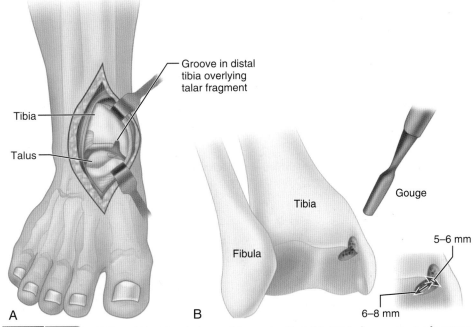

FIGURE 10.46 Flick and Gould technique of "grooving" of distal tibia for exposure of postero-medial lesions without osteotomy of medial malleolus. **A,** Groove used to expose posterior lesions better. **B,** Gouge used on medial tibia to avoid osteotomy of medial malleolus.

More recent reconstructive methods for large lesions (>5 mm) involve transplantation of autogenous osteochondral grafts into the defect. A single plug of bone is obtained in the osteochondral autograft or allograft transplantation (OATS) procedure; *mosaicplasty* refers to harvesting and transplanting multiple smaller plugs. For very large lesions (>12 mm), a "mega-OATS" fresh talar allograft is often needed. Several authors have shown good results using talar allograft (Fig. 10.51), which avoids the risks associated with harvesting from the ipsilateral femur or talus. The allograft usually can be obtained from the same-side talus to allow for matched grafts. Fresh allografts are typically harvested within 24 hours after death, and testing of the graft is undertaken to assess for disease and sterility.

Although often not possible, fresh allografts should be implanted within 1 week. There is no clear evidence that fresh allografts provide superior results to fresh-frozen allografts. Fresh-frozen allografts are processed and kept refrigerated.

A mosaicplasty technique can be performed for defects larger than 10 mm. Osteochondral cylindrical grafts from the ipsilateral knee were delivered into the talar defect using specially designed tube chisels. Good-to-excellent results have been reported in as many as 94% of patients with this technique; however, some have emphasized the technical challenge of reproducing a smooth articular surface with the protruding plugs. Latt et al. noted increased contact pressure when the graft is left elevated. These authors recommended

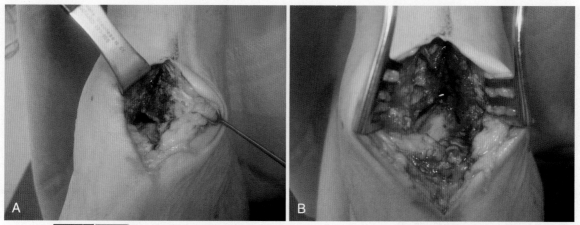

FIGURE 10.47 **A,** Osteochondral lesion on lateral border of talus extending posteriorly. Even with maximal plantarflexion, access is suboptimal for microfracture. **B,** After grooving of distal lateral tibia, access is significantly improved.

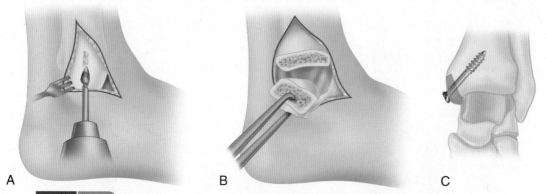

FIGURE 10.48 **A,** Drill hole through medial malleolus into tibia. **B,** Oblique osteotomy of medial malleolus to expose tibiotalar joint. **C,** Reattachment of osteotomy fragment with malleolar screw.

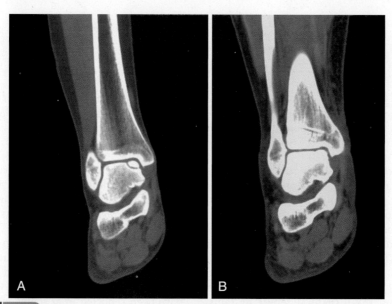

FIGURE 10.49 Osteochondritis of talus. **A,** CT of grade IIB lesion. **B,** Medial malleolar osteotomy and talar lesion healed 6 months after surgery. Screws were used for fixation and were subsequently removed.

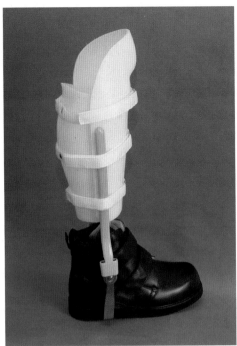

FIGURE 10.50 Patellar tendon–bearing brace used after surgery to decrease pressure on defect.

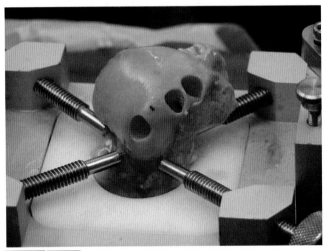

FIGURE 10.51 Harvest of allografts for large talar defects. **SEE TECHNIQUE 10.10.**

making as much of the graft flush as possible, but slight recess was noted to be better than elevation.

Autologous chondrocyte transplantation has been used more often in the knee, but good results in the ankle have been reported at up to 5-year follow-up. An arthroscopic technique for placement of autologous chondrocytes also has been described. The matrix-associated chondrocyte implantation (MACI) technique has shown promising results, but studies are limited. With this arthroscopic technique, autologous chondrocytes are cultured in a biologic matrix that doubles as both the delivery system for the chondrocytes and the scaffold for repair. For large lesions, cancellous bone grafting may be placed in the defect followed by two periosteal patches with the chondrocytes placed between the patches ("sandwich technique").

MEDIAL MALLEOLAR OSTEOTOMY

TECHNIQUE 10.7

(COHEN ET AL.)

- Make a 6- to 8-cm apex-posterior curved incision centered over the medial malleolus (Fig. 10.52A).
- Open the posterior tibial tendon sheath at the level of the mortise. The posterior tibial tendon must be retracted and protected at all times.
- Predrill the medial malleolus with a 2.5-mm drill and tap it.
- Incise the periosteum but do not reflect it.
- Use a microsagittal saw to create a chevron-type osteotomy with the apex directed proximally (Fig. 10.52B). In the anteroposterior plane, angle the osteotomy toward the junction of the medial malleolus and tibial plafond articular surface (Fig. 10.52C). It is beneficial to obtain a fluoroscopic image at the start of the osteotomy to ensure the correct angle. It is important to angle neither too obliquely and enter the weight-bearing surface of the tibia nor too vertically and limit visualization. Also, direct visualization is obtained from the anteromedial gutter.
- Complete the osteotomy with a fine hand osteotome.
- Reflect the medial malleolus inferiorly.
- Release capsular attachments as necessary for visualization, maintaining the attachments of the superficial and deep deltoid.
- At the conclusion of the procedure, stabilize the osteotomy with two 4.0-mm partially threaded cancellous screws.

POSTOPERATIVE CARE A plaster splint is worn for 10 to 14 days. Range of motion is begun while maintaining non–weight-bearing status until radiographs confirm maintenance of reduction (approximately 6 weeks).

POSTEROMEDIAL ARTHROTOMY THROUGH ANTEROMEDIAL APPROACH

TECHNIQUE 10.8

(THOMPSON AND LOOMER)

- Make a 10-cm curved incision, convex posteriorly, centered posterior to the medial malleolus, and expose the medial capsule.
- Make a 2-cm longitudinal incision in the anteromedial capsule extending from the tibia to the talus (Fig. 10.53A).
- Maximally plantarflex the foot, and inspect the anterior half to two thirds of the superomedial rim of the talus.
- If the defect cannot be completely inspected, curetted, and drilled from this approach, make a curved incision directly over the posterior tibial tendon.
- Retract anteriorly and make an incision in the deep surface of the flexor retinaculum (Fig. 10.53B).

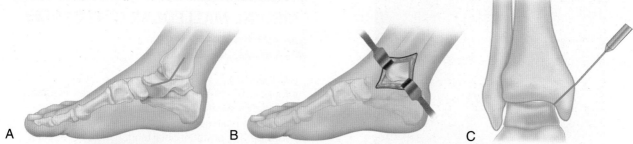

FIGURE 10.52 Chevron transmalleolar osteotomy. **A,** Incision. **B,** Orientation of osteotomy in lateral plane (apex proximally and limbs of chevron extending from mortise level). **C,** Orientation of osteotomy in anteroposterior plane (angled toward junction of medial malleolus and tibial plafond articular surface). (From Cohen BE, Anderson RB: Chevron-type transmalleolar osteotomy: an approach to medial talar dome lesions, *Tech Foot Ankle Surg* 1:158, 2002.) **SEE TECHNIQUE 10.7.**

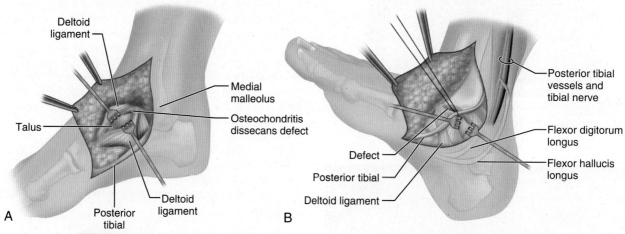

FIGURE 10.53 **A,** Anteromedial exposure of talus with foot in maximal plantarflexion. **B,** Posteromedial exposure through same skin incision with foot in maximal dorsiflexion. **SEE TECHNIQUE 10.8.**

- Do not expose or examine but gently posteriorly retract the remainder of the contents of the tarsal tunnel.
- By maximally dorsiflexing the foot, observe the posterior one half of the superomedial border of the talus, inspect the lesion, and treat it appropriately by excision and curettage.

POSTOPERATIVE CARE A soft dressing is used with immediate range-of-motion exercises, weight bearing as tolerated, and return to function as soon as tolerated.

APPROACH TO POSTEROMEDIAL ANKLE THROUGH POSTERIOR TIBIAL TENDON SHEATH

TECHNIQUE 10.9

(BASSETT ET AL.)

- Place the patient either prone, to allow access to the posteromedial ankle, or supine with the hip and knee flexed and externally rotated; the latter position is more commonly used.
- Palpate the medial malleolus and the Achilles tendon.
- Make a 5- to 8-cm incision immediately overlying the posterior tibial tendon behind the medial malleolus (Fig. 10.54A) and curve it distally and slightly anteriorly, following the contour of the medial malleolus.
- Deepen the incision through the subcutaneous tissue down to the flexor retinaculum overlying the posterior tibial tendon. Do not damage the long saphenous vein and nerve, which lie anteriorly, during the dissection.
- Palpate the posterior tibial tendon posterior to the medial malleolus. Make a 5- to 8-cm longitudinal incision in the flexor retinaculum, and follow the contour of the posterior tibial tendon (Fig. 10.54B).
- Retract the tendon posteriorly to expose the deep flexor retinaculum and the joint capsule. This also protects the posterior neurovascular bundle from injury.
- Make a 3- to 5-cm longitudinal incision in the deep layer of the posterior tibial tendon sheath and joint capsule; this is crucial to the precise entrance into the joint.
- Place a retractor through this incision and retract the capsule and the posterior tibial tendon (Fig. 10.54C).
- Move the foot into dorsiflexion and plantarflexion and inversion and eversion to allow complete examination of the articular surface of the posterior talus and tibia

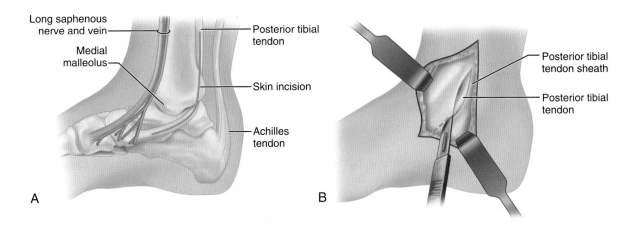

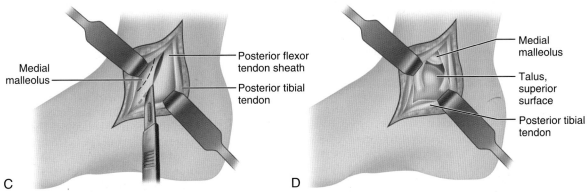

FIGURE 10.54 Approach to posteromedial ankle. **A,** Skin incision posterior to medial malleolus and in line with posterior tibial tendon. **B,** Incision in posterior tibial flexor tendon sheath. **C,** Retraction of posterior tibial tendon and deep layer of flexor tendon sheath and incision of joint capsule. **D,** View of superior articular surface of talus as seen through posteromedial approach. **SEE TECHNIQUE 10.9.**

and the posterior joint capsule (Fig. 10.54D). In this manner, approximately 60% of the posterior talar dome and 50% of the posterior tibial surface can be exposed, whereas the posterior fibers of the deltoid ligament are spared.

OSTEOCHONDRAL AUTOGRAFT/ ALLOGRAFT TRANSPLANTATION

TECHNIQUE 10.10

(HANGODY ET AL.)

- With the patient under general anesthesia, prepare the affected lower extremity from the ankle to the knee. Examine the ankle arthroscopically to delineate the chondral lesion further.
- Harvesters are made for lesions 5 to 11 mm (larger sizes also are available).

- Approach lateral lesions through an anterior sagittal incision, and perform a medial malleolar osteotomy for medial lesions (see Technique 10.7) (Fig. 10.55A-D). Rarely, a lateral malleolar osteotomy is needed to access posterolateral lesions.
- Use a commercially available recipient sizer and harvester to create a recipient hole for the donor osteochondral plug. Extract the plug to a depth of 10 mm (Fig. 10.55E,F). Place the harvester perpendicular for dome lesions (Fig. 10.55G-I) and at 45 degrees for talar shoulder lesions (Fig. 10.51).
- Drill multiple holes into the subchondral bone of the recipient hole (Fig. 10.55J).
- Obtain a graft from the ipsilateral knee, arthroscopically from the medial femoral condyle or lateral femoral condyle (Fig. 10.55K,L). For talar shoulder lesions, obtain a graft from the lateral trochlea. Alternatively, a talar allograft has been shown to be effective and removes the risk of iatrogenic injury during harvesting.
- Use the specially designed donor harvester to obtain osteochondral grafts that measure 5 to 11 mm in diameter and 10 to 12 mm in depth (slightly deeper than the recipient hole).
- Insert the cylindrical grafts carefully into the recipient hole using the designed extruder or collared pin through the donor harvester (Fig. 10.55M,N). If the defect is large

(>11 mm in diameter), it is best to use an allograft. A mosaicplasty may be needed in which multiple grafts are used (Figs. 10.56 and 10.57). Do not remove the OATS harvester before completion of full graft extrusion. Do not allow the harvester to deviate from the insertion angle. Either of these may cause fracture of the donor core.

- Use the sizer-tamp to tamp the core gently flush with the surrounding cartilage.
- Test range of motion of the ankle to ensure that the graft is well seated and secured.
- Close the incision and secure the osteotomy in the usual fashion (Fig. 10.55O). Place one drain in the knee and apply a compressive dressing to the ankle. Apply a posterior splint with strips.

POSTOPERATIVE CARE The patient is kept non–weight bearing for 10 weeks. At 2 weeks, the sutures are removed and a short leg non–weight bearing cast is applied. At 4 weeks, a boot is fitted; the patient is kept non–weight bearing, and range-of-motion exercises are begun. At 6 to 8 weeks, pool therapy and stationary biking can be instituted.

■ ARTHROSCOPIC TREATMENT

Arthroscopic treatment of transchondral fractures (osteochondritis dissecans) of the talar dome consists of partial synovectomy, debridement of the osteochondral lesion with removal of any loose fragments, curettage, abrasion, and occasionally drilling of the lesion. Excellent and satisfactory results have been reported with minimal complications. Arthroscopic excision was recommended because of decreased morbidity, brief hospitalization, and rapid recovery by avoiding long skin incisions, deep soft-tissue dissection, grooving of the distal tibia, and osteotomy of the medial malleolus. Ogilvie-Harris described arthroscopic treatment that consisted of removal of the osteocartilaginous

fragments, debridement of disrupted cartilage, and abrasion of the base to bleeding subchondral bone that produced significant improvement of pain, swelling, stiffness, limp, and activity level.

Arthroscopy of the ankle is technically difficult and requires considerable expertise to work in such a tight space. The dome of the talus also is difficult to work over and around. A well-done arthrotomy is superior to a poorly done arthroscopy. We routinely place the patient supine with the knee and ankle in extension and follow the principles of knee arthroscopy (Fig. 10.58). A 4-mm arthroscope with 30- to 70-degree angles generally should be used; however, we have used a larger 4.5-mm scope. We routinely begin by using a large-bore needle to distend the joint and make an anteromedial portal (Fig. 10.59A). When this portal is established, an anterolateral portal can be made (Fig. 10.59B). The light from the anteromedial portal against the skin laterally outlines the dorsal cutaneous nerve, allowing it to be avoided when making the anteromedial portal. The posterolateral portal often is used to gain exposure to posterior structures or for more efficient inflow by having this dedicated portal. Because so much synovium is present in the anterior portion of the ankle joint, we routinely remove much of it with a motorized shaver. Lateral lesions are more easily exposed because the lateral malleolus is more posterior than the medial malleolus. The use of invasive ankle distractors is discouraged. Complications can occur with the use of a noninvasive ankle distractor as well because much force can be exerted across the ankle joint during distraction, causing neurovascular complications. We routinely excise the area of osteochondritis dissecans, contour the sides of the crater, and drill multiple holes in the crater to promote vascularization. These holes can be drilled transmalleolarly under direct vision through the arthroscope or with image intensification. Multiple holes can be drilled in the crater in the talus through one hole drilled through the malleolus, combined with dorsiflexion and plantarflexion of the ankle (Fig. 10.60).

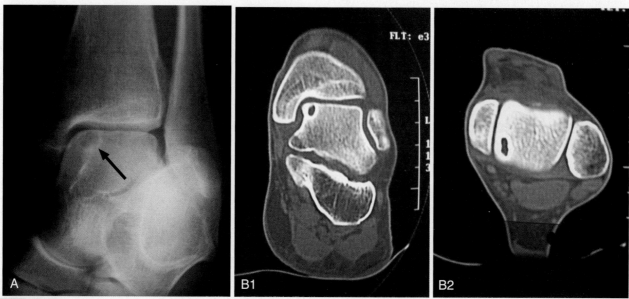

FIGURE 10.55 Osteochondral autograft/allograft transplantation (see text). **A,** Posteromedial osteochondral lesion of talus *(arrow).* **B,** Coronal and axial plane CT images.

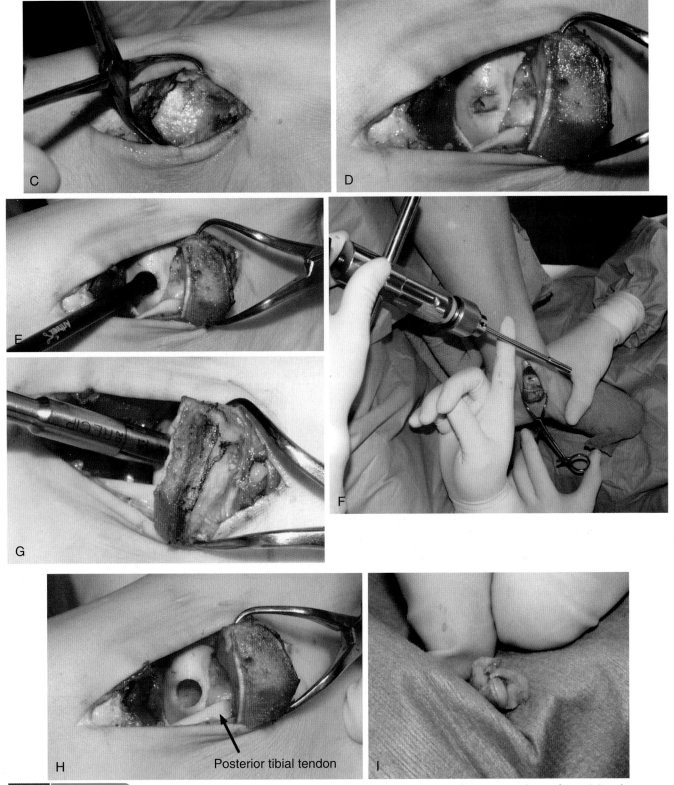

FIGURE 10.55 Cont'd **C,** Medial malleolar chevron-type osteotomy. **D,** Shoulder lesion of talus. **E,** Trial sizer for recipient harvester. **F,** Recipient harvester. **G,** Plug 10 to 12 mm in depth removed from recipient hole. **H,** Prepared recipient hole. **I,** Excised osteochondral lesion.

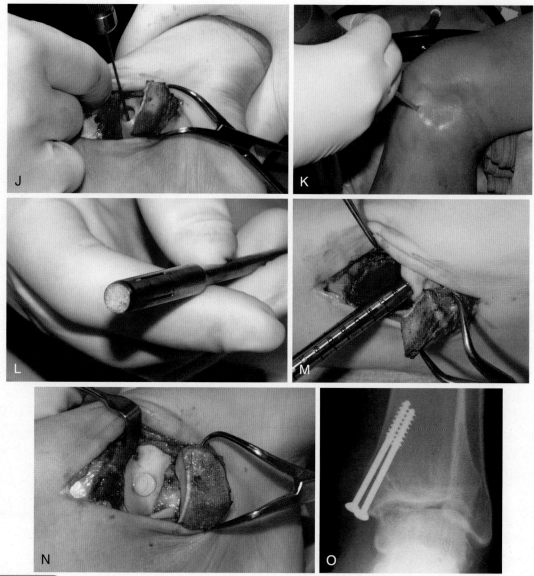

FIGURE 10.55, Cont'd   **J,** Multiple holes drilled at base of lesion. **K,** Autograft obtained from femoral condyle using donor harvester (for talar shoulder lesions, graft is obtained from corner of trochlea). **L,** Donor graft in harvester. **M** and **N,** Graft placed in recipient hole. **O,** Osteotomy secured with two partially threaded cancellous screws (holes predrilled before osteotomy). (Courtesy Robert B. Anderson, Charlotte, NC.) **SEE TECHNIQUE 10.10.**

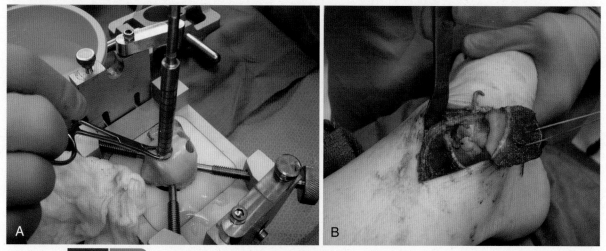

FIGURE 10.56   **A,** Multiple osteochondral allografts are harvested when large defects are encountered. Note two plugs obtained from shoulder of talus for closer morphology. **B,** Overlapping allograft placed to avoid leaving damaged tissue between plugs.

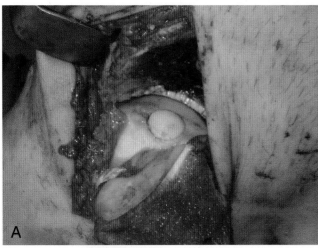
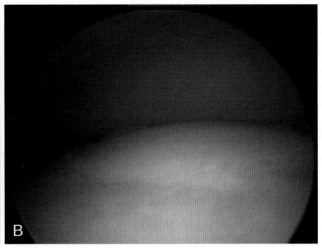

FIGURE 10.57 **A,** Note slight mismatch after osteochondral implantation. **B,** Second-look arthroscopy 15 months after the index position. Note slight irregularity of the articular surface.

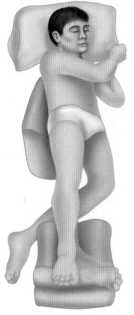

FIGURE 10.58 Positioning of patient for ankle arthroscopy.

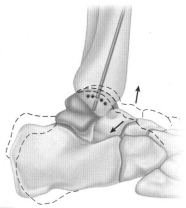

FIGURE 10.60 Arthroscopic drilling of osteochondritis dissecans of talus. Single Kirschner wire through hole drilled in malleolus produces multiple holes in crater of talus when ankle is flexed at different degrees.

Bryant and Siegel described an arthroscopic technique that avoids a transmalleolar portal by using meniscal repair instrumentation for accurate arthroscopic localization and drilling of osteochondral lesions. The preattached suture is removed from a 25-cm trocar point needle, and the needle is tightened on a power drill. With arthroscopic observation through the anterolateral portal, a curved cannula is inserted into the joint through the anteromedial portal and placed on the posteromedial defect. The needle is inserted through the curved cannula, and the lesion is drilled. Additional drill holes are created by moving the cannula to other sites on the lesion. Bleeding usually is observed from the multiple perforations in the subchondral bone. After arthroscopic drilling is completed, the wounds are closed and a sterile dressing is applied.

Whether open or arthroscopic techniques are used, the best results are obtained with excision and drilling of the crater. In the Campbell Clinic series, 87% of patients had satisfactory results with this procedure and recurrences were rare. Transmalleolar drilling (proximal to distal) can be done arthroscopically or percutaneously with the aid of image intensification. Multiple drill holes crossing the physis should be avoided if the distal tibial physis is open.

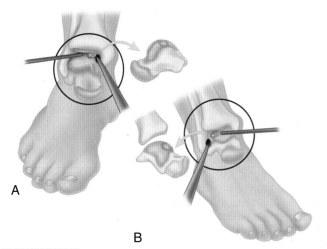

FIGURE 10.59 Anteromedial **(A)** and anterolateral **(B)** portals for arthroscopic excision of osteochondritis dissecans of ankle.

REFERENCES

ACUTE ANKLE LIGAMENT INJURIES, CHRONIC ANKLE INSTABILITY

Acevedo JI, Mangone B: Arthroscopic Broström technique, *Foot Ankle Int* 36:465, 2015.

Akoh CC, Phisitkul P: Anatomic ligament repairs of syndesmotic injuries, *Orthop Clin North Am* 50(3):401, 2019.

Alshalawi S, Galhoum AE, Alrashidi Y, et al.: Medial ankle instability: the deltoid dilemma, *Foot Ankle Clin* 23(4):639, 2018.

Amendola A, Williams G, Foster D: Evidence-based approach to treatment of acute traumatic syndesmosis (high ankle) sprains, *Sports Med Arthrosc* 14:232, 2006.

Anderson RB, Catanzariti A, Hollawell S, et al.: Ankle instability, *Foot Ankle Spec* 4:46, 2011.

Ashfraf A, Murphree J, Wait E, et al.: Gravity stress radiographs and the effect of ankle position on deltoid ligament integrity and medial clear space measurements, *J Orthop Trauma* 31(5):270, 2017.

Aynardi M, Pedowitz DI, Raikin SM: Subtalar instability, *Foot Ankle Clin* 20:243, 2015.

Barg A, Tochigi Y, Amendola A, et al.: Subtalar instability: diagnosis and treatment, *Foot Ankle Int* 33:151, 2012.

Bava E, Charlton T, Thordarson D: Ankle fracture syndesmosis fixation and management: the current practice of orthopedic surgeons, *Am J Orthop* 39:242, 2010.

Bell SJ, Mologne TS, Sitler DF, Cox JS: Twenty-six-year results after Broström procedure for chronic lateral ankle instability, *Am J Sports Med* 34:975, 2006.

Buchhorn T, Sabeti-Aschraf M, Dlaska CE, et al.: Combined medial and lateral anatomic ligament reconstruction for chronic rotational instability of the ankle, *Foot Ankle Int* 32:1122, 2011.

Burn A, Buerer Y, Chopra S, et al.: Critical evaluation of outcome scales assessment of lateral ankle ligament reconstruction, *Foot Ankle Int* 34:995, 2013.

Burrus MT, Werner BC, Hadeed MM, et al.: Predictors of peroneal pathology in Broström-Gould ankle ligament reconstruction for lateral ankle instability, *Foot Ankle Int* 36:268, 2015.

Chan KW, Ding BC, Mroczek KJ: Acute and chronic lateral ankle instability in the athlete, *Bull NYU Hosp Jt Dis* 69:17, 2011.

Cho BK, Hong SH, Jeon JH: Effect of lateral ligament augmentation using suture-tape on functional ankle instability, *Foot Ankle Int* 40(4):447, 2019.

Cho BK, Park JK, Choi SM, SooHoo NF: A randomized comparison between lateral ligaments augmentation using suture-tape and modified Broström repair in young female patients with chronic ankle instability, *Foot Ankle Surg* 25(2):137, 2019.

Cho BK, Shin YD, Park HW: Outcome following a modified Broström procedure with arthroscopic debridement of medial gutter osteoarthritis combined with chronic ankle instability, *Foot Ankle Int* 39(12):1473, 2018.

Chun TH, Park YS, Sung KS: The effect of ossicle resection in the lateral ligament repair for treatment of chronic lateral ankle instability, *Foot Ankle Int* 34:1128, 2013.

Clanton TO, Campbell KJ, Wilson KJ, et al.: Qualitative and quantitative anatomic investigation of the lateral ankle ligaments for surgical reconstruction procedures, *J Bone Joint Surg* 96A:e98, 2014.

Clanton TO, McGarvey W: Athletic injuries to the soft tissues of the foot and ankle. In Coughlin MJ, Mann RA, Saltzman CJ, editors: *Surgery of the foot and ankle*, ed 8, Philadelphia, 2007, Elsevier.

Crim JR, Beals TC, Nickisch F, et al.: Deltoid ligament abnormalities in chronic lateral ankle instability, *Foot Ankle Int* 32:873, 2011.

de César PC, Avila EM, de Abreu MR: Comparison of magnetic resonance imaging to physical examination for syndesmotic injury after lateral ankle sprain, *Foot Ankle Int* 32:1110, 2011.

de Vries JS, Krips R, Sierevelt IN, et al.: Interventions for treating chronic ankle instability, *Cochrane Database Syst Rev* 8:CD0004124, 2011.

Emre TY, Ege T, Cift HT, et al.: Open mosaicplasty in osteochondral lesions of the talus: a prospective study, *J Foot Ankle Surg* 51:556, 2012.

Espinosa N, Smerek J, Kadakia AR, Myerson MS: Operative management of ankle instability: reconstruction with open and percutaneous methods, *Foot Ankle Clin* 11:547, 2006.

Haytmanek CT, Williams BT, James EW, et al.: Radiographic identification of the primary lateral ankle structures, *Am J Sports Med* 43:79, 2015.

Hsu AR, Lareau CR, Anderson RB: Repair of acute superficial deltoid complex avulsion during ankle fracture fixation in National Football League players, *Foot Ankle Int* 36:1272, 2015.

Hubbard-Turner T, Wikstrom EA, Guderian S, Turner MJ: An acute lateral ankle sprain significantly decreases physical activity across the lifespan, *J Sports Sci Med* 14:556, 2015.

Hunt KJ, Pereira H, Kelley J, et al.: The role of calcaneofibular ligament injury in ankle instability: implications for surgical management, *Am J Sports Med* 47(2):431, 2019.

Jones CR, Nunley 2nd JA: Deltoid ligament repair versus syndesmotic fixation in bimalleolar equivalent ankle fractures, *J Orthop Trauma* 29:245, 2015.

Jung HG, Kim TH, Park JY, Bae EJ: Anatomic reconstruction of the anterior talofibular and calcaneofibular ligaments using a semitendinosus tendon allograft and interference screws, *Knee Surg Sports Traumatol Arthrosc* 20:1432, 2012.

Ko KR, Lee WY, Lee H, et al.: Repair of only anterior talofibular ligament resulted in similar outcomes to those of repair of both anterior talofibular and calcaneofibular ligaments, *Knee Surg Sports Traumatol Arthrosc*, 2018.

Kubo M, Yasui Y, Sasahara J, et al.: Simultaneous ossicle resection and lateral ligament repair give excellent clinical results with an early return to physical activity in pediatric and adolescent patients with chronic lateral ankle instability and os subfibulare, *Knee Surg Sports Traumatol Arthrosc*, 2019.

Lee DJ, Shin HS, Lee JH, et al.: Morphological characteristics of os subfibulare related to failure of conservative treatment of chronic lateral ankle instability, *Foot Ankle Int* 30:1071100719884056, 2019.

Lee JH, Lee SH, Jung HW, Jang WY: Modified Broström procedure in patients with chronic ankle instability is superior to conservative treatment in terms of muscle endurance and postural stability, *Knee Surg Sports Traumatol Arthrosc*, 2019.

Lee KM, Chung CY, Kwon SS, et al.: Relationship between stress ankle radiographs and injured ligaments on MRI, *Skeletal Radiol* 42:1537, 2013.

Lee K, Jegal H, Chung H, Park Y: Return to play after modified Broström operation for chronic ankle instability in elite athletes, *Clin Orthop Surg* 11(1):126, 2019.

Lee KT, Park YU, Kim JS, et al.: Long-term results after modified Broström procedure without calcaneofibular ligament reconstruction, *Foot Ankle Int* 32:153, 2011.

Li X, Killie H, Guerrero P, Busconi BD: Anatomical reconstruction for chronic lateral ankle instability in the high-demand athlete: functional outcomes after the modified Broström repair using suture anchors, *Am J Sports Med* 37:488, 2009.

Mabit C, Tourné Y, Besse JL, et al.: Chronic lateral ankle instability surgical repairs: the long term prospective, *Orthop Traumatol Surg Res* 96:417, 2010.

Maffulli N, Del Buono A, Maffulli GD, et al.: Isolated anterior talofibular ligament Broström repair for chronic lateral ankle instability: 9-year follow-up, *Am J Sports Med* 41:858, 2013.

Maffulli N, Ferran NA: Management of acute and chronic ankle instability, *J Am Acad Orthop Surg* 16:608, 2008.

Markolf KL, Jackson S, McAllister DR: Force and displacement measurements of the distal fibula during simulated ankle loading tests for high ankle sprains, *Foot Ankle Int* 33:779, 2012.

Miller AG, Raikin SM, Ahmad J: Near-anatomic allograft tenodesis of chronic lateral ankle instability, *Foot Ankle Int* 34:1501, 2013.

Miyamoto W, Takao M, Matsushita T: Hindfoot endoscopy for posterior ankle impingement syndrome and flexor hallucis longus tendon disorders, *Foot Ankle Clin* 20:139, 2015.

Miyamoto W, Takao M, Yamada K, Matsushita T: Accelerated versus traditional rehabilitation after anterior talofibular ligament reconstruction for chronic lateral instability of the ankle in athletes, *Am J Sports Med* 42:1441, 2014.

Morelli F, Perugia D, Vadalá A, et al.: Modified Watson-Jones technique for chronic lateral ankle instability in athletes: clinical and radiological mid- to long-term follow-up, *Foot Ankle Surg* 17:247, 2011.

Nelson OA: Examination and repair of the AITFL in transmalleolar fractures, *J Orthop Trauma* 20(9):637, 2006.

Nery C, Raduan F, Del Buono A, et al.: Arthroscopic-assisted Brostrom-Gould for chronic ankle instability: a long-term follow-up, *Am J Sports Med* 39:2381, 2011.

Nielson JH, Gardner MJ, Peterson MG: Radiographic measurements do not predict syndesmotic injury in ankle fractures: an MRI study, *Clin Orthop Relat Res* 436:216, 2005.

O'Neill PJ, Van Aman SE, Guyton GP: Is MRI adequate to detect lesions in patients with ankle instability, *Clin Orthop Relat Res* 468:1115, 2010.

Pakarinen H, Flinkkilä T, Ohtonen P, et al.: Intraoperative assessment of the stability of the distal tibiofibular joint in supination-external rotation injuries of the ankle: sensitivity, specificity, and reliability of two clinical tests, *J Bone Joint Surg* 93A:2057, 2011.

Park HJ, Cha SD, Kim HS, et al.: Reliability of MRI findings of peroneal tendinopathy in patients with lateral chronic ankle instability, *Clin Orthop Surg* 2:237, 2010.

Park CH, Park J: Effect of modified Brostrom procedure with periosteal flap augmentation after subfibular ossicle excision on ankle instability, *Foot Ankle Int* 40(6):656, 2019.

Pefanis N, Karagounis P, Tsiganos G, et al.: Tibiofemoral angle and its relation to ankle sprain occurrence, *Foot Ankle Spec* 2:271, 2009.

Pesquer L, Guillo S, Meyer P, Hauger O: US in ankle impingement syndrome, *J Ultrasound* 17:89, 2013.

Petersen W, Rembitzki IV, Koppenburg AG, et al.: Treatment of acute ankle ligament injuries: a systematic review, *Arch Orthop Trauma Surg* 133:1129, 2013.

Pihlajamäki H, Hietaniemi K, Paavola M, et al.: Surgical versus functional treatment for acute ruptures of the lateral ligament complex of the ankle in young men: a randomized controlled trial, *J Bone Joint Surg* 92A:2367, 2010.

Pijnenberg AC, Bogaard K, Krips R, et al.: Operative and functional treatment of rupture of the lateral ligament of the ankle: a randomized, prospective trial, *J Bone Joint Surg* 85B:525, 2003.

Porter DA, Kamman KA: Chronic lateral ankle instability: open surgical management, *Foot Ankle Clin* 23(4):539, 2018.

Porter M, Shadbolt B, Ye X, Stuart R: Ankle lateral ligament augmentation versus the modified Brostrom-Gould procedure: a 5-year randomized controlled trial, *Am J Sports Med* 47(3):659, 2019.

Ramdass RS, Grierson KR: A comparison of split peroneus brevis tendon and semitendinosus allograft tendon for lateral ankle ligament reconstruction, *J Foot Ankle Surg* 58(6):1197, 2019.

Redfern D, Myerson M: The management of concomitant tears of the peroneus longus and brevis tendons, *Foot Ankle Int* 25:695, 2004.

Rodriguez-Merchan EC: Chronic ankle instability: diagnosis and treatment, *Arch Orthop Trauma Surg* 132:211, 2012.

Roemer FW, Jomaah N, Niu J, et al.: Ligamentous injuries and the risk of associated tissue damage in acute ankle sprains in athletes: a cross-sectional MRI study, *Am J Sports Med* 42:1549, 2014.

Schmidt R, Benesch S, Friemert B, et al.: Anatomical repair of lateral ligaments in patients with chronic ankle instability, *Knee Surg Sports Traumatol Arthrosc* 13:231, 2005.

Schottel PC, Baxter J, Gilbert S, et al.: Anatomic ligament repair restores ankle and syndesmotic rotation stability as much as syndesmotic screw fixation, 30(2):e36, 2016.

Slater K: Acute lateral ankle instability, *Foot Ankle Clin* 23(4):523, 2018.

Sman AD, Hiller CE, Refshauge KM: Diagnostic accuracy of clinical tests for diagnosis of ankle syndesmotic injury: a systematic review, *Br J Sports Med* 47:620, 2013.

Spiga S, Vinci V, Tack S, et al.: Diagnostic imaging of ankle impingement syndromes in athletes, *Musculoskelet Surg* 97(Suppl 2):S145, 2013.

Strauss JE, Forsberg JA, Lippert 3rd FG: Chronic lateral ankle instability and associated conditions: a rationale for treatment, *Foot Ankle Int* 28:1041, 2007.

Takao M, Miyamoto W, Matsui K, et al.: Functional treatment after surgical repair for acute lateral ligament disruption of the ankle in athletes, *Am J Sports Med* 40:447, 2012.

Tochigi Y, Takahashi K, Yamagata M, et al.: Influence of the interosseous talocalcaneal ligament injury on stability of the ankle-subtalar joint complex—a cadaver experimental study, *Foot Ankle Int* 21:486, 2000.

Tohyama H, Yasuda K, Ohkoshi Y, et al.: Anterior drawer test for acute anterior talofibular ligament injuries of the ankle: how much load should be applied during the test? *Am J Sports Med* 31:226, 2003.

van den Bekerom MP, Kerkhoffs GM, McCollum GA, et al.: Management of acute lateral ankle ligament injury in the athlete, *Knee Surg Sports Traumatol Arthrosc* 21:1390, 2013.

Ventura A, Terzaghi C, Legnani C, Borgo E: Arthroscopic four-step treatment for chronic ankle instability, *Foot Ankle Int* 33:29, 2012.

Viens NA, Wijdicks CA, Campbell KJ, et al.: Anterior talofibular ligament ruptures, part 1: biomechanical comparison of augmented Brostrom repair techniques with the intact anterior talofibular ligament, *Am J Sports Med* 42:405, 2014.

Vuurberg G, Pereira H, Blankevoort L, van Dijk CN: Anatomic stabilization techniques provide superior results in terms of functional outcome in patients suffering from chronic ankle instability compared to non-anatomic techniques, *Knee Surg Sports Traumatol Arthrosc* 26(7):2183, 2018.

Wainright WB, Spritzer CE, Lee JY, et al.: The effect of modified Brostrom-Gould repair for lateral ankle instability on in vivo tibiotalar kinematics, *Am J Sports Med* 40:2099, 2012.

Waterman BR, Belmont Jr PJ, Cameron KL, et al.: Epidemiology of ankle sprain at the United States military Academy, *Am J Sports Med* 38:797, 2010.

Waterman BR, Belmont Jr PJ, Cameron KL, et al.: Risk factors for syndesmotic and medial ankle sprain: role of sex, sport, and level of competition, *Am J Sports Med* 39:992, 2011.

Wickstrom EA, Hubbard-Turner T, McKeon PO: Understanding and treating lateral ankle sprains and their consequences: a constraints-based approach, *Sports Med* 43:385, 2013.

Williams BT, Ahrberg AB, Goldsmith MT, et al.: Ankle syndesmosis: a qualitative and quantitative anatomic analysis, *Am J Sports Med* 43:88, 2015.

Williams GN, Jones MH, Amendola A: Syndesmotic ankle sprains in athletes, *Am J Sports Med* 35:1197, 2007.

Wortmann MA, Docherty CL: Effect of balance training on postural stability in subjects with chronic ankle instability, *J Sport Rehabil* 22:143, 2013.

Yasui Y, Takao M, Miyamoto W, et al.: Anatomical reconstruction of the anterior inferior tibiofibular ligament for chronic disruption of the distal tibiofibular syndesmosis, *Knee Surg Sports Traumatol Arthrosc* 19:691, 2011.

Youn H, Kim YS, Lee J, et al.: Percutaneous lateral ligament reconstruction with allograft for chronic lateral ankle instability, *Foot Ankle Int* 33:99, 2012.

Xu HX, Choi MS, Kim MS, et al.: Gender differences in outcome after modified Brostrom procedure for chronic lateral ankle instability, *Foot Ankle Int* 37:64, 2015.

Zhan Y, Yan X, Xia R, et al.: Anterior-inferior tibiofibular ligament anatomical repair and augmentation versus trans-syndesmosis screw fixation for the syndesmotic instability in external-rotation type ankle fracture with posterior malleolus involvement: a prospective and comparative study, *Injury* 47(7):1574, 2016.

OSTEOCHONDRAL LESIONS, IMPINGEMENT SYNDROMES

Adams Jr SB, Viens NA, Easley ME, et al.: Midterm results of osteochondral lesions of the talar shoiulder treated with fresh osteochondral allograft transplantation, *J Bone Joint Surg* 93A:648, 2011.

Ahmad J, Jones K: Comparison of osteochondral autografts and allografts for treatment of recurrent or large talar osteochondral lesions, *Foot Ankle Int* 37:40, 2016.

Al-Shaikh RA, Chou LB, Mann JA: Autologous osteochondral grafting for talar cartilage defects, *Foot Ankle Int* 23:381, 2002.

Amendola A, Panarella L: Osteochondral lesions: medial versus lateral, persistent pain, cartilage restoration options and indications, *Foot Ankle Clin* 14:215, 2009.

Badekas T, Takvorian M, Souras N: Treatment principles for osteochondral lesions in foot and ankle, *Int Orthop* 37:1697, 2013.

Baltzer AW, Arnold JP: Bone-cartilage transplantation from the ipsilateral knee for chondral lesions of the talus, *Arthroscopy* 21:159, 2005.

Baums MH, Heidrich G, Schultz W, et al.: Autologous chondrocyte transplantation for treating cartilage defects of the talus, *J Bone Joint Surg* 88A:303, 2006.

Baums MH, Heidrich G, Schultz W, et al.: Autologous chondrocyte transplantation of the talus with use of a periosteal graft. Surgical technique, *J Bone Joint Surg* 89A(Suppl 2 pt 2):170, 2007.

Berlet GC, Hyer CF, Philbin TM, et al.: Does fresh osteochondral allograft transplantation of talar osteochondral defects improve function? *Clin Orthop Relat Res* 469:2356, 2011.

Bohl DD, Frank RM, Lee S, et al.: Sensitivity of the saline load test for traumatic arthrotomy of the ankle with ankle arthroscopy simulation, *Foot Ankle Int* 39(6):736, 2018.

Buda R, Castagnini F, Cavallo M, et al.: "One-step" bone marrow-derived cells transplantation and joint debridement for osteochondral lesions of the talus in ankle osteoarthritis: clinical and radiological outcomes at 36 months, *Arch Orthop Trauma Surg* 136:107–116, 2016.

Bugbee WD, Khanna G, Cavallo M, et al.: Bipolar fresh osteochondral allografting of the tibiotalar joint, *J Bone Joint Surg* 95A:426, 2013.

Cadossi M, Buda RE, Ramponi L, et al.: Bone marrow-derived cells and biophysical stimulation for talar osteochondral lesions: a randomized controlled study, *Foot Ankle Int* 35:981, 2014.

Calder JD, Sexton SA, Pearce CJ: Return to training and playing after posterior ankle arthroscopy for posterior impingement in elite professional soccer, *Am J Sports Med* 38:120, 2010.

Choi WJ, Kim BS, Lee JW: Osteochondral lesions of the talus: could age be an indication for arthroscopic treatment? *Am J Sports Med* 40:419, 2012.

Choisne J, Hoch MC, Bawab S, et al.: The effects of a simi-rigid ankle brace on a simulated isolated subtalar joint, *J Orthop Res* 31:1869, 2013.

Coetzee JC, Giza E, Schon LC, et al.: Treatment of osteochondral lesions of the talus with particulated juvenile cartilage, *Foot Ankle Int* 34:1205, 2013.

Cohen BE, Anderson RB: Chevron-type transmalleolar osteotomy: an approach to medial talar dome lesions, *Tech Foot Ankle Surg* 1:158, 2002.

Cuttica DJ, Smith WB, Hyer CF, et al.: Osteochondral lesions of the talus: predictors of clinical outcome, *Foot Ankle Int* 32:1045, 2011.

Dahmen J, Lambers KTA, Reilingh ML, et al.: No superior treatment for primary osteochondral defects of the talus, *Knee Surg Sports Traumatol Arthrosc* 26(7):2142, 2018.

D'Ambrosi R, Maccario C, Ursino C, et al.: The role of bone marrow edema on osteochondral lesions of the talus, *Foot Ankle Surg* 24(3):229, 2018.

D'Ambrosi R, Villafane JH, Indino C, et al.: Return to sport after arthroscopic matrix-induced chondrogenesis for patients with osteochondral lesion of the talus, *Clin J Sport Med* 29(6):470, 2019.

D'Hooghe P, Murawski CD, Boakye LAT, et al.: Rehabilitation and return to sports: proceedings of the international consensus meeting on cartilage repair of the ankle, *Foot Ankle Int* 39(1_Suppl):61S, 2018.

Dombrowski ME, Yasui Y, Murawski CD, et al.: Conservative management and biological treatment strategies: proceedings of the international consensus meeting on cartilage repair of the ankle, *Foot Ankle Int* 39(1_Suppl):9S, 2018.

Donnenwerth MP, Roukis TS: Outcome of arthroscopic debridement and microfracture as the primary treatment of osteochondral lesions of the talar dome, *Arthroscopy* 28:1902, 2012.

Dunlap BJ, Ferkel RD, Applegate GR: The "LIFT" lesion: lateral inverted osteochondral fracture of the talus, *Arthroscopy* 29:1826, 2013.

Easley ME, Latt LD, Santangelo JR, et al.: Osteochondral lesions of the talus, *J Am Acad Orthop Surg* 18:616, 2010.

Easley ME, Vineyard JC: Varus ankle and osteochondral lesions of the talus, *Foot Ankle Clin* 17:21, 2012.

El-Rashidy H, Villacis D, Omar I, Kelikian AS: Fresh osteochondral allograft for the treatment of cartilage defects of the talus: a retrospective review, *J Bone Joint Surg* 93A:1634, 2011.

Elias I, Zoga AC, Morrison WB, et al.: Osteochondral lesions of the talus: localization and morphologic data from 424 patients using a novel anatomical grid scheme, *Foot Ankle Int* 28:154, 2007.

Fansa AM, Murwski CD, Imhauser CW, et al.: Autologous osteochondral transplantation of the talus partially restores contact mechanics of the ankle joint, *Am J Sports Med* 39:22457, 2011.

Ferkel SD, Scranton Jr PE, Stone JW, Kern BS: Surgical treatment of osteochondral lesions of the talus, *Instr Course Lect* 59:387, 2010.

Ferkel RD, Zannoti RM, Komenda GA, et al.: Arthroscopic treatment of chronic osteochondral lesions of the talus: long-term results, *Am J Sports Med* 36:1750, 2008.

Garras DN, Santangelo JA, Wang WW, Easley ME: A quantitative comparison of surgical approaches for posterolateral osteochondral lesions of the talus, *Foot Ankle Int* 29:415, 2008.

Gaul F, Tirico LEP, McCauley JC, et al.: Osteochondral allograft transplantation for osteochondral lesions of the talus: midterm follow-up, *Foot Ankle Int* 40(2):202, 2019.

Gautier E, Kilker D, Jakob RP: Treatment of cartilage defects of the talus by autologous osteochondral grafts, *J Bone Joint Surg* 84B:237, 2002.

Georgiannos D, Bisbinas I, Badekas A: Osteochondral transplantation of autologous graft for the treatment of osteochondral lesions of talus: 5- to 7-year follow-up, *Knee Surg Sports Traumatol Arthrosc*, 2014, [Epub ahead of print].

Giannini S, Battaglia M, Buda R, et al.: Surgical treatment of osteochondral lesions of the talus by open-field autologous chondrocyte implantation: a 10-year follow-up clinical and magnetic resonance imaging T2-mapping evaluation, *Am J Sports Med* 37(Suppl 1):112S, 2009.

Giannini S, Buda R, Mosca M, et al.: Posterior ankle impingement, *Foot Ankle Int* 34:459, 2013.

Giannini S, Buda R, Pagliazzi G, et al.: Survivorship of bipolar fresh total osteochondral ankle allograft, *Foot Ankle Int* 35:243, 2014.

Giannini S, Buda R, Vannini F, et al.: Arthroscopic autologous chondrocyte implantation in osteochondral lesions of the talus: surgical technique and results, *Am J Sports Med* 36:873, 2008.

Giannini S, Buda R, Grigolo B: Autologous chondrocyte transplantation in osteochondral lesions of the ankle joint, *Foot Ankle Int* 22:513, 2001.

Giannini S, Vannini F, Buda R: Osteoarticular grafts in the treatment of OCD of the talus: mosiacplasty versus autologous chondrocyte transplantation, *Foot Ankle Clin* 7:621, 2002.

Giza E, Delman C, Coetzee JC, Schon LC: Arthroscopic treatment of talus osteochondral lesions with particulated juvenile allograft cartilage, *Foot Ankle Int* 35:1087, 2014.

Giza E, Sullivan M, Ocel D, et al.: Matrix-induced autologous chondrocyte implantation of talus articular defects, *Foot Ankle Int* 31:747, 2010.

Gobbi A, Francisco RA, Lubowitz JH, et al.: Osteochondral lesions of the talus: randomized controlled trial comparing chondroplasty, microfracture, and osteochondral autograft transplantation, *Arthroscopy* 22:1085, 2006.

Görmeli G, Karakaplan M, Görmeli CA, et al.: Clinical effects of platelet-rich plasma and hyaluronic acid as an additional therapy for talar osteochondral lesions treated with microfracture surgery: a prospective randomized clinical trial, *Foot Ankle Int* 36:91, 2015.

Görtz S, De Young AJ, Bugbee WD: Fresh osteochondral allografting for osteochondral lesions of the talus, *Foot Ankle Int* 31:281, 2010.

Griffith JF, Lau DT, Yeung DK, Wong MW: High-resolution MR imaging of talar osteochondral lesions with a new classification, *Skeletal Radiol* 41:387, 2012.

Gross AE, Agnidis Z, Hutchison CR: Osteochondral defects of the talus treated with fresh osteochondral allograft transplantation, *Foot Ankle Int* 22:385, 2001.

Haene R, Qamirani E, Story RA, et al.: Intermediate outcomes of fresh talar osteochondral allografts for treatment of large osteochondral lesions of the talus, *J Bone Joint Surg* 94A:1105, 2012.

Hahn DB, Aanstoos ME, Wilkins RM: Osteochondral lesions of the talus treated with fresh talar allografts, *Foot Ankle Int* 31:277, 2010.

Haleem AM, Ross KA, Smyth NA, et al.: Double-plug autologous osteochondral transplantation shows equal functional outcomes compared with single-plug procedures in lesions of the talar dome: a minimum 5-year clinical follow-up, *Am J Sports Med* 42:1888, 2014.

Hangody L, Dobos J, Baló E, et al.: Clinical experience with autologous osteochondral mosaicplasty in an athletic population: a 17-year prospective multicenter study, *Am J Sports Med* 38:1125, 2010.

Hannon CP, Bayer S, Murawski CD, et al.: Debridement, curettage, and bone marrow stimulation: proceedings of the international consensus meeting on cartilage repair of the ankle, *Foot Ankle Int* 39(1_Suppl):16S, 2018.

Hannon CP, Smyth NA, Murawski CD, et al.: Osteochondral lesions of the talus: aspects of current management, *Bone Joint Lett J* 96B:164, 2014.

Hess GW: Ankle impingement syndromes: a review of etiology and related implications, *Foot Ankle Spec* 4:290, 2011.

Higashiyama I, Kumai T, Takakura Y: Follow-up study of MRI for osteochondral lesions of the talus, *Foot Ankle Int* 21:127, 2000.

Hintermann B, Wagener J, Knupp M, et al.: Treatment of extended osteochondral lesions of the talus with a free vascularised bone graft from the medial condyle of the femur, *Bone Joint Lett J* 97B:1242, 2015.

Hirtler L, Schellander K, Schuh R: Accessibility to talar dome in neutral position, dorsiflexion, or noninvasive distraction in posterior ankle arthroscopy, *Foot Ankle Int* 40(8):978, 2019.

Imhoff AB, Paul J, Ottinger B, et al.: Osteochondral transplantation of the talus: long-term clinical and magnetic resonance imaging evaluation, *Am J Sports Med* 39:1487, 2011.

Hurley ET, Murawski CD, Paul J: Osteochondral autograft: proceedings of the international consensus meeting on cartilage repair of the ankle, *Foot Ankle Int* 39(1_Suppl):28S, 2018.

Jiang D, Ao YF, Jiao C, et al.: Concurrent arthroscopic osteochondral lesion treatment and lateral ankle ligament repair has no substantial effect on the outcome of chronic lateral ankle instability, *Knee Surg Sports Traumatol Arthrosc* 26(10):3129, 2018.

Jones MH, Amendola A: Syndesmosis sprains of the ankle: a systematic review, *Clin Orthop Relat Res* 455:173, 2007.

Kim YS, Park EH, Kim YC, et al.: Factors associated with the clinical outcomes of the osteochondral autograft transfer system in osteochondral lesions of the talus: second-look arthroscopic evaluation, *Am J Sports Med* 40:2709, 2012.

Kim TY, Song SH, Baek JH, et al.: Analysis of the changes in the clinical outcomes according to time after arthroscopic microfracture of osteochondral lesions of the talus, *Foot Ankle Int* 40(1):74, 2019.

Klammer G, Maquieira GJ, Spahn S, et al.: Natural history of nonoperatively treated osteochondral lesions of the talus, *Foot Ankle Int* 36:24, 2015.

Kono M, Takao M, Naito K, et al.: Retrograde drilling for osteochondral lesions of the talar dome, *Am J Sports Med* 34:1450, 2006.

Koulalis D, Schultz W, Heyden M: Autologous chondrocyte transplantation for osteochondritis dissecans of the talus, *Clin Orthop Relat Res* 395:186, 2002.

Kubosch EJ, Erdle B, Izadpanah K: Clinical outcome and T2 assessment following autologous matrix-induced chondrogenesis in osteochondral lesions of the talus, *Int Orthop* 40:65, 2016.

Kumai T, Takakura Y, Kitada C, et al.: Fixation of osteochondral lesions of the talus using cortical bone pegs, *J Bone Joint Surg* 84B:369, 2002.

Lambers KTA, Dahmen J, Reilingh ML, et al.: Arthroscopic lift, drill, fill, and fix (LDFF) is an effective treatment option for primary talar osteochondral defects, *Knee Surg Sports Traumatol Arthrosc*, 2019.

Lambers KTA, Saarig A, Turner H, et al.: Prevalence of osteochondral lesions in rotational type ankle fractures with syndesmotic injury, *Foot Ankle Int* 40(2):159, 2019.

Latt LD, Glisson RR, Montijo HE, et al.: Effect of graft height mismatch on contact pressures with osteochondral grafting of the talus, *Am J Sports Med* 39:2662, 2011.

Lee JC, Calder JD, Healy JC: Posterior impingement syndromes of the ankle, *Semin Musculoskelet Radiol* 12:154, 2008.

Lee KB, Bai LB, Chung JY, Seon JK: Arthroscopic microfracture for osteochonral lesions of the talus, *Knee Surg Sports Traumatol Arthrosc* 18:247, 2010.

Lee KB, Bai LB, Park JG, et al.: Efficacy of MRI versus arthroscopy for evaluation of sinus tarsi syndrome, *Foot Ankle Int* 29:1111, 2008.

Lee KB, Bai LB, Yoon TR, et al.: Second-look arthroscopic findings and clinical outcomes after microfracture for osteochondral lesions of the talus, *Am J Sports Med* 37(Suppl 1):63S, 2009.

Lee M, Kwon JW, Choi WJ, Lee JW: Comparison of outcomes for osteochondral lesions of the talus with and without chronic lateral ankle instability, *Foot Ankle Int* 36:1050, 2015.

Lee KB, Park HW, Cho HJ, Seon JK: Comparison of arthroscopic microfracture for osteochondral lesions of the talus with and without subchondral cyst, *Am J Sports Med* 43:1951, 2015.

Lee KB, Yang HK, Moon ES, Song EK: Modified step-cut medial malleolar osteotomy for osteochondral grafting of the talus, *Foot Ankle Int* 29:1107, 2008.

Lektrakul N, Chung CB, Lai YM, et al.: Tarsal sinus: arthrographic, MR imaging, MR arthrographic, and pathologic findings in cadavers and retrospective study data in patients with sinus tarsi syndrome, *Radiology* 219:802, 2001.

Maquirriain J: Posterior ankle impingement syndrome, *J Am Acad Orthop Surg* 13:365, 2005.

McCollum GA, Myerson MS, Jonck J: Managing the cystic osteochondral defect: allograft or autograft, *Foot Ankle Clin* 18:113, 2013.

McGahan PJ, Pinney SJ: Current concept review: osteochondral lesions of the talus, *Foot Ankle Int* 31:90, 2010.

Mei-Dan O, Carmont MR, Laver L, et al.: Platelet-rich plasma or hyaluronate in the management of osteochondral lesions of the talus, *Am J Sports Med* 40:534, 2012.

Miller TL, Skalak T: Evaluation and treatment recommendations for acute injuries to the ankle syndesmosis without associated fracture, *Sports Med* 44:179, 2014.

Mitchell ME, Giza E, Sullivan MR: Cartilage transplantation techniques for talar cartilage lesions, *J Am Acad Orthop Surg* 17:407, 2009.

Muir D, Saltzman CL, Tochgi Y, Amendola N: Talar dome access for osteochondral lesions, *Am J Sports Med* 34:1457, 2006.

Murawski CD, Kennedy JG: Operative treatment of osteochondral lesions of the talus, *J Bone Joint Surg* 95A:1045, 2013.

Myerson MS: Osteochondral lesions of the talus, *Foot Ankle Clin* 18:vi, 2013.

Nakasa T, Ikuta Y, Sawa M, et al.: Relationship between bone marrow lesions on MRI and cartilage degeneration in osteochondral lesions of the talar dome, *Foot Ankle Int* 39(8):908, 2018.

Nguyen A, Ramasamy A, Walsh M, et al.: Autologous osteochondral transplantation for large osteochondral lesions of the talus is a viable option in an athletic population, *Am J Sports Med* 31:363546519881420, 2019.

Niemeyer P, Salzmann G, Schmal H, et al.: Autologous chondrocyte implantation for the treatment of chondral and osteochondral defects of the talus: a meta-analysis of available evidence, *Knee Surg Sports Traumatol Arthrosc* 20:1696, 2012.

Noguchi H, Ishii Y, Takeda M, et al.: Arthroscopic excision of posterior ankle bony impingement for early return to the field: short-term results, *Foot Ankle Int* 31:398, 2010.

Odak S, Ahluwalia R, Shivarathre DG, et al.: Arthroscopic evaluation of impingement and osteochondral lesions in chronic lateral ankle instability, *Foot Ankle Int* 36:1045, 2015.

Orr JD, Dutton JR, Fowler JT: Anatomic location and morphology of symptomatic, operatively treated osteochondral lesions of the talus, *Foot Ankle Int* 33:1051, 2012.

Paul J, Sagstetter A, Lämmle L, et al.: Sports activity after osteochondral transplantation of the talus, *Am J Sports Med* 40:870, 2012.

Paul J, Sagstetter A, Kriner M, et al.: Donor-site morbidity after osteochondral autologous transplantation for lesions of the talus, *J Bone Joint Surg* 91A:1683, 2009.

Raikin SM: Fresh osteochondral allografts for large-volume cystic osteochondral defects of the talus, *J Bone Joint Surg* 91A:2818, 2009.

Rathur S, Clifford PD, Chapman CB: Posterior ankle impingement: os trigonum syndrome, *Am J Orthop* 38:252, 2009.

Reilingh ML, Murawski CD, DiGiovanni CW, et al.: Fixation techniques: proceedings of the international consensus meeting on cartilage repair of the ankle, *Foot Ankle Int* 39(1_Suppl):23S, 2018.

Roche A, Calder JD, Lloyd Williams R: Posterior ankle impingement in dancers and athletes, *Foot Ankle Clin* 18:301, 2013.

Rogers J, Diikstra P, McCourt P, et al.: Posterior ankle impingement syndrome: a clinical review with reference to horizontal jump athletes, *Acta Orthop Belg* 76:572, 2010.

Rothrauff BB, Murawski CD, Angthong C, et al.: Scaffold-based therapies: proceedings of the international consensus meeting on cartilage repair of the ankle, *Foot Ankle Int* 39(1_Suppl):41S, 2018.

Sammarco GJ, Makwana NK: Treatment of talar osteochondral lesions using local osteochondral graft, *Foot Ankle Int* 23:693, 2002.

Schachter AK, Chen AL, Reddy PD, Tejwani NC: Osteochondral lesions of the talus, *J Am Acad Orthop Surg* 13:152, 2005.

Schneider TE, Karaikudi S: Matrix-induced autologous chondrocyte implantation (MACI) grafting for osteochondral lesions of the talus, *Foot Ankle Int* 30:810, 2009.

Schuman L, Struijs PA, Van Dijk CN: Arthroscopic treatment for osteochondral defects of the talus: results at follow-up at 2 to 11 years, *J Bone Joint Surg* 84B:364, 2002.

Seow D, Yasui Y, Hurley ET, et al.: Extracellular matrix cartilage allograft and particulate cartilage allograft for osteochondral lesions of the knee and ankle joints: a systematic review, *Am J Sports Med* 46(7):1758, 2018.

Shimozono Y, Hurley ET, Myerson CL, Kennedy JG: Good clinical and functional outcomes at mid-term following autologous osteochondral transplantation for osteochondral lesions of the talus, *Knee Surg Sports Traumatol Arthrosc* 26(10):3055, 2018.

Smyth NA, Murawski CD, Adams Jr SB, et al.: Osteochondral allograft: proceedings of the international consensus meeting on cartilage repair of the ankle, *Foot Ankle Int* 39(1_Suppl):35S, 2018.

Sofka CM: Posterior ankle impingement: clarification and confirmation of the pathoanatomy, *HSS J* 6:99, 2010.

Steman JAH, Dahmen J, Lambers KTA, Kerkhoffs GMMJ: Return to sports after surgical treatment of osteochondral defects of the talus: a systematic review of 2347 cases, *Orthop J Sports Med* 7(10):2325967119876238, 2019.

Tanaka Y, Omokawa S, Fujii T, et al.: Vascularized bone graft from the medial calcaneus for treatment of large osteochondral lesions of the medial talus, *Foot Ankle Int* 27:1143, 2006.

Thordarson DB, Kaku SK: Results of step-cut medial malleolar osteotomy, *Foot Ankle Int* 27:1020, 2006.

Toale J, Shimozono Y, Mulvin C, et al.: Midterm outcomes of bone marrow stimulation for primary osteochondral lesions of the talus: a systematic review, *Orthop J Sports Med* :7(10):2325967119879127, 2019.

Valderrabano V, Leumann A, Rasch H, et al.: Knee-to-ankle mosaicplasty for the treatment of osteochondral lesions of the ankle joint, *Am J Sports Med* 37(Suppl 1):105S, 2009.

Valderrabano V, Miska M, Leumann A, Wiewiorski M: Reconstruction of osteochondral lesions of the talus with autologous spongiosa grafts and autologous matrix-induced chondrogenesis, *Am J Sports Med* 41:519, 2013.

Van Berger CJA, Baur OL, Murawski CD, et al.: Diagnosis: history, physical examination, imaging, and arthroscopy: proceedings of the international consensus meeting on cartilage repair of the ankle, *Foot Ankle Int* 39(1_Suppl):3S, 2018.

van Bergen CJ, Tuijthof GJ, Sierevelt IN, van Dijk CN: Direction of the oblique medial malleolar osteotomy for exposure of the talus, *Arch Orthop Trauma Surg* 131:893, 2011.

van Dijk NC: Anterior and posterior ankle impingement, *Foot Ankle Clin* 11:663, 2006.

Vaseenon T, Amendola A: Update on anterior ankle impingement, *Curr Rev Musculoskelet Med* 5:145, 2012.

Verghese N, Morgan A, Perera A: Osteochondral lesions of the talus: defining the surgical approach, *Foot Ankle Int* 18:49, 2013.

Wang C, Kang MW, Kim HN: Arthroscopic treatment of osteochondral lesions of the talus in a suspended position with the patient in a prone position, *Foot Ankle Int* 40(7):811, 2019.

Wiewiorski M, Barg A, Valderrabano V: Autologous matrix-induced chondrogenesis in osteochondral lesions of the talus, *Foot Ankle Clin* 18:151, 2013.

Wikstrom EA, Hubbard-Turner T, McKeon PO: Understanding and treating lateral ankle sprains and their consequences: a constraints-based approach, *Sports Med* 43:385, 2013.

Winters BS, Raikin SM: The use of allograft in joint-preserving surgery for ankle osteochondral lesions and osteoarthritis, *Foot Ankle Clin* 18:529, 2013.

Wood JJ, Malek MA, Frassica FJ, et al.: Autologous cultured chondrocytes: adverse events reported to the United States Food and Drug Administration, *J Bone Joint Surg* 88A:503, 2006.

Yang HY, Lee KB: Arthroscopic microfracture for osteochondral lesions of the talus: second-look arthroscopic and magnetic resonance analysis of cartilage repair tissue outcomes, *J Bone Joint Surg Am*, 2019.

Yoon HS, Park YJ, Lee M, et al.: Osteochondral autologous transplantation is superior to repeat arthroscopy for the treatment of osteochondral lesions of the talus after failed primary arthroscopic treatment, *J Sports Med* 42:1896, 2014.

Young KW, Deland JT, Lee KT, Lee YK: Medial approaches to osteochondral lesion of the talus without medial malleolar osteotomy, *Knee Surg Sports Traumatol Arthrosc* 18:634, 2010.

Zengerink M, Struijs PA, Tol JL, van Dijk CN: Treatment of osteochondral lesions of the talus: a systematic review, *Knee Surg Sports Traumatol Arthrosc* 18:238, 2010.

FOOT INJURIES

Anderson RB, Hunt KJ, McCormick JJ: Management of common sports-related injuries about the foot and ankle, *J Am Acad Orthop Surg* 18:546, 2010.

Chinn L, Hertel J: Rehabilitation of ankle and foot injuries in athletes, *Clin Sports Med* 29:157, 2010.

Fowler JR, Gaughan JP, Boden BP, et al.: The non-surgical and surgical management of tarsal navicular stress fractures, *Sports Med* 41:613, 2011.

Guettler JH, Ruskan GJ, Bytomski JR, et al.: Fifth metatarsal stress fractures in elite basketball players: evaluation of forces acting on the fifth metatarsal, *Am J Orthop* 35:532, 2006.

Hudson Z: Rehabilitation and return to play after foot and ankle injuries in athletes, *Sports Med Arthrosc* 17:203, 2009.

Kaplan LD, Jost PW, Honkamp N, et al.: Incidence and variance of foot and ankle injuries in elite college football players, *Am J Orthop* 40:40, 2011.

McCormick JJ, Anderson RB: Rehabilitation following turf toe injury and plantar plate repair, *Clin Sports Med* 29:313, 2010.

McCormick JJ, Anderson RB: The great toe: failed turf toe, chronic turf toe, and complicated sesamoid injuries, *Foot Ankle Clin* 14:135, 2009.

Niva MH, Sormaala MJ, Kiuru MJ, et al.: Bone stress injuries of the ankle and foot: an 86-month magnetic resonance imaging-based study of physically active young adults, *Am J Sports Med* 35:643, 2007.

Pearce CJ, Brooks JH, Kemp SP, Calder JD: The epidemiology of foot injuries in professional rugby union players, *Foot Ankle Surg* 17:113, 2011.

The complete list of references is available online at expertconsult.inkling.com.